Anglo-European Science and the Rhetoric of Empire

Anglo-European Science and the Rhetoric of Empire

Malaria, Opium, and British Rule in India, 1756–1895

Paul C. Winther

LEXINGTON BOOKS
Lanham • Boulder • New York • Oxford

LEXINGTON BOOKS

Published in the United States of America
by Lexington Books
A Member of the Rowman & Littlefield Publishing Group
4501 Forbes Boulevard, Suite 200, Lanham, Maryland 20706

PO Box 317
Oxford
OX2 9RU, UK

Copyright © 2003 by Lexington Books

All rights reserved. No part of this publication may be reproduced, stored
in a retrieval system, or transmitted in any form or by any means, electronic,
mechanical, photocopying, recording, or otherwise, without the prior permission
of the publisher.

British Library Cataloguing in Publication Information Available

Library of Congress Cataloging-in-Publication Data
Winther, Paul C., 1937–
 Anglo-European science and the rhetoric of empire: malaria, opium,
and Brisith rule in India, 1756–1895 / Paul C. Winther.
  p. cm.
Includes bibliographical references and index.
 ISBN 0-7391-0584-1 (hardcover : alk. paper)
 1. Opium trade—India—History. 2. Opium trade—China—History. 3.
Malaria—Prevention—History. I. Title.
 HV5840.I4W56 2003
 382'.4561532335—dc21
                                                                    2002154763

Printed in the United States of America

∞™ The paper used in this publication meets the minimum requirements of
American National Standard for Information Sciences—Permanence of Paper
for Printed Library Materials, ANSI/NISO Z39.48-1992.

Contents

Map	Regions of India with Opium and Malaria Witnesses	vii–viii
List of Tables		ix
Preface		xi
Acknowledgments		xv
List of Abbreviations		xvii
1	Introduction	1
2	The Missionaries' Lament in a Milieu of Indifference, 1773–1874 C.E.	33
3	The Gathering Storm: Protest, Politics, and Science, 1874–1893 C.E.	75
4	The Serendipitous Nature of "Except for Medical Use" and Participants in the Royal Commission Hearings	115
5	Hope for the Anti-Opiumists: Witnesses' Perspectives about Why People in India Eat Opium	157
6	More Hope for the Moralists? Witnesses' Observations about Who Eats Opium in India	203
7	Sir William Roberts' Evaluation of the Opium and 'Malaria' Evidence	231
8	The Anti-Opiumists' Nightmare	273

9	The Wider Context: Anglo-European Science and the Rhetoric of Empire	323
Appendix A	Opium Only Relieves Pain	343
Appendix B	Opium Prevents and Cures Just About Everything, Including 'Malarial Fever,' 'Fevers,' and the Diverse Detrimental Consequences of 'Miasmatic Influences'	345
Appendix C	Cinchona Cultivation and Quinine Production in South Asia During the Nineteenth Century	349
Appendix D	Anarcotine and Crude Opium Requirements (in Pounds) Using the Three Alkaloid Extraction Ratios for More than One Million Sufferers	357
Appendix E	Alternative Format for Contents of Tables 12, 13, and 14	359
Appendix F	Nineteenth- and Early Twentieth-Century Anarcotine/Narcotine Research and the Alkaloid's Irrelevance for 'Malaria' and Fever, and Subsequent Research	363

Tables	369
Selected Bibliography	381
Index	409
About the Author	429

MAP: REGIONS OF INDIA WITH OPIUM AND MALARIA WITNESSES

Convenience determines regional classification and terminology for witnesses providing information about opium and malaria to the Royal Commission. Witnesses often had different postings during their careers. Other respondents lived in various parts of the country before testifying. Placing provinces and administrative entities in geographic groups enables a reader unfamiliar with nineteenth-century Indian politics to quickly comprehend approximately what part of India the witness is discussing. "Middle India" refers to a large area consisting of the "Central India Agency," "Central Provinces" Berar and Bastar. Quasi-independent native states and territories comprise the "Central India Agency." The "Central Provinces" pertains to the native states and territories that were permanently administered by the British. Most of these were south of "Central India."

"West India" consists of native states of various sizes, the Northwest Frontier Agency, Delhi and its environs, the province of Punjab, and Rajputana Agency. Rajputana Agency is designated in the "west" region although its location permits inclusion in "Middle India." Proximity of parts of Rajputana to adjacent locations could also qualify it as "Western Coast;" this is the author's decision.

Location on the Gangetic plain is a defining feature of "North India." The United Provinces plus the western districts of Bihar province comprise the region.

"East India" refers to the east and northeastern part of the subcontinent. It includes the provinces of Bengal, Orissa (also referred to in the literature as one of the "Lower Provinces" because it was in the southern part of the region), as well as Assam, neighboring territories, Chota Nagpur, and Burma. Eastern Bihar province is included in the "East India" region because several witnesses' comments pertain to eastern districts in Bihar and to adjacent western districts of Bengal (East India.)

Bombay Presidency, Gujerat, Sind, Kathiawar, Surat, Baluchistan Agency, and several other locales constitute the "Western Coast." Sind and the Baluchistan Agency are designated "Western Coast" because a coastline is part of their boundaries. Both, especially the Baluchistan Agency could also be grouped in the "west" region since part of each area was next to territories categorized as "West India." Again, this is the author's decision.

"South India" refers to the provinces, native states, and minor administrative entities in peninsular India. It includes Madras Presidency, Mysore, Hyderabad, Travancore, and other areas in the region.

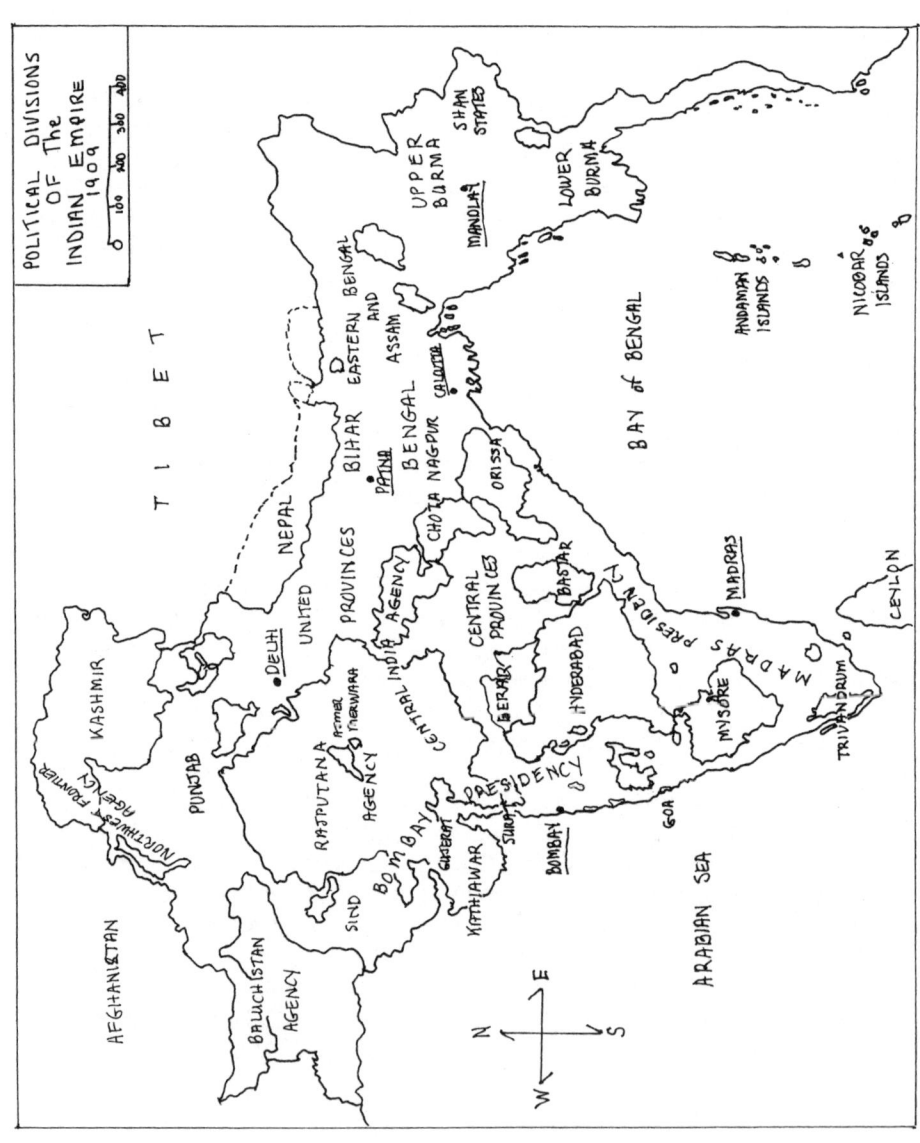

Tables

1 Occupational Category of Witnesses with Opium and
   Malaria Testimony   369
2 Patients Receiving Anarcotine During the Two Periods of
   Dr. Garden's Nine-Month Study   370
3 Condensation of Statistics in Dr. Garden's Table 4: "Shewing
   [sic] the Number of Paroxysms After the First Administration of
   Anarcotine with Percentage"   370
4 Statistics in Dr. Garden's Table 5: "Shewing [sic] Average Amount
   of Anarcotine Taken Before and After Cessation of Fever
   According to the Numbers of Paroxysms"   371
5 Estimate of Anarcotine and Opium Requirements for Quotidian
   and Tertian Fever Patients Based upon Dr. A. Garden's 1859–1860
   Ghazipur Experiment   372
6 Bengal and Malwa Opium Exports   373
7 Statement Showing Quantities of Excise Opium Manufactured at
   the Bihar and Benares Agencies and the Quantities Supplied to
   the Several Local Governments during the Last 20 Years   374
8 Chests of Malwa Opium Weighed/Taxed at All Stations and
   Number of Chests Manufactured for Sale in British Territory and
   Native States   375
9 Total Population Grouped by Provinces, with Average Yearly
   Consumption of Licit Opium per Head   376
10 Population and 'Fever' Mortality Statistics in Five British Provinces
   Compiled by Mr. S. E. J. Clarke, Secretary to the Bengal Chamber
   of Commerce, 4 December 1893 and Submitted to the Royal
   Commission on Opium   377

11	Anarcotine and Bengal Excise Opium Requirements Using the Three Ratios for More than One Million Sufferers	377
12	[116.9:1 Ratio]: Quantity of Bengal Abkari (Excise) Opium Chests Required to Extract Sufficient Anarcotine for 'Cure' and 'Convalescence' of Four Groups of 'Malarial Fever' Sufferers. Entries Are Expressed as Percentage of Bengal Chests Prepared for Domestic Consumption During the Twenty-Year Period from 1873/74 to 1892/93	378
13	[24:1 Ratio]: Quantity of Bengal Abkari (Excise) Opium Chests Required to Extract Sufficient Anarcotine for 'Cure' and 'Convalescence' of Four Groups of 'Malarial Fever' Sufferers. Entries Are Expressed as Percentage of Bengal Chests Prepared for Domestic Consumption During the Twenty-Year Period from 1873/74–1892/93	379
14	[16:1 Ratio]: Quantity of Bengal Abkari (Excise) Opium Chests Required to Extract Sufficient Anarcotine for 'Cure' and 'Convalescence' of Four Groups of 'Malarial Fever' Sufferers. Entries Are Expressed as Percentage of Bengal Chests Prepared for Domestic Consumption During the Twenty-Year Period from 1873/74 to 1892/93	380

Preface

One task confronting an author is presenting information as clearly as possible. The style followed in this book reflects the concern. It is a blend of several traditions. The *American Anthropologist* format for citing a source in a chapter narrative (author-date-page) is used because it is simple and the author is an anthropologist. The *Chicago Manual of Style* is preferred for everything else. Some of its rules, however, are not followed because the kind of data in several chapters and sources used necessitate amendments.

This writer appreciates complete bibliographic information if an author cites old government documents that are rare and difficult to access. The discussion in sections of the book is based almost exclusively upon data taken from this type of material. The *American Anthropologist* and the *Chicago Manual of Style* formats are modified to enable readers to quickly identify these sources if they so desire. The task is tedious in the absence of format change because data are sometimes drawn from enclosures that are part of larger enclosures. These in turn are sections of still more inclusive documents. Such is the nature of many Session Papers, Command Papers, and Reports of Standing and Select Committees that comprise the British Parliamentary Papers. The complexity also characterizes the content of Royal Commission documents. Commissions were created periodically to investigate specific, diverse problems confronting England and the Commonwealth throughout its many decades of existence. The Royal Commission on Opium, whose activities are central to this book, was one of these temporary institutions. There also is a wealth of information found in Session and Command Papers, and in the deliberations of Parliament's Standing and Select Committees. Much of the information is difficult to find without a little help from the writer.

This author errs by commission rather than omission. The Parliamentary Papers section of the Selected Bibliography provides detailed information about all documents mentioned in the book. Citation of any government publication in a chapter contains sufficient information (more than often found in material published in or about India) to quickly find its more complete rendition in the Selected Bibliography.

The reader occasionally will find a key word, phrase, or specific location (enclosed within brackets) inserted between an author's name and the document's year of publication. An example found in this book is: GBO [Lyall] 1894:II:317. This indicates the material referred to in the discussion involves what Lyall says on page 317 of an 1894 publication. In this case, Lyall's entire commentary is located on pages 315–18 in volume II of the Royal Commission on Opium multivolume series. The bracketed information minimizes time spent searching for data verification in the Selected Bibliography. The first paragraph of the Parliamentary Paper section explains the bracket format in more detail. GBO is the abbreviation for the longer title: Great Britain. Royal Commission on Opium. See the List of Abbreviations for other codes.

A name, word, or phrase within brackets, however, does not determine where a source appears in the Selected Bibliography for Parliamentary Papers. Location follows standard bibliographic format, this being author or institution (in alphabetical order), year of publication for works by the same author, title of publication, page location, and other *Chicago Manual* stipulations. Please note that the Royal Commission on Opium documents are entered according to the volume in which they appear. Separate sections within the Select Bibliography for government documents such as the Royal Commission material also contributes to quick source identification. Other sections are Command Papers [GBC], Reports of Standing and Select Committees [GBR], Session Papers [GBS], and the Irish University Press Series of Parliamentary Papers [IUP/PP].

Complete bibliographic information for all source material cited in appendices A–F are found in the book's Selected Bibliography for Books/Articles, Parliamentary Papers, or Witnesses. The sources are not listed separately for each appendix.

Several chapters have citations mentioned only in a chapter's endnotes. Full particulars for many of these sources appear only in the Selected Bibliography. The endnote entry, therefore, is shortened or abbreviated. A publisher's name and location frequently is omitted to save space. Books, articles, and documents with long names often are abbreviated: either the title is shortened or the author uses the source code (found in the List of Abbreviations). For example, *AJMS* identifies the source as the *American Journal of Medical Science*.

Complete information about a source is given in the endnote if it an integral part of the commentary. The data reappear in the Selected Bibliography. Convenience to the reader, nature of the material, and author's preference dictate the endnote format. It also governs document citation found in appendices A–F.

Several publications consulted for this study have authors with the same last name. Citation of these people includes their first names or initials if confusion is a possibility when discussing a topic. The author prefers the format because it is a convenience to readers. It expedites finding bibliographic information although date of publication and title usually suffice to differentiate one individual from another.

Locations, titles, and names of people mentioned in the book are spelled as found in source documents. This means, for example, the very few English-language transliterations of Chinese names for people, cities, and geographic locations do not always conform to the pin-yang system. The manner in which they appear is the style deemed proper when the document was created during the eighteenth or nineteenth century. The same format applies to individuals, locations, and so forth in other countries or regions discussed in the study. Obvious spelling errors have been corrected (and noted), as have changes in citations a reader might have difficulty locating or understanding today. Other instances of inconsistency are noted when necessary. This also is done for older books and articles.

References to 1861/62, 1893/94, and so forth often appear in nineteenth-century East India Company and Government of India documents. It also is common in British Parliamentary Papers. The slash separating dates signifies a growing and manufacturing season spanning several months in each year, not to a twelve-month period when presented as 1856, 1888, 1889, or 1894. An entry such as 1885/86–1894/95 denotes a ten-year period of successive growing or manufacturing seasons.

Modification of the American Anthropological Association format for identifying source of "run in" quotations and partial quotations keeps repetitious citations to a minimum. A paragraph containing only quoted material from the same page of one source will have the author/date/page number identified at the conclusion of the paragraph rather than at the end of each sentence within the paragraph in which the quotation appears. The American Anthropological Association style is followed if a quotation in a single paragraph is taken from a different source, or from the same source but found on a different page. This format also applies to a paragraph containing a "blocked quotation" (i.e., indented material containing as many as eight to ten sentences). This atypical format enhances readability and conforms to preferences for source citation of quoted material.

A word or phrase enclosed by single vertical marks indicates historical usage. 'Malaria,' for example, signifies this author (or the person discussed) is referring to nineteenth-century interpretations of the term whereas malaria (with no vertical slashes) is used when discussing contemporary understanding of the disease. The same applies to such terms as 'fever,' 'malarial conditions,' and so forth; all had diverse meanings in past centuries and often quite different from present-day definitions. Terms demarcated by vertical marks are most often found in the second half of the book. Sometimes words or short phrases appear within quotation marks, such as "malaria." This only signifies that the person, people, or institution being discussed used that term or phrase in the source document.

A few books consulted for this study were published in more than one volume. In this case, the volume from which information is obtained is included in the citation. For example, the number between the two colons in "(Wootton 1910:2:116)" signifies volume two. The page number (116) in the volume providing the data follows the second colon. Roman numerals to identify volumes, however, are used for the Royal Commission on Opium material. This is how these primary sources were printed.

Acknowledgments

This book could not have been written without help from some people. To Ernest Weyhrauch, former director of Eastern Kentucky University's Crabbe Library, thank you for seeing merit in this endeavor. A thank you is extended to Ken Barksdale (Director of Crabbe Library's Collection Development) for his diligence in procuring rare documents. It is difficult to express the gratitude I have for the staff of Crabbe Library. Without their help, few sources that are cited in this book (and the many not mentioned) would have been available to me. To Pat New, Linda Witt, Peggy Flaherty, Mary Dewey, and many others—thank you. A thank you is also extended to Dean Dominick Hart.

Data concerning the distribution of malaria in nineteenth-century India are difficult to find. Dr. V. P. Sharma (director of the Malaria Research Center, Indian Council of Medical Research, Delhi, India) provided this information. Several chapters in this book benefit from his insight.

One pleasure in visiting Chicago is roaming the stacks at the University of Chicago's libraries. I have done this on several, albeit too brief, occasions. The staff of each library visited has been exceptionally helpful. I am particularly indebted to several university personnel; they truly made these visits fruitful. To James Nye (director of the Southern Asia collection) and William Alsbaugh (East Asian collection) at Regenstein Library: your hospitality and ability to answer many questions will not be forgotten. Christa Modschiedler (reference librarian at John Crerar Medical Library) was always helpful when I was in Chicago or calling from somewhere in the country. Another valued resource at the institution was Joan Anderson and her colleagues at Harper Library. Ms. Anderson allowed me to search the many rows of stored documents in the Harper basement. It was a hot, dusty experience, but the data I found years ago eventually inspired this book. To Joan Anderson and everybody else affiliated with the University of Chicago, many, many thanks.

I also express gratitude to the library staff at the University of Wisconsin (Madison), and to their counterparts at the Library of Congress and the State Department Library in Washington, D.C. The time spent at these institutions was brief compared to the University of Chicago but the help given was no less valuable.

I wish to say thank you to the research committee at Eastern Kentucky University for several grants enabling me to visit the aforementioned libraries. To Angel and Gwyn Rubio, your encouragement has always been appreciated. The same sentiment is felt for Lori Pierelli, Rebecca Brooks, and Jason Hallman of Lexington Books.

Last, but most definitely not least, there are the quiet ones who always are supportive. Monique, Max, Pepper, and Ernie, you made everything worthwhile.

Abbreviations

AJMS	*American Journal of Medical Science*
AOSSOT	Anglo-Oriental Society for the Suppression of the Opium Trade
APA	American Pharmaceutical Association
B.C.E.	Before Christian Era
BFMR	*British and Foreign Medical Review*
BMJ	*British Medical Journal*
C.E.	Christian Era
DIB	*Dictionary of Indian Biography*
DNB	*Dictionary of National Biography*
EB	*Encyclopædia Britannica*
GBC	Great Britain Parliament Command Papers
GBO	Great Britain Royal Commission on Opium
GBOW	Great Britain Royal Commission on Opium Witness Testimony
GBR	Great Britain Parliament Reports of Standing or Select Committees
GBS	Great Britain Parliament* Session Papers [*"East India" replaces "Parliament" in some library catalogs for several documents. Material is often referred to as "Ordinary" Session Papers.]
IAMS	*The Indian Annals of Medical Science*
IDR	India Department of Revenue
IDRA	India Department of Revenue and Agriculture
IDFC	India Department of Finance and Commerce
IFCD	India Finance and Commerce Department
IJMPS	*Indian Journal of Medical and Physical Science*
IMG	*Indian Medical Gazette*
IMR	*Indian Medical Record*
IMS	Indian Medical Service
IUP/PP	Irish University Press Series of Parliamentary Papers

JAMA	*Journal of the American Medical Association*
JIMA	*Journal of the Indian Medical Association*
JTM	*Journal of Tropical Medicine*
LAN	*Lancet*
MR	*Medical Reporter*
MTG	*Medical Times and Gazette*
NEBma	*New Encyclopædia Britannica (Macropædia)*
NEBmi	*New Encylcopædia Britannica (Micropædia)*
PuID	Publications and Information Directorate
PJT	*The Pharmaceutical Journal and Transactions*
PJ	*The Pharmaceutical Journal*
PMJ	*The Provincial Medical Journal (Leicester)*
RSTM	Royal Society of Tropical Medicine
RSY	Royal Society Yearbook
SG	Surgeon General (United States)
SSOT	Society for the Suppression of the Opium Trade
WNID	*Webster's New Intercollegiate Dictionary*
WWW	*Who Was Who*

1
Introduction

One of my mentors in graduate school said that the study of British imperialism is the study of controversial events. He was right. The India-China opium trade during the eighteenth, nineteenth, and the early part of the twentieth century was one of the most controversial. The commerce has been the subject of many books, articles, monographs, unpublished studies, government reports, private letters, and other correspondence. Authors include actual participants and observers during the era. Some of these people opposed the trade; others supported it. Few were neutral.

In subsequent decades, journalists and nonacademicians offered their perspective. Academicians in diverse disciplines have added to an impressive body of knowledge. We now know a lot about this seminal event in the history of contact between Asia and the west. Scholars continue to explore the economics and politics of the trade. So, it is not hyperbole to say that our understanding will increase in the years to come. This sounds good. But listen carefully. You will hear a scream from some dead missionaries. For too long, they tell us, something has been overlooked.

Dr. Wilbur F. Crafts and his wife were still enraged seventeen years later. So were Mary and Margaret Leitch. The event had "whitewashed a stinking sepulcher of 'infernal revenue' and given to the world the verdict that opium was hardly worse than tea and coffee" (Crafts & Leitch 1911:287). This was their published, public opinion. What they said in private was probably laced with a bit of profanity. Several of the people they include in the 1911 diatribe come close to doing just that.[1]

These missionaries were condemning the 1895 Royal Commission decision not to end the India-China opium trade, and not to change policy regarding opium consumption within India. Decades of missionary and nonmissionary anti-drug agitation in Asia had come to naught. Wilbur and his wife, and Mary and Margaret had good reason to complain.

COMMON AGENDA, DIFFERENT EMPHASIS

If there is any "theme" that emerges from immersing oneself in the pronouncements of the British defenders of opium during the nineteenth century, it is that *they* were convinced of the morality of *their* stance. The same attitude is evident from the literature of their opponents; the anti-opiumists believed that *they* were the righteous people.

The Crafts and Leitch condemnation indicates that the conviction continued for several decades after 1895. Apologists for the Royal Commission ruling were no different. They express no doubt about its rectitude.

Despite their rhetoric, participants in this bitter struggle were really not opposed to each other. Virtually all Anglo-Europeans who voiced concern about the drug trade were not protesting the western presence in Asia.[2] The Christian missionaries who labored in China and their fellow worshippers back home, for example, did not reject the *idea* of western intrusion in China or elsewhere in the world. Nobody condemned the expansion and consolidation of British domination in India.

The anti-opiumists and defenders of the trade articulated a perspective about imperialism that contemporary scholars contend was prevalent among most nineteenth- and early twentieth-century citizens in Great Britain (Burton 1994).[3] Imperialism was viewed "as a civilizing mission based upon both commerce and Christianity" (Grant 2001:53). And for the anti-opiumists during the era, "religious motivations and humanitarian concerns [were] not an alternative to imperial control [but rather] the best means of securing it" (Thorne 1999:9).[4] Their strategy for saving souls did not include enslavement to opium. Participants in this decades-long controversy were arguing about the content of imperialist activity. They were upset about unbecoming behavior, not about grand design. Commerce should be, must be, governed by Christian principles of proper conduct. The drug policy of the East India Company and its successor, the Government of India, was the antithesis of this ideal. Other commentators confirm the assessment.

For Hilary Beattie, the 1895 Royal Commission decision demonstrated that moral suasion was "evidently powerless against imperialist interests, which could not contemplate risk to the Indian Empire." Furthermore, the "ardent Christians" were themselves practicing "a kind of cultural imperialism." They wanted to spread the word of Jesus. The British rulers of India could care less. They wanted to make money, and lots of it. Neither group was a stranger to "imperialist expansion" (Beattie 1969:124–25). In fact, their success depended upon it.

J. B. Brown agrees. The year 1874 was a watershed for the Christian evangelists. The "simple negativism of earlier" efforts was abandoned, and these people proceeded to develop "an enthusiastic programme of empire" (Brown,

J. B. 1974:97). They were, however, concerned with preaching, not profit. The export of Indian opium to China, these evangelists insisted, "was blamed for retarding the progress of Christianity—on the premise that the Chinese could not be expected to distinguish between the white missionary and the white opium peddler" (Brown, J. B. 1974:102). For the missionaries and their supporters, the British Empire was "a laboratory for moral legislation" (Brown, J. B. 1974:106). They were not against commerce per se, but they did object vehemently to immoral trade. This was opium.

Look beyond the rhetoric, Brown tells us, and you find that the anti-opiumists "desired a more thoroughgoing interference with Eastern culture than did the imperial bureaucracy against which [they] fought for almost fifty years" (1974:110).

Kathleen Lodwick (1976) describes the predicament that missionaries in China found themselves in during these decades. One of her sources is an editorial from an 1894 issue of the *Chinese Recorder*, an influential missionary periodical. The editors had previously expressed concern that "outside" forces would prevent the Chinese government from ending poppy cultivation in the country. Now, they said that

> it behooves [us] to redouble [our] prayers in this important matter, and beseech God to grant them deliverance from the stigma of offering salvation with one hand while with the other they hold out opium. (Lodwick 1976:43)

The metaphor reveals more than was intended. From the perspective of the Chinese native, or from any Asian experiencing the British presence, the hands were attached to one body. These appendages represented two manifestations of the same intrusion, the same form of insidious domination. Furthermore, many Chinese associated "Christianity and opium, due to the unfortunate coincidence that the missionaries and the opium had arrived in China at about the same time" (Lodwick 1976:46–7). The Chinese, as well as all people in Asia, were guilty of no sin when they ignored the evangelists' message about salvation. The only deliverance many of them undoubtedly wanted was for the missionaries to get out of the country.

The message from contemporary scholars is clear: Anglo-European participants in the opium controversy were arguing about whose version of exploitation would prevail in Asia. They were, metaphorically speaking, two sides of the same coin; they were cut from the same cloth.

SCIENCE IN THE SERVICE OF EMPIRE

Another trait is obvious in the participants' literature. Both groups of antagonists appropriated facets of Anglo-European science to advance their agendas. Sometimes the facts they cited were correct. Sometimes their interpretation of theoretical material was valid. Sometimes neither quality was present. For the most prominent activists on both sides, science was an instrument that bestowed a veneer of objectivity upon what they were arguing about.

Berridge and Edwards (1981), Kurland (1978), Parsinnen (1983), Peters (1981), Miskel (1973), Musto (1973), Sonnedecker (1963), and others provide information about the anti-opiumists' appropriation of medical data to attack the trade. This is good.

Nothing equivalent exists for the other side. That is not so good. It also is a paradox. Defenders of the status quo "won" the "battle" and they used Anglo-European science to do it. Yet, there is no extensive commentary of the pro-trade activists' selection of facts and theory to nullify their opponents' medical arguments.

This book is a modest attempt to rectify the omission. It is a case study of sorts, and it is modest because the focus is upon one argument. This was the pro-traders' contention that eating the drug prevents and cures malaria. Members of the Royal Commission accepted this notion as valid medical evidence. It became a very important part of their rationale for doing nothing. And it infuriated the hapless missionaries in 1911, those people who can be heard if you listen carefully.

You now have the skeleton of a book about "western" science and British imperialism. The rest of the chapter puts some flesh and blood on its bones.

THE ARGUMENT

The British rulers of India during the late nineteenth century faced two serious problems concerning opium. First, they confronted mounting criticism of the ethical and health implications of the drug trade. The second problem was the continuing, albeit declining revenue from opium sales; the third pillar that sustained the British Raj was crumbling. Anti-opiumists' success in mobilizing opposition in the British Parliament and segments of the Anglo-European public threatened to accelerate the decline and to exacerbate existent political instability in south Asia. It also meant an encroachment upon British officials' autonomy to govern India in a manner that they deemed fit.

The controversy culminated in the creation of the Royal Commission on Opium during 1893–95. Members of the Commission reviewed the political, economic, moral, and medical aspects of the Government of India's involvement in the drug trade. All of the anti-opiumists' proclamations were refuted. Central to the Government of India's triumph was medical evidence that supported the continuation of the commerce in opium. Much of this material simply rejected what the anti-opiumists had claimed.

Another argument took the anti-opiumists by surprise. Their rebuttal was ineffective. They said too little, too late, too infrequently. The Government of India and its supporters asserted that eating the drug prevents and cures malaria, and that narcotine, one of the drug's components, was responsible for this capability. Opium and narcotine do neither. The pronouncement was a tactic to preserve British hegemony in South Asia. The following chapters illuminate the contribution of this medical misconception to nineteenth-century British imperialism.

The early part of the book traces the emergence of the anti-opiumists' moral position and their use of medical data. This material describes their vision of imperialism: what Anglo-Europeans of good conscience had to do for unenlightened inhabitants of distant societies. The latter chapters present the belated medical defense mustered by defenders of India's opium commerce. The sections include a description of what happened when the Royal Commission endorsed the drug and disease correlation. It was a political and economic windfall for the Government of India. And it ended anti-opium agitation in the country. The significance of this book for contemporary studies of imperialism is the subject of the final chapter.

The remainder of this introduction provides more exposition about the factors that gave rise to the drug and disease argument: historical context, imperial finance, and the Royal Commission on Opium, its composition, mission, and the evidence that its members heard and reviewed.

The chapter concludes with a discussion about the *actual* status of malaria and opium in Anglo-European medical theory and practice during the nineteenth century. This material describes what antagonists should have assumed, known, and said about the drug and disease argument. Some of them obliged. Others did not. The discussion reveals how big a gap existed between science and something other than science.

HISTORICAL CONTEXT

No discussion about eighteenth, nineteenth, and twentieth century contact between Asian and European society is complete without appreciating the role of opium in opening China to English, European, and American merchants. *Papaver somniferum Linn* (the opium poppy's botanical name) was especially vital for British rule in South Asia, in particular India, from the mid-1700s and the nineteenth century. Satisfying demand for opium capable of yielding a smoking extract that was acceptable to Chinese consumers, the largest market, required technical skill and political acumen. The British struggled for more than a century to acquire and to retain both.

Opium obtained from poppies grown in territory under direct English control in India soon earned a worldwide reputation for yielding a high-quality smoking extract. Protecting and enhancing profits from the China market involved delicate negotiations with diverse parties. This necessitated political skill no less sophisticated than the expertise required for the careful preparation of the exported drug. Great Britain prevented other opium-producing nations, as well as the European and American merchants who transported the product, from seriously contesting its import monopoly in China and elsewhere in the Far East.

Great Britain also protected its domination of the Asia trade by regulating opium commerce within India. The threat came from the quasi-independent native (or princely) states capable of producing opium. During the first half of the nineteenth century, the East India Company negotiated treaties that prohibited poppy cultivation in some of these entities. The Company compensated rulers for estimated losses. Military force ended other native states' unfettered access to seaports on India's western coast. The Company now controlled the amount of opium shipped overseas. Its administrators proceeded to raise or lower taxes imposed on the native states' commodity, or the number of chests permitted for export, whenever they deemed it necessary. The East India Company, and its successor, the Government of India, also dictated how much opium from the native states could be legally sold in British territory. The British administration, however, refrained from interfering in the opium commerce within native states not under its direct control. No restrictions applied to cultivation or manufacture. Citizens were free to consume as much as they desired. British policy for the quasi-independent native states translated into an uninterrupted source of revenue from exported as well as domestically sold and consumed opium. For the Raj, this income during the nineteenth century was not only uninterrupted, it was crucial.

Great Britain's domination of the China market and an ability to impose its will upon India's indigenous rulers quickly led to the enduring status of opium as one of the three most important sources of revenue for the British Indian Empire. The drug's salience began early in the era. It ended in the first decade of the twentieth century. Furthermore, sales of opium anywhere in the world depended upon the drug's ability to engender physiological and psychological responses. This fact dominated commerce regardless of which nation produced the commodity and how a consumer actually ingested the substance.

The Asian drug trade was never free from controversy. Opposition began in the late 1700s. It continued until the trade was halted between 1907 and 1917. Antagonists demanded either an end to, or a drastic decrease in, exports to China and elsewhere in the Far East. Other opponents implored Great Britain to voluntarily cease, or at least immediately reduce, opium production within India. Many groups agitated for both programs. Protestant missionaries and Quaker reformers dominated their ranks. With varying degrees of participation throughout the nineteenth century, other anti-opiumists included Chinese nationals as well as British, American, and European medical personnel with much experience in India, China, and elsewhere. Prominent religious personalities in western nations, and some secular leaders, joined them. The premise of their collective argument was the immorality of making money by encouraging drug addiction and ensuring human degradation. They were not alone. Officials of the East India Company and its post-1857 successor, the Government of India, periodically voiced reservations about the drug commerce.

Apologists for the trade said the condemnation was nonsense. They offered no medical justification to support their political and economic rationalizations. They did not have to. The anti-opiumists' lament fell on deaf ears and British politicians simply ignored them. Nonetheless, the protests and warnings from overseas observers did not stop. Religious and secular sympathizers at home continued to educate the public about detrimental aspects of the trade. It was slow going. An important factor for the indifference was massive opium consumption within the British Isles. There was no stigma associated with the habit so there was no problem linked to consumption elsewhere in the world.

Health professionals' increasing alarm about opium abuse in England finally ended this era of complacency and silence. The accumulation of scientific knowledge about the drug, including its effect upon the human body, and what gave opium its power, strengthened their argument. Commencing in the mid- to-late 1860s, a remarkable change in attitude about unrestricted use of opium occurred among influential segments of the British public and members of Parliament. The new awareness extended to opium-based medicines of all kinds. The drug was now officially classified as a poison. Anti-opiumists used this cognizance in Great Britain to press for termination of the India-China drug trade. Their demands remained the same, and their logic was unambiguous; opium was dangerous regardless of who used it or where they lived. Evidence from laboratory research and clinical observation seemed to support these proclamations. The public began to elect anti-opiumists to Parliament.

By the mid-1870s, the literature that demanded an end to the trade was substantial and vitriolic. Leaders of the movement spoke loudly, clearly, and often. Their influence in Parliament was increasing. The public was listening to them. Well-known agitators now included members of a new organization called the Anglo-Oriental Society for the Suppression of the Opium Trade. Quakers were prominent in its creation. The literature usually refers to the organization as the Society for the Suppression of the Opium Trade (SSOT). The number of respected secular and religious leaders in the major western nations increased. The rank and file in these countries also participated in the movement. More natives in China were joining indigenous anti-opium organizations. The Imperial government helped. It denounced all people and all governments involved in the trade. These proclamations were issued infrequently, and they did not stop the commerce.

Many Anglo-European activists remained equally hostile to British administrators' lenient attitude about consumption of the drug within India itself. Great Britain, the principal exporter to Asia and chief beneficiary of profits during the era, received most of the criticism. Apologists for the trade continued to be condemned for initiating two wars over opium, and they were blamed for creating unending misery among the Chinese people. Although ardent anti-opiumists' yearning for an immediate end to the India-China opium trade never wavered, tactics changed in this new decade. They tailored pronouncements to refute pro-traders' counterattacks, as well as to circumvent the unexpected decision of leaders of China not to end imports of the Indian drug when given this opportunity in 1885. The anti-opiumists' interpretation of medical data was sobering. It also was frequently self-serving. Consumption of the drug always led to addiction. It made no difference why opium was used, or the amount ingested. Some advocates asserted that chronic dependence resulted in death or generated serious anti-social behavior such as crime and licentiousness.

The anti-opiumists now targeted poppy acreage in India. Cultivation, they demanded, should be prohibited throughout the country. The only exception was the acreage that produced the opium necessary for legitimate medicinal use. Everything else should be stopped. Great Britain's domestic distribution policy could be, and should be, emulated. The anti-opiumists proposed that only qualified, licensed people were to be permitted to dispense the drug in India. It must be given solely for medical purposes; no other rationale qualified. Other steps that were proposed for India at this time were responses to the conditions of cultivation and production that were unique to South Asia.

The SSOT and its supporters were truly ambitious and incredibly ingenuous. They had no doubt that this program would end the moral and physical degradation of millions of citizens in India. The benefits would extend beyond the country's borders to China and elsewhere in Asia. The good news did not end with Asia. They wanted a drastic reduction of opium available to anybody in the world, a world in which people who used the drug had a credible reason for doing so. The evils of addiction would then be only a painful memory. What these anti-opiumists got was something else.

Anti-opium agitation had minimal effect upon the sale of India's opium for most of the nineteenth century. Consumers' preference for the country's exports determined the percentage contribution of opium to British India's general revenue. Additional profits came from selling the substance within India. The exported drug that was manufactured in British India was called Provision opium. The domestic commodity was known as Excise (Abkari) opium.

A change was underway by the beginning of the last decade of the nineteenth century. Profits from the exported commodity had fallen, and income from Abkari opium was increasing. Although the anti-opiumists were not responsible for the change, these people were doing something else during the 1890s that would make the situation worse. They were influencing more members of Parliament. The SSOT's successful lobbying promised two things. Both were ominous. The first effect was to accelerate the Provision drug's declining profitability. The second consequence was to curtail sales of the domestic commodity. Statistics reveal just how bad things were for the Government of India.

OPIUM AND IMPERIAL FINANCE

Opium in the Total Gross Revenue of the East India Company and the Government of India, 1720–1893

The first time that the East India Company sent opium to China was in 1720. The amount was negligible. About twenty chests were sent during 1767. The Company made no profit from this commerce until 1773. The trade then rapidly expanded. By 1793, the drug had become the East India Company's third principal branch of revenue. It held that position during the Royal Commission on Opium hearings (GBO [Clarke] 1894:II:440–41, 495).[5]

Overseas sales provided most of the money earned from opium between 1793 and 1893. Any change in this export activity had enormous repercussions for both the general opium revenue and total earnings for the Company. In 1842/43 "percentage on total gross revenue" for opium was 9.2 percent (Great Britain. Parliament [East India] [Statement–Opium] 1891–92:244). The manufacture and distribution of opium within and beyond the country ten years later (in

1852/53) now accounted for 18 percent of the East India Company's total revenue from all sources.[6]

The end of the decade brought the end of good times. There was more competition from Persian and Turkish opium. Indigenous production in China was increasing. Both factors made exports of the Indian commodity to the Asian mainland and the Straits settlements (Singapore, Penang, and native states on the Malay Peninsula) a progressively less profitable enterprise. By 1862/63, the declining monetary contribution of *Papaver somniferum Linn* to the economic solvency of the British Raj was evident when its share of the total gross revenue dropped to 17.4 percent. The trend continued for the remainder of the century. The exported and domestically consumed drug accounted for 15.4 percent in 1872/73.[7] In 1880, the opium revenue comprised 14 percent of the Government of India's budget (Richards 1981:69). And in 1882/83 the drug's share had fallen to 13.5 percent. Ten years later (1892/93) opium amounted to 8.9 percent of the Government of India's total gross revenue (Great Britain. Parliament [East India] [Statement–Opium] 1891–92:244).

Other documents provide net, as well as gross, Provision opium revenue data from the second half of the nineteenth century. The figures in these sources differ slightly. The discrepancies are the result of different time spans covered within the fifty-year period, and what expenditures were deducted in calculating net revenue.

Nevertheless, the documents confirm two facts: the continuing importance of exports to Government of India revenue during the latter decades of the nineteenth century, and the consequences of a diminution in overseas commerce.

Gross and Net Earnings from Provision (Exported) Opium

A 1904 Parliamentary paper lists gross revenue from provision chests in 1880/81 as 10.48 million rupees. As of 1893/94, the sum had fallen to 6.63 million. The decline was not an aberration; it continued during the Royal Commission's existence and thereafter. By 1897/98 and 1898/99, the contribution of the exported drug to the general revenue fund was 5.18 and 5.73 million rupees in 1897/98 and 1898/99 respectively (GBC [Statistical Abstract–Population] 1904:58).

Other sources reveal the same trend for net revenue. The 1896 issue of *Statistical Abstracts*, for example, documents a rapid and dramatic decrease in the amount of money earned after deducting all expenses. "Total net receipts" minus "total expenditures" in 1889/90 amounted to 6,977,949 (in tens of rupees.) By 1893/94, the statistic had fallen to only 4,750,964 (GBC [Statistical Abstract–No. 42] 1896a:95). The difference represents about a 30 percent decline in the net revenue that was derived from the export of Indian opium. It occurred within a period of only five years.[8]

The data clearly indicate a gradual decline in the contribution of India's *Papaver somniferum Linn* to the financial well-being of the British Raj. The trend began in the 1860s. And within this long-term diminution, the gross and net revenue of the domestically consumed drug was becoming an increasingly important component of the Government of India's general opium revenue.

Changing Status of the Excise (Abkari) Drug in India's General Opium Revenue

Net Revenue from Excise Opium, 1867/68 through 1889/90

Statistics for a twenty-one year period, from 1867/68 through 1889/90, reveal the change. Excise opium represented only 4.6 percent of the total net Indian opium revenue in 1867/68. It rose to 5 percent for the next two seasons (1868/69 and 1869/70) and then reached 5.6 percent during 1870/71. After accounting for a mere 3.2 percent in 1871/72, contribution of the excise commodity increased almost every season. Eleven years later, in 1882/83, it had risen to 10.2 percent followed by a slight decline to 9.9 percent during 1883/84. The percentage thereafter remained in double figures. By 1888/89 domestic sales of *Papaver somniferum Linn* represented 13.4 percent of total net opium revenue (GBS [Watt] 1891:72).[9] The contribution of domestic sales of the mother drug to total net opium revenue in India was in double digits when members of the Royal Commission conducted their investigation, and it retained this position for the rest of the century.

W. S. Meyer's Calculations of Excise Earnings Compared to Provision Opium Gross and Net Revenue from 1878/79 through 1898/99

W. S. Meyer's 1900 analysis of data from 1878/79 through 1898/99 furnishes more evidence for declining revenues of exported opium compared to the increasing importance of the domestic commodity. In 1878/79 the Government of India realized a gross profit of 940 lakhs of rupees from Provision opium. Since one lakh = 100,000, the exported commodity during that year earned an impressive total of 94 million rupees for the Government of India. Twenty years later, gross profits had fallen to 573 lakhs or 57.3 million rupees (IFCD [Meyer] 1900:2). A decrease of 36.7 million rupees, or more than 39 percent, over two decades was a sufficient reason for British administrators to be concerned.

Net revenue statistics for the drug that was shipped overseas were no better. After "deducting expenses of production, etc.," Meyer calculated a net profit of 770 lakhs, or 77 million rupees, for 1878/79. As of 1898/99, the tally for this category was only 23.7 million rupees, or 237 lakhs (IFCD [Meyer] 1900:1–2). A decline of 53.3 million rupees (69.22 percent) over twenty-one years was irrefutable and sobering evidence that the third pillar sustaining the economy of British rule was eroding. The exported drug's shrinking contribution was one problem confronting the Government of India when the Royal Commission on Opium was conducting its inquiry.

The receipts from Excise opium, in contrast, increased from sixty lakhs in 1878/79 to 100 lakhs in 1898/99. This represented a 40 percent gain in two decades. Meyer states that the excise revenues (Abkari opium) were "shared with the various provincial governments according to the proportions fixed for excise revenue generally," whereas profits from overseas sales (Provision opium) were credited to the central government in New Delhi. This means that any change in the domestic use of opium had serious ramifications for these

British India administrative entities (IFCD [Meyer] 1900:1–2). The SSOT agenda guaranteed disruption.

THE ROYAL COMMISSION ON OPIUM

Anti-opiumists eventually succeeded in mobilizing public concern about opium use in Great Britain and linking it to reservations about foreign policy. In 1893, Parliament recommended the creation of a Royal Commission on Opium. The Commission was to investigate the economic, political, and moral issues associated with India's poppy cultivation, collection of crude opium, and its processing for domestic consumption and export. British India officials sent documents that they thought germane for the investigation to the Royal Commission. The anti-opiumists submitted far fewer items. One reason for the discrepancy is that anti-opiumists lacked statistics that quantified the amount of consumption in India. Many anti-opiumists also were confident that the righteousness of their cause precluded the need for numerous supporting documents. Health professionals' awareness about opiate abuse in Great Britain reinforced this conviction; the danger of opium use was not a hypothesis, it was a fact requiring no additional confirmation.

Members of the Royal Commission had access to almost all material submitted by both sides in the argument. They also heard testimony, virtually all of it in India, from more than 700 witnesses. The Government of India avowed that the people it selected to testify on its behalf possessed a wide range of experience and expertise in South Asia. Completion of the formidable task of interviewing and reviewing documents enabled members of the Royal Commission to ascertain the importance of opium to the status of Great Britain as a world power. The Commission also formulated policy after comprehending the ramifications of continuing, or terminating, the reliance of the Government of India upon opium as a source of revenue. Its recommendations, therefore, shaped the future character of British rule in the subcontinent. Part of this perspective was the financial stability of the poppy-cultivating native states on the Malwa plateau that exported their drug beyond India.[10]

The Royal Commission's proceedings were published in seven volumes during 1894 and 1895. The conclusions outraged anti-opiumists. None of their moral and medical arguments were accorded credibility. The Commission saw no need to diminish production and distribution of the drug in India. Furthermore, Commission members provided the British Parliament with a medical justification to augment opium activities in the subcontinent.

The Royal Commission used two types of information in its decision. Each one consisted of oral depositions, memorials (petitions), and a smattering of technical literature. The first type alleged that eating opium was the prevalent form of ingestion in South Asia, that the practice was long-standing, and that natives themselves defended eating opium as a way to prevent and cure disease. Acceptance of *Papaver somniferum Linn*, therefore, was so engrained in Indian natives' consciousness that any interference with consumption of the drug constituted an unjustified assault upon individual liberty and disrespect for tradition. The Indian public simply would tolerate no prohibition. Policy that ignored this fact was an insult to the intelligence of India's natives. A habit that had marginal value, or no value whatsoever, would have ended long ago. Restricting *Papaver somniferum Linn*'s availability in South Asia meant dooming people to unnecessary suffering.

The Royal Commission called the second type of information medical evidence. This information, it claimed, was a paramount factor in determining the content of the final report. Their interpretation of this medical evidence was unequivocal; the drug had a remarkable capability to reduce disease mortality and alleviate human misery throughout Asia. The Commission concluded that moderate opium consumption in India was beneficial for numerous human ailments and disease. This was true regardless of how the substance was introduced into the human body. Even the ingestion of prodigious amounts of the drug was, in most cases, harmless or advantageous.

One body of data, compelling because of the terror and suffering it addressed, portrayed opium as being able to prevent and to cure malaria. Some witnesses testifying before the Royal Commission and several Government of India documents both praise and analyze the drug's prophylactic and curative effects upon the physiology and psychology of 'malaria' victims in the subcontinent. Most people asked to comment or interjecting an opinion, however, said the correlation was spurious.

In the past, supporters of the drug commerce had ignored the connection between opium and malaria. Political and economic issues dominated their defense before the SSOT's creation in the mid-1870s. A British physician working in India then recognized the linkage as a way to refute anti-opiumists' allegations about the dangers of unrestricted availability. Defenders of the status quo, however, articulated the notion only when the anti-opiumists' medical arguments had changed public opinion in Great Britain about the drug-induced misery in Asia. By 1890 the opium and 'malaria' correlation appeared periodically in pro-defense arguments; by 1892 it was commonplace.

The severity of malaria in South Asia, and prevalence of other diseases in the subcontinent, permitted the Commission to phrase its opposition to substantial cuts in production and public accessibility to the drug in India as a refusal to contribute to human suffering. The people who did not want Great Britain to stop being involved in the cultivation, processing, and distribution of opium had interpreted the Commission's findings as a moral imperative. An abrupt end to the domestic trade was tantamount to the Crown denying an obligation to Indian subjects for fair and humane rule.

The Royal Commission's acceptance of data concerning opium's status in malaria eradication and prevention, as well as evidence of the drug's prophylactic functions for other diseases, devastated the SSOT. Membership declined drastically. The Commission's stance also lessened the effectiveness of anti-opiumists' subsequent proclamations for terminating British involvement in any aspect of the trade. Most of their arguments continued to focus on the immorality of the drug trade, not on challenging the validity of medical evidence and testimony regarding opium and disease that the Commission utilized.

What Did the Royal Commission on Opium Accomplish?

In the decade after 1895, the South Asian drug once again competed with Persian and Turkish imports into China. India, however, still accounted for approximately 95 percent of the country's foreign opium (Reins 1991:114). The most serious challenge was the

> rapid expansion of China's own opium production. Amounts of [Persian and Turkish imports] were small, but China's domestic production was enormous; by 1905 China manufactured over eight times as much as she imported and Szechuan province alone produced more than India. (Newman 1989:530)

The Royal Commission had no control over production in China. Hence, it was unable to halt the continuing decrease of the exported drug's percentage contribution to the financial and political stability of the British Raj.

The Commission's *real* success was domestic. First, it provided the Government of India with an economic opportunity of immense proportions. The Commission's pronouncement about the medical benefits of eating opium condoned a dramatic increase in poppy cultivation and the amount of opium manufactured for use within India. The domain of eligible recipients for the drug, as defined by anti-opiumists, extended beyond South Asia. Second, and most important, the decision to expand acreage and output, as well as determining future policy regarding the China trade, would remain the prerogative of British India's administrators, not the moralistic evangelists, whom they chastised as knowing nothing about imperial governance. In other words, the Royal Commission had succeeded in eliminating the SSOT in the battle over whose version of imperialism would be the future of India.

Chinese nationalists, not Christian moralists, were prime catalysts in galvanizing western concern about the commerce in opium after 1895. Outraged by the decadence associated with massive addiction in the early twentieth century, the Chinese demanded curtailment of poppy cultivation within their country. They also wanted imports of opium to cease. Their protest about foreign opium culminated in a 1907 treaty involving the Governments of India, Great Britain, and China. It stipulated annual reductions of opium exports from India over a ten-year period. The India-China drug trade formally ended in 1917, and a tumultuous episode in relations between Asia and western society became history.

Another series of events had transpired during the previous century. They also demarcate the end of an era. The epoch that came to a close concerned misconceptions in medical science. Anglo-European scientists during the 1800s produced seminal revelations about malaria. By the end of the century, they knew much about what caused the disease and how to cure it. The discoveries about opium were even more impressive. The reasons for its fabled powers were no longer a mystery.

Some comments about this work reveal what the SSOT and its opponents appropriated to further their respective imperialist agendas. What did they say that was true, that was false, that was hyperbole? The other chapters in the book present their arguments. The comments in the rest of this chapter help evaluate what the antagonists were talking about. What did they have in mind when they mentioned opium, when they referred to malaria, and when some of them disparaged quinine? This discussion is brief.

NEW EXPLANATIONS, FADING PARADIGMS, ENDURING FALLACIES

Malaria and 'Malaria' in Late Nineteenth Century Anglo-European Science

The definition and understanding of malaria in Anglo-European medical circles changed drastically during the nineteenth century. The transformation was obvious by 1893–1895. No longer was the term only a synonym for the lethal effects of a noxious gas (a miasm or vapor) produced by rotting corpses and decaying vegetation.

Monocausal interpretations that had dominated western thought for centuries were also discredited. Medical theoreticians did not blame malevolent supernatural entities. Trees, soil types, elevation above sea level, and other terrestrial (tellurian) characteristics were not principal culprits. Damp climate alone did not produce the disease. Neither did excessive exposure to the sun's heat followed by the coolness of night guarantee sickness. For knowledgeable western commentators, wrathful deities, bad air ("mal' aria") that conveyed harmful emanations and toxic vapors, or other earthly vicissitudes external to the victim, had become or were becoming inadequate explanations of human sickness.

Equally implausible was humoral theory, a conception that dated back to the early Greeks, Romans, and the enduring legacy of Galen. Proponents of this explanation and its variations through the centuries portrayed ill health as a manifestation of ephemeral imbalances within the human body. The paradigm's inadequacies were evident to Western medical practitioners during the Renaissance. Their disenchantment with this explanation of misery, including interpretations of malaria, accelerated thereafter.

Furthermore, filthy habits of human beings, popular among some western observers, especially in Great Britain, during the earlier decades of the nineteenth century, did not suffice as the principal, or only cause, for the malady's presence. A lack of sanitation among a population or the absence of personal hygiene was one, but only one, variable accounting for the presence and mortality associated with the disease, or any disease.[11]

This is not to say that by the end of the nineteenth century, Anglo-European medical investigators had dismissed factors that were external to the victim to explain poor health and death. The environment was indeed implicated: it created conditions conducive to the appearance of disease; it was the midwife to serious maladies, an incubator that spawned episodes of human tragedy (Richmond 1980:84).

Many western scientists also accepted the long-held notion that entities within the human body caused misery. It was not, however, humoral imbalance, or an excess of heat or coldness within an individual. The entity was microbes inhabiting a person, with different kinds of tiny living organisms affecting different parts of the body and disrupting different body processes. These investigators had assimilated the germ theory of disease propounded by Louis Pasteur during the 1860s. They also heeded what Robert Koch and others said in subsequent years. The result was a tenable paradigm to explain disease causation (Crellin 1968:57; Harrison, Gordon 1978:4; Marcovich 1988:109).

One of the maladies was malaria. Perceptive Anglo-European researchers disenchanted with theories of humoral imbalance and noxious vapors then recognized the significance of Alphonse Laveran's 1880 identification of peculiar protozoa in the blood of patients suffering from the disease. The microbes were plasmodium.[12]

Other researchers confirmed Laveran's controversial observation and provided new revelations in the decade after the discovery. By 1885, the Italian researchers Ettore Marchiafava and Angelo Celli had described in detail the "parasite's feeding, accumulation of black pigment, and gradual enlargement almost to fill the host cell, by that time emptied of itself." In the same year, Camillo Golgi, another Italian, discovered that Laveran's parasites periodically divide in human blood, and that the event "coincided with the onset of fever" (Harrison, Gordon 1978:14).

Golgi had demonstrated that cell division, not ephemeral imbalances within the body or a tellurian variable external to the victim, was specifically linked to episodes of elevated temperature. He also identified the different microbes that were responsible for the long-noted peculiar characteristics of malarial paroxysms (Hehir 1913:683; Hehir 1927:3).

This observation enabled Golgi to correctly conclude that a new generation of a certain kind of parasite also appeared during the seventy-two hour period. The new generation coincided with the predictable appearance of quartan fever. He also deduced the significance of individuals who suffered from irregularly occurring fevers. Their paroxysms did not follow a three-day or four-day cycle. They were victims of "double or triple infections by either quartan or tertian parasites" (Harrison, Gordon 1978:15). This meant that a person could host more than one kind of plasmodium, and that one species of parasites in different stages of its life cycle can simultaneously attack the same individual. Human beings, therefore, can suffer from multiple infections at the same time. These achievements prompted one twentieth-century commentator to say that in 1885, Golgi had "formulated a series of laws which may be looked upon as classical" (Hehir 1927:3).

Mark Boyd claims that Laveran's 1880 observation of microbes finally discredited the "fallacious doctrine of miasma" (1949:13). The labor of Marchiafava, Celli, and Golgi during the next five years and thereafter confirmed the optimistic assessment. Even Dr. William Osler of Baltimore, Maryland, the most eminent blood specialist at the time and suspicious of Laveran's veracity, was converted. At the end of the 1880s, he "knew of no qualified pathologist working in a region where malaria was prevalent who still doubted Laveran's findings" (Harrison, Gordon 1978:16; see also Haynes 2001:86–95; Scott, H. H. 1939:149).

Seminal discoveries and empirical data about the clinical course of malarial microbes continued to accumulate for the remainder of the century and beyond. Research validating humoral theory during the same period was nonexistent.

Participants in the Anglo-European quest to understand why people got sick had also established the credibility of an idea that Egyptian, Greek, and Roman physicians had articulated so long ago.[13] The conviction had been a part of European folk beliefs for centuries. Giovanni Maria Lancisi and other commentators during the Renaissance and thereafter were convinced of its veracity. The unorthodox thought they held in common was that small flying insects were a factor in ill health; they were transporting something lethal to people. In other words, the animals were vectors and vector identification is the third component of contemporary malariology. The Anglo-European study of disease had matured and this sophistication included impressive progress in illuminating the cause, the clinical course, and the animate, conveying mechanism responsible for what we now call malaria.[14]

The emergence of germ theory as a viable paradigm facilitated greater accuracy in disease classification. Two changes express this nosological erudition. Most western researchers and medical practitioners now refrained from portraying diseases possessing obvious, or subtle, differences as points along a continuum of miasmatic emanations, or intensities of dampness, variations in sea level, and so forth. Physicians now had the opportunity to classify diseases according to the miniscule organisms that are the primary cause. Many health practitioners chose to do so. Using only symptoms to categorize episodes of human sickness, a trait dating back to Greek physicians, had become passé (Jones, W. H. S. 1909:67).

Associated with this development was a disinclination to view fever as a disease unto itself. Fever was now construed as a trait shared by many etiologically distinct or separate maladies. It was a phenomenon that accompanied a phase, or several stages, of a specific disease in a human victim. An instance of elevated body temperature, or paroxysms with varying intensities and duration, indicated the presence of something more fundamental. Fevers, then, were hints or clues; they were symptoms but nothing more. Furthermore, preventing the appearance of a symptom did not mean that the underlying cause had been eliminated.

This emerging exactitude had profound consequences for determining the presence of malaria in a person. The ancient Greeks' referred to the disease as fever and chills. They also identified the periodic episodes of pyrexia as quotidian, tertian, and quartan (Jarcho 1980:134; see also Jones, W. H. S. 1909). Despite these observations, they had no "dependable way of distinguishing such cases from the recurring fevers and chills that might occur in other diseases, except that fever and chills happening in the presence of an obvious focus, such as osteomyelitis or puerperal sepsis, were easy to identify" (Jarcho 1980:134). The inability to differentiate among separate maladies characterized nosology in western societies for many centuries.

The appearance of the term malaria in Anglo-European medical literature during the 1500s did not signify diagnostic precision. As late as the 1820s, prominent western commentators portrayed this pathogenic, sometimes malodorous, substance as the cause of a group of diseases. The maladies were variously known as:

... autumnal fever, intermittent fever, bilious fever, congestive fever, swamp fever, and ague ... [and by] ... a natural extension, fevers which were thought to result from exposure to noxious effluvia could be designated as malarial or malarious. (Jarcho 1970:36)

A coterie of Anglo-Europeans during the middle third of the nineteenth century then contended that the noxious gas was responsible for more than just intermittent fever. The role of miasma in cholera, yellow fever, and typhoid fever was extensively debated (Jarcho 1970:36).

The work of Pasteur and his associates challenged this speculation. Acceptance of Laveran's achievement would almost end it. The detection of plasmodia had "given the concept of malaria increased precision because it made possible the differentiation between malaria and other tropical and subtropical fevers such as kala-azar and brucellosis" (Jarcho 1980:135). Some investigators after 1880 now used the word "malaria" to designate a specific, devastating disease caused by protozoa. For others, malaria remained a hypothetical vapor that produced intermittent fevers.[15] By 1890, however, a substantial—and increasing—number of members of the scientific community recognized the numerous, separate diseases formerly subsumed under 'malaria' were actually the product of different species of microorganisms. For these theoreticians, the misamatic paradigm had become an anachronism (Jarcho 1970:38). The few proponents of humoral theory had even less support from reputable investigators. The nosological confusion dominating ancient Greek disease therapy, and almost two thousand years thereafter in western societies, was coming to an end.

Nineteenth-century discoveries about causation, clinical course, vectors, and disease identification were indeed remarkable. By 1899, according to R. N. Chaudhuri, "the etiology of every tropical disease known to humankind at that time had been explored, and in many cases, understood" (1954:423).[16] The information accumulated throughout the century was available to any health professional and interested citizen. Most Anglo-Europeans circa 1893–1895 accepted the new perspective. Some did not. Still others incorporated elements of the emerging orientation into old paradigms.

The Prevention and Cure of Malaria and 'Malaria' in Late Nineteenth Century Anglo-European Science

By 1893–1895 the medical personnel and lay people who accepted the veracity of germ theory realized there was no panacea for the prevention and cure of human sickness. Solutions tended to be disease-specific. A drug or therapy that eliminated one kind of microbe might be ineffective for another type of harmful organism. The prescription could even exacerbate misery or kill the patient.

Proponents of nineteenth-century interpretations of humoral and tellurian theories rarely expressed this level of awareness. Humoral theoreticians, for example, continued to view health as a body in equilibrium and a cure was a substance or procedure that restored balance. A prophylactic was something that prevented change in internal equilibrium.

Elevated body temperature was an overt expression of humoral disruption. Clues to the extent of imbalance included when a fever began, how long it lasted, when and if it reappeared, its severity, and how the person behaved after the paroxysm's abatement. A substance that eliminated this manifestation of sickness qualified as a cure. "Sickness" comprised those elevated temperatures with discernible and unique patterns. Since fever is common to many diseases and minor ailments among humans, we now know that people who espoused variants of humoral theory defined a cure as any plant or chemical that suppressed the overt expression of something more fundamental. A more realistic assessment is that the substance administered to the patient did not cure the disease. The plant or chemical most often prevented an observer from detecting the obvious signs of high temperature. A corollary is that the substances interfered with a person's consciousness of having a fever. Most likely both events occurred. In other words, the few proponents of humoral theory and its variants in the late nineteenth century construed symptom management as cure. These people viewed vegetable material or chemicals capable of suppressing fevers generated by distinct diseases and many ailments as very good cures indeed. It also made sense to use the item to preclude internal disequilibrium before the condition even became a problem.

Tellurian proponents contended that removing people from negative environmental conditions was a prophylactic and a febrifuge for 'malaria.' If excessive heat and sun caused the malady, encourage people to minimize such exposure. If the culprit was a type of soil or trees, then get rid of the trees and avoid contact with the former. The list of procedures and techniques that tellurian theoreticians recommended for the disease in diverse regions of the world is almost endless. They also were receptive to substances that people could ingest to ensure continued internal equilibrium despite living in 'malarious' locales.

Medical personnel and lay people articulating some variant of humoral theory, therefore, were predisposed to accepting a substance as a febrifuge or prophylactic, or both, if it 'controlled' or suppressed a symptom common to many maladies. Germ theorists thought otherwise, as did the Anglo-European scientists who accepted Laveran's plasmodia. They did not glibly confuse the absence of a sign of sickness with proof that health had been restored.

The Mystery of Opium's Power Revealed

The ambiguity that characterized what was known about malaria during the early 1890s was far less pronounced in opium research. By 1893, the drug was neither mysterious nor its powers vaguely understood. Western scientists had literally taken the substance apart and analyzed its components. One consequence of this work was skepticism. Members of the Anglo-European medical community had rejected the opium-based remedies that had been inherited from the distant past. These concoctions were not a reliable way to exploit the drug's potential. They felt the same way about eating opium.

Participants in the Royal Commission deliberations did not argue the merits or demerits of the ancient recipes. That was a nonissue. They did, however, debate the wisdom of eating the crude drug. The SSOT and its supporters agreed with the western medical community. So did many people who otherwise defended the trade during the 1890s. Both groups were very aware of some facets of drug research, and their statements prove it. For these people, opium did not do many of the things that defenders of the trade had claimed. Furthermore, eating it hindered people from obtaining whatever benefit the drug might possess.

The Royal Commission disagreed. So did other defenders of the Government of India. These people either ignored the discoveries or they were blissfully unaware of what the western chemists were doing. Their minds were made up. Opium *did* wondrous things; it prevented and cured many diseases, and eating the drug was a nonproblematic mode of ingestion. They were wrong.

What Is Opium?

The nineteenth century was truly the golden age of discovery for opium. Researchers, early on, confirmed that the drug consisted of two things: alkaloid and nonalkaloid substances.

Nonalkaloids were "inert." They amounted to approximately 66 percent (by volume when dried) regardless of where the opium came from. The body absorbed this nonnarcotic material when a person ate the crude or "prepared" drug. These components exerted little or no change in the normal functioning of organs and body processes. This was not the case if adulterating agents had been added to the drug before its ingestion. This often was done in India. Cultivators tried to alter the weight, color, texture, smell, and water content (consistency) of the crude drug. These attributes determined how much money the cultivators received for their raw latex. If undetected, the varied substances that had been added could harm the consumer. This occasionally was a problem for the opium that was sold and consumed within India. The development of quality control technology in the 1900s helped to minimize the problem.

The "active" ingredients of opium were its alkaloids. They were responsible for the diverse physiological and psychological effects in human and nonhuman recipients. Anglo-Europeans also knew that several alkaloids in the drug were highly toxic to humans. A person eating opium in any form, therefore, could not avoid being simultaneously exposed to all components. A consumer might experience discomfort until the body eliminated or neutralized noxious ingredients. Excessive consumption could debilitate or kill people.

Chemists had isolated seventeen opium alkaloids before 1879.[17] By 1891, the number of known alkaloids of opium had increased to eighteen, and before the end of that year the tally was nineteen. The number of discovered alkaloids had risen to twenty in 1893. The twenty-fourth substance was isolated in 1894 (GBS [Watt] 1891:68; Taylor 1929:354). The last two were identified in the twentieth century.[18]

Anglo-European researchers had also detected differences among opium alkaloids. This awareness dates back to 1833, when the word 'alkaloid' became part of the scientific lexicon. The term was consistently used after 1844 to refer only to a "class of naturally-occurring nitrogenous organic compounds, possessing basic properties" (Henry 1929:1). All alkaloids were kindred entities having physiological and psychological properties. They ranged from subtle to sublime. And virtually all alkaloids were procurable from a variety of sources in the animal, mineral, and plant world. By mid-nineteenth century, scientists recognized that some alkaloids produced physiological and psychological effects that were different from other alkaloids even though given to the same experimental subject. Alkaloids, therefore, were not identical; they were composed of families whose members induced similar responses in animal organs. Furthermore, alkaloids that were in different families might come from the same plant source. Many of these early organic chemists concentrated upon analyzing the different alkaloids. They wanted to know what was common to a family of these entities.

Researchers investigating opium at mid-century shared this interest in identifying the alkaloid families. They wanted to know what groups were present in *Papaver somniferum Linn* and to which family each opium's alkaloids belonged. The answers came in 1885. Narcotine, papaverine, and several other opium components were confirmed as belonging to the Benzylisoquinoline group (Wootton [1910] 1972:2:270).[19] This discovery also confirmed nineteenth-century chemists' long-held, but unsubstantiated suspicion, about the distinctiveness of morphine, codeine, and thebaine. They were members of the Pyridinphenethrane family of alkaloids. Chemists during the late nineteenth and early part of the twentieth centuries often shortened the terms to isoquinoline and phenethrane. The abbreviations appear in this book. The phenethrane entities produced the most dramatic physiological and psychological effects in animals and humans. Chemists had long warned that two phenethrane members should be used with caution. For many people, morphine and thebaine were especially lethal if ingested in more than very small amounts.

Twentieth century research validated the 1885 revelations. Enhanced experimental sophistication also resulted in the recognition of other, subtle distinctions. This generated differences of opinion about the classification of several minor constituents of the drug.[20] A few chemists discerned additional properties that were possessed by alkaloids within one family. The purported family members lacked these attributes. These groups of minor alkaloids in the two families, the researchers proposed, were sufficiently distinct to warrant a separate category.

Several members from the alkaloid families in opium were removed. The most physiologically and psychologically significant alkaloids in the drug (morphine, codeine, and thebaine) however, retained their family classification although some twentieth-century investigators changed the previously used family names. Morphine, codeine, and thebaine were now referred to as the "Morphine Group" instead of "Phenethrane." Furthermore, the isoquinoline alkaloids constitute one of the largest families. Henceforth, they were designated as the "Papaverine Group." Opium has several of them. Narcotine and papaverine are the members that are found in greatest abundance in the mother drug. Although papaverine is the most "active" alkaloid in this family, its physiological and psychological capability is modest. The alkaloid is a weak base with mild narcotic properties (Flückiger & Hanbury 1879:59; Leake 1975:121; Jaffe & Martin 1985:491).

The Rise and Fall of Narcotine in Anglo-European Science

The Royal Commission on Opium was wrong about narcotine. It ignored a mistake that had been made in the early 1800s. The problem was a misconception about what the alkaloid did to the human body. Anglo-European scientists had resolved the issue long before 1893–1895.

In 1804, Charles Louis Derosnè proclaimed that he had isolated the substance that was responsible for opium's physiological and psychological effects. They were crystals which quickly became known as Derosnè's narcotic salts (Leake 1975:12; Wootton [1912 1972:2:244). And just as fast, these crystals became central to the argument of the eminent French chemist Francois Magendie. Magendie did not share his colleagues' belief that opium functioned as a sedative. His colleagues also claimed that the newly discovered morphine (morphia) was the agent most responsible for tranquilization. Although Magendie did not dispute the significance of morphine, he refused to change his mind about the principal effect of opium in the human body. The drug was, basically, a stimulant, and Magendie insisted that Derosnè's narcotic salts (renamed narcotine in 1817) was responsible for the characteristic.

The stimulant/sedative argument continued for several decades albeit in different guises. Nonetheless, most members of the Anglo-European scientific community soon recognized morphine as the most important active ingredient of opium. They also concluded that opium's most prominent effect upon the human body seemed to be sedation. Nonetheless, a few people clung to Magendie's interpretation. They believed that ingestion of the mother drug and its inherent narcotine increased the activity of some organ or vital process. The effect was temporary.

Magendie's critics were correct about narcotine. It was not as "important," or as active as morphine. In other words, the consequences of morphine upon human physiology and psychology were far more dramatic. And as the decades passed, the acclaim given to narcotine continued to wane. Researchers extracted hitherto unknown alkaloids from Magendie's crystals. This signified that all alleged capabilities were really the result of several alkaloids that existed in combination with narcotine.[21] There was even a possibility that narcotine did nothing at all, or, at best, that it contributed very little to what had been observed or hypothesized.

The reevaluation began in 1844. A chemist by the name of Blyth claimed success in calculating a chemical formula for the alkaloid. No one challenged his contention about its unique molecular structure for twenty-four years.

Then, in 1868, J. C. Brough's analysis of six samples of opium from different parts of the world prompted a modification of the formula. He extracted opianic acid and cotarnine from the samples' inherent narcotine. These alkaloids had been previously discovered, albeit not in combination with narcotine. Chemists had long suspected their presence in Blyth's material, and Brough's work now confirmed the speculation. Subsequent analyses resulted in modification of the formula for cotarnine, and confirmation for the composition of opianic acid (Brough 1868–69:211). This was another indication that the people who had proclaimed that narcotine was capable of doing something were actually describing the effects of several alkaloids.

Additional justifications for narcotine's diminished status appeared during the 1870s. In 1876, C. R. Alder Wright discovered a "community of 'structure'" between it and narceine. Both were closely related to the aforementioned oxynarcotine, an alkaloid that had been recently separated from narceine (1876:246).[22] And during the same year, D. B. Dott reviewed the opium alkaloid research literature. He concluded that morphine, codeine, and narceine were indeed the drug's most physiologically and psychologically significant entities. The idea was already commonplace among members of the western scientific community. Dott does not mention narcotine (1876:239–40). The omission denotes its minor status among leading researchers in the mid-1870s.

One of these authorities was Frederick Flückiger. His name is synonymous with the evaluation of opium and its components during the 1870s. Two observations are especially germane for the opium/malaria controversy. One was made in 1875. The other was included in his 1879 discussion about the best method for assaying the morphine content of opium from Turkey. He then expanded the analysis to include the drug that came from other parts of the world. The physiological effects of each alkaloid in these samples were measured. Flückiger concluded that the "action assigned to narcotine . . . appears to be not considerable at all" (1879:25). This German scientist, in fact, was so unimpressed that he suggested narcotine might not be an alkaloid.

Flückiger's 1875 comment clearly identifies the problem that still confronted the rulers of India twenty years later. The growing stature of morphine and the devalued importance of narcotine made opium from India much less attractive to the Western pharmaceutical market. The South Asian product had an abundance of the wrong alkaloid. Its inherent low morphine and high narcotine content was, however, ideal for opium smokers because a preparation provided sedation without the lethal effects of too much morphine. Indian opium's morphine deficiency, therefore, was an advantage in China (Flückiger 1875:845).[23] The chemical composition of the South Asian drug simply required a market like China. And India faced a financial disaster if it lost this clientele.[24]

Early twentieth-century narcotine research confirmed Flückiger's 1879 assessment. Frank O. Taylor demonstrated that the substance is only "feebly narcotic, exhibiting poisonous effects only in somewhat large doses (1.5 to 3.0 grm)" (1929:710).[25] Magendie's acclaimed stimulant had turned out to be a very weak base. It possessed meager narcotic and tetanizing capabilities, whereas morphine, codeine, and thebaine were strong bases having "strongly marked basic characters" (Taylor 1929:661).

Charles Lawall was more dismissive. Two years before Taylor's 1929 pronouncement, he said that narcotine was misnamed because it had no narcotic properties whatsoever (1927:454). Anglo-European chemists agreed. They eventually dropped the old name to reflect the absence of narcotic capability. It is now called noscapine (gnoscopine). Twentieth-century western physicians described the alkaloid as a mild anti-tussive for people; it reduces the severity of coughing.

The Problem with Oral Ingestion

The Royal Commission compounded its mistake about narcotine. It accepted no testimony or evidence that questioned the prevailing mode of drug ingestion in the subcontinent. Yet, the oral consumption of the substance by itself, or in solution, had been subjected to extensive criticism for centuries in western societies. Critics during the nineteenth century merely had more sophisticated tools to challenge archaic ideas. And by the 1890s, the Anglo-European medical community had no doubt that the traditional modes of ingestion were woefully inadequate. They were inefficacious, potentially unsafe, and unnecessary.

The list of targets included the ancient galenicals and officinal capitals. These were the complicated, often bizarre, concoctions associated with the era of polypharmacy in western science. Their Greek and Roman creators believed that any therapeutic capability *Papaver somniferum Linn* possessed was released or strengthened only in the presence of other substances. Eighteenth century scientists and clinicians such as William Heberden, Charles Harvey, William Boyle, and others succeeded in challenging most tenets of polypharmacy. However, they did not eliminate some of its basic ideas. That task fell to nineteenth century chemists.

The emergence of Paracelsian essences during the Renaissance, and their continuing popularity in the post-Renaissance decades, did not dispel the belief that the "power" of opium to prevent or cure ailments was enhanced by the presence of other ingredients in a formula. This orientation spawned products containing different amounts of the drug's "essence," its "essential kernel." In the 1820s, opium's essence was morphine that was only crudely distilled from the mother drug. Other opium-based concoctions flooded the western market in ensuing decades. No different from the past, their creators promised miracles. And a skeptical buyer was told that a medicine contained consistent amounts of opium or its important alkaloids.

Astute nineteenth-century chemists disagreed. They dismissed the Paracelsian elixirs, infusions, and nostrums as nonsense. Popular items such as Dover's Powder, the several varieties of laudanum, and numerous other opium-based "medicines" were criticized as not being what they claimed to be. Eating pieces of the mother drug also did not escape condemnation.

An early nineteenth-century attack upon the veracity of oral ingestion came from Richard Battley in 1823/24. He discovered that opium prepared for the western market produced effects that differed from those generated by any of the drug's individual components known to exist at that time (Matthews 1962:246). Eating opium or ingesting one of its alkaloids, therefore, were not merely alternate modes of introduction. Physicians who substituted one method for the other were mistaken if they predicted identical or similar reactions in a patient. In other words, alkaloids such as morphine and narcotine were not clones of the mother drug. People should not expect a recipient to derive full benefits from any alkaloid unless that substance is ingested alone.[26]

Battley's experiments (1823/24a; 1823/24b) also revealed that samples of crude opium obtained in the marketplace did not have consistent percentages of morphine. This was an early recognition that the quantity of active ingredients in a recipe that contained opium from several countries could differ from year to year. Pharmacologists and chemists later realized that the only thing consistent about raw latex and the *Papaver somniferum Linn* prepared for export from the poppy-cultivating countries was the variability of inherent alkaloids. Furthermore, the percentage of each alkaloid fluctuated within a range determined by the genetic structure of the variety of poppy.[27] This meant the actual contents of the galenicals, the officinal capitals, the Paracelsian essences, and the more recent opium-based nostrums available to the public, deviated from their assumed or declared contents. The implications were startling. The composition of traditional opium-based popular medicines might partially, or wholly, lack the active ingredients that the public assumed they contained and that some members of the medical profession proclaimed they possessed. A preparation also might have too much of one ingredient. A possible consequence was the consumer's incapacitation or worse.

Eating the mother drug did not circumvent the problem. The opium used to create the traditional nostrums had at least been subjected to some form of distillation, albeit modest, after importation of the drug. Some irrelevant ingredients and substances moderating the effects of the important alkaloids might have been eliminated. The attention given to crude opium before its export, however, was minimal. It was limited to the steps that guaranteed arrival at the port of destination in a form acceptable to the purchase and nothing more.[28] The destination might be overseas or someplace in the country where the poppy had been cultivated.

Anglo-European scientists such as Battley had good reason to question the ability of the ubiquitous opium-based commodities to perform specific physiological and psychological tasks. Skepticism about the benefits of eating crude opium that had not been subjected to distillation and content analysis was even more justified. Other nineteenth-century researchers joined Battley in critiquing modes of oral ingestion (Jaffe & Martin 1985:491).[29] They also succeeded in removing dubious entries enshrined in the *Materia Medica* of allopathic medicine and the pharmacopoeias of Anglo-European societies. Some researchers addressed the preparations directly. Other people challenged the reigning assumptions about any crude opium that was used to extract alkaloids.

The warning from Edward Squibb (1860:115–20), D. B. Dott (1876:239–40), John Woodland (1882/83:275–76), Henry Napier Draper (1885:546–47), and their colleagues, was unequivocal. The ubiquitous 'medicines' guaranteed inexactitude. So did eating small pieces of opium (or dissolved in water.)[30] They all lacked uniformity and consistency of therapeutic ingredients. They were vestiges of another era; unneeded anachronisms in modern science unless their deficiencies were recognized and corrected. The best way to resolve this problem was to stop using them. Since alkaloids, at least some alkaloids, were the mother drug's active ingredients, dispense them, and get rid of everything else.

A technology that was capable of introducing alkaloids into a human subject had been available since the mid-1850s. It was the subcutaneous (intra-arterial) hypodermic injection. This mode of delivery prohibited the use of crude or semi-processed opium. The drug contained insoluble material that could not pass through needles. Furthermore, the mother drug contained nonalkaloidal substances (as much as the aforementioned 66 percent) that were unnecessary and possibly harmful if they were ingested by mouth and entered the stomach. Carefully measured, pure solutions of opium alkaloids circumvented the problems. The message was clear. Prior to the 1890s, western medical practitioners knew that the quickest way to benefit from opium's alkaloids was to inject them directly into the bloodstream. This approach bypassed the stomach, and digestive complications were avoided. Another mode was a pill or liquid solution that contained a precise amount of the therapeutic substance(s). The list of useful alkaloids for introduction via injection and other forms of delivery did not include narcotine.

The Status of Quinine in Nineteenth-Century Anglo-European Science

In 1640, the introduction of bark from several varieties of the South American cinchona tree changed Anglo-European medicine in three ways. Practitioners had to rethink the concept of sickness, how to cure it, and how to prevent it. The bark was first pulverized, and then dispensed in several ways, to ill people. The patients were suffering from the various maladies that many people still referred to as 'malaria.' Other individuals had certain types of 'fever.' The results were startling. According to Lyons and Petrucelli,

> since cinchona cured quickly and acted specifically on only a certain kind of fever, the belief in fever as a general manifestation of unbalanced humours received a severe blow. It was then felt that each fever could be a different disease. (1978:454)

Cinchona seemed to cure the form of 'malaria' and 'fever' that was caused by plasmodia. The western medical community finally had an effective treatment for people who harbored these microbes. Physicians also soon realized that cinchona was a prophylactic. A healthy person who consumed it most often did not suffer from the 'sickness' that plagued nonconsumers. No one yet knew why this South American vegetation ameliorated and "cured" the dreaded periodic fevers. But the work of researchers such as Thomas Morton, Francisco Torti, and Thomas Sydenham did prompt many health professionals to doubt the old paradigm. And that, as discussed earlier in the chapter, was progress toward a more accurate diagnosis of disease.

Then, in 1820, the French chemists Pelletier and Caventou isolated quinine. This alkaloid is the prime reason for the reputation of cinchona. And cinchona bark is the only plant source for quinine.

In subsequent decades, other alkaloids in the bark were extracted. They were cinchonidine, cinchonine, and quinidine. The substances also had value for treating victims of malaria caused by plasmodia. However, none of them were as effective as quinine. They were dispensed infrequently to citizens in western society. The same thing happened in India and elsewhere in the world. The alkaloids were distributed for only a few decades.

Quinine was the alkaloid that Anglo-European physicians and lay people wanted. But great demand and scarcity meant exorbitant prices for the substance. Few people could afford to buy it. Slightly less than forty years after Pelletier and Caventou, several western nations attempted to ensure an ample supply of quinine and its sister alkaloids. They planted varieties of the cinchona tree in locales under their control. With one exception, these efforts failed during the nineteenth century. South Asia was not the exception.

By the early 1890s, and most certainly during the remaining years of the century, western medical researchers knew a great deal about the "nature of the disease [malaria], [and] the various forms of fever." They also recognized "the action of quinine as a therapeutic in suppressing the multiplication of the asexual forms" (Harrison, Gordon 1978:81).[31] This erudition disappeared en route to India. Anti-opiumists and pro-trade activists *did* debate the merits of cinchona, quinine, and the other alkaloids. The following chapters describe what they said. Here, it suffices to repeat what has already been stated: quinine was the cure of choice for many Anglo-European medical practitioners. But "many physicians" is not "all physicians," and most certainly not all of the people who were practicing western medicine in India. Some of these dissenters were very influential.

NOTES

1. A less vitriolic assessment of opium use in India by a missionary appeared thirteen years later. See William Paton (1924).

2. The author uses Anglo-European as a synonym for western. Terms such as metropolitan, center, metropolis, and periphery also are found in the literature. Contemporary students of imperialism use them to identify locations of western scientific activity. Metropolitan denotes theory and practice originating or conducted "in the homeland" (center or metropolis). Periphery designates the content of Anglo-European science found in regions beyond metropolitan locales. It refers to activities in European and British colonies and possessions located in Asia, Africa, and other parts of the world. The thesis of this volume is that the content of prevailing medical theory and practice concerning malaria and its prevention and cure in one region of the periphery circa the 1890s differed radically from dominant ideas evolving in the metropolis. The Government of India's preference for an analysis based on fading paradigms and a selective interpretation of data was not accidental. The predilection protected British hegemony and guaranteed increased revenue from poppy cultivation in South Asia.

3. See Antoinette Burton (1994) for an analysis of middle-class British feminists' acceptance of imperialist ideology to advance their own agenda.

4. Thomas D. Reins (1991:101–42) also discusses perspectives about imperialism among nineteenth and early twentieth century British citizens at home and abroad.

5. S. E. J. Clarke cites the number of exported opium chests for 1781, 1790, 1820, 1820–1830, 1840, and every ten year interval thereafter, beginning with 1850 and ending with 1880, plus the amounts for 1884, 1886, 1890, and 1892 (GBO [Clarke] 1894:II:440–41). As of 1893, the two most lucrative sources of imperial finance for British India were land revenue and railway income.

6. The 18 percent share of opium in the East India Company's total gross revenue from all sources as of 1852/53 resulted from several events earlier in the century. One of the most important was the Company's defeat of the Maharajah of Sind (or Sindh) and its subsequent control of the country's entire western coast during the 1840s. Other significant events were England's triumph in the "opium war" with China, and treaties negotiated even earlier in the century with opium-producing native states. The Company was now able to tax production, and to some extent consumption, in many parts of India.

7. Martin Booth says inhabitants of Great Britain and elsewhere in the West were appalled upon learning that "17 to 20 percent of the gross national product of the Indian subcontinent was entirely due to the demoralization of millions of Chinese" (1996:152). This apparently occurred during the early 1870s. Official documents indicate Booth's statistics for the decade are too high. Booth might have obtained the data from a document written by Sir John Strachey. In the sentence immediately preceding these percentages, the author quotes Strachey as saying that "'[n]ext to the land revenue, the most productive source of the public income [in India] is opium.'" Salt, not opium, was the Government of India's second most important source of revenue during the 1870s. Opium ranked third early in the 1800s and before the 1857 uprising. It retained the position after Great Britain assumed control from the East India Company.

Booth's very readable introduction to the topic is marred by at least one other mistake (or unsubstantiated data) regarding India. He contends that during the 1870s "[p]ublic opinion in Britain against opium had started to gain a voice, spurred on by devastating effects of the trade in China and upon the native population of India which was such that, at times, the amount consumed in India exceeded the amount exported" (1998:151).

The first part of Booth's statement is credible: a factor in raising awareness in Great Britain about the detrimental effects of opium indulgence were the allegations of harm to the Chinese people. The comment concerning opium use in India lacks veracity. Booth does not identify a source for his comments about these countries. He most likely is using SSOT estimates of consumption in India. Many of these statistics should be accepted with caution. All members of the organization were not neutral observers in this decades-old argument, and both sides in the controversy exaggerated numbers in their efforts to persuade people.

Another commentator's statistics for the same period also present a problem. In his excellent article about the SSOT, J. B. Brown says that "opium still yielded enormous profits for the Government in India" despite revenue fluctuations. In 1870/71, for example, the administration earned £51 million. Opium had contributed more than £8 million and "British administrators treasured opium funds as the only source of direct taxation other than the politically explosive salt tax" (1973:99). Brown does not identify the source for these statistics. He also fails to indicate if the amounts pertain to both Provision and Abkari sales or only to the exported commodity.

8. The 1896 *Statistical Abstracts* document itemizes the "cost of production," and net receipts for "Bengal, including all opium other than Bombay." Statistics for Bombay (i.e., the Malwa drug) minus "charges of collection" and "net receipts" also are cited as well as "total revenue" for both Bengal and Bombay. The 1889/90 and 1893/94 figures cited in the discussion are "total revenue" from Bengal and Bombay minus expenditures incurred for both in India as well as "[i]n England, including exchange" (1896a:95).

For supplementary data regarding Excise opium revenue, including the "Duty on Opium Consumed in India" for 1890, see IDFC 1891:30–31, 35. Miscellaneous categories relating to Excise opium for the remainder of the decade and the early years of the twentieth century are scattered throughout the yearly issues of the Revenue Accounts. Titles and contents of category topics are inconsistent.

S. E. J. Clarke also provides Government of India opium revenue figures for the Bengal and Bombay product. The period covered is 1882/83 through 1891/92, and amounts are calculated in tens of rupees. The document has statistics regarding yield, cost of production, and cost of collecting latex plus totals for the ten-year period. According to Clarke, the "total net receipts during ten years 1882/83–1891/92" amounts to "in tens of rupees, Rs. 63,748,717" (GBO [Clarke] 1894:II:447). And on page 448, he says the net opium revenue for 1862 was £4 million.

9. These percentages are calculated using two sets of statistics for the period 1867/68 through 1889/90. These are on page seventy-two in George Watt's table entitled "Revenue Derived from Opium." The columns are "Approximate Net Revenue from Excise Opium (i.e., Consumption in India)", and "Approximate Total Net Opium Revenue" (Excise and Provision). Watt also says "a few minor details of revenue and expenditure [have] been purposely left out of account" but he does not indicate their contents. The omission is unimportant because other documents and commentary support the trend illustrated by his data (GBS [Watt] 1891:72). The net Excise revenue percentage contributions to the total net opium revenue for the twenty-year period that are not cited in the chapter narrative are as follows: 1872/73 (5.7 percent); 1873/74 (6.1 percent); 1874/75 (7.0 percent); 1876/77 (8.1 percent); 1877/78 (8.2 percent); 1878/79 (7.9 percent); 1879/80 (7.8 percent); 1880/81 (8.8 percent); 1881/82 (9.3 percent); 1884/85 (12.6 percent); 1885/86 (12.5 percent); 1886/87 (12.2 percent); and 1887/88 (12.6 percent). Each percentage is rounded off to the nearest tenth.

10. Thomas D. Reins describes the native states' position when the Government of India agreed to phase out its opium exports over a period of ten years, commencing in 1907. He declares that the "decline of the China trade endangered many of the princely economies. Gwalior [State] had much to lose, since it had more than 100,000 bighas under poppy and an annual income of nearly 1.4 million rupees from opium, but some of the smaller states, such as Partabgarh with 21 percent of its revenue from opium, were in the most difficulty" (1991:537).

11. The emergence of new paradigms in metropolitan science did not preclude different or older explanations from dominating theories of human sickness articulated by western or western-trained medical practitioners working in the periphery. This was especially true for India during the second half of the nineteenth century. The subcontinent's severe climate elevated environmental variables to paramount importance in explaining the occurrence, duration, and elimination of diseases. The maladies include malaria. British officials' dismay about hygienic practices among India's indigenous population resulted in sanitation theory's popularity long after its limitations were recognized in Great Britain. The two interpretations of disease causation, and how each influenced the opium–malaria controversy, are discussed in the last chapter.

12. Laveran was not the first nineteenth-century Anglo-European investigator to detect these microbes. For comments about the achievements of Heinrich Meckel (1847), T. Frerichs (1858), Karl Binz (1867), Delafield (1872), and Achille Kelsch (1875), see Boyd 1949:11–13; Hehir 1927:1; Harrison, Gordon 1978:8, 10; and Warshaw 1947. Giovanni Maria Lancisi's earlier speculations were prescient. His conception of the disease appeared in a 1717 volume entitled *De Noxiis Paludum Effluviss Eorumque Remediis* (Noxious Emanations of Swamps and Their Cure). Lancisi accepted swamps as the final

abode of the disease, but the inhalation of bad air or organic substances floating in air did not produce fever (Boyd 1949:12; Hehir 1913:683; Warshaw 1947:42). His observation about numerous mosquitoes breeding in swampy regions associated with malaria prompted him to hypothesize that mosquitoes and other insects transmit disease-causing organisms. Tiny worms or bugs entered the human bloodstream where they multiplied. The act of reproduction produced unique characteristics in a victim (Bass 1926:855; Warshaw 1947:42).

13. Numerous publications describe the sophistication of Greeks and Romans. See, for example, Boyd 1949:12; Hehir 1913:681, 683; Hehir 1927:1; Scott, H. Harold 1939:159–68; and Warshaw 1947:58 for comments about the Romans' astute awareness of insect vectors.

14. The well-known status of Patrick Manson and the work of Ronald Ross in India during the 1890s in malarial vector theory need no documentation. Other nineteenth-century pioneers have lower profiles but are almost as significant. Prominent in this group is John Crawford, an American physician practicing in Baltimore in the late 1700s and early 1800s (Harrison, Gordon 1978:29; Warshaw 1947:61). Crawford's colleagues in vector analysis were an individual whose last name was Bright (1831), and James K. Mitchell (1849), Josiah Clarke Nott (1850), Louis Beauperthy (1854 & 1858), Albert Freeman Africanus King (1882 & 1883). The following sources provide commentary: Boyd 1949:13; Harrison, Gordon 1978:29; Thin 1899:1; Warshaw 1947:61–3. Also see Nuttall 1900: 2:March:198–200, April:231–33, May:245–47; June:275–77, July:302–07, & 3:August:11–13:198–99. Giovanni Maria Lancisi's remarkable 1717 observation about flying insects and disease transmission is mentioned in a previous endnote.

15. Nineteenth century Western physicians laboring in the colonial periphery were susceptible to terminological ambiguity and faulty categorization. A cursory reading of Anglo-European commentary about disease causation in overseas possessions suggests the number and kind of entities capable of generating the dangerous vapor was limited only by the imagination of the theoretician. Different kinds of topography spawned different kinds of malarial afflictions, as did climatic zones. Seasonal changes in the latter affected the composition of miasma, which in turn produced additional gradations of sickness.

In India, for example, Douglas Haynes says that "in the absence of a specific causal agent, practitioners purported to find malarial poisons virtually everywhere . . . in hot and cool climates, in deserts and lush landscapes, and in undeveloped and developed regions" (2001:43).

Nomenclature invented to designate malaria in India and elsewhere in the world was equally inventive—and confusing. Jarcho says that clinical characteristics provided the majority of terms. Examples were "tertian fever, quartan fever, pernicious fever, intermittent fever, and—favored by laymen—ague (from the Latin *acuta*)" (Jarcho 1970:39). Medical theory generated another group of names that included bilious fever and congestive fever. Swamp fever, lake fever, hill fever, as well as other local and geographical associations were a third source of nomenclature (Jarcho 1970:39). Since many diseases produce fever having similar patterns, the terms did not guarantee that the malady being discussed was the product of plasmodia.

16. Chaudhuri is almost correct. Proponents of the germ theory of disease during the 1890s were not completely free from misdiagnosis. There is evidence that a few diseases having very similar overt symptoms were placed in one category. For example, some otherwise perceptive investigators in malaria-plagued locales still had difficulty distinguishing

between kala-azar, enteric fever, "tropical anemia," and so on, and the plasmodia-induced malaria. They classified these etiologically separate afflictions under one term: 'malaria.' Furthermore, one form of the plasmodia-induced disease might escape detection. Cerebral malaria could be mistaken for Parkinson's disease, meningitis, encephalitis, or some form of brain injury. Symptoms of these afflictions include delirium, disorientation, excitement, convulsions, somnolence, and coma.

For discussions of the identification problem in the post-1895 era and procedures to eliminate it, see deKorte 1900:178–81; Hodgson & Vardon 1926–27:14:779–84; and Plehn 1899: October: 72–4; December: 121–23; January: 141–45.

Numerous publications describe related problems confronting malariologists during the late 1800s and early 1900s. Many of them also discuss the favorable response from members of the medical establishment and from the public to the new explanation of malaria. Commentary about both topics is found in Bass 1915:2:12:735–37; Bass 1915–16: 15: June–July: 298–303; EB. 1911:17:461–65; Guiart 1900: July:300–05; Giles 1899: October:62–5; *JIMA*. 1980:74:8 (April):156–57; Kitchen 1949:2:995–1016 & 2:1027–45; Knab 1913:1:1 (July):33–43; Lyons & Petrucelli 1978; Maxwell 1899: November:90–91; MacGregor 1900: October:63–71; Russell 1943:19:9: September:599–630; Talbott 1970; Thayer 1897; and Winchester & Mertens 1983.

17. For details, see Taylor 1929:655–758.

18. They were hydrocartinine, morphine, pseudomorphine, codeine, thebaine, protopine, laudanine, codamine, papaverine, rhoeadine, opianine, meconidine, crytopine, laudonosine, narcotine, lanthopine, narceine, papaveramine, and gnoscopine. For more details, see GBS [Watt] 1891:3–79. The discovery of opium alkaloids continued with tritopine and followed by xantholine in 1893. The isolation of laudanidine in 1894 increased the number to twenty-four and by 1949 it was twenty-six (Taylor 1929:354; Watt & Johnson 1949:98–105, 108–116).

19. While individual alkaloids are members of an alkaloid family and specific alkaloids might be found in different plants, some alkaloids in a family might be obtainable from only one source. The alkaloids of *Papaver somniferum Linn* are in the last category. They are unique despite shared membership with other alkaloids in a larger family, these being either the phenethrane or isoquinoline group.

20. The twenty-four opium alkaloids found by 1929 were initially classified as belonging to either the phenethrane or isoquinoline families. Six of the alkaloids were "major," which means they were pharmacologically significant. The designation of major was not altered after 1929, when researchers found one more alkaloid and the total rose to twenty-five. Debates revolved around inclusion and exclusion of the minor opium alkaloids in either category. Other people argued that advances in determining the atomic structure of chemicals warranted a change in the nineteenth-century's twofold classification system. These highly technical discussions are in various locations of Wootton [1910] 1972; Watt & Johnson 1949; Taylor 1929; Thorpe 1950; Jaffe & Martin 1985; and Schlittler 1950.

21. Some westerners in India during the 1830s shared the Anglo-European scientific community's earlier enthusiasm about narcotine. In later decades, metropolitan practitioners and scientists, as well as their counterparts in India, eventually relegated narcotine to an insignificant status compared to other alkaloids. The Royal Commission on Opium, however, accepted data that reflected the misplaced fervor of these British nationals who were living in India decades before the inquiry.

22. Improved technology is responsible for Wright's contribution. The Robertson-Gregory method of morphine extraction was a modification of Gregory's original tech-

nique. Perfected by the MacFarland Company of Edinburgh, Scotland, the modified technique was used to obtain oxynarcotine. Later research revealed that narcotine exposed to oxidizing agents underwent "a kind of hydrolysis into base and acid." The process of decomposition produced cotarnine and opianic acid (Henry 1929:46). That the same 'new' alkaloids can be obtained from two different 'old' alkaloids indicates their shared, common chemical affinity.

Wright's 1876 observation about the structural similarity between narcotine, narceine, and oxynarcotine implied that other opium alkaloids had the same characteristics. His statement also suggested that careful alteration of alkaloid structure might yield something analogous to oxynarcotine. Wright was particularly interested about the relevance of his discovery to morphine and quinine, the most valuable alkaloids in opium and cinchona, respectively. Their creation in the laboratory as of the mid-1870s remained a "prospect . . . still far off" (Wright 1876:246). However, Wright implies that alkaloids structurally similar to morphine and quinine might be changed, as was narceine, to yield items of medical importance.

23. Although Flückiger's stature in nineteenth-century opium research is impressive, the man was not infallible. Research conducted in the post-1879 era confirmed his opinion about the minor therapeutic significance of narcotine compared to morphine. His contention about narcotine's questionable status as an alkaloid, however, was wrong. As indicated above, narcotine is in the isoquinoline family of vegetal alkaloids.

24. Except for an occasional shipment of the Malwa product, no Indian opium was shipped to western markets during the nineteenth century (*EB* 1911:20:130–37).

25. Taylor also found that narcotine decomposes at temperatures above 200 degrees (Centigrade or Fahrenheit are not specified) to produce coarnine and meconin. When in the form of a solid base, narcotine has virtually no taste. It is bitter when in solution. Taylor's 1929 discussion about a concoction from which narcotine had been removed is indicative of the alkaloid's minor status during the first third of the twentieth century (1929:710).

26. Human beings and other animals react differently to opium. Furthermore, the drug's alkaloids affect human organs and body processes in different ways. One alkaloid might sedate an organ, whereas another component might generate a reaction akin to stimulation. Ingested by itself, an alkaloid "performs' its sedative or stimulative function. This "work" might be compromised when the mother drug (with its inherent nonalkaloidal and numerous alkaloids) is "eaten." The performance of each alkaloid is modified by the presence of all other substances. Some alkaloids are more affected by this admixture than other ingredients. The effects of morphine, for example, will be slightly different when the mother drug is ingested compared to the consequences that are observed when the alkaloid is introduced by itself. The alkaloid's effect upon the organ or process might be accentuated or decreased. In any case, a modification occurs. One of the lessons from Battley's 1823/24 experiments was that the method of introduction was not irrelevant. The mode of ingestion did affect the "behavior" of an alkaloid. It also meant that any proclamation about eating opium doing something and that one of its alkaloids administered in isolation doing the same thing was, at best, questionable. David Macht and his associates investigated this topic at length in the early 1900s. They confirmed Battley's pioneering observations. For details about processes and specific organs, see Macht (1915a, 1915b, 1917a, 1917b, and Macht & Issacs (1917).

Another explanation of what Macht, and Macht & Issacs observed is that the alkaloid's capability is not changed in the presence of the mother drug's other active ingredients.

Rather, it is the organ or the body process that is modified. For example, assume that morphine tends to "calm" some function in the body. It does this if administered by itself. Other substances in the mother drug might have the opposite effect upon the process. An observer might then detect a reaction in an opium eater that is a blend of both reactions; the body process is a bit agitated, or it is slightly sedated. Each interpretation is valid.

27. Nineteenth-century researchers documented this characteristic of *Papaver somniferum Linn*. Excellent sources of information, especially for the poppy in India, are Flückiger & Hanbury (1879); John Scott (1877); and GBS [Watt] 1891:3–79.

28. Sometimes not even that. Poppy cultivators who shipped the raw latex to private or government factories and the merchants who sold the substance were creative about adulterating crude opium exports. The practice was perpetrated in the belief that additives increased or enhanced the preferred color, consistency, texture, and aroma of the drug. Items used to adulterate the drug differed among the opium-producing countries. And, within any society, the agent (or agents) might change from year to year. The list of substances is long, and in some regions they included human saliva and urine. Adulteration began early in *Papaver somniferum Linn*'s career as a commodity of world importance. See Flückiger & Hanbury (1879:46–48) for comments about practices after mid-nineteenth century. Elijah Impey's 1848 monograph is an excellent source of information for adulteration techniques that cultivators and merchants in central India used before 1850.

29. A brief review of achievements in facets of *Papaver somniferum Linn* research as of 1896 is found in APA 1896:44:609–13.

30. Pro-trade statements about the effects of opium eating were therefore, at best, crude estimations. The predictions were based upon assumptions that were unproven, tenuous, or false. The way to avoid imprecision was to administer the alkaloid that produced the desired result. But this meant that a person had to know precisely what the substance did in the human body, exactly how much of the substance to dispense, and that a pure or uncontaminated alkaloid had to be administered. The Royal Commission and defenders of the trade demonstrated no awareness of this requirement.

31. Fevers erupt during the phase of asexual reproduction.

2

The Missionaries' Lament in a Milieu of Indifference, 1773–1874 C.E.

INTRODUCTION

The dominant theme in early western opposition to the India-China opium trade was the inevitable moral degeneration of Asian natives. The idea remained prominent throughout the era. Early opponents assimilated no medical data into arguments decrying the negative consequences of opiate indulgence because the material did not exist. The deficiency gradually disappeared and so did western indifference to protest from people in Asia and their supporters back home. By the early 1890s, the anti-opiumist ethical and medical argument exerted decisive influence upon members of the British Parliament.[1] The amalgamation of laboratory insights about opiate addiction in western societies and statements of moral outrage forced politicians to reevaluate the Asian drug trade. But much to their dismay, anti-opiumists' realization that opium also had medical utility became their Achilles heel.

The next two chapters document the evolution of the anti-opiumists' argument and its inherent weakness. Chapter 2 describes events shaping the content of protest regarding consumption in Asia and the West, especially in Great Britain, from the earliest years of the China-India drug commerce through 1874. Chapter 3 covers activities from 1875 through 1893. This is the period in which public and scientific attitudes about opiates changed dramatically in Great Britain. By 1893, the Anglo-European research community had enough facts to challenge the status quo regarding drug use at home. The anti-opiumists used this information to attack Great Britain's drug policy in India.

Chapter 2

THE EVOLUTION OF DISCONTENT

Pre-Trade Chinese Attitudes about Opium Use

The rulers of China tolerated opium use before prolonged European involvement in East Asia. The drug was an ingredient in several herbal medicines taken for dysentery, diarrhea, and several other maladies. Leniency ended when Dutch merchants introduced tobacco smoking to the Chinese during the 1600s. These Europeans encouraged tobacco use by claiming smoking was beneficial to health. The Chinese added arsenic to give the tobacco more "kick" as well as to enhance its medicinal value. Opium in turn replaced tobacco when the latter became expensive and scarce in the Empire. The Chinese then deleted arsenic and they soon smoked only opium. Imperial leniency ended when increasing numbers of Chinese began processing the drug shipped from India into an extract used only for pleasure (GBO [Baines] 1895a:VI:163; Lowes 1966:59).

Emperor Yung Cheng issued the first edict prohibiting opium smoking in 1729. Authorities periodically attempted to curtail the practice with varying degrees of urgency and success. The imperial court outlawed imports in 1796 and again in 1799. The penalty for smoking the extract was banishment or imprisonment for life, or death (Inglis 1975:73–4; Kuo 1935:28–9; Lowes 1966:25–7; Moorhead & Tobin 1931:471; Stelle 1981:3, 5; O'Brien & Cohen 1984:XVI; Willoughby 1925:8; GBS [Watt] 1891:14–15; Holmes 1894:17:788; EB 1911:20:130). The edicts were ineffectual. Authorities discovered the drug being imported from the interior of the country less than a decade later. Local officials were either unwilling or unable to stop the illegal trade (Inglis 1975:74; Kuo, 1935:29). Then in 1813, China's emperor found that his own bodyguards and court eunuchs "had become enslaved by the habit." His disgust prompted issuance of another mandate in 1815 (Inglis 1975:74).

"Western" Secular and Religious Opposition to the India-China Opium Trade

The Chinese who voiced alarm about their fellow citizens' attraction to opium were not alone. Consternation among some westerners living in India, China, and elsewhere in East Asia about selling Indian opium to Asian citizens existed from the trade's inception. Charles W. King, an American merchant living in Canton at the beginning of the nineteenth century, for example, refused to have anything to do with the drug despite its profitability. He condemned the East India Company for encouraging British businessmen to violate "the highest laws and the best interests of the Chinese empire" (King, cited in Inglis 1975:80; see also Fay 1976:85–5). And in 1820, Stamford Ruffles declared that opium was destroying the character and sapping the energies of the people of Java (Inglis 1975:77).

East India Company Officials' Misgivings During the Early Decades about the India-China Opium Trade

The directors of the East India Company living in England during the late 1700s and early 1800s were not oblivious to Chinese protests about illegal drug shipments. They said they would gladly stop all involvement in the trade "out of compassion for mankind" if India's development was not hindered (Inglis 1975:75). The money earned from increased Chinese demand for the Indian drug made this altruistic option impossible. The East India Company then offered to help resolve the problem by limiting expansion of poppy cultivation and keeping export prices high. Restrictions on poppy cultivation and export quotas would be lifted only if the policy proved detrimental to India. The regulations were disadvantageous and they ended.

Warren Hastings exemplified the disquietude that some East India Company officials felt during the very early decades of English involvement in the trade. Upon becoming director for Company activities in India in 1773, Hastings established control over poppy cultivation and opium production in Indian territories that the English governed directly (Eisenlohr 1934:213). This architect of the drug monopoly, ambivalent about the accomplishment, declared opium was a "vile drug [that] should be tolerated for the purposes of foreign commerce only" (Hastings, quoted in Crafts & Leitch 1911:66; also see Inglis 1975:73, and Tinling 1876:83). Consumption within India, however, should be discouraged. Lieutenant-Colonel James Tod, the East India Company representative at the Court of Maharajah Rana of Udaipur, a native state in Rajasthan province of western India, was more specific in 1820.

> This pernicious plant (the poppy) has robbed the Rajpoot of half his virtues; and while it obscures these it heightens his vices, giving to his natural bravery a character of insane ferocity, and to his countenance which otherwise beam with intelligence, an air of imbecility. Like all stimulants, its effects are magical for a time; but the reaction is not less certain, and the faded form, or amorphous bulk, too often attest to the debilitating influence of a drug which alike debases mind and body. (Tod, quoted by Turner 1876:240; Scott, James Maurice 1969:97)

The British government ignored protests from overseas missionaries and others during these early years. A Select Committee created by Parliament to review the operations of the East India Company typifies the response. Their reports, published between 1805 and 1813, contain virtually no recognition of European and English consternation about the detrimental effects of opium consumption for the morals and health of people in China, India, or anywhere elsewhere in Asia. The topic was a nonissue for members of Parliament.

Western missionaries living in China during the opening decades of the new century, consequently, had few channels to express their objection to an audience wider than their respective congregations back home. Citizens without institutional support in their native country faced even greater difficulty in finding an audience. And before the 1830s, all accusations were questionable because information about the drug's effects upon the Chinese was scarce and unreliable (Inglis 1975:78–9). The situation began to change in 1832 when E. C. Bridgeman and S. Wells Williams, two American missionaries in China, published the first issue of *The Chinese Repository* (Bridgeman & Williams [1831] 1968; Inglis 1975:79; Owen [1934] 1968:374; Kuo 1935:202). Bridgeman and Williams were sympathetic to Chinese citizens opposing opium imports. Although antagonistic to the trade, their comments did not have the outraged moral tone that characterized many other critiques during the era (Owen [1934] 1968:374). The periodical ceased publication in 1851.

Bridgeman, Williams, and other anti-opiumists scattered throughout Asia were finding common cause during the early 1830s. Greater numbers of Chinese nationals and foreigners in that country, joined by concerned Europeans in India, were becoming more antagonistic and vocal about the penchant of Great Britain's leaders for exploiting a colony's wealth but doing little or nothing to help its indigenous people (Johnson 1975:307). The problem was that by the beginning of the fourth decade of the nineteenth century only a small segment of the British public thought what anti-opiumists in Asia were decrying was cause for alarm. The British Parliament was more responsive.

The Parliamentary Committee and Debates: 1830–1833

In the latter part of 1831 a House of Commons Select Committee reviewed all phases of opium production in the subcontinent as well as trade relations between China, India, and Great Britain. And for the first time, committee members investigated opium's alleged harmful effects upon consumers (GBO [Baines] 1895a:VI:163; see also Lowes 1966:59).

The volumes of oral testimony and supplementary material collected by the Select Committee offered little solace to the anti-opiumists. Ethical issues raised in the House of Commons between 1830 and 1832 focused upon the trade's illegality. Apologists admitted opium was contraband but they proclaimed Chinese authorities knew what was occurring and tacitly condoned imports. Again, a rationale for inaction was that ending the trade would impede India's development (GBO [Baines] 1895a:VI:163; Lowes 1966:59).

Sir Henry Pottinger illustrates the disdain some high-ranking British officials felt for anti-opiumists' accusations about inducing misery among the Chinese. In a Foreign Office report circa 1831, Pottinger, the British Governor-General Minister Plenipotentiary in China at the time, said he could not

> admit in any manner the idea adopted by many persons, that the introduction of opium into China is a source of unmitigated evil of every kind and a cause of misery. Personally, I have been unable to discover a single case of this kind, although I admit that, when abused, opium may become most hurtful. Besides, the same remark applies to every kind of enjoyment when carried to excess; but . . . from what Mandarins themselves say, I am convinced that the demoralisation [sic] and ruin which some person attributes to the use of opium, arise more likely from imperfect

knowledge of the subject and exaggeration, and that not one hundredth part of the evil arises in China from opium smoking which one sees daily arising in England, as well as in India, from the use of ardent spirits, so largely taken in excess in those countries. (Pottinger, quoted in GBO [Batten] 1894:I:140)

Pottinger rejected the image of the wretched, degraded, and depraved opium user "enfeebled in mind and body, unfit for the active duties of life-thieves, vagabonds, and beggars" as a ridiculous scenario. It was, he asserted, obtained exclusively from opium dens. He complained that the anti-opiumists refuse to acknowledge that moderate use of opium is, or even might be, helpful to consumers (Pottinger, quoted in GBO [Batten] 1894:I:140). For Pottinger and others of like mind, England was engaging in normal and moral trade with a foreign nation. It was supplying needy people with a substance that had medicinal value.

One of the East India Company's own officials, however, discredited humanitarian concern as a rationalization for British involvement in the commerce. Mr. Hugh Stark, director of the Revenue Department of the Indian Board and testifying before the Select Committee, admitted the Bengal government had never even attempted to produce opium for medical purposes. The administration's sole aim was to satisfy Chinese demand for a superior smoking extract, a luxury product, and nothing else (GBR [Stark] 1831–32:25).[2]

The 1833 House of Commons did not deny the negative moral and health consequences of opium consumption among the Chinese. It was, however, a topic they preferred not to address, and the only member who brought it up for discussion during the session was ignored. The attitude was due in no small part to influential people like Pottinger.

One year later Lord Palmerston sent Lord Napier to China. The purpose was to convince the emperor to open ports other than Canton to foreign trade and to legalize opium imports (Inglis 1975:78). British merchants wanted to make money, but profit in a Christian country should be earned in a moral way. China's agreement to Napier's entreaty would protect the self-image of England. Undeterred by what they viewed as British hypocrisy, anti-opiumists continued to voice concern about the plight of the Chinese people (Lowes 1966:59).

Reverend W. H. Medhurst was one of the earliest missionary protestors. As early as 1816, Medhurst had concluded opium was injurious to the health and morals of the Chinese people, and in 1840 he published a book detailing his observations. The man alluded to drug dependence and claimed that opium smuggled into China had demoralized nearly three million people. The smoking habit also was impossible to end once begun. There was no such thing as moderate consumption and the victim was progressively susceptible to all forms of temptation. A weakened body and mind accompanied moral laxity. This rendered the person unable to earn a wage for supporting a family. People who attempted to stop the habit invariably died (Inglis 1975:90).

Medhurst's depressing prognosis of inevitable moral and physical degeneration culminating in premature death among the Chinese was a prominent theme in future anti-opiumist arguments. However, the portrayal motivated few people other than those already committed to ending the trade.

The Missionaries' Lament and the Environment of Indifference in Great Britain Prior to 1830

Parliament felt no compulsion to criticize the East India Company's drug export policy in response to the lamentations of Christians in Asia because the latter had no mass support at home. The vast majority of citizens in the British Isles before and during the 1830s simply were unconcerned. The Anglo-European medical establishment extolled the drug. The attitude dated to the Renaissance and before. There is another indication of the drug's nonproblematic status. Eighteenth and early nineteenth century entrepreneurs successfully cultivated the poppy in England and Scotland. The fledgling industry died because labor costs were too high. People who preferred self-medication also could purchase inexpensive opium-based concoctions. Some of these "medicines" were created during the early 1800s. Other preparations were ancient recipes.

Eminent literary figures also contributed to the British public's indifference. The most famous was Thomas DeQuincey (1785–1859).[3] DeQuincey described opiate habituation in provocative detail in a sensational 1822 book, *Confessions of an English Opium-Eater*. He explained addiction as the result of a type of artistic temperament, of which he was an example. Furthermore, the trait required no medical justification and anyone decrying the detrimental physical effects of the opiate was wrong (Peters 1981:465–66). The book's popularity ensured DeQuincey's status as a "noble self-experimenter" and an opium expert among the nonmedical public for years (Parssinen 1983:8, 61–3).[4]

Samuel Taylor Coleridge (1772–1834) is another, and unfortunate, example. The man purportedly composed the poem *Kubla Khan* with its famous description of a "stately pleasure dome" while under the drug's influence. Coleridge paid a high price for creativity; he faced "progressive physical and intellectual debilitation from his well-documented addiction to opium in the form of laudanum" (O'Brien & Cohen 1984:XIII; see also Peters 1981:465). The poet's fate caused no alarm among the general population.

The absence of concern was typical even among the clinicians and toxicologists who were writing many papers about the drug during the 1700s. Some of them recognized and investigated "patient dependence, physiological tolerance, and withdrawal pains" (Parssinen 1983:85). They found nothing alarming (see Musto 1973:69; Sonnedecker 1963:11–12; Terry & Pillens 1928:58–9; Peters 1981:465; and Clausen 1968:269 for commentary and details about specific explorations). A clearer description of opiate dependence emerged by the beginning of the 1790s, but physicians still did not view the phenomenon as a threat or as a sickness with physiological origins (Berridge 1977a:276; Brill 1969:8, 15). Samuel Crumpe, the first person to use the term "addiction" in the late 1700s, "employed the term to indicate it was merely 'a bad habit'" and others portrayed the trait as a simple vice (Kurland 1978:2).

The perception of opium habituation as benign continued into the next century. Furthermore, the scant technical literature published during the early 1800s that alluded to the negative dimension of indulgence blamed the consumer, not the drug. Dependency was the result of moral deficiency, a self-inflicted disease of the will, an intemperate habit, a consequence of bad character and so forth (Berridge 1978:456; Sonnedecker 1963:11–4). The collective message of this eighteenth- and early nineteenth-century research was unequivocal: abnormal psychological and physiological attributes of human beings, not chemical substances, were the source of moral laxity and other unfortunate qualities among a population. The presence of many peculiar and most likely inherently defective individuals, therefore, sufficed to explain widespread chronic habituation in an entire society. China was an example.

The few Anglo-Europeans who acknowledged a possible problem linked to opium consumption in China embraced a racial theory to explain the alleged plight of men, women, and children in a country so far away. For example, the Chinese looked different from western people and these unusual physical features were the ultimate cause of misery. Traits such as eating different foods or speaking a different language intensified the peculiar mental and physiological problems ostensibly generated by opium consumption. In other words, the Chinese had problems because they were born Chinese.

Using a racial theory to "understand" the Chinese was not new. During the late 1700s, for example, the renowned Samuel Crumpe of the Royal Irish Academy proclaimed "Orientals were much more resistant or susceptible to opium than Occidentals" (Musto 1973:69). Other intellectuals said there was some undiscovered quality about Asians that made them react to the pleasurable effect of a narcotic in a way different from Europeans (Lodwick 1976:34, 297). Nonetheless, if the effects of excessive consumption were virtually unrecognized or viewed as benign in Great Britain, it is understandable that few of its citizens were upset about similar behavior in a distant country inhabited by peculiar people.

Intimations of Concern about Opium Use in Great Britain Before 1830

Some eighteenth-century physicians believed addiction was not the only reason for cautious use of the drug. These doctors, like people in preceding centuries, argued about opium's dominant trait. They also debated the merits of Samuel Crumpe's diverse, and conflicting, statements about the drug's function as a "stimulant or depressant" in the human body (Sonnedecker 1963:11–14). In Philadelphia during 1791–1792, Mr. Hast Handy claimed that opium enabled a person to exert considerable "mental energy" over long periods of time. This made the person think clearly. At the same time another American by the name of Valentine Seaman challenged Handy's thesis about the capability of opium to enhance cognition. Seaman said sedation was the principal function and he provided examples of pain relief and the alleviation of other ailments to prove it (Terry & Pillens 1928:59–60). Both interpretations are correct. Opium, or more accurately its alkaloids, has a sedative effect upon some organs and processes. The mother drug and some of its components function as a stimulant for other organs and processes. And, as cited in the preceding chapter, Francois Magendie continued the discussion about the drug's principal "action" in the early 1800s.

The Anglo-European debate about *Papaver somniferum Linn*'s status as a stimulant or a sedative was not limited to the laboratory. The issue also became part of the embryonic ethical controversy in Great Britain during the first half of the nineteenth century. People who stressed its role as a stimulant argued with each other about the 'goodness' or 'badness' of being stimulated. Others accorded the sedative interpretation more credibility. They debated the morality of inducing passivity in people regardless of the rationale for doing so. Some members of this second group did not even consider sedation a moral issue. The opiate was dangerous because its pain-relieving capability prevented the detection of maladies that required other kinds of treatment (Musto 1973:69).[5] The intellectual discord indicates that by 1800, a few western medical doctors were giving serious and spirited attention to the clinical use of *Papaver somniferum Linn*. Most of the medical community and public in Great Britain at the time, however, continued to ignore early warnings from the religious community. The complacency was both enhanced and challenged thirty years later.

Great Britain's opium imports escalated in the early 1830s. At first glance each factor responsible for increased consumption appears to diminish the credibility of anti-opiumist declarations about the dangers of ingesting the drug. By the end of the decade, however, the combined effect was different; opium abuse emerged as a problem articulated by some health professionals and politicians in the commonwealth. Overindulgence also was about to be associated ever so slightly with the Asian experience.

The salience of opium as a therapeutic agent in English medicine during the decade exacerbated anti-opiumists' difficulties (Parssinen 1983:22). As alluded to above, one of several factors accounting for its prominence was the medical profession's typical portrayal of the drug. Few commentators between 1820 and 1830 published articles about the negative physiological and psychological effects of consumption.[6] Most commentators either extolled the drug's virtues for all kinds of ailments or said it was harmless.[7] The second factor was the influence of former East India Company officials. They suggested opium might benefit victims of the great cholera epidemic in Great Britain during 1831–1832. The drug distributed to sufferers came from Turkey and other locations in the Middle East, not from India. It was mixed with calomel and the concoction seemed to help. The medical establishment was so impressed that the medication became "one of the most frequently used and successful cholera remedies in nineteenth century Britain" (Parssinen 1983:23).

A prolonged crisis in English medicine also contributed to the salience of opium. Homeopaths, hydropaths, and other "irregular" practitioners who appeared in the 1830s, and were present during the 1840s, appealed to a clientele that patronized traditional medical doctors. While the latter no longer subscribed to Galenic medical views, they still relied upon old "heroic treatments" such as bleeding and blistering in combination with "harsh drugs like calomel" (Parssinen 1983:24). English physicians initially condemned these "irregulars." These charlatans administered placebos because their therapy was much less painful, therefore not efficacious. Some of these upstarts were part of "noninterventionist medical practice" and opium was admirably suited to their agenda. Ingestion of the drug involved no torture and it relieved symptoms such as diarrhea, 'fever,' and pain. The newcomers' growing popularity by mid-century was a "deathblow to heroic therapies" such as bloodletting. In contrast, consuming opium was, in most cases, a gentle way to feel better although the patient had most likely not eliminated the underlying cause of misery.

Manufacturers of patent or proprietary medicines, whose formulas were kept secret from the public, also contributed to opium's prominent place in therapeutic practice during the 1830s. Entrepreneurs created numerous new concoctions. Each one ostensibly had great power and all of them contained varying amounts of the drug (Parssinen 1983:31).[8] The desire for medical self-reliance, the herbalist legacy, and orthodox doctors continuing to charge high prices that common folk could not afford, also played a role. Combined with imports of inexpensive opium in post-1830 Great Britain, these factors resulted in local chemists, pharmacists, and grocers in hamlets, villages, towns, and cities of the commonwealth becoming popular sources of free medical advice and cheap medications that relieved simple aches and pains.[9] Indeed, opium became a staple in their business. Customers did not have to spend time traveling to a physician, and they could avoid a consultation fee. People also needed no prescription to buy patent medicines, inexpensive homemade elixirs, and crude opium (Parssinen 1983:x, 17, 28, 30).[10]

The medical profession denounced local chemists as unfit and unqualified to dispense medical expertise. The latter responded by declaring they were performing a valuable service for people who did not need, did not trust, or could not pay for the advice of a professional doctor. And for more than half of the nineteenth century, grocers throughout the country confronted no government regulations for selling crude opium and opium-based products.[11] Physicians' contempt for a working-class grocer's right to distribute the drug in any form was most likely intense and probably unprintable.

Growing Awareness in Great Britain During the 1830s about the Negative Consequences of Opium Use

Who was qualified to distribute opium and opium-based products was not the only issue raised during the decade. A climate more hospitable to moralists such as Medhurst in distant China was slowly evolving. The death of the Earl of Mar in 1828 was the first of several events undermining English confidence about the benign nature of opiate indulgence. The Earl bought an expensive insurance policy but the company refused to pay after discovering he had been consuming laudanum for thirty years. In a highly publicized trial between 1830 and 1832, the firm successfully argued that the contract did not cover the cause of death. Some people said it was addiction. Lawyers for both parties needed valid facts, not conjecture, about the consequence of habitual opiate use upon human longevity. In 1832 they asked Sir Robert Christison, a prominent expert, to testify. Acknowledging the meager amount of empirical evidence and its dubious quality, Christison concluded that opium was not automatically fatal and that a consumer could live to a ripe old age if the quantity ingested each time was modest. Furthermore, the link between habituation and inevitable bad behavior was merely conjecture. For Christison, the public's fear of narcotics generated by the Earl's demise was unnecessary and irrational (Peters 1981:467–68).

Christison deplored the absence of reliable data about topics related to opium for a country in which use of the drug was so pervasive. He thought no statistics were available because many consumers died young and the "better classes . . . were able to conceal their use from physicians, while the lower classes destroyed the opportunity for accurate observation of the habit because they combined it with excessive drinking" (Peters 1981:468). He also believed his statements would be verified if the government kept better records.

The case had implications beyond who benefited from an insurance policy. Members of the Temperance Movement viewed citizens' anxiety about narcotics as a godsend and used it in the effort to ban any kind of 'stimulant.' Their list of taboo articles included opium. Public concern also was a boon to those anti-opiumists who objected to opium consumption only within Great Britain. Both groups dismissed or ignored Christison's conclusions regarding the harmless long-term effects of ingesting opiates. They claimed the Earl's fate was to be expected because dosage increase and chronic dependence were the inevitable consequences of indulgence. Some medical practitioners, while less strident, were equally influential in influencing public opinion. Physicians began to doubt the assumed benign status of opium products. Other kinds of health care professionals voiced concern about the wisdom of continuing a policy of unrestricted public access to the increasing volume of opium imports (Berridge & Edwards 1981:192).

All parties, however, agreed with Christison about one thing. They needed more reliable statistics regarding consumption among the different socioeconomic classes. They also criticized the underreporting of substance abuse. Subsequent documentation indicated the amount of opium imported per annum into the commonwealth for home consumption rose from 23,000 pounds to 41,100 pounds between 1829 and 1839. Consumption per thousand, calculated as two pounds per person in the 1830s, would increase to three pounds by the late 1850s (Berridge 1977a:276; Berridge 1978:442; Peters 1981:462, 466; Parssinen 1983:10).[12]

The general public and the medical community had reason for alarm about opiate use among Great Britain's laboring classes (Berridge 1978:442). Citizens apparently used the drug "in all but the most serious cases of childhood illnesses" and more cases of overindulgence were inevitable (Parssinen 1983:x, 30). Differences in urban and rural patterns of consumption also were beginning to emerge. The contrast was obvious by midcentury. The homemade opiates and poppyhead tea that were prevalent in the countryside had been replaced in urban locations by laudanum and the abundant, commercially prepared opium commodities (Berridge 1978:443, 447; Austin 1978:156).

The number of deaths throughout the country attributed to opium in 1840 was five per million (Berridge 1978:443). And the Office of the Registrar General, plus other agencies created during the 1830s and early 1840s, discovered high death rates among the opium-consuming agricultural workers in the Fens district of England. The tragedy was not confined to adult proletarians. Particularly sobering was the extremely high infant mortality rate in the region. Women with babies were absent from families for long periods of time because they had to work outside the home to supplement their husbands' meager incomes. Elder children often had to care for the very young or an older woman was responsible for as many as thirty-five children. Opiates and opium-based remedies were a blessing to both groups; the drug kept infants quiet and easy to manage. Excessive dosage resulting in opium poisoning was frequent. It explained the striking increase in infant deaths compared to past decades (Berridge 1977a:276–77; Parssinen 1983:49).

The habit of giving opium to children in the Fens was not always benevolent. Commentators say the practice also was a form of euthanasia. It was easy to explain the crime as an accident (Berridge 1977a:280; Parssinen 1983:50–1). According to Berridge, "[t]wins and illegitimate children almost always die" due to intentional excessive, hence fatal dosage of the opiate (Berridge 1977a:280). Data for 1837–38 pertaining to the entire country indicated approximately 543 children perished from opium poisoning. Another report estimated 200 infant deaths (Miskel 1973:4; Lomax 1973:170–72).[13] Many of these fatalities probably were accidental, the result of busy mothers or caretakers giving daily doses of the drug with varying amounts of morphine, thebaine, and other alkaloids to pacify children. The number of deaths from intentional overdosing is unknown. The same question applies for locales beyond the Fens and other rural regions of Great Britain. And in a classic 1842 report about England's factory system, William Dobb told of factory workers using opiates, most often laudanum, to keep babies quiet (Brecher 1972:5).[14]

The people who argued about the ethical consequences of opium ingestion did not remain passive when confronted with this kind of evidence. The data reaffirmed the convictions held by one faction about all stimulants being morally and physiologically detrimental. These people wanted all of these substances, including opium, banned to the public. In England, the Temperance Movement used the material to strengthen their already passionate argument that featured the Earl of Mar's legal case. They demanded no public availability to stimulants of any kind. A similar response came from those people preoccupied with opium. This group insisted the Earl's death from an uncontrollable habit was proof that the drug was a dangerous stimulant. The accumulating and alarming statistics about consumption among the common folk confirmed the accusation. Some physicians agreed, as did lay people unaffiliated with either the Temperance Movement or any anti-opiumist organization. And all aforementioned groups categorized opium as a stimulant that did negative things to users. They believed habituation was a perilous, contaminating moral disease that diminished economic productivity. It destroyed the "individual effort and hard work seen as necessary for the industrial work force" (Berridge 1978:447). The drug's seductive allure also threatened the stability of middle-class society by exciting guileless members of these "better classes" (Berridge 1978:448).

Two categories of people opposed the pessimistic "stimulation is bad" interpretation. The group that considered sedation as either the only or primary function of opium dismissed the controversy as irrelevant. The people who accepted the stimulant scenario but rejected the idea of inherent negativity assumed that stimulation was one of the universal needs of humankind. The latter group believed that depriving people of opium, especially the working class, would only increase the consumption of alcohol and liquor, the other two stimulants. Compared to alcohol and liquor, opium also had far less pernicious consequences for an individual and for society. Serious problems were avoided by keeping opium inexpensive and accessible to the masses because the drug satisfied their natural desire to feel good. The people who were antagonistic only to the Temperance Movement's effort to eliminate alcohol used the same logic. They said restricted access to liquor would increase the public's consumption of opium because both were necessary stimulants. Furthermore, opium's negative effects were a greater danger to society than alcohol (Berridge 1978:448). The arguments went back and forth, around and around. While 'dispassionate' science had yet to provide unequivocal proof for any particular theory, one thing was definite; some people in England were now echoing the China missionaries' lament about a correlation between opium, morality, health, and longevity. By the end of the decade, doubts about the relevance of warnings from influential segments of Great Britain's population about a possible relationship between the Asian drug situation and the welfare of British society had waned.

The First Opium War and Its Consequences, 1839–1850

The decade ended with Commissioner Lin's confiscation and destruction of 20,000 chests of opium near Canton, China, during 1839. This was one of a series of events leading to the 1840–42 Opium War. The conflict demarcates a new era in anti-opium activities. During the 1840s numerous observations from Asia and more medical data added credibility to some of the anti-opiumists' issues. The politicians hostile to Christian 'do-gooders' in the Orient also noticed that respected individuals were investigating opium abuse at home. What they found was disturbing. The 'problem' in China was emerging as a 'problem' in Great Britain. Starting in the 1840s, members of Parliament were listening, and listening intently, to the anti-opiumist message from Asia.

Defenders of the Asian opium commerce responded cautiously to Commissioner Lin's confiscation of opium chests in Canton during 1839. Mr. Jardine, of Jardine & Matheson Co., Ltd., urged infuriated English merchants to temper their outrage and moderate their demand for compensation. This was necessary to avoid Parliament raising questions about the immorality of opium exports (Collis 1947:263).

Jardine's plea for restraint yielded a dividend. The first prolonged debate about British involvement in the commerce took place just before the declaration of war. Sir James Graham raised a question concerning the negative effects of opium upon the Chinese. The query generated little discussion. Lord Stanton and Sir George Staunton also contemplated introducing a resolution condemning British involvement in the trade. They decided not to bring it forward because Sir Robert Peel's speech persuaded them that more subtle chastisement would garner support for ending involvement. Peel said the English Government was remiss in not giving bureaucrats an incentive to "provide against the growing evils connected with the contraband traffic in opium" (Peel, quoted in GBO [Baines] 1895a:VI:163). This failure, he continued, led to Commissioner Lin's outrageous behavior. The 533 members of the House of Commons defeated the resolution in which Peel's comment appeared. It lost by only nine votes (GBO [Baines] 1895a:VI:163).

In January 1840 Parliament denounced Commissioner Lin as a 'bandit.' It called for the formation of an international naval force of French, American, and British ships to halt Chinese aggression (Collis 1947:286). The aforementioned Mr. Jardine's Tory allies in Parliament labored to persuade the Whig government to sanction a war against the Chinese. The Tories emphasized the illegal status of the confiscation. They insisted the matter be resolved to protect Great Britain's prestige. The Whigs feared public opinion might turn against them if national pride was not restored. Pro-war members of Parliament narrowly won the ensuing vote and the first Opium War began.

Approximately one month later Lord Stanhope wanted to denounce both the conflict and the trade in the House of Lords. He planned to send a translation of the document to the Chinese court. Lord Melbourne, the head of government, opposed Stanhope's proposal. A young Mr. Gladstone, who later helped to create the Royal Commission on Opium, in turn disagreed with Melbourne (GBO [Baines] 1895a:VI:163; Lowes 1966:59–60). In March of 1840, Gladstone rallied against the "infamous and atrocious traffic in the drug," calling it a "pernicious article" (Hess 1965:24; Berridge & Edwards 1981:174). Few members of Parliament defended opium during the 1840 debate. Nonetheless, most participants, the exception being Gladstone, thought the allegations about the drug being evil were exaggerated. They contended that effects of consumption really "were no worse than those of overindulgence in ardent spirits, all too familiar in the West" (Inglis 1975:91). The anti-opiumists might be overwrought and unduly concerned, and Gladstone might be misled and lapsing into hysteria, but these politicians had finally associated problems in China with those in Great Britain.

Anti-opiumists condemned the war as a conspiracy to ensure massive subjugation of the Chinese people (Kurland 1978:2). The earliest publication of one anti-opium group in existence before 1840 even cited the "principles of Christianity and commercial opposition" as reasons to oppose the war. The group's pronouncements were reiterated three years later in the first anti-opium resolution in Parliament that condemned the war on religious, moral, commercial, and political grounds (Lowes 1966:60). Another organization, the Society for the Suppression of the Contraband Trade in Opium, sent a petition to Lord Palmerston during the conflict. Its members beseeched him to persuade Her Majesty's plenipotentiaries to discourage poppy cultivation in India. This change would decrease the volume of drug exports to China (Owen [1934] 1968:230). Palmerston ignored the memorial and the conflict continued.

British, French, and American military forces were victorious in China. The 1842 Treaty of Nanking formally ended hostilities. The pact forced the Chinese to open the seaports of Ningpo, Shanghai, Foochow, Amoy, and Canton to foreign trade (Owen [1934] 1968:156–57, 192). Interrupted for two years, the flow of Indian opium to the Empire resumed. It soon became a flood. The influx of Anglo-Saxon Protestant missionaries also escalated, thereby increasing the ranks of potential antagonists in China. The anti-opiumists' resolve to halt exports to China intensified. The reformers who were already in the country were aided by the presence of more opium and additional missionaries. First, there were more people to document *possible* abuse. Second, all of them had numerous opportunities to report *actual* cases of excessive indulgence. They hoped these incidents might generate greater awareness at home.

Aftermath of the First Opium War: Parliamentary Debate in 1843

In 1843, the London, the Baptist, and the Wesleyan Missionary Societies in China sent petitions to several members of Parliament. The entreaties called for termination of the trade. In April of the same year and acting on behalf of Samuel Gurney and William S. Fry (two prominent anti-opiumists), Lord Shaftesbury introduced the petitions to Parliament (Lowes 1966:60–1; Owen [1934] 1968:230–31; GBO [Baines] 1895a:VI:164; Berridge & Edwards 1981:174; Tinling 1876:vi). Parliament implied it was agreeable to ending export and the Board of Trade favored it. Shaftesbury was delighted. He then proclaimed that opium destroys all goodwill between England and China. It is an obstruction to "legitimate commerce [and] utterly inconsistent with the honour and duties of a Christian kingdom; and steps [must] be taken as soon as possible, with due regard to the rights of Government and individuals, to abolish the evil" (GBO [Baines] 1895a:VI:164).

Lord Shaftesbury then became the first anti-opiumist member of Parliament to publicly acknowledge the dual nature of the substance and to use medical data to support the contention. He cited the opinions of twenty-five British medical administrators and physicians. Shaftesbury's list included Anthony White (President of the Royal College of Surgeons), Sir Henry Halford (President of the Royal College of Physicians), and Sir Benjamin Brodie, a prominent surgeon. Brodie said opium was a valuable medicine but he qualified the statement. Any moderately informed person, he proclaimed, knows that use of the drug leads to destructive habituation. This results in a destroyed digestive system and a weakened mind and body. The person is now "worse than [a] useless member of society" (Brodie, quoted in Berridge & Edwards 1981:175). Others whom Shaftesbury cites articulate similar opinions. Henceforth, Shaftesbury and fellow anti-opiumists deemed opium to be a valuable albeit dangerous medicine. This stance implies that control over distribution was necessary to ensure the well-being of society.

The support of Sir George Staunton, a veteran of many years in China, enhanced the credibility of Shaftesbury's attack. Shaftesbury's eloquent, convincing argument then turned scathing. It was replete with firsthand observations and statistics that emphasized the most negative aspects of opiate use in China. Staunton became increasingly hesitant. Shaftesbury's "righteous indignation or his unfamiliarity with conditions in China led him into lamentable overstatement and a use of authorities that was less than critical" (Owen [1934] 1968:230).

Sir Robert Peel, the Head of Government, wanted Shaftesbury to withdraw the resolution because it would interfere with current tariff negotiations between China and England. His rebuttal of Shaftesbury's argument was weak but the latter agreed (GBO [Baines] 1895a:VI:164; Johnson 1975:307, 309; Owen [1934] 1968:231; Berridge & Edwards 1981:174). There would be no serious anti-opium activity in Parliament until 1855 and no formal debate until 1870. Nonetheless, animosity about the drug expressed during the 1843 session disturbed members of the British government (Owen [1934] 1968:231).

The administration also responded to the English abolitionists' accusation of moral laxity. The aforementioned Sir Henry Pottinger, Great Britain's plenipotentiary in Hong Kong and no friend to the anti-opiumists, was told to issue an anti-smuggling proclamation in the early 1840s. Pottinger had no intention of enforcing the order and he never did (Hess 1965:24; Inglis 1975:85–9). Despite Pottinger's actions, the defenders of the trade unaffiliated with Government remained upset by the anti-opiumists' growing influence (GBO [Baines] 1895a:VI:164; Johnson 1975:307, 309; Berridge & Edwards 1981:174). Observations reported during the decade confirmed their fears. The next decade was no different.

Beyond Parliament: Public Debate about Opium, 1839–1843

Most apolitical medical practitioners in Great Britain and Europe during the war remained indifferent to the physiological and moral consequences of opium use in Asia. Other physicians expressed only modest interest in the subject. China was, after all, a distant country and consumers in the Orient who had problems were neither English nor European. They also expressed little concern about another issue. It was the continuing increase of consumption in Great Britain during the 1830s despite warnings of health professionals regarding effects upon the working classes.[15]

A few physicians, however, thought otherwise and viewed opium indulgence by people of any nationality with concern. At the 1840 Westminster Medical Society symposium on opium indulgence in Great Britain and China, two individuals denounced the substance as "both extremely dangerous and addictive" (Miskel 1973:4). One of them, a Dr. Charles Toogood Downing, attempted to describe the negative similarities between opium eating and alcohol consumption, thereby linking the two substances in the minds of members of the audience (Peters 1981:468). Some attendees agreed with Downing. Other people said opium was much more harmful than alcohol. Still other conference participants labeled Downing and his colleague as extremists because opium simply was not as dangerous as they claimed. Some of these people identified alcohol as the worst offender (Miskel 1973:4, 8).

Debate about the similarities between opium and spirits spread beyond the confines of Westminster to Great Britain's medical establishment. Most physicians preferred either the "opium and alcohol are equally harmful" scenario or the "alcohol is the worst offender" interpretation (Miskel 1973:8). For example, in 1846, a Dr. Basham, prompted by his experience at Westminster Hospital, declared there was no difference between the habitual use of opium and alcohol. Both were detrimental (Peters 1981:468–69). Other physicians said alcohol was worse because heavy drinkers committed more crimes and had a greater propensity to engage in antisocial behavior compared to opium addicts (Miskel 1973:8).

Regardless of what position a medical practitioner embraced, the centuries-old diffident attitude toward indulgence was no longer ubiquitous in the West. The Westminster conference was a precursor to comparisons soon to be made between opium eating in England and opium smoking in China. There also was increasing dialogue in Great Britain about the dangers of addiction to opium and liquor, plus the differences and similarities associated with the two substances. And by mid-decade at the latest, people were seriously investigating the effect of opium habituation upon people's health (Miskel 1973:4). These events added credence to the kinds of comments and data from Asia and intensified the discomfort felt by the trade's defenders. The latter group found it increasingly difficult to evoke a variant of racial theory to explain chronic opium habituation among people in distant countries. Anti-opiumists condemned pro-trade individuals as being part of the problem; they were suppliers who exploited vulnerable populations.

Missionary and Secular Lament from Asia, 1840 to 1850

Chinese officials' negative proclamations about the English encouraging drug consumption was no help in converting natives to Christ (Lowes 1966:58; Moorhead & Tobin 1931:473). The experience of Reverend George Smith in the Chinese seaport of Amoy during 1840 was typical. After telling opium addicts he was an English missionary, "they exposed the inconsistency of my rebuking their habit of smoking opium, while my countrymen brought them the means of indulging it" (Smith, quoted in Hess 1965:23).[16]

Although Christian proselytizers such as Smith rejected Chinese accusations of hypocrisy, virtually all evangelists agreed with Chinese opinions about drug use in the Empire. A depressing missionary refrain with statistical data appeared in the same year. It was the influential tract entitled *Facts and Evidence Relating to the Opium Trade with China*. William S. Fry, the previously cited anti-opiumist activist, was the author (Berridge & Edwards 1981:175). Other diatribes followed. English and American missionaries in China during the rest of the decade and the 1850s unanimously agreed that smoking opium was a serious social evil, the trade was unbecoming to a Christian nation and it was a serious impediment to spreading the gospel (Lowes 1966:61).

The portrayals were dismal. The infamous drug generated unimaginable misery among the Chinese. The terrible syndrome got worse because users were unable to satisfy their craving. These hopeless people lingered near opium shops begging for more of the drug. Shopkeepers, already having taken all their money, ignored them. Relatives or landlords cast the forlorn souls out of their own homes. Their future was certain; they would die in the street, despised and untouched by pity. The opium habit also destroyed health and it reduced life expectancy by about ten years. It also ruined the moral foundations of Chinese families, an estimated population of at least ten million per annum (Inglis 1975:90–1; Muirhead 1870:118). Opium consumption was unmitigated evil and encouraging the habit was Satan's work. And in 1847, Dr. George Smith complained that 50 percent of the poor people in the Chinese seaport of Amoy smoked opium. He lamented meeting men who spent three-quarters of their daily wage on the drug (Tinling 1876:19).

Still other observers recorded their objections at great length, and with impressive conviction and detail. James Pegg's 1846 book was a compelling argument for ending the trade. Pegg described the pernicious consequences of opium ingestion in India as well as in China. He said that continuing poppy cultivation, then exporting and encouraging the consumption of the demoralizing and degrading processed latex, was not the kind of enterprise that a civilized state should be promulgating. The work of this missionary, a veteran of long service in Cuttack, India, was different from other tirades during the 1840s. Pegg presented negative reactions from government officials and native observers from the two Asian societies. He also included Christian missionaries' commentaries.

Nonmissionaries working in China also expressed concern about the prevalence of opium in the Empire. At least one critic was a high-ranking British official. In 1847, Robert Montgomery, a former treasurer of Hong Kong, published a book about his experience. The volume included testimonials from important Chinese statesmen who condemned the drug as destructive and demoralizing (Tinling 1876:5–6).[17] And in 1850, the merchant Nathan Allen expressed his opinion about why people began the habit. He also presented a theory about the physiological and psychological effects of smoking the opium extract. Indulgence was a bad habit and a moral failing, but Allen did not condemn the Chinese for their self-inflicted misery. He declared that the drug has "a fatal fascination which needs almost superhuman powers of self denial, and also capacity for the endurance of pain, to overcome" (Allen, quoted in Kuo 1935:31–2). The physiological consequences for the Chinese opium smoker were sobering; a smoker's blood receives inadequate amounts of oxygen and this produces a "most destructive influence" (Allen, quoted by Tinling 1876:13). Furthermore, the way people smoke opium differs greatly from that of tobacco. The former produces a poison that enters the human body in a "purer and more concentrated [sic] form, and its deadly effects fall more directly upon the vital organs of the system" (Allen, quoted by Tinling 1876:13).

Missionaries in China and other locations in Asia also were using what they thought were scientific data to support subjective assessments. Surgeon Little's 1850 study of the effects of opium eating and smoking upon life spans of 250 Singapore addicts challenged Sir Robert Christison's conclusions about consumption and longevity. Dr. Christison, the expert in the Earl of Mar legal case, had just published his article in an 1850 issue of the *Journal of Medical Science*. Other anti-opiumists, such as Dr. Julius Jeffreys in his 1858 book, also used Asian evidence to debunk what they considered an erroneous notion about opium consumption prolonging human life. Jeffreys believed the behavior resulted in premature death (Berridge & Edwards 1981:175; Miskel 1973:5).

Some missionaries were not content to document their moral outrage with astute, long-term field observations. They also prescribed therapies for alleviating the misery of habituates. The medical missionary Dr. D. J. MacGowan, for example, recorded the prevalence and consequences of addiction while working near Ningpo, China, between 1845 and 1851. He found that the amount of opium must constantly increase to attain the level of pleasure derived from a previously consumed, smaller quantity. Moderation, therefore, was impossible. Furthermore, initiating consumption was as devastating to the destitute as it was to the wealthy because anyone taking the drug, be it for pleasure or pain relief, experienced moral and physical decay.

The only bright spot, if it can be called that, in MacGowan's gloomy scenario was that the habit was more entrenched among officials and the literati than among the poor and working classes. The latter rarely had time to indulge and often had insufficient money to buy the smoking extract. Physiological and moral degeneration, consequently, was not as prevalent among the agricultural classes as it was among the wealthier echelons of Chinese society. This class distinction in opiate use and abuse would continue only if the price of the drug remained high (MacGowan 1859:48 [comments from excerpt about Missionary Hospital visit at Ningpo, 1845] and 1847).

MacGowan, however, did not believe that controlling the price of opium and confining addiction to one socioeconomic class was a permanent cure for drug-induced misery. He agreed with Chinese officials who advocated abstinence plus the eating of licorice and honeysuckle flowers and other "equally inert" items (MacGowan 1859:49 [comments from 1847]). The therapy might help a few "miserable opium-smokers" if they could endure many aches and pains for twenty-four hours after stopping consumption. The discomfort of these "truly wretched" souls might be lessened by giving them "appropriate remedies—wine, ammonia, iron, quinine, hyoscyamus, and Dover's powder, according to circumstances" (MacGowan 1859:50 [in 1849 excerpt]). Emancipating oneself from the opium habit required a near superhuman effort, and the success rate of restoring an opium smoker to a productive life, and to remain productive, was low. Lasting freedom required something more powerful than medicine and abstinence.

MacGowan believed the only permanent cure for opium smoking was Christianity. The symbolic act of giving oneself to God was such a fundamental, preliminary step that he admitted having "ministered to the 'diseased minds of his patients before attending to their physical ailments'" (MacGowan, quoted in Miskel

1973:10). The results, he asserted, were remarkable: "no class of patients are [sic] so grateful for cure, and none receive exhortations to faith and repentance better, than reformed opium-smokers" (MacGowan 1859:50–1 [excerpt from 1849]).

What was good for the addicted individual also was good for the addicted nation. MacGowan proclaimed that the ultimate solution to the plague of opium smoking in China, indeed for all social problems in that troubled land, was neither politics nor medicine; it was Jesus Christ (Miskel 1973:9–10). His remedy was common among Anglo-Saxon Protestants in China who believed their "hopes are fixed upon the successful prosecution of the missionary enterprise, which is the only effectual antidote to the bane, and which of itself can improve their moral and physical condition" (MacGowan 1859:52 [from excerpt of 1851]). Other missionaries felt the same way but refrained from putting their thoughts down on paper as extensively as MacGowan.

Opposition to the Anti-Opiumists from China and India During the 1840s and the Early 1850s

Some westerners with medical training who were in China and India during the 1840s took issue with the anti-opiumists. In 1842, a Dr. MacPherson's own experience with a "few pipefuls" plus service in the Madras Army sent to China during the war prompted him to conclude the problems attributed to opium-smoking had been exaggerated (Miskel 1973:4–5). In a book published during 1843, he declared that if the habitual opium use was so debilitating, people in China should be a "shriveled, and emaciated, and idiotic race." They were not. Although MacPherson acknowledged that opium smoking was "universal among the rich and poor, [he] found them to be a powerful, muscular, and athletic people, and the lower orders more intelligent and far superior in mental acquirements to those of corresponding rank in our own country (MacPherson, quoted in GBO [Batten] 1894:I:145).

Government of India officials and experts also had entered the fray. In 1841, Dr. W. B. O'Shaughnessy drew upon his experience as a medical practitioner in Bengal Presidency. He had concluded that habitual opium eaters lived to a very old age. This, he claimed, refuted the anti-opiumist accusation about drug use resulting in premature death. Harmless if consumed in small amounts, even moderate consumption produces "no greater evil that the proportionate indulgence in wine or other spirituous liquors" (O'Shaughnessy, quoted in GBO [Batten] 1894:I:145; see also Miskel 1973:4–5). And in 1848 Dr. Elijah Impey, an influential opium inspector from the Central India administrative territory, declared that opium was addictive but its effect was ethereal (Miskel 1973:4–5; Impey 1848:1 (appendix), and also see Impey 1848:2, 6–9).

Reactions of Western Protagonists and Antagonists in China and India between 1850 and 1860

Opponents and supporters of the drug trade continued to agitate between midcentury and 1860. Their respective arguments remained the same and so did the circumstantial evidence that prompted the debate. The purported evils of unfettered opiate consumption in Asia were debated in Parliament, in popular magazines, in newspapers, and in the pages of scholarly and not so scholarly journals. Representatives for Great Britain in the Far East defended the commerce. Missionaries in the same countries rejected these declarations as nonsense. The trade's most prominent defenders continued to be employees of government institutions engaged in the actual production of opium or they worked for agencies associated with the drug. Both situations made them susceptible to accusations of being biased (Miskel 1973:7). For these people and other officials during the period, the real danger was not the drug; it was the harm done by irrational anti-opiumists who insisted otherwise. The same charge of bias exemplified by overzealous proselytizing could be and was made about Christian antagonists to the trade. But the consequences of debates about *Papaver somniferum Linn* in the 1850s differed from those of the 1840s in one important aspect. Despite energetic responses from apologists for the trade, the prevailing reason that encouraged Parliamentarians during the 1840s not to consider a re-examination of opium policy in Asia, as well as in Great Britain, was becoming increasingly untenable. The edifice of indifference, first challenged during the previous decade, was further undermined in the new decade. The opposition responded accordingly.

In a detailed 1851 description about how opium for the China market was manufactured in government-run factories of India, W. C. B. Eatwell declared the substance was harmless to consumers (Eatwell 1851–52:364; Miskel 1973:6). A long career as the Opium Examiner in British India and a three-year visit to China had provided sufficient proof for the evaluation. Eatwell echoed other British officials in saying that habitual use had no visible deleterious consequences. There also were no data demonstrating that moderate opium ingestion was more harmful than the moderate use of liquor. Furthermore, it was "certain that the consequences of the abuse of [opium] are less appalling in their effect upon the victims, and less disastrous to society at large, than are the consequences of the abuse of the latter" (GBO [Batten] 1894:I:140).

Other high-ranking government apologists during the decade supported Eatwell's implicit condemnation of the anti-opiumists as irrational and ignorant. They also published their opinions. In 1856, John Crawfurd, the former Governor of the Straits Settlement, author of a history of the East Indies, and long familiar with Southeast Asia and India, declared that people used opium extensively in Malaysia, China, and Indo-China. They experienced no bad effects other than moderate amounts of the drug being "very seductive." The anti-opiumists, Crawfurd admonished, were wholly unfamiliar with real conditions in Asia. They were opposed to any form of seducement, be it from fellow humans or from substances (Crawfurd, in GBO [Batten] 1894:I:139; Tinling 1876:4–5).[18] The 1858 publications of Dr. Sinibaldo de Mas also supported apologists like Crawfurd. Dr. de Mas, the former Envoy Extraordinary and Minister Plenipotentiary of the Court of Spain at Peking and fluent in Chinese, had traveled widely in China, India, Java, Borneo, and Malacca. He never heard of opium smoking blamed for a single death or serious illness (GBO [Batten] 1894:I:140).

Sinibaldo de Mas and the missionary Donald Matheson seem to be writing about different countries. In his 1856 publication entitled *What Is the Opium Trade?*, Matheson condemned the commerce as a scourge and the greatest obstacle to the spread of Christianity among the Chinese (Bhattacharya 1971:246).[19] Matheson expressed the frustration experienced by Anglo-Saxon missionaries who confronted Chinese accusing them of hypocrisy. The Christians preached salvation and redemption. At the same time they encouraged an insidious form of moral enslavement for this "weak and heathen nation, whose moral feelings are, nonetheless, outraged by our act" (Matheson, quoted in Bhattacharya 1971:246). And in the same year a critic by the name of Malcolm Lewis said that all monopolies were inherently bad and that the opium monopoly was the worst of all of them (Bhattacharya 1971:246).

Researchers in Great Britain very early in the new decade and most certainly before 1857, however, had collected sufficient data to lend credence to questions about morality and health raised by opium consumption in China. The English public heard stories of disreputable characters in their own country using opium for immoral and criminal purposes. Beginning in the early 1850s, allegations appear in the media about prostitutes surreptitiously adding laudanum to beer consumed by sailors. The seamen claimed they were completely stupefied when these women robbed them. The scenarios might have been excuses proffered by embarrassed males to protect their self-esteem. Nonetheless, there is one authenticated case of opium being used to commit a crime. In 1856, Henry Tipper, a cab driver accused of robbing old people, tried to poison witnesses for the prosecution by giving them beer containing forty-five grains of opium (Berridge 1978:445). The amount was alarming, as were tales of nefarious activities of prostitutes and miscellaneous bad characters. Public alarm finally forced Parliament to respond. In 1861, passage of the "Offences Against the Person Act" made giving laudanum with intent to rob a criminal offense (Berridge 1978:445–46).

There was other evidence about opium use during these years. Most of the material justified citizens' concern. Some of it indicated otherwise. One person in the latter category was uninvolved in the dispute about the morality and wisdom of the India-China opium trade. In a pioneering survey entitled *The Chemistry of Common Life* (1854), James Johnston estimated 400 million people in the world used opium. The number of habituates in Europe was increasing (Inglis 1975:117; Miskel 1973:3; Terry & Pillens 1928:53). Such a great number, for Johnston, suggested the drug was not as bad as doomsayers were declaring because people were not stupid, and opium's detrimental consequences would have precluded the substance from ever becoming so popular. Instead of condemning narcotics and stigmatizing users, he believed one of the more enlightening examples of human accomplishments was the recognition and use of opiates (Inglis 1975:116–17).

Even a good thing for James Johnston in 1854 was easily abused with serious consequences for unsuspecting people. He admitted that eating as well as smoking opium were dangerous. At approximately the same time a Dr. John Wilson and colleagues were advocating that eating the drug was the greater danger. Another faction, of which Robert Christison was a member, was convinced that smoking produced the greatest harm (Miskel 1973:6–7).

These conflicting opinions indicate that during the early to mid-1850s, there still was no unanimity in the British medical establishment concerning the consequences of opium smoking and opium eating. For some members, the distinction between the two was irrelevant. Regardless of the mode of ingestion, habitual opium use was a disease no less pernicious than chronic inebriation. Two sources provided them with evidence. The first one was a Royal Commission created in 1834 to study alcohol consumption in Great Britain. The second came sixteen years later when the British medical profession said that chronic inebriation was a dangerous 'disease'. Some of the 1834 Commission's findings were used in making the evaluation.

Alcoholism now had physiological origins and the condition could not be explained solely as a moral deficiency or character defect. Anti-opiumists were delighted. From 1850 and thereafter, they proposed a "disease model of opiate addiction . . . [so] they could extend to the nonmedical use of opium the logic that condemned alcoholism" (Peters 1981:478). The anti-opiumists had no pathological evidence verifying the profound physical deterioration of opium users compared to the quality and amount of data available for alcoholics, but they remained convinced empirical evidence was forthcoming.[20]

Anti-opiumists now also imitated the medical establishment's proclivity to classify alcohol as an injurious stimulant to strengthen their similar claim about the drug. Opium habituation became a disease, and promoting opium imports into China was tantamount to promoting involuntary exposure to a dangerous malady with tragic social and physiological consequences. The most radical anti-opiumists perceived encouragement of opium consumption anywhere in the world for any purpose whatsoever as a deliberate introduction of misery.

A respected physician's ambivalence toward the drug added credibility to the anti-opiumist argument. In an influential 1854 textbook about therapeutics, Dr. Pereira recognized opium as the most important remedy in all *materia medica*. But it also was dangerous because consumption corrupted morals, injured a human being's internal organs, and hindered child development. The drug's popularity in England prompted him to alert the British medical profession about the probable increase in antisocial behavior, especially likely among the lower classes. Poor people's penchant for smoking the drug was damaging their moral and physical character. The cure was almost as dangerous because withholding opium would probably kill the habituates (Musto 1975:5, 70–2, 75). And Pereira's belief in the "concept of inheritance of acquired characteristics and damage to germ cells by disease or excesses" meant that the addicted also harmed future generations (Musto 1973:1). Dependence, therefore, could be passed from one generation to the next. This resulted in "'weak, stunted, and decrepit'" children born to opium smokers (Pereira, quoted in Musto 1973:71). Opium indulgence now was a doubly dangerous threat because adults become habituated and innocent infants are damned through no fault of their own. Doubts about indiscriminate use of the drug expressed by Pereira and other scientists were reflected in Parliament's debates one year later.

The Parliamentary Debate of 1855

In 1855, Lord Shaftesbury introduced a resolution demanding an end to the opium trade. And, in a speech to the House of Commons on 7 August of the same year, a Mr. Bright assailed the traffic in opium as an evil second only to the slave trade between Africa and the Americas. Shaftesbury then raised the issue in a memorial to the Foreign Secretary but the man's penchant for overstatement weakened the anti-trade argument (Owen [1934] 1968:230; Berridge & Edwards 1981:174–75; Bhattacharya 1971:245; Stelle 1981:117). Nonetheless, anti-opiumists' appeal again worried government apologists. John Bowring, the British plenipotentiary in China, rejected most of Shaftesbury's accusations. Bowring said that chastising only Great Britain was both unfair and indefensible because other nations were involved in the trade. He also dismissed Shaftesbury's contention about the money spent for opium leaving the Chinese unable to buy British manufactured goods. Bowring said these people wanted virtually nothing produced in Great Britain (Owen [1934] 1968:232).

The well-intentioned Shaftesbury continued to harm the anti-opiumist cause. He then claimed that England was responsible for twenty million Chinese enslaved by the opium smoking habit. The anti-trade missionaries Drs. Hobson and W. M. Medhurst reluctantly admonished him for the excessively high calculation. They said approximately two million might be affected and admitted their estimate was probably high (Owen [1934] 1968:232–33). The fortunes of the anti-opiumist cause in Parliament improved two years later.

1857/58–1860: The Second Opium War, Parliamentary Debate, and Its Aftermath

The second Opium War erupted between China and the western powers during 1857 and Parliament again debated the morality of involvement. Anti-opium organizations, such as the Edinburgh Committee for the Suppression of the Indo-Chinese Opium Traffic and the Quaker's Society of Friends, were especially vocal in attempting to persuade Parliament to reverse policy in Asia. In 1858, the Quaker group beseeched the Prime Minister, Lord Derby, to insist that any provision legalizing opium imports be excluded from peace treaty negotiations conducted by British officials (Berridge & Edwards 1981:175). Anti-opiumist sympathizers in Parliament added their own voice. They attacked the party in power for even contemplating not to include such a provision in the treaty. By a majority of sixteen in the 510-member House of Commons, Parliament again created a Select Committee to investigate trade relations between China and Great Britain. The report did not help the anti-opiumists. The only objection were several witnesses urging the Government to distance itself from obvious and intimate association with opium production and sales (GBO [Baines] 1895a:VI:165; Johnson 1975:307).

Shaftesbury then claimed that the 1833 Parliamentary Act prohibited the East India Company from manufacturing opium for export to China. The Company's behavior, therefore, was illegal as well as unfriendly. Judges appointed to resolve the issue ruled in favor of the monopoly. Shaftesbury realized the government was deaf to the argument about morality. Undeterred, in 1857 he voiced his opposition in the House of Lords (Owen [1934] 1968:233).

The Lord of Albemarle used medical data to attack Shaftesbury. He claimed that Sir Benjamin Brodie, and other prominent authorities, had long ago concluded opium did not excite the nervous system upon entry into the stomach. The drug soothed and was therefore beneficial. This proved that Shaftesbury's worries were groundless.

Lord Albemarle was correct; Brodie did say this and participants did use his ideas in the 1843 Parliamentary debate. But the Earl of Albemarle was as selective as Shaftesbury was prone to hyperbole. The Earl failed to acknowledge Brodie's implicit distinction between medical and nonmedical use of the drug. He also neglected to mention Brodie's acknowledgment that unrestricted availability of opium was not good for society. Brodie thought opium functioned as a sedative only up to a point; prolonged use produced a very different and very adverse effect. Albemarle also failed to say that Brodie, and "twenty-five of the most distinguished physicians of England" who signed the man's document, regarded "those who promote the use of opium as an article of luxury as inflicting a most serious injury on the human race" (Brodie [1857], quoted in Tinling 1876:5). In contrast to Lord Albemarle, these authorities (and Pereira) also recognized a difference between immediate and long-term consequences of drug use. Their observations bestowed legitimacy upon Shaftesbury's insistence and upon the admonishments from other anti-opiumists. They all agreed that restricting opium acquisition, no matter how it was consumed, benefited society. For the anti-opiumists, medical illuminati had established the danger of using opium under most conditions. The only acceptable situation was closely supervised distribution for valid medical purposes (Tinling 1876:5). Other experts who portrayed opium use in Asia as benign, however, influenced members of the House of Lords. The Lords chose to overlook Albemarle's selectivity and they resisted Shaftesbury's pleas to request a judicial ruling (Tinling 1876:5; Berridge & Edwards 1981:174; Owen [1934] 1968:233).

The years of 1857 and 1858 were not all gloom and doom for anti-opiumists. Events occurring at home forced policy makers to question the drug's benign status. The death of Augustus Stafford, a member of Parliament, in 1857 shocked the public. His expiration "was said to have been accelerated . . . by the incautious use of laudanum" (Berridge 1978:444). Politicians could not ignore the data indicating accidental overdosing was killing other people in the country. The British public also was becoming aware of the intentional nature of still other fatalities; people contemplating suicide preferred the drug because it was a gentle way to end life (Berridge 1978:444). And if members of Parliament failed to notice their colleague's demise from overdosing and ignored the same thing happening to the common folk, they could not fail to notice something else that occurred in May 1857. Drug abuse in Great Britain so alarmed health professionals that they petitioned Parliament to pass a Pharmacy Act to restrict and regulate poisonous substances. They wanted opium classified as a "dangerous poison," which in turn would restrict the public's use of the drug and opium-based commodities.

Proponents of the new legislation faced formidable obstacles. They incorrectly assumed there was a generally accepted basis for defining what habituation was "beyond its component element of mere habit" (Peters 1981:464). Members of the embryonic Pharmaceutical Society immediately objected to the Act. They claimed there was no coherent theory of addiction accepted by everybody. There also was no agreement about how the phenomenon differed, if at all, from habitual use. Last, but not least, some pharmacists still did not recognize an unequivocal distinction between medical versus nonmedical use of opiates. Other opponents of the 1857 Pharmacy Act relegated the "undesirable effects of habitual use," such as the stupor and heightened sensual pleasures noticed among consumers in Asia and the Fens district of England, "to the realm of the exotic, and thus not considered a standard phenomenon of opiate use" (Peters 1981:464).

Opponents also offered practical reasons for preventing passage of the bill. The original had two classification schedules. The first, Schedule A, contained fifteen drugs categorized as poisons. This label required documentation about who bought the item and for what purpose (Berridge 1978:452). Classification in Schedule A, which included opium, meant the chemist had to keep the items under lock and key. These articles could be sold only to adults in the presence of someone who knew both the vendor and the buyer. The sale also had to be recorded (Lomax 1973:173). Drugs included in Schedule B were far less regulated. They required only a label (Berridge 1978:452).

Pharmacists said the legislation was unrealistic and ridiculous because of the tedium and expense of keeping extensive documentation (Lomax 1973:173; Parssinen, 1983:29). Furthermore, editors of the *Pharmaceutical Journal* had serious reservations about the consequences of labeling. They believed "no careful chemist would suffer laudanum to leave his shop without its name and the word 'Poison' being affixed to the bottle containing it, we can quite see the depreciation which that same word must suffer if it be applied indiscriminately to all preparations of poppies" (PJ, quoted in Peters 1981:463). The editors also doubted the syrup of red poppies required a poison designation and concluded that the labeling would create more problems than it solved. They merely recommended that dispensers of drugs honor their civic duty through common sense and care when dispensing dangerous drugs (Peters 1981:461). The reluctance of this influential professional journal to support legislation was reiterated by *The Times*, an equally influential newspaper. The editors believed the "sales of poisons should not be hedged in by unnecessary restrictions, but instead be regulated by ensuring the competence of the vendors" (Lomax 1973:173). A qualified vendor would be a member of the Pharmaceutical Society who had passed an examination approved by the society (Lomax 1973:173).

Pharmacists and chemists were motivated by profit as much as they were by concern for public safety. They said opium and opium-based products were one of their most important items of trade. The articles were sold so frequently that excessive regulation in the form of minute record keeping would hurt business (Lomax 1973:173; Berridge 1978:452). Furthermore, druggists and consumers would ignore the Act if they considered it too restrictive (Lomax 1973:175).

Antagonists also said Schedule A ensured creation of a black market. Demand for opiates was so great, they warned, that nonqualified vendors would enter the market despite the Pharmaceutical Society's regulations to satisfy demands of people who were legally prohibited from buying opium products (Lomax 1973:173). But the fear expressed by pharmacists and chemists about the loss of sales and money was not as justified as they wanted the public to believe. Section sixteen of the Act excluded patent medicines, including many that contained opium, from regulation. Druggists and chemists simply wanted to retain control of their activities, and to eliminate any threat to making money (Berridge 1978:452). Lobbyists for chemists and druggists in different parts of the country immediately petitioned supporters of the bill in Parliament to strike opium from Schedule A. They wanted the drug in Schedule B.

Representatives of the medical profession disagreed. They shared the pharmaceutical profession's desire to stop unqualified people from selling the drug, and were hostile to self-medication. They were, however, aware of opium's liabilities. They also had nothing to lose by discrediting the Pharmaceutical Society. Physicians argued for opium being kept in Schedule A because it would enable government to identify druggists who, in their desire to maximize profits, were responsible for unwarranted distribution of a toxic entity. It would force chemists and druggists to honor their self-proclaimed professional ethics. The arguments of pharmacists and chemists were persuasive, however, and their influence continued for more than ten years thereafter (Lomax 1973:176). For example, in 1857, Dr. A. S. Taylor, a professor of medical jurisprudence at Guy's Hospital, had insisted that opiates be strictly controlled because they caused one-third of all deaths by poisoning. By 1865, however, he "agreed that this requirement was impracticable, although still desirable" (Lomax 1973:173).

Parliament did not pass the 1857 Pharmacy Act but its members took notice of the spirited debate that the legislation engendered. The issue of opium use at home and abroad would not go away. Furthermore, most parliamentarians were probably aware of a prominent British official's reaction to his recent experience in China.

China's defeat in the second 1858 Opium War forced its rulers to open more ports formerly closed to foreign trade to European, American, and British merchants. The Chinese were also compelled to legalize opium imports. Lord Elgin, one of the negotiators responsible for the 1860 Treaty of Tientsin that ended the conflict, was appalled by what he had helped to create. Two years later he bemoaned the "emaciation and wretchedness of the opium smokers" on Chinese streets (Elgin, quoted by Lowes 1966:45–6). Legalization of the trade also did not deter anti-opiumists at home and missionaries in Asia from continuing to protest.

One example from that year was Reverend James Johnstone's almost poetic lament. Johnstone, a missionary in China, described the "bright and pleasant scene" of an Indian family going out together in the early morning to collect poppy juice. He appreciated the skill required to manufacture the product that was popular in China and the drug's commercial importance for the British Empire. Yet, he implored Parliament to admit that "the whole trade [is] a foul blot on the fair name of England, as well as a curse to India, and a deadly wound in the heart of China" (Johnstone, quoted in Scott, James Maurice 1969:86–8). An opium smoker will do anything to satisfy his craving, including selling sons into slavery and assigning "a wife and daughters to fate far worse" (Johnstone, quoted in Scott, James Maurice 1969:89).

Opponents to the trade remained relatively inactive in Parliament during the 1860s because official government policy toward opium was "[now] based upon an unchallenged commercial morality" (Johnson 1975:306). Other politicians assumed the issue was resolved and that they would hear no more of it. Pragmatic supporters of the trade within Parliament and beyond were not so confident. Although victory in the second Opium War removed the threat of Chinese retaliation against British merchants, future opinions of Parliamentarians and the British public might be less agreeable. The merchants had cause to worry; the era of Palmerston's influence in Parliament was ending and the Conservative party had never been sympathetic to the trade. Lord Shaftesbury and fellow anti-opiumists continued to condemn the Treaty of Tientsin as the continuation of a crime against humanity abetted by the Government of India. It was an unforgivable sin that a drug sold as a poison in England could be exported, without any stigma, to a foreign country with full knowledge of the British government (Rowntree 1905:268; Johnson 1975:306). Members of Parliament might be indifferent, but anti-opiumists were attracting increasing support from influential members of British society and other segments of the population. Reluctant politicians could be forced to reconsider the status quo if their constituencies objected to the trade. And public perceptions were indeed changing, albeit slowly.

Anti-opiumists in Asia added credibility to their unending moral lamentations by providing disquieting observations about addiction and sobering physiological consequences. Medical evidence documenting the detrimental aspects of opiate use in Great Britain also kept accumulating. Scientific data from Great Britain and Europe and elsewhere in the world available during the 1850s did not end debate about specific arguments associated with opiate use to the satisfaction of prominent participants in the controversy. The data, however, did not bode well for pro-opiumists. Their argument for continued, unfettered availability of opium products for people in China, India, Great Britain, and anywhere else in the world was moot. The old rationale for maintaining the status quo would lose still more credibility during the next decade and beyond.

PRELUDE TO A CHANGE: 1860–1874

Westerners' statements about opium use in China and elsewhere in Asia remained dismal. Travel throughout China enabled Thornville T. Cooper to declare that among the poorer classes, females as well as little boys and girls above the age of eleven smoked opium extensively. Rickshaw coolies spent 60 percent of their salaries on the drug. Manual laborers and "boatmen on the great waterways" were the greatest consumers (Cooper, quoted in Tinling

1876:20). Cooper also admitted that alleviation of misery in the country created a dilemma. One-third of China's adult addicts would die if prevented from satisfying the need created by their sickness. This was unethical and cruel. For Cooper, the humanitarian way to minimize premature death was to make the drug accessible to those individuals already addicted (Scott, James Maurice 1969:94). Many westerners and Asian citizens rejected the idea.[21]

The Chinese continued to embarrass westerners about the contradiction between Christian proselytizers' noble intentions and the other-than-noble behavior of their respective governments. For example, when Sir Robert Alcock departed from Peking in 1869, Prince Kung told him to "[t]ake away your opium and your missionaries and you will be welcome" (Kung, quoted in Lowes 1966:63; also see Beattie 1969:104; Lodwick 1976:44). The sentiment was responsible for William Rowntree's comment that Christian missionaries and opium "came together, spread together, have been fought for together, and finally legalized together" (Rowntree, quoted in Lowes 1966:62–3). A similar lament came from the Reverend W. K. McKibbin of the American Baptist Missionary Union in Swatow, China, in 1872. The Chinese citizen's ubiquitous greeting to English-speaking missionaries, he noted sarcastically, was that it "is your country that sent us the opium" (McKibbin, quoted in Crafts & Keitch 1911:110). The China missionary William Muirhead echoed these sentiments. Opium was a formidable barrier for the Christians trying to minister to the heathens' spiritual need, which was acceptance of salvation through Christ. For Muirhead, Thomville Cooper and people like him were misguided because their good intentions actually perpetuated pain and human degradation. But people who chose to be involved in the trade, be they Chinese or Anglo-European, were dangerously close to being enemies of God (Muirhead 1870:119).

Anti-opiumists back home struggled to end the contradiction. Motions to condemn the trade were presented to the House of Commons in 1868, two in 1869, again in 1870, 1871, and for the three next years. All were soundly defeated (Bhattacharya 1971:245, 278; Berridge & Edwards 1981:177; GBO [Baines] 1895a:VI:165; Johnson 1975:307; Lowes 1966:61–2; Tinling 1876:vi–vii).

Despite these setbacks, anti-trade activity did prompt inclusion of the opium question in the 1871 *Select Committee on East India Finance* agenda. Its report contained information about the negative aspects of indulgence and the consequences of drug policy in Asia. Past and present British government officials, unaffiliated citizens, and supporting documents provided critiques. Sir R. N. C. Hamilton claimed opium eaters quickly became "unfit" and died prematurely (Tinling 1876:6). A Mr. Winchester, Her Majesty's Consul at Shanghai until 1870, said there was no doubt about opium being a stimulant that created great hardship for a consumer's family. Sir Rutherford, another witness, said opium users sold all their property for money to buy the drug, and in so doing condemned their families to poverty. An addict also would commit any crime to satisfy his craving for the drug, including murder and theft. Desperate males even sold wives and children to satisfy their needs.

Members of the 1871 Select Committee also heard sobering words from Sir Rutherford Alcock, the aforementioned British official who reported Prince

Kung's disparaging comment in 1869. Alcock said he knew of no substance affecting the nervous system as totally as opium. Furthermore, many missionaries and nonmissionaries believed a person required ever-increasing amounts of opium to satisfy desire. In other words, increased consumption was inevitable once a person started the habit. Alcock also said the Chinese officials he knew concurred with the missionaries' negative views, and he indicated that addicted individuals "always consider themselves as moral criminal[s]" (Alcock, quoted in Tinling 1876:6). Alcock was cognizant of the related phenomena of addiction and tolerance. He suggested both Christian proselytizers and Chinese were aware of it as well. Anti-opiumists welcomed what they thought was support from this influential British citizen.

Other people now voiced negative comments about the consequence of opium indulgence in south Asia. According to Mr. C. A. Bruce, superintendent of a tea plantation in Assam, the people of this region were physically and morally ruined by what the British government hailed as "one of the blessings of British rule." And Dr. George Smith, referring to consumption of the drug in nearby Burma, said that before English domination the punishment for opium use in at least one area of the country was death. The contemporary British policy of encouraging consumption was scandalous (Tinling 1876:6). Mr. Hind, who spent most of his life in Burma, declared the British were responsible for depravity in the society. The administration initially enticed impressionable young Burmese males into addiction by charging nothing for opium. The drug was later sold to all people at low cost. The price was then raised as people became addicted. Although the British made a handsome profit, the practice had appalling consequences; the physical and mental powers of consumers soon wasted away and there was a "fearful increase in gambling and dacoity" (Tinling 1876:7).[22]

There also were criticisms about the situation in locations other than Burma and Assam. J. F. B. Tinling, for example, disagreed with people who claimed the drug possessed far less negative potential than the public had been led to believe. He claimed opium ingestion in India caused violence just as serious and widespread as any antisocial act attributed to alcohol. Rajput caste males, Tinling asserted, gained their remarkable courage from the opium they consumed on the day of battle. Since the drug enabled them to become ardent killers in time of war, ingestion of the drug in peacetime could lead, and has led, to the same kind of behavior.

Opium consumption generated other kinds of behavior unsuited to civilized society. Tinling alluded to a pamphlet written by a Mr. Sym, who had lived for many years in the opium-producing districts of India. Sym discovered that opium consumption was responsible for half of the rapes, murders, and other crimes committed in these locations (Tinling 1876:13). Other critics voiced similar ideas. Dr. Wilson, a Christian missionary in western India, proclaimed "opium eating might properly be spoken of as a national evil" (Wilson [1871], quoted in Tinling 1876:24).[23] Still another western commentator posited a link between opium purchases and famine in India. Money spent on the vice should have been used to buy tools, equipment, seeds, and other items needed for survival. The failure to do so contributed to twenty-seven million people starving to death during the twenty-one famines plaguing India between 1770 and 1879 (Brown, cited in Crafts & Leitch 1911:80).[24]

Many members of Parliament ignored the reservations articulated by witnesses appearing before the 1871 Select Committee on East India Finance. They also paid scant attention to other complaints from China and India. Nonetheless, one politician had heard enough. On 3 June 1870, Lord Mayo condemned the moral indignation articulated by some members of Parliament, missionaries, their friends at home and abroad, and all sympathizers unaffiliated with any of these groups. He labeled their comments an "absurd . . . senseless outcry [of] philanthropists' twaddle" (Mayo, quoted in Bhattacharya 1971:249, 279; see also Scott 1969:87, 196). Anti-opiumists still had cause for optimism despite Mayo's castigation. The man admitted that the opium monopoly and profits derived from it was "one of the deepest blots on our escutcheon" (Mayo, quoted in Bhattacharya 1971:249, 279).

Reports from Asia after 1871 continued to challenge Mayo's contention about the stupidity of anti-opiumist consternation, as did statistics from Great Britain itself. And western scientists' investigations into the effects of opium and opium alkaloids upon the human body had already indicated the correct target for Mayo's accusation of "philosophical twaddle" just might be the man's own intemperate comment of 1870.

Supporters of the Asian opium traffic disagreed. They continued to cite Parliament's legalization of the trade after the second Opium War in 1855 as proof that the drug posed no serious threat to the inhabitants of these countries. Opium's purported benign effect upon Asians, however, did not lessen anxiety felt by British health professionals and citizens. They objected to the growing prominence of their own nation in the international drug market. They also were distressed by the amount of crude opium being imported for processing and subsequent reexportation, and were equally concerned about increased consumption of opiates in their homeland. Great Britain had imported 41,000 pounds of opium per annum during the 1830s. The amount increased to an average of 151,000 pounds during the 1860s. By 1870, the volume of opium reexports, primarily processed crude opium in the form of opiate-based drugs and alkaloids, had made England the center of the world's opium commerce (Parssinen 1983:10). Import levels remained essentially the same for the next four decades and beyond. This permitted the nation to retain its "predominance in the world market for drugs in general, and opium in particular" through the second decade of the twentieth century (Parssinen 1983:18).[25] British statistics from the 1860s were far more disturbing than data from the previous decade. Behavior attributed to the opium habit had become both increasingly obvious and onerous (Berridge 1978:443–44). In 1864, the Government published its Report of Medical Officer of the Privy Council. Investigators had concluded that the paramount goal of some ambitious wholesale merchants had not changed. They wanted druggists to buy more opiates. The druggists, in turn, still considered these opiates as their most important commodities. Popularity of the drug resulted in more accidental and intentional tragedies among the British. By 1863 there were

126 deaths from opiates . . . out of a total of 403 poisoning fatalities, with eighty deaths in that year and ninety-five in 1864 from laudanum and syrup of poppies alone. Around a third of all poisoning deaths in the decade were the result of the administration of opiates, and the relatively high accidental, rather than suicidal, death rate from opiates bore witness to the drug's easy availability. Prior to 1868, at least two-thirds of these deaths, and often a higher portion of the general narcotic death rate, comprised accidental deaths: 5.1/million in 1863 from a total of 6.1/million for all violent opium deaths, 4.3/million in 1866 out of a total of 5.3/million living. (Berridge 1978:443)[26]

Infant mortality also remained an unpleasant reality confronting working class people. Between 1863 and 1867, 292 children died from narcotic poisoning compared to only 254 people thirty-five years or older in the same period (Berridge 1978:448; also see Peters 1981:461, Parssinen 1983:42–46, and Miskel 1973:4). Ignorant working class midwives and mothers were overdosing children with their own concoction or with commercially-produced laudanum. The women used crude opium (pieces from a "cake" of opium) if they could not afford the former (Berridge 1978:449).

Parliament again responded to the accumulating data about opiate abuse in Great Britain. The Pharmacy Act, originally introduced in 1857 and defeated by strenuous opposition from chemists and pharmacists, was reintroduced in 1868. It became law. Pragmatic promoters of the legislation admitted they had removed opium from Schedule A and put it in the less restrictive Schedule B to pacify chemists from Cambridgeshire, Norfolkshire, and Lincolnshire (Lomax 1973:175). Now only registered chemists or druggists and qualified apothecaries could sell opiates. The substance also must be sold in a container labeled "poison" with the vendor's name and address included. Furthermore, the 1868 version deleted the onerous paperwork that the 1857 bill had required. And no regulations were imposed on patent medicines (Lomax 1978:174; see also Parssinen 1983:71–2). Anyone could sell the drugs if they paid the annual vendor's fees and put the required tax stamp on each bottle sold. A "poison," therefore, could still be sold legally as long as the government obtained its share of the profit. Pharmacists were both displeased and poorer because "[i]n the last third of the century, . . . sales of patent medicines soared, [and] the cost to pharmacists of this exemption became painfully apparent" (Parssinen 1983:71).

More physicians now deplored opium use even though they disagreed about how dangerous the drug was to peoples' health and social stability (Miskel 1973:7). Consternation prompted some practitioners to participate in the antiopiumist effort to restrict the availability of all opiates to the general public (Berridge 1978:443). The difference of opinion during the 1860s was not exclusive to Great Britain. The influential Dr. George Bacon Wood, affiliated with the University of Pennsylvania and president of the American Philosophical Society, expressed one view about the conditions determining who suffered and the nature of harm done. Wood had praised opium in an 1868 book but his enthusiasm contained a caveat. The withdrawal process might result in death even though opium had less addictive capability than alcohol (Musto 1973:71). For

Wood, possible death resulting from abstinence was a problem that only inferior people confronted. The individual's moral constitution determined if this physiologically powerful drug was harmless or a minor threat to ethics or life itself. People of strong character either abstained or controlled their intake of this pleasurable intoxicant. Individuals with "weak character," however, could not avoid chronic dependence. They inevitably abused the substance. This culminated in addiction which in turn led to anti-social behavior and self-abasement (Musto 1973:72).

Wood's perspective was a blend of old and new ideas. He construed chronic habituation as a personality defect; moral constitution was the prime variable for starting the habit.[27] Nonetheless, this influential American physician's recognition that some people "inevitably" succumbed to addiction was a significant event. It signified awareness that continuation of the vice was more complicated than only a voluntary act. However, even for Wood and others during the decade, relying exclusively upon a lack of moral constitution to explain why a person continued to use opium despite negative consequences was becoming an unconvincing scenario. The drug could damage people, but how much, in what way, and why was the behavior difficult to end? Investigating the effects of one of the opium alkaloids helped to answer these questions.

THE PROMISE AND THE PROBLEM OF SUBCUTANEOUS INJECTIONS OF MORPHIA/MORPHINE

Deaths attributed to the mother drug were not the only reason for alarm among members of the medical establishment and the public in Great Britain. Morphine was another problem. Available to the public since the early 1800s, the alkaloid was ingested orally. This mode of introduction was unpleasant and sometimes dangerous; accidental overdosing killed people. Consequently, few people consumed the substance. The infrequent use of morphine seduced many members of the medical profession and the wider population during the 1850s and early 1860s into assuming the alkaloid was not habit-forming (Brill 1969:16; Carlson & Simpson 1963:15; Kurland 1978:3).

The hypodermic syringe and needle altered that perception. The medical community initially thought the technology offered "vague hope that the small, controlled dosage of morphine might largely obviate the habituation risk of opiates in oral dosage forms" (Sonnedecker 1963:19).[28]

Other medical practitioners during the decade were more than vaguely hopeful. The well-known physicians Edward Wilson and Arthur Evershed were euphoric. They thought morphine injections were "more effective than ingested opium and [the method avoided] . . . opium's most unpleasant side effects, such as constipation and stupor" (Parssinen 1983:80). They were partially correct. Colleagues also concluded that injections seemed to avoid digestive tract troubles caused by swallowing opium-based medications and opium itself.[29] The alkaloid was soon administered for many illnesses. The list included neuralgia and headaches. In Great Britain and Europe the mode of ingestion was so popular it "began to replace opium and laudanum as a sedative and a painkiller" (Inglis 1975:122; see also Clausen 1968:299; O'Brien & Cohen 1984:xiv; Terry & Pillens 1928:69–70; Terry 1931:244). Health professionals also hailed subcutaneous introduction of the alkaloid as a cure for addiction to the mother drug.

The only serious note of caution about morphine injection coming from the medical establishments of Great Britain, the United States, and the European nations during the period between 1854 and before 1870 was the danger of poisoning through carelessness and overdosing (Parssinen 1983:80). The prevailing belief was that the amount introduced at any one time was the sole factor determining toxicity. It was benign for the general public if used in moderation and it was invaluable for handicapped segments of the population. The American Civil War, for example, demonstrated the benefits of morphia injection. The problem was that many wounded veterans exposed to the alkaloid during the conflict never stopped using it.[30]

The "morphine habit" spread quickly throughout the United States and should have cast doubts about the assumed nonaddictive status of the alkaloid. However, even as late as 1868, the aforementioned American Dr. George Wood remained even more oblivious to the addictive potential of the alkaloid than he was about opium. Morphia, he claimed, was easier to use and "cured" more rapidly than the mother drug (Musto 1973:73). For Wood, the harm a person experienced was largely self-inflicted. The reason for succumbing to "intoxication" offered by the alkaloid was moral weakness. "Weak" people will be harmed by morphia just as they will suffer from opium. For Wood, the addiction of Civil War veterans to morphia was symptomatic of their innate inferiority or something akin to it. Proponents of one German school of thought during the late 1860s and 1870s had a similar idea. They claimed the craving for morphine was "a psychological hunger related to the personality or constitution of the addict . . ." (Musto 1973:74; see also Sonnedecker 1963:19, 21). The Germans were a minority. The association of morphia with inherent character traits lost credibility early in the next decade. Other members of the medical community realized that injections of the alkaloid did not circumvent addiction (Peters 1981:455).

In 1870, Thomas Clifford Allbutt, one of Great Britain's most respected physicians, declared his "uncomfortable fear of mischief is growing rather than diminishing" (Allbut, quoted in Sonnedecker 1963:19). He chastised the medical profession for not recognizing the danger posed by the rapid rise in morphia use and the absence of warnings about using it. The alkaloid, for Allbut, was as dangerous as opium, regardless of the mode of ingestion. This meant that the purported cure was no less detrimental than the malady it was supposed to eliminate (Brill 1969:16). The hypodermic syringe did not circumvent habitual dependence and the instrument was irrelevant in determining the level of toxicity in the human body. The method enabled the introduction of more precise amounts but nothing more. At the same time, another researcher had confirmed Allbut's reservations about the relation between habituation and technology. Sewall's brief comments about his case studies are revealing. They indicate that hypodermic syringe injections of morphia did not cure people who were addicted to eating opium (1870:137). Both men had sullied the reputation of morphine injection as a remedy for opium addiction, whereas several Europeans' investigations of the alkaloid led to a new perspective about the more inclusive problem of chronic indulgence.

Edward Levinstein, Albrecht Erlenmeyer, and S. Laehr were the first Europeans to write about narcotic addiction using a disease model. For Laehr in 1872, the dominant explanation of addiction was antiquated. Addiction was not a bad habit or a manifestation of moral deficiency; it was a serious illness. Furthermore, the idea of self-curing was a myth because people addicted to morphine required hospitalization and control. Laehr's most important contribution was his insistence upon consistent and strict therapy (Sonnedecker 1963:20).

Edward Levinstein's scenario was similar. The difference between them is that Levinstein explored other dimensions of addiction and its cure and he was better known among the public. Levinstein was, as Sonnedecker suggests, a pioneer in every sense of the term because he studied the condition methodically and objectively. The man succeeded in giving the phenomenon a "new and definite meaning [and elevated] informed medical discussion, henceforth, beyond the level of curious speculation and armchair moralizing" (Sonnedecker 1963:22, see also 19).

As of 1875, Levinstein's analysis of the clinical course of morphia habituation and its cure was complementing French investigations of compulsive consumption of the substance. The combined effort enabled scientists to distinguish between a mere habit and degrees of genuine addiction (Peters 1981:455; Sonnedecker 1963:21). English-speaking researchers now used such terms as "morphinomania" or "morphiomania." These classifications conveyed a sense of "mania" or mental condition that was more complicated than a simple addiction and certainly not a mere habit (Brill 1969:16–7). Levinstein discovered that some people ingested the alkaloid and remained addiction-free. Other consumers succumbed. From this he concluded that susceptibility to addiction induced by regular doses of morphia had a physiological basis (Musto 1973:74). Although society might still label the inclination to use the alkaloid as a vice initiated by the user, some perceptive commentators now realized that the need to keep ingesting the substance once started was involuntary. Levinstein's interpretation, even more so than Laehr's contention, was controversial among a declining number of members of the medical establishment and the public. These people preferred to view addiction strictly as a matter of personal choice.

Levinstein echoed Laehr in criticizing as unrealistic and unworkable any therapy that assumed addicts chose to become habituated. These people, therefore, were incapable of curing themselves by merely deciding to abstain. The old approaches relied upon vague notions of moral character that alluded to quality of child rearing and socioeconomic class affiliation to explain continued dependence. Levinstein thought these notions hindered the understanding of addiction propensity.

Although Levinstein's compelling evidence revealed the fallacy of viewing addiction exclusively as a question of individual character, the data also suggested the idea was not completely erroneous. He studied the discouraging rate of relapse among former addicts, as much as 75 percent, and concluded their psychic disturbances were a symptom, but not a cause of addiction. This observation, according to Sonnedecker, demonstrates that Levinstein had initiated "the long and elusive search for definitive understanding of the size and nature of the psychic component of the addiction concept" (1963:23). Levinstein was implying that some assumed character defect might have a role in explaining long-term morphia usage. The idea was an unproved hypothesis at the time, and a general theory of opiates predicated upon the notion was equally speculative.[31]

Levinstein's Cure for Opiate Addiction

This 75 percent patient relapse rate also enabled Levinstein to invalidate the belief that using one alkaloid could end dependence upon another. The statistics also indicated that administering the substitute as a cure for opiate addiction was equally worthless.[32] The only way to end enslavement to morphine and opium was abrupt, unyielding deprivation accompanied by careful, managed care of the patient. He admitted the patient would suffer, but rejected the immediate, inevitable death predicted by others (Kurland 1978:3–4; Musto 1973:74; Peters 1981:483; Berridge 1978:457).

THE END OF AN ERA

Implications of Alkaloid Addiction Research During the 1870s for the India–China Opium Trade Controversy

The data accumulated during the late 1860s and 1870s revealed the inadequacy of attributing morphine addiction to a personality defect or moral deficiency. Mortality rates attributed to the alkaloid exacerbated the medical community's dissatisfaction with the notion. The number of deaths fluctuated during the 1860s through the 1890s. Nonetheless, incidents during each year were always sufficiently high to generate alarm about the country being in the midst of a morphine epidemic. The intellectual consequences were profound. In fewer than forty years, the British medical community had a complete change of mind. What had been initially viewed as a "promising new therapy" came to be seen as a deadly pathogen (Parssinen 1983:79).

Other research during the 1870s explored the human body's reactions to the mother drug and to alkaloids other than morphine. This resulted in the British medical profession finally recognizing the emerging pharmacological concept of addiction (Peters 1981:456). An extreme case of human susceptibility to opium and its numerous alkaloids was now construed as a disease having a physiological foundation. The change in thinking had ramifications beyond the laboratory.

Dispassionate clinical observation had replaced subjective assessment in the study of morphine addiction in the 1870s. Anglo-European scientists now had a far more accurate understanding of a very complicated phenomenon. The achievement affected the debate between anti-opiumists and defenders of the

Asian drug traffic in at least two ways. It invalidated the impressionistic declarations that relied exclusively upon nonphysiological foundations for either defending or castigating the status quo regarding opiate use in Great Britain, Asia, and elsewhere in the world.

The second consequence of studying the effect of morphine was to provide British anti-opiumists with what they thought was compelling evidence that justified their condemnation of government drug policy at home and abroad as nothing less than unqualified irresponsibility. Some scientists during the decade were "agreeing independently . . . that although morphine (unlike alcohol) produced no bodily deterioration, a decline of moral character was associated with chronic opiate use and that the prolonged use of opiates endangered anyone who indulged and could lead to immoral and criminal actions and social ineffectiveness" (Kurland 1978:3).[33]

This was good news for anti-opiumists. They had always claimed a correlation existed between the use of the drug and moral degeneration. Comments about social order from respected scientists now added credibility to a major contention: one probable consequence of habituation was an addict's disinclination to comply with the moral dictates of contemporary society. Behaving in this manner earned one the label of a reprobate. This was unfair because the disinclination to honor society's standard of proper behavior was beyond the person's ability to control (Musto 1973:75). For many anti-opiumists, the addict deserved sympathy, not derision. Contempt was reserved for the people or agency responsible for the victim's involuntary misery and depravity.

The China missionaries' lament about dissipated morality, therefore, was not ridiculous. They could now argue that opium produced a weakened character that was ultimately a consequence of metabolic imbalance. And since the mother drug contained morphine, any form of opium ingestion or its principal alkaloid guaranteed moral decline and antisocial behavior. The missionaries' most prescribed cure for the addict was deprivation of the drug and a heavy dose of religion. Professional addiction therapists such as Laehr and Levinstein shared the idea minus the religion.

Anti-opiumists wanted to eliminate the possibility of anyone ever becoming addicted by preventing hapless individuals from succumbing to the drug's allure. Stopping Chinese importation of opium from India was one way. This did not eliminate the root of the problem because the dangerous commodity was manufactured in South Asia. A better solution was termination of poppy cultivation in India altogether, thereby ending the association of Great Britain and the Government of India with a nefarious substance. Realization of this grandiose ambition was decades away, but the anti-opiumist recognition of the contributions of laboratory science in the 1870s was part of the foundation for successful agitation.

Other factors contributed to and reflected the changing attitude toward opium and its alkaloids in the medical community and the British public during the early 1870s. Opium's status in the Fens region (or Fenland), where the habit had been most firmly entrenched in England, indicated what was happening throughout the country. Inhabitants and commentators at the time thought the rate of opium consumption was increasing during the 1850s and 1860s (Parssinen 1983:51). The British Medical Association provided an estimate. In 1867, people in the Fens districts of Norfolk and Lincolnshire used 50 percent of England's imported opium. Import data for 1859, the last year for which home consumption data were available, reveals this quantity was "at least 30,000 lbs, and possibly more" (Berridge 1977a:280).

The 1868 Pharmacy Act regulations were rarely enforced in the malaria-plagued Fens region. Nonetheless, beginning in the 1870s and continuing throughout the 1880s, grocers and other traditional vendors had increasing difficulty in selling the drug in its various forms. Opiate consumption had declined so dramatically that by the early 1890s there were "few opium eaters in existence" (Parssinen 1983:51). One reason for the remarkable change is that inhabitants no longer considered the drug to be indispensable to health. The attitude is significant because defenders of the Asian drug trade used the previous disease/drug correlation in this part of England to justify unrestricted opium consumption in India. They ignored the region's past two decades. They also disregarded what had occurred throughout the country.

Opium consumption in England was now associated with something very different from what the early nineteenth-century literary celebrities had done so much to foster. DeQuincey's public image as a "noble self-experimenter" and the romanticism pervading the literary depiction of opiate use in the early decades of the century had given way to literature, first appearing in the 1870s, that reflected the stern morality of the late Victorian era. Charles Dickens' unfinished serialized tale, *The Mystery of Edwin Drood* (1870), Oscar Wilde's *The Picture of Dorian Gray* (1890), and Arthur Conan Doyle's well-known short story "The Man with the Twisted Lip" (1892:Story 6:126–52) were instrumental in altering images about opium use. This literature was especially influential in associating Chinese people living in Great Britain with the nefarious opium den (Parssinen 1983:63–6). The stereotype raised awareness about narcotic addiction. It also increased xenophobia among the English about suspected antisocial behavior of alien minorities present in their society (Berridge 1978:460; Mitchell 1988:560). Regardless of ethnicity, a person who smoked a watery extract of *Papaver somniferum Linn* was a "secret degenerate" lurking in "darkened opium dens" seeking refuge from the company of respectable people (Parssinen 1983:61–3). Good people, once tempted by the seductive delights of the drug, could not prevent eventual moral depravity and physical deterioration. Consumption of the drug for medicinal reasons was either condoned or tolerated as morally ambiguous albeit worthy of sympathy. Hedonistic overindulgence, however, earned disdain. The public's attitude concerning opium use in Great Britain had indeed gone full circle—from indifference to curiosity to disquietude—in less than a century.

Some anti-opiumists between 1860 and 1874 concentrated upon convincing influential segments of British society that opiate indulgence had ramifications as serious as the acknowledged negative social effects of alcohol abuse. Other activists focused upon incorporating opium and alkaloid research discoveries into their agenda. For them, opiate addiction was a disease. It was sufficiently compelling to justify remedial action regardless of whether or not the condition shared characteristics with chronic habituation induced by other substances. Still other anti-opiumists tried to do both. Their collective ability to change government policy improved in mid-decade. Opium research was gradually eroding Anglo-European indifference to the missionaries' lament.

NOTES

1. Anglo-Saxon Protestant missionaries in China were the earliest and most vocal occidental anti-opiumists. The number of missionaries in China increased during the nineteenth century, as did nonmissionaries hostile to opium consumption. This resulted in anti-opium societies composed of assorted Christian denominations in Great Britain. Some organizations evolved elsewhere in the West. There also were secular groups with diverse membership. Anti-opiumists gradually became politically active. By the 1830s, a few influential members of Parliament supported the movement.

Henceforth, the term 'anti-opiumist' is used with the understanding that the 'movement' ebbed and flowed. This fluctuation refers to membership in a group or groups, the number of functioning organizations, and the degree to which the public acknowledged anti-opiumists' efforts. Their common theme in all decades, however, was the danger and immorality of peoples' use of opium regardless of where they lived.

2. In 1876 the missionary J. F. B. Tinling used Stark's testimony to chastise the Government of India's claim that South Asian opium production is necessary for the manufacture of medicine. Tinling said this was nonsense. Opium imported into Great Britain for medicinal purposes comes from Turkey, and "little, if any, . . .[is] supplied from our Indian possessions" (Tinling 1876:vii). Tinling was correct. And the 1911 edition of the *Encyclopaedia Britannica* states that it "was a remarkable fact that the only Indian opium ever seen in England is an occasional sample of the Malwa sort . . . indeed, the whole of the opium used in medicine in Europe and the United States is obtained from Turkey" (1911:20:134). Joshua Rowntree's condemnation of the trade more than seventy years later supports Stark's statement. The drug was "especially prepared to minister to the weakness of the Chinese [and] has been poured into their country at the rate of a ton an hour for twelve hours a day for sixty years" (1905:268).

3. There are several excellent sources of information about literary celebrities' experiences with opium. See Berridge 1977a:276; Berridge 1978:437; Brill 1969:15; Hayter 1968; Inglis 15:110–15; O'Brien & Cohen 1984:XIII; Peters 1981:465–66; Parssinen 1983:1–8, 61–7; Scott, James Maurice 1969:46–82; Sonnedecker 1963:17; and Terry & Pillens 1928:62–4. Austin (1978:155) provides a brief comment.

4. The Victorian conception of an "opium eater" is misleading. People such as Coleridge and DeQuincey did not consume the crude or unprepared latex and they usually did not ingest the semi-processed opium in the dry form typical of consumers in India. The Victorian "opium eater" ingested the substance in liquid form, most often laudanum or "other opiate liquids" (Brecher 1972:5). The term as found in the medical literature and popular press of the era only refers to a penchant for using the substance. The phrase is another way of referring to addiction that results from several modes of ingestion.

Earlier comments in the book about opium indicate the form in which *Papaver somniferum Linn* was introduced affected the range of typical reactions in consumers. Alcohol could dissolve some alkaloids. It was useless for others. There was no guarantee that the insoluble material in a mixture distributed among many customers would be consumed in equal proportions. And the amount one individual actually ingested often was very different from the quantity that another person consumed. The same thing was true for opium pills and for eating small pieces of an opium cake. Differential exposure to unsuspected toxic levels of alkaloids and other material, regardless of the particular mode of ingestion, could be disastrous for a person's health.

The same qualification applies to the "morphine eater" mentioned in medical literature. The alkaloid was introduced into the body by injection or some way other than by mouth. Nonetheless, nineteenth century publications often depict morphine consumption as "opium eating" (Brecher 1972:5).

5. The opium debate in the United States in following decades also had class and gender overtones. In 1832 a W. G. Smith warned about unseemly stimulation and sedation because of its "every day's use . . . particularly among the better circles of society, and by the softer sex" (Smith, quoted in Terry & Pillens 1928:61). The relation between opiate consumption and class affiliation also was a significant component of the controversy in Great Britain by the 1830s.

6. Opium use also became commonplace in nineteenth-century psychiatry, although English, French, German, and American doctors administered the drug in different ways. Some of their experiences contributed to the post-1830 evolution of awareness about the detrimental consequences of excessive opiate use (Carlson & Simpson 1963:114).

7. Prescribing opium-based medicines continued to be common practice in Great Britain for several decades during the nineteenth century (Berridge 1978:441; Mitchell 1988:559; Peters 1981:576–7). According to Peters, some concoctions were construed as a specific remedy for diabetes, consumption, cholera, syphilis, and rheumatism. Other items were occasionally used to treat smallpox, dysentery, whooping cough, dropsy, and gout. The capability to sedate, according to Peters, also prompted physicians to prescribe opium for chest disease, delirium tremens, and fever (1981:457). See Berridge 1978:441; Mitchell 1988:559; Peters 1981:576–77; Brecher 1972:5 for additional comments about the ubiquity of opiates. This material also provides sales statistics during the 1830s through the 1860s. In the 1830s, for example, opium was used to alleviate pain, stop spasms, encourage sleep, reduce nervousness, induce sweating, and "check profuse mucous discharge from the bronchial tubes and gastrointestinal canal" (Pereira, II, 1301, quoted in Berridge 1978:441). Opium's status as a panacea continued for at least two more decades with "[u]p to 20 percent of all prescriptions dispensed by pharmacists in Islington and Holloway in the period between the 1840s and 1860s contain[ing] opium" (Berridge 1978:441). For information about poppy cultivation in Great Britain from 1740 to 1823, see Berridge 1977b:90–4.

8. Patent or proprietary rights had existed for centuries in Great Britain, but the Crown did not issue the first patent until 1698. More than 200 patent medicines existed by 1748. The British government imposed a 12 percent stamp duty on all of them in 1798 (Parssinen 1983:31). Popularity of the article increased dramatically in the late nineteenth century; from "1855 to 1905, the period of greatest growth, sales of patent medicines increased nearly tenfold, while the population just about doubled" (Parssinen 1983:31; also see his discussion on pages 32–3). The pharmaceutical industry, therefore, had a vested interest not to lobby for regulation of opium sales because it endangered patent medicine profits. It was to their advantage to agitate for elimination of a grocer's ability to dispense the opiate, and they expended much time and money in doing so during the second half of the nineteenth century.

9. Several sources have abundant information about the kinds of opium-based medicines available to the public, who sold them, who bought them, for what purpose, and the sobering consequences of widespread availability. Consult Berridge 1978:438–40; Brecher 1972:6; Lomax 1973:169; Miskel 1973:3–4; Mitchell 1988:559; Parssinen 1983:28–32, and Peters 1981:457.

10. Parssinen says that for most of the nineteenth century, opium was "the Victorian's aspirin, Lomotil, Valium, and Nyquil, which could be bought at the local chemist's for as little as a penny" (1983:36).

11. The emergence of pharmacology as a profession during the second half of the nineteenth century contributed to ending grocers' distribution of opium products. The pharmacists promoted passage of government regulation of opium sales during the late 1860s. Members of the association, many of them local chemists, now were legally entitled to sell opium-based medicines.

12. Domestic consumption of opium in Great Britain increased 2 percent per capita per year between 1831 and 1859. The rate of increase probably continued through the 1870s. The amount of opium imported escalated during the same period. From an average of 91,000 pounds annually during the 1830s, imports rose to an average of 280,000 pounds in the 1860s. The figure continued to rise for the next four decades, although at a more modest rate of increase. "Reexports" of opium, meaning opium imported for processing and then sold abroad, also rose from only 41,000 pounds during the 1830s per annum to an average of 151,000 pounds by the 1860s (Parssinen 1983:10).

13. Lomax (1973:170–72) discusses medical profession and government explanations for the amount of abuse as well as for infant mortality during the 1830s. Details about opium consumption in the Fens and embryonic awareness of opiate overindulgence elsewhere in the country during the decade are provided by Berridge 1977a:275, 277–80, 281, 283; Berridge 1978; Brecher 1972:5; Mitchell 1988:559; Parssinen 1983:48–51; Austin 1978:156, and Tinling 1876:16–7.

14. The lack of standardization was a growing problem. So was the inability of a manufacturer to guarantee consistent amounts of ingredients in their products. The public eventually protested. Reformers demanded government legislation to regulate the availability and use of opiates. Berridge and Lomax provide additional examples of researchers circa midcentury who were finding unacceptable deviations between purported and actual contents of these opium-based remedies (Berridge 1978:445–46). Lomax says the tragic rate of infant deaths due to opium poisoning was mostly unintentional; overdosing by mistake was easy because opium was one of the most commonly adulterated drugs. In 1855, only five out of fifty-five samples were found to be pure. Mistakes in preparing mixtures by pharmacists or anyone else were to be expected. There were grave consequences; if "Godfrey's Cordial was prepared with insufficient alcohol to dissolve all the opium, a sediment of narcotic would settle at the bottom of the bottle, with potentially disastrous consequences when the last spoonfuls were taken" (Lomax 1973:170). A child might die from inanition, a condition produced by constant opiate sedation. Lomax says physicians misdiagnosed many infant deaths because the cause of death was identified as "lack of breast milk," starvation, or "failure to thrive," whereas the real cause was addiction (1973:171). Opium, therefore, was probably responsible for higher infant mortality in England during the nineteenth century than official records indicate. These documents alone indicate the number was tragically high. Also see Lomax's discussion of the serious problem of infant mortality due to opiate consumption. He also discusses explanations of the calamity offered by physicians and government officials (1973:170–72).

15. Berridge and Edwards suggest one of the long-term consequences of the 1839–1842 Opium War and interruption of drug imports into China was "comment made about the apparent increase in opium being brought into England and the consequent dangers of increased use of the drug, in particular among the working class." At the same time, ideological issues about opium being debated at home were merged with the "moral opposition to opium in the Far East" (1981:174).

16. See Craft and Keitch (1911) and Park (1899) for numerous other examples of missionary complaints with similar content. Park's volume also provides illustrations of moral outrage supported by some medical data collected by people laboring in China, India, other British-dominated regions of South Asia, and elsewhere in the Far East.

17. See pages 191–253 of R. M. Martin (1847) for the Chinese testimonials. Tinling (1876) provides excerpts from British documents supporting his assertion about high-ranking officials having doubts about opium accessibility to various publics because of its detrimental effects upon morality and physical condition. Tinling's discussion complements Martin's statements, and are found on pages 5–6. Scattered throughout the 1847 Thomas Taylor Meadows publication are comments suggesting the levels of government bureaucracy that Tinling and Martin were castigating.

18. Peters also mentions the divergent observations as of 1857. There were descriptions of the opium-smoking Chinese coolie's depraved countenance offset by portrayals of the robust Rajput caste male in India eating opium. Yet, British physicians "with similar educational preparation, located in the same region of India, presented flatly contradictory accounts of the effects of opium eating among the same group of people" (Peters 1981:465).

19. The correct date is 1856, not 1857 as cited in Bhattacharya.

20. Peters says "the search for structural change as conclusive evidence of a specific disease of opiate addiction remained fruitless. Anti-opiumist medical men were slow to abandon their belief that pathological evidence was forthcoming" (1981:479). They retained this belief even after the Royal Commission on Opium published its conclusions in the mid-1890s (Peters 1981:479–80).

21. For example, see William Lockhart (1861).

22. Dacoity is robbery perpetrated by five or more individuals.

23. Wilson is referring to the "Mahratta country," Gujerat, Kathiawar, and Rajputana.

24. The Crafts and Leitch (1911) book is useful for gauging the intensity of missionary hostility to opium use and the diversity of their observations. It contains numerous statements from missionaries. They describe the varied and negative consequences of opium indulgence for both sexes. These missionaries also provide commentary for all socio-economic strata, and all ages in China, India and elsewhere in Asia. Few of their observations are cited because Crafts and Leitch infrequently provide dates regarding when the comments were first uttered, and for what year or years comments are applicable.

25. Reexports declined earlier (by about fifteen years) than the decrease in opium consumption among the British public. The United States was Great Britain's biggest market during the second half of the nineteenth century. Americans bought almost one-half of the reexported commodity. Most opium imported into England beginning in the 1890s and thereafter was converted into morphine and then reexported (Parssinen 1983:104).

26. Berridge says these figures might not be as alarming as they seem. Deaths due to opium were five per million in 1840. The number increased to six per million by the early 1860s (1978:443). Also see Parssinen's conclusions about accidental poisonings, murders, and suicides based upon available statistics for the era. Data also reveal high

opium consumption in the Fens district of England during the decade. The British Medical Association estimated the population of Norfolk and Lincolnshire to be consuming half of the opium imported into England in 1867. On the basis of import numbers for 1859, the last year for which home consumption data were available, Berridge says this translates into "at least 30,000 lbs, and possibly more" (1977a:280).

27. Horace Day, another American, presents essentially the same idea as Wood. Day's 1868 book *The Opium Habit; with Suggestions as to the Remedy* is a tract with religious overtones discussing the evils of the drug. Its main thesis is that Christianity is the only enduring cure. Other therapeutic endeavors should incorporate the idea. See especially "Outlines of a Cure" on pages 285–335.

28. People who accepted morphine's physiological and psychological capabilities, but doubted its purported nonaddictive nature, were mollified. They also believed technology, not inherent chemical composition, was the prime variable determining what the alkaloid did to a person. The hypodermic syringe eliminated any residual potential for chronic habituation and did the same thing for toxicity. Others refused to invest the new technology with magic; subcutaneous hypodermic injection was only a more efficient way of introducing chemicals into the human body. This was true for people postulating morphine as neither toxic nor addictive and for those viewing the alkaloid as both toxic and habituating.

29. Although the hypodermic syringe made it possible for people to inject themselves, they had difficulty in obtaining the alkaloid because it was included in Schedule A of the 1868 Pharmacy Act. Trained individuals such as physicians frequently injected people and they were most likely to detect addiction.

30. The same thing occurred among Europeans during the 1870s after the Franco–Prussian War.

31. Future researchers postulated "some nervous instability often predisposed [a person] toward addiction" (Sonnedecker 1963:23). This suggested some facet of individual personality might lead to both initiating and continuing the habit, but only for some people and only to some degree. It was not, therefore, an acceptable explanation for all cases of addiction. Theoreticians were engaging in dubious science if they proposed this possible link as an explanation for the behavior of masses of people defined by socio-economic class, ethnicity, or religion.

32. The idea of using one alkaloid to cure addiction to opium, the mother drug, was analogous to the misconception about heroin (diacetylmorphine) after its synthesis from morphine in 1874. Heroin was first made available to the public in 1898. The medical community hailed it as the cure for morphine addiction. Similar to the career of the alkaloid from which it was derived, the consequences of using heroin were soon discovered to be worse than the affliction it was supposed to cure. See Kramer 1977:9:3 (July–September):193–97; Kurland 1978:3–4; and Weil & Rosen 1983:82, 86. These scholars discuss the public image of heroin during the late-nineteenth and early-twentieth centuries.

33. Anti-opiumists found merit in what scientists were discovering. They incorporated many of these facts into the anti-trade argument. Supporters of the drug commerce did not share this enthusiasm. Careful reading of the pro-trade evidence from 1884–1845 through 1895 indicates that they found 'valid proof' elsewhere. In most cases, they ignored laboratory research conclusions. What these people dismissed, what they selected, and their reasons for doing so, are discussed in later chapters.

3
The Gathering Storm: Protest, Politics, and Science, 1874–1893 C.E.

INTRODUCTION

The era of resolute individuals and short-lived anti-opiumist organizations with limited success in influencing Parliament ended in the autumn of 1874 with the formation of the Anglo-Oriental Society for the Suppression of the Opium Trade in London (Brown 1973:97). Founded by Quakers, the SSOT's major ally for the remainder of the century and beyond was the "[r]adical nonconformist wing" of the Liberal Party (Berridge & Edwards 1981:177, 179; see also Brown, J. F. 1973:101).

The SSOT, Addiction Experts, and Addiction Data Commencing in 1874

Edward and Arthur Pease of Yorkshire, Thomas Hansbury, a pharmaceutical merchant with business interests in China, and the Birmingham merchant Arthur Albright provided most of the funding for the organization. These four wealthy Quakers also occupied prominent positions during the early years (Lowes 1966:63; Owen [1934] 1968:262, 311; Berridge & Edwards 1981:176). F. Storrs Turner, a veteran of ten years of missionary work in China, was the only non-Quaker highly prominent during this period. He was appointed editor of the *Friend of China*, the society's journal. Lord Shaftesbury became the SSOT's first president because of his anti-trade efforts in Parliament (Johnson 1975:309; Lowes 1966:63). Sir Joseph Pease, another prominent Quaker, assumed the presidency after Shaftesbury's death. Active in the Liberal Party and elected to Parliament, Pease represented Barnard Castle in County Durham (Berridge & Edwards 1981:179).

Most of the SSOT's non-Quaker religious support during the remaining years of the century came from British evangelical groups, the Church of England, other Protestant sects, Catholics, "nonconformists," and notables such as the Bishop of Durham. They supplemented the cadre of English and American missionaries in East Asia and elsewhere (Lowes 1966:58, 63; Berridge & Edwards 1981:176; Lodwick 1976:76–8).

Soon after the organization's creation, the SSOT's treasurer went on a world tour. He was told to become familiar with the 'opium problem' and to give advice to embryonic anti-opiumist organizations anywhere they existed. He encouraged Christian missionaries in English colonies to submit articles, to compose letters for the SSOT journal, to make anti-opium speeches, and to write books.

Missionaries in Asia and secular anti-opiumists also responded to the SSOT message with commentaries and statistics contained in articles appearing in periodicals other than the *Friend of China*. They also wrote books and monographs published by firms independent from SSOT management (Johnson 1975:309; Lowes 1966:63).

The SSOT effort provided people with abundant information about the negative consequences of opium smoking, opium eating, and morphine abuse in Great Britain and other occidental nations. It also raised awareness, especially among the educated middle class, about opiate use and addiction in Asia. Combined with increasingly successful agitation in Parliament, the SSOT in less than two decades had forced the Government of India to confront the contradictions of its opium policy.

The Past and the Present: The Same Fight, Better Ammunition

The SSOT's platform was essentially the same as the pre-1874 anti-trade perspective. Opium was dangerous to human health and morality. Encouraging its consumption in any form without supervision was irresponsible, if not criminal behavior. The Government of India's drug policy was the antithesis of commerce befitting a Christian nation. Exports of Indian opium to China and elsewhere in Asia were poisoning innocent, unsuspecting people. British administrators in India were not governing natives in the subcontinent; they were encouraging depravity and promoting premature death.

The SSOT differed from its predecessors because it had more medical data amenable to an interpretation that supported its argument. Furthermore, the group's leadership recruited medical experts as valuable allies in its attempts to persuade Parliament to classify all nonmedical use of opiates as harmful (Peters 1981:475). These renowned professionals provided a "cross fertilization between medical and moral views in the formulation of the disease model" (Berridge 1978:458–59). Dr. Risdon Bennett, president of the Royal College of Physicians, became a SSOT vice president and delivered the election address in 1880. The SSOT council also included "addiction specialists" such as Professor Arthur Gamgee, Benjamin Ward Richardson, Brigade Surgeon Dr. Robert Pringle, and Dr. Norman Kerr. Gamgee, director and dean of the Medical School at Owen's College in Manchester, was designated by the SSOT to refute Sir George Birdwood's influential early 1880s articles published in *The Times* (London).[1] Some commentators credited Benjamin Ward Richardson as the first English physician to write extensively about therapy for morphine addiction. He later became the SSOT's president and organized a conference in 1892 devoted to discussing the medical aspects of the opium question. Brigade Surgeon Dr. Robert Pringle, a paid official of the SSOT and author of many publications about addiction, complemented Richardson's effort. Pringle was "equally at home addressing an anti-opiumist gathering, or one organized by the Society for the Study of Inebriety [and] he was a regular speaker at the latter's meetings" (Berridge & Edwards 1981:191). In 1894, Pringle testified on behalf of the SSOT before the Royal Commission on Opium.

Norman Kerr is another example of this amalgamation. Before his affiliation with the SSOT, some members of the medical establishment had disparaged anti-opiumists' insistence upon the analogy between opium and alcohol use. In 1873, for example, the *Medical Times and Gazette* editors were ecstatic about the benevolence of opium use in contrast to the disaster from liquor. Alcohol consumers were prone to violence and often threatened social order whereas opium use defused aggression. The former "say 'damn,' [but opium eaters] say 'blessed' [and enter] a state in which people dream of virtue, and goodness, and piety, and do nothing" (Editor[s], quoted in Berridge 1977a:282). Kerr challenged this interpretation. He had become an advocate for total abstinence from liquor very early in his career. Years later his interest in morphine habituation enabled him to develop a "model of alcoholism into a disease of inebriety which encompassed the process of narcotic habituation" (Peters 1981:475). The perspective was institutionalized in 1884 when he established the British Society for the Study and Cure of Inebriety.

For Kerr, inherited physical conditions caused alcohol addiction. A complete absence of will power and moral control signified an advanced stage of the disease. He then used the hypothesis to examine other forms of substance abuse, including opiate dependence. In 1877, he concluded that these addictions, which at the time were called opiomania, morphinomania, and chorodynomania, depending upon the substance involved, were not vices. They were "diseases with predisposing and exciting causes" (Berridge 1978:457). The etiology of narcotic addiction, for Kerr, became a physiological phenomenon over which the individual had minimal control, rather than some personality defect the individual chose to affect. These people were not malcontents; they were victims afflicted by a "physical crave," an "involuntary morbid craze," and a "functional neurosis" (Peters 1981:476).[2] Kerr confirmed what Allbutt and the German researchers had concluded during the previous decade. The consequence of Kerr's alcoholism studies was to enhance the political power of the temperance, or liquor prohibition, movement by providing its members with clinical data. His laboratory experience with opium and morphine did the same thing for anti-opium agitation in Great Britain and elsewhere in the west (Berridge 1978:457).

Addiction specialists such as Kerr also helped to diminish the credibility of patent medicines advertised as providing cures for substance dependence. Eucomen and Orphine, two products sold in 1880 for treating "opiomania" or 'addiction to opium,' were themselves addictive. Eucomen contained 41 percent alcohol and 1.5 percent morphine. Orphine, a "permanent cure for drug addiction," provided a daily dose of eight grains of morphine per day if taken as prescribed (Parssinen 1983:34).

The proliferation of discussion in the Anglo-European scientific community about the benefits and liabilities of morphine use, about opium and opiates in general, added authenticity and urgency to the anti-opiumist argument. They now had impressive data to support their insistence upon ending unfettered public use of both the mother drug and its alkaloids in Great Britain and everywhere in Asia. Participation of renowned medical professionals in years after 1874 made it even more difficult for any but the most adamant pro-trade advocate to dismiss SSOT members as reincarnations of pre-1874 bible-spouting, unrealistic do-gooders misinformed about reality in their own country and obsessed with Asia. Less than one year after the SSOT's founding, and much to the dismay of defenders of the status quo, more members of Parliament were listening to the message.

THE ARGUMENTS

Parliamentary Debates from 1875 to the Early 1880s

In June 1875, Sir Mark Stewart called for the House of Commons to demand the Government of India terminate poppy cultivation and opium sales. Stewart's petition was defeated by only thirty-seven votes from Parliament's 151 members (GBO [Baines] 1895a:VI:165; Johnson 1975:309; Lowes 1966:64).

The second SSOT-inspired event occurred in June 1880. Sir Joseph Pease reiterated the 1875 demand. He also wanted a provision for opium exports to be excluded from any future treaty with China. Pease was attacking British refusal to sign the Chefoo Convention of 1876 which reconsidered aspects of the 1860 Treaty of Tientsin. The Chinese wanted a high import duty on opium but British merchants, and the Government of India in particular, objected because poppy cultivation was increasing in several parts of China. Indigenous Chinese merchants and cultivators might be able to undersell the Indian product. The motion was withdrawn. Pease introduced it again in 1881 (GBO [Baines] 1895a:VI:165–66; see also Lowes 1966:61–2; Owen [1934] 1968:263; Johnson 1975:209–10).

Pease's 1881 effort was not a total failure. In the autumn of that year, prominent members of the Society, including the Lord Mayor of London, Cardinal Manning, and the Archbishop of Canterbury, met to reformulate the SSOT position (Lowes 1966:65; Owen [1934] 1968:262–63; GBO [Baines] 1895a:VI:166; Berridge & Edwards 1981:181; Scott, James Maurice 1969:106). *Hansard*, the publication containing deliberations of the House of Lords, referred to the event as "a triumvirate which might well overawe evil itself" (Owen [1934] 1968:263). Members of this eminent group wanted the trade to end immediately because it was antagonistic to the commercial interests of England and contrary to

"Christian and international morality." They also demanded that England help the Chinese suppress the drug's importation, and that poppy cultivation in India be terminated "except for strictly medical purposes" (GBO [Baines] 1895a:VI:166; Owen [1934] 1968:302).

The provision "except for strictly medical purposes" formally signified the SSOT's recognition of the therapeutic utility of opium and some of its components. Shaftesbury and other early agitators also were aware of the drug's potency. The difference between the past and present, however, is that the SSOT now wanted to regulate production at its source and to dictate for what purpose manufacturing was to be undertaken.

This demand was predicated upon the assumption that British authorities would encounter no resistance in areas under their control and in the quasi-independent native states that cultivated poppy. The SSOT's principal rationale for this provision was the disgraceful consequence of opium sales in parts of Burma under British jurisdiction (SSOT declaration of 1881, in GBO [Baines] 1895a:VI:166). The proposed remedy consisted of British officials prohibiting sales of the drug and providing sufficient and reasonable aid to the Government of India to compensate for the loss of the opium revenue from Burma. Compensation also should be extended to all parties in India involved in cultivation. A delegation of participants from the meeting presented the memorial on behalf of the SSOT to Mr. Gladstone, the head of Her Majesty's government.

Pro-Trade Reaction to SSOT Initiatives of the Early 1880s

Defenders of the opium trade retaliated during the early 1880s. The trade was still legal, but for how long was becoming a moot point. They needed support from physicians such as a Dr. Elliot. In his 1881 letter to the *British Medical Journal*, Elliot categorized the opium and alcohol analogy as erroneous (Berridge 1978:459–60). Many years of experience in a region where the opium habit was prevalent and consumption was high had convinced him the drug was virtually harmless (Berridge 1977a:282). His opponents' preoccupation with documenting opiate abuse was unfortunate and foolish. Unlike opium, alcohol taken in excess

> . . . ruins the health and fills our jails and workhouses. We should be inclined rather to class opium with tobacco in its ill-effect (in excess) as regards the body. (Elliot, quoted in Berridge 1977a:282)

Another attack upon the SSOT during the decade involved sex. Some anti-opiumists believed the drug was an aphrodisiac and that its consumption encouraged lewd behavior—hence immorality—among the Chinese. Sir George Birdwood, a staunch defender of the trade, disagreed. In a 20 January 1882 article published in *The Times* (London), he said opium was no more an aphrodisiac than other substances. Furthermore, people claiming it caused bad behavior "can have little idea what morality means in Eastern Asia—much less immorality" (Birdwood 1882a:1; also quoted in Scott, James Maurice 1969:95).

Pro-trade documents in subsequent years frequently cited Birdwood's dismissal of the sexual appetite argument as proof of the nonharmful nature of opium.[3]

Sir Rutherford Alcock was also of no help to the anti-opiumists in 1881. Alcock, whom anti-opiumists praised after he expressed doubt about the opium monopoly while a member of the 1871 *Select Committee on East Indian Finance*, now incurred their wrath. In 1871 he suggested that a gradual—not an abrupt—end of the trade would create little animosity and travail for the governments and citizens of China and England. Anti-opiumists were delighted to find a sympathetic British official, and they construed these statements as a desire for a quick resolution that he simply did not have (Berridge & Edwards 1981:182). They were infuriated by the contents of two articles Alcock wrote in 1881 and 1882. The first, entitled "Opium and Common Sense," appeared in the periodical *Nineteenth Century*. The second piece, according to Berridge and Edwards, was published in the *Journal of the Society of Arts*. Both articles called upon the SSOT to moderate its demands. Anti-opium readers interpreted this sentiment as support for the trade. Their dismay intensified when, in 1882, he agreed to be the leading speaker for the India section of the Royal Society of Arts, which was the "main forum for the pro-opium response" (Berridge & Edwards 1981:182). Alcock and Sir George Campbell, another participant speaking early in the conference, stressed economic aspects of the trade (Parssinen 1983:90). The SSOT was now convinced that Alcock was a turncoat.

An entire book challenging the SSOT argument about opium in China also appeared in 1882. William H. Brereton, a retired Hong Kong solicitor and former legal adviser to opium farmers in Hong Kong, published *Truth about Opium, Being a Refutation of the Fallacies of the Anti-Opium Society and a Defense of the Indo-China Opium Trade*. The volume contains chapters written by Brereton and previously published documents authored by fellow defenders of the trade. The latter pieces include discussions about the benign consequences of eating crude opium among various castes in India, and why eating the substance cannot be compared to the Chinese practice of smoking a watery extract of the drug. There also are commentaries about the 'actual' nonlethal effects of the smoking extract, and other issues. (Also see comments of Brereton's book in Inglis 1975:92 and Berridge & Edwards 1981:182.)

A lesser-known but equally impressive document refuting SSOT claims about China also circulated in 1882. Mr. W. Donald Spence, the acting consul for Great Britain in Ichang, a city in Szuchuan [sic] province of western China, sent an urgent report to the Government of India's Finance and Commerce Department in 1881. The department forwarded the document to London for distribution among policy makers in Parliament in 1882. Spence said arguments circulating back home about opium use in Asia came from people, specifically the "National Church and to men of activity in Parliament" who had absolutely no knowledge about reality in China. Spence claimed the report was intended to help his "countrymen to sober and intelligent views of a question more than ordinarily obscured by rhetorical misrepresentation . . ." (GBO [Spence] 1894:II:383). Spence's document is long but its message is clear: anti-opiumists' reports about the nefarious consequences of opium use in China are unfounded. Anglo-European observers such as Colborne Baber and the legendary Baron Richthofen are cited to "prove" the harmless, even beneficial, consequences of opium use among the Chinese. Both men, and Spence as well, attest to the direct correlation between consumption and high standards of living and quality of life. For example, the smoking of opium was prevalent in Szuchuan [sic] province. The amount ranged from moderate to monumental. Yet during a four month tour, Spence encountered only "stout able-bodied men, better housed, better clad, better fed, and healthier looking than the Chinese of the lower Yangtse, and I did not see amongst them more emaciated faces and wasted forms that disease causes in all lands" (GBO [Spence] 1894:II:386). He also addresses anti-opiumists' complaints that the Chinese government is forcing its peasants to cultivate the poppy and that the bureaucracy profits handsomely from encouraging substance abuse. The allegation, Spence tells us, is ignorant hyperbole from ill-informed religious zealots. The government does not tax poppy and its leniency about consumption is a response to the peoples' will. This, for Spence, is evidence that Chinese officials were guilty only of being democratic (GBO [Spence] 1894:II:386).

The SSOT Response to Pro-Trade Critiques

The pro-trade counteroffense did not deter Sir Joseph Pease and his SSOT colleagues. They now attempted to influence imminent treaty renegotiations. In April 1883, Pease's resolution permitted China to set import quotas on opium free from British interference. It lost in the House of Commons by sixty-six votes. A total of 192 members voted (GBO [Baines] 1895a:VI:166; Johnson 1975:310; Lowes 1966:64; Owen [1934] 1968:263; Berridge & Edwards 1981:180).

The setback was temporary. Pease's insistent lobbying for the issue was rewarded in 1885 despite vigorous protests from the Government of India. The India Office under the direction of Lord Kimberley finally accepted the right of the Chinese government, as stipulated in the Chefoo Convention, to impose high taxes on imported opium if it so desired (GBO [Baines] 1895a:VI:167; GBO [Baines] 1895b:VI:175; Lowes 1966:65, 67; Owen [1934] 1968:311). In a letter to the Viceroy, Kimberley, the secretary of state for India, credited SSOT activities as one reason for the policy change (Lowes 1966:65; Johnson 1975:310).

Although SSOT members were pleased that the Chefoo convention was now a reality, they mistakenly assumed the Chinese would quickly eliminate drug imports by imposing prohibitive tariffs. Chinese officials instead immediately raised duties albeit not to a level that discouraged exports from India. To the disgust of many anti-opiumists, the Chinese were now demonstrating as much interest as the British in making money from opium. The nation's leaders would be no help in ending the trade. Other anti-opiumists were content to declare a moral victory because the Chinese at least had been offered a chance to decide opium policy themselves (Johnson 1975:310). Many people who expressed this sentiment ceased participating in SSOT activities.

The Turning Point (July 1885): Changing the Target from China to India

Other SSOT participants remained determined to save the Chinese people from destruction despite the indifference of their government. The society's leadership met in July 1885 to discuss strategy but there was no unanimity in how to proceed. Some attendees said the organization should continue in the same form. Other members wanted the organization to adopt a less confrontational approach to change drug policy (Berridge & Edwards 1981:183–84). The focus of activity was another issue. Should it remain China or be redirected toward South Asia? The SSOT leadership opted for the latter (Owen [1934] 1968:311; Berridge & Edwards 1981:180, 183).[4] India, the ultimate source of outraged morality because it produced the poison killing the Chinese, became the principal SSOT geographical target after 1885.

The most vigorous leader in forging consensus for the new focus was the Quaker barrister Joseph Grundy Alexander. He became secretary of the SSOT in 1889 (Lowes 1966:65–6; Owen [1934] 1968:311; Scott, James Maurice 1969:106). Like other anti-opiumists, Alexander was disappointed by the Chinese decision not to end drug imports when given the opportunity to do so. But he was encouraged by the SSOT's success in enabling China to exert some control of imports.

Alexander then concentrated on what he defined as the fundamental task: eliminate all poppy cultivation in Bengal that was not intended for medical use (Lowes 1966:65–6; Owen [1934] 1968:311–12). He was referring to acreage in regions over which the British had direct control.

In contrast to the recent past, the SSOT leadership now strenuously objected to issuing licenses for poppy cultivation. The provision, according to Alexander, was designed to transfer operations in British India to private individuals. This would end direct government involvement in primary production. It was, in effect, an initial step toward full disengagement.

The SSOT also was opposed to any individual or government agency that planted poppy for unspecified purposes. This meant that the native states of India must stop cultivating the plant. Implementation of this demand would end the Government of India's ability to earn money from taxes imposed on the native states' drug when it entered British territory. The SSOT's model for regulating public access to the drug in India was Great Britain's 1868 Pharmacy Act. Sir Joseph Pease again performed his duty in Parliament on 4 May 1886. The anti-opiumists remained unsuccessful (GBO [Baines] 1895a:VI:167; Lowes 1966:66).

1889 (May) Parliamentary Debate

Mr. Samuel Smith raised the opium question yet again in May 1889. It lost by seventy-seven votes (GBO [Baines] 1895a:VI:167; Lowes 1966:66; Scott, James Maurice 1969:107; Owen [1934] 1968:312). Despite dismaying defeats experienced during the late 1880s, anti-opiumists had reason for optimism; greater numbers of Conservatives and Liberal Unionists were changing their minds about policy. The margin of defeat was becoming narrower (Lowes 1966:66).

The SSOT Resolution and Memorial of 3 June and 30 June 1890

The SSOT had a reason to worry. Aware that indigenous production of opium in China was increasing, it now accused the Government of India of encouraging consumption within south Asia to compensate for losses in the China revenue. The issue was the subject of a SSOT meeting on 3 June 1890. Resolutions adopted at the parley were incorporated into a memorial presented on 30 June to Viscount Cross, Her Majesty's Secretary of State. The SSOT demanded three things:

1. British officials should persuade the Chinese government to halt opium production in China itself;
2. The Government of India must ensure that poppy cultivation in the quasi-independent native states of Central India, the source of Malwa opium, would not be expanded in order to compensate for diminished poppy cultivation in British India; and
3. The Chinese should be strongly encouraged not to import the Malwa drug to offset the decreased amount of the commodity manufactured in British India. (GBO [Batten] 1894:I:143)

The memorial included data from various parts of India revealing an increase in opium smoking and consumption of drug preparations. According to the SSOT, the government's granting of licenses to entrepreneurs who sell the drug to the public had created the nefarious opium dens. These establishments should be closed because they caused "great demoralization" throughout the country, including Burma. Anti-opiumists again urged passage of a bill similar to the 1868 Pharmacy Act to halt the commerce (GBO [Baines] 1895a:VI:167). They still believed that in Great Britain the bill had effectively restricted the use of dangerous substances such as opium. The memorial stipulated that trained personnel were responsible for distributing the drug in India, and that these people dispense it only for "legitimate medical use." The last criterion would dictate the annual acreage of opium poppy cultivation (GBO [Batten] 1894:I:143).

Viscount Cross's acceptance of the document in 1890 revitalized existing anti-opium organizations. It also encouraged the creation of new ones. Benjamin Broomhall, Secretary of the China Inland Mission and SSOT executive board member, had founded the National Righteousness in 1888 after the SSOT decided to concentrate on India. He claimed SSOT tactics for changing the status quo were ineffective. Broomhall now established a group called the Christian Union for the Severance of the Connection of the British Empire with the Opium Traffic. And in 1891, the Woman's Anti-Opium Urgency Committee appeared. Rachel Braithwaite, its secretary, edited a series of pamphlets under the title of *Britain's Opium Harvest*. Other groups were the Friends' Anti-Opium

84   Chapter 3

Committee for Suffering, the Anglican Anti-Opium Committee, and the Edinburgh Committee for the Suppression of the Indo-Chinese Opium Traffic. An organization called the Anti-Opium Urgency Committee was created during the March 1891 National Christian Anti-Opium Convention held in London (Johnson 1975:310; Berridge & Edwards 1981:184).

The SSOT's effort was very impressive. As of 1891, it had sponsored more than 100 meetings each year in Great Britain that specifically addressed the drug issue. The organization had also issued more than 40,000 anti-opium tracts, and members had collected 192,000 signatures in approximately 3,000 anti-opium petitions (Johnson 1975:310–11; Austin 1978:157).

This Foolishness Must End: The Definitive Pro-Trade and Government of India Rebuttal of the Entire SSOT Argument

Public reaction to the 30 June 1890 memorial sent to Viscount Cross alarmed pro-traders. Eight months later they launched the harshest and most influential attack upon the movement thus far in the controversy. The assault, a precursor of the Government of India defense during the Royal Commission investigation three years later, came from G. M. Batten in the form of a paper entitled "The Opium Question." He presented it to attendees at the 24 March 1891 meeting of the Society of the Arts (GBO [Batten] 1894:I:133–46). Batten, a former member of the Bengal Civil Service in India, condemned the 1890 SSOT memorial as a misguided effort based upon falsehoods. Demand for this foolish proposal "is made not by the people of India, not by the people of China, not by the responsible administrators of those countries, but by an irresponsible party of philanthropists seeking to obtain their ends by the despotic action of the Parliament of the United Kingdom, in which India has no representatives" (GBO [Batten] 1894:I:136). The SSOT was the antithesis of reason. Its members in China mistakenly focused on collecting the rare exceptional abuse in coastal towns. They conveniently ignored people in the country's interior "to whom the use of opium is as common, as moderate, and as beneficial as that of beer is to the people of England (GBO [Batten] 1894:I:146).

The zeal of the SSOT leadership did not excuse a lamentable ignorance about such rudimentary facts as geography. The authors of the document, Batten asserted, "had the most elementary knowledge of India, or if there were such a person [present] he could not have read the memorial" (GBO [Batten] 1894:I:144). For Batten, ignorance about geography was indicative of the SSOT's superficial scenario. It was unforgivable to print

> Lucknow as being in the Punjab, and Lahore as being in the North-Western Provinces! This blunder is as stupendous as would be that of persons memorialising for the suppression of alcohol in Europe, should place Paris in Scotland and Dublin in Holland. (GBO [Batten] 1894:I:144)

Batten also took issue with trade defenders who were preoccupied with economic aspects of the trade. Their focus upon the pecuniary value of the poppy crop and its products was insignificant when considering "the well-being and happiness of hundreds of thousands of the people of India [whose health] would be greatly affected by its extinction." Batten intended to demonstrate to his audience the "real value" of the crop. He wanted to expose the kind of sacrifice the anti-opiumists were demanding from India "in order to satisfy the theories of a party of English philanthropists, whose excellent intentions in the cause of morality are only equaled by their determination to ignore all but one side of the question, on which they have fixed their attention, and which serves their purpose" (GBO [Batten] 1894:I:133).

Batten's paper is lengthy, far longer than Spence's seminal 1882 report, and at first reading, it is convincing.[5] But the kind of evidence he used was similar to his predecessors' material. It has many testimonials, including a substantial number decades old, from "important" witnesses. Many of them were affiliated in some way with the production and distribution of opium in India and elsewhere.

Batten's document, however, lacks the kind of medical data that anti-opiumists were using with increasing effectiveness in presenting their case to the public and to Parliament. The standard of what constituted credible proof had now changed. Laboratory research conducted by addiction specialists, and from pharmacologists whose interest in international politics was most likely minimal, gave some anti-opiumist arguments the quality of believability. Their statements were now supported by something akin to "science," something other than subjective evaluation. Granted, much of the scientific work generated more questions than answers. Many issues had not been addressed, and decades of research in the new century revealed that some of these "scientific findings" were only crude approximations of reality. But the material available at the time did provide a fund of facts (or information that passed as facts) for anti-opiumists to use if so inclined. Some activists did so.

Many anti-opiumists refrained from using the information because they did not think it was necessary. This luxury was not available to defenders of the trade. Nonetheless, people supporting the drug commerce launched no sustained laboratory effort specifically designed to refute the scientific observations and conclusions that anti-opiumists were citing to educate members of Parliament and the British public. The 'science' of pro-traders, Batten's diatribe being an example, had a large component of anecdotal comments by nonnatives about habitual behavior being equivalent to "proof." Old customs and traditional beliefs about drugs, merely because they were old and traditional, confirmed the positive contribution of opium to society.

Batten reiterated the ideas of many pro-traders from the past. His arguments reappear in different guises and varying detail in subsequent debates during the 1890s. They were prominent in the Royal Commission on Opium hearings. The kind of evidence Batten used to support his perspective is as predictable as anti-opiumists' earlier expressions of outraged morality; there is a numbing repetitiousness to both. The great majority of individuals Batten cited offered opinions derived from assumptions about opiates and from firsthand or secondhand observations in the field. The absence of recent laboratory discoveries about addiction and drugs in their statements did not discourage Batten. He declared his conclusions reflected "a great consensus of opium arrived at by a number of independent persons of high character and reputation; gentlemen of ability and integrity, who have attained responsible positions, in which they have had the best opportunities of ascertaining the truth; whose duty it has been to state the truth; and who have had no personal interest in perverting it" (GBO [Batten] 1894:I:146). Batten was oblivious to the possibility of his authorities having a vested interest in the outcome of the controversy, and that even people of "high character" are sometimes wrong.

Batten did not totally exclude 'science' based upon something other then customary behavior. He does mention "eminent" authorities and researchers of past decades to support proclamations from nonscientists. But 'facts' from nonscientists dominate his critique. These two sources of information enabled him to ask questions that anti-opiumists had to address. In most cases they did so. However, anti-opiumists' inability or reluctance to answer other queries, and their dismissal of some of these questions as unimportant or irrelevant, enabled the Government of India to construct an effective defense for the future Royal Commission hearings. The witnesses Batten used, and the observations they provided to advance the pro-trade position, are briefly mentioned below. The remainder of the Batten discussion describes the scant medical evidence he selected to attack anti-opiumists.

Batten used two kinds of authorities. The first were well-known individuals from the past. Almost all had no medical training and are introduced earlier in the chapter. W. C. B. Eatwell, the British India Opium Examiner, author of the aforementioned 1851–1852 article appearing in the *Pharmaceutical Journal and Transactions*, was the India expert. Batten's "proof" of the benign consequences of opium smoking for habitual users in China was taken from W. Donald Spence's (1881) document for Szechuan province (Spence's 'Szuchuan'). Batten then uses the 1858 commentary of Dr. Sinibaldo de Mas, the former Envoy Extraordinary and Minister Plenipotentiary of the Court of Spain at Peking. Other China authorities were Baron Richthofen and Colborne Baber, the same people whom Spence cited. Batten's citation of some comments in the 1831 report by Sir Henry Pottinger, the British Governor/General Minister Plenipotentiary in China, provided additional "proof" as did John Crawfurd's 1856 brief comment about the drug's status in the Straits settlements. Batten also cited William Brereton's *Truth About Opium* book (1882) as authoritative and he mentioned a Dr. D. B. Ayres' assertion that opium smoking is a "luxury of a very harmless description." Ayres' comments are from an 1881 Hong Kong Government report (GBO [Batten] 1894:I:146).

THE OBVIOUS AND IRREFUTABLE BENEFITS OF OPIUM CONSUMPTION FOR PEOPLE IN INDIA

Lest he be accused of using outdated observations by dead, or almost dead, people and ignoring more contemporary data, Batten included responses to Government of India questionnaires. The queries had been forwarded to regional officers in the subcontinent after the SSOT submitted the 1890 memorial to Viscount Cross.[6] Physicians or scientists contributed virtually none of the data in this official document. It consisted of "the opinions of experienced officers engaged in the administration of the country, writing from their own personal knowledge, which it was a part of their duty to acquire, as to the effects of opium consumption on the people of India" (GBO [Batten] 1894:I:140). Batten proclaims these opinions completely refute the SSOT allegation of increased consumption in the country. The organization's assumption about the ability of English authorities to tell Indian subjects to do anything compounded the folly. The Government of India, he admonished, is not a despotic entity, and treaties and contracts honored for many years cannot be ignored.

Batten cites officials from Assam, Burma, Bengal, the Central Provinces, Madras, the Northwest Provinces, Punjab, Bombay Presidency, Gujerat, and Sind Province. All of them spoke about the foolishness of anyone being upset by use of the drug anywhere in British India. The only regional administrator reporting anything negative about opium, and it was a very mild reservation, was an unnamed Commissioner of Excise from the Central Provinces. He believed moderate opium consumption was usually benign but natives tended to consider opium eaters disreputable and the habit a vice (GBO [Batten] 1894:I:141). Reports from other locations of drug consumption were very positive.

Good, hardworking people living in "damp and malarious" locales in Assam used opium. According to the Excise commissioner for the province, the habit was not increasing, consumers did not abuse the drug, and they would die if supplies were terminated (Driberg, cited in GBO [Batten] 1894:140–41). The situation was much the same in neighboring Burma. The financial commissioner said the Chinese living in two very "malarious regions" indulged themselves. Hill tribes also used the drug and like the Chinese, they inhabited "feverish tracts" (GBO [Batten] 1894:I:141). Sir Charles Aitchison, a former Chief Commissioner of Burma, made a similar observation. Non-Burmese people ingested opium as did the "most thriving and industrious section of the population, to whom the drug is a necessity of life, and by whom it is rarely abused" (Aitchison, quoted in GBO [Batten] 1894:I:141). Mr. Copleston, a former Excise commissioner, said Chinese and natives of Madras consumed the drug in Burma. They did not think the habit was a "special evil either to individuals or to society. . . ." The Chinese were so healthy that Copleston concluded opium use "may almost be called a legitimate luxury." The few Burmese who complained about the drug were abstainers. For Copleston, abstinence made their statements suspect (Copleston, quoted in GBO [Batten] 1894:I:141).

Batten included the testimony of only one person from Bengal. This was Sir Charles Elliott, the lieutenant governor. Elliott, enthusiastic about the benefits of opium for many things, said it restored strength to exhausted people. It also was a wholesome stimulus even in a hot, dry climate. Elliott claimed that opium was "especially beneficial in moist and marshy countries like eastern Bengal [particularly] in the malarious alluvial tracts which forms a great proportion of the area of these provinces." It was no surprise, therefore, that opium is consumed everywhere in the country. The many positive functions opium performed made it "not so much a vice as a necessity [because] [t]heir vegetable diet would not keep them alive without stimulants" (Elliott, quoted in GBO [Batten] 1894:I:141).

The report from Madras asserted that few people smoked opium and still fewer opium dens existed. Furthermore, customers patronizing these establishments exhibited none of the sordid characteristics so luridly portrayed in anti-opiumist writings (GBO [Batten] 1894:I:141–42). The situation was different in the Northwest Provinces. No data existed for the region precisely because there was widespread cultivation of poppy. Consumption was so common and the consequences so benign that "absence of any mention in the government reports of any marked evil effects on the population is, at any rate, negative evidence that no glaring abuses exist" (GBO [Batten] 1894:I:141).[7]

The Government of Punjab echoed officials from the Northwest Provinces. The drug was used, and in some districts the amount was great, but nowhere was consumption detrimental to health and morality (GBO [Batten] 1894:I:142). People living in locales of above average consumption are merely following a custom of long standing. They believe opium protects them against fever (GBO [Batten] 1894:I:142). R. M. Dane, the Excise commissioner for Punjab, identified Sikhs, Hindus, and Muslims as major consumers and warned that any attempt to force them to curtail use would fail (GBC [Consumption] 1892:62–3; GBO [Batten] 1894:I:142). Dane also said issuance of licenses for poppy cultivation in the Punjab was neither "contrary to the elementary principles of morality [nor] inconsistent with the gospel of Christ" (GBC [Consumption] 1892:62–3). The SSOT demand might be justified for opium smoking, but the population of Punjab avoided the practice; they ate the drug and this did no harm whatsoever. Furthermore, the Government of India already recognized the dangers of smoking opium. The administration had taken steps to prevent this mode of ingestion from ever becoming a serious problem by denying licenses to shops wanting to manufacture the smoking extract (GBC [Consumption] 1892:64). The misinformed SSOT was concerned about a "problem" that did not even exist in Punjab. Batten said the official also stated that "memorialists [i.e., anti-opiumists] themselves admit that in malarious tracts opium is useful as a prophylactic" (Punjab Commission of Excise, quoted in Batten in GBO [Batten] 1894:I:142).[8] The situation was similar farther south.

The unidentified Collector of Nasik district said that natives in this part of Bombay Presidency used the drug only in moderation. The habit, consequently, was no more harmful than moderate use of liquor. Indeed, the opium "sot" was much less a social problem than the person drunk from alcohol. Furthermore, no one should even contemplate reducing accessibility to the drug because no form of prohibition will work (GBO [Batten] 1894:I:142). Responding to the SSOT lament about opium hindering missionary proselytizing, the official said that in his twenty-three years of work in India, he never once heard of a

> "single missionary—and I have met dozens—specially refer to or quote the opium trade as interfering with his endeavours. The proposition is true in the abstract, no doubt, but in the same manner that the abstract proposition is true that the existence of public-houses in the slums of London interferes with Christian efforts there. (Collector of Nasik, quoted in Batten, in GBO [Batten] 1894:I:142)

Mr. Campbell, another collector in Bombay, said the anti-opiumists' descriptions of opium dens were "overdrawn and misleading" (Campbell, quoted in Batten, in GBO [Batten] 1894:I:142). The wretched physical descriptions of these opium smokers existed only in the minds of anti-opiumists. These patrons were not lowlife derelicts. They were only tired laboring men seeking relaxation. Reports of little boys and girls being found in such places were also erroneous. Campbell had never heard of such a thing because parents would be appalled if their children smoked opium (GBO [Batten] 1894:I:142–43).

The original document from which Batten selected his data also contained the comments of an official from Gujerat, a province close to Bombay. The administrator accused the SSOT of being wildly imaginative and slightly hysterical. The "gentlemen who penned the highly coloured accounts of opium dens must have been shown the worst haunts in large towns, and that they and those who think with them inveigh against the use of opium as much as teetotalers at home attack the use of spirits and beer and wine because of the evils of the gin palaces of our great cities. . . ." This unidentified government worker was reluctant to admit that "the use of opium in moderation is more harmful than the use of whisky" (GBC [Consumption] 1892:92). He believed opium abuse was not increasing in Gujerat or anywhere else. There also was no comparison between opium consumption in India and alleged alcohol abuse in Great Britain. The anti-opiumists who worried about India were suffering from a sour attitude concerning harmless relaxation.

Mr. A. C. Trevor, the commissioner in Sind, submitted the last Government of India questionnaire that Batten cited. Sind was a province north of Gujerat. Trevor said the SSOT contention about a moderate intake of the drug being detrimental to physical and mental health was a discredited, outdated notion. He was familiar with "whole tribes" in the region that have consumed opium for generations. Rajputs and Bhils were cited as examples. These peoples' "energy, endurance, and bravery cannot be said to have been affected by their addiction to opium" (GBC [Consumption] 1892:100; Commissioner of Sind, quoted in GBO [Batten] 1894:I:143). The Commissioner, therefore, acknowledged the existence of addiction but SSOT consternation about Sind was much ado about nothing. Smoking opium could lead to abuse and the presence of opium dens might even encourage bad behavior. The easiest way to halt this tendency was to deny licenses to sell the locally produced smoking extract. Anything else was unrealistic and counterproductive. This measure also was unnecessary in Sind because people in the province, indeed throughout the country, consume opium in moderation just as the "English gentleman of the present takes his wine" (Commissioner of Sind, quoted in GBO [Batten], 1894:I:143; GBC [Consumption] 1892:100–01).

THE BRITISH ARE NOT THE CAUSE OF DEGENERACY AND DEGRADATION IN INDIA OR CHINA

Batten portrayed British India officials as virtually unanimous about the beneficial, even lifesaving, status of opium in South Asia. And he was adamant in denying that the administration had compelled Chinese citizens to endure the drug's destructive consequences. These people simply wanted opium. Great Britain and the Government of India had little to do with stimulating demand at any time in China's history.

Elementary common sense and an understanding of Chinese history also discredited the SSOT argument about opium consumption leading to degradation. Batten used a study written in May 1889 by Dr. Edkins of the Chinese Customs Service in Shanghai to refute the charge. Some of Edkins' statements are accurate. The others are an interpretation of events written by a British official trying to condone his country's involvement in a controversial activity.

Edkins claimed the Chinese had consumed opium long before the British presence in India. Chinese documents from 763 C.E. first mention the drug (GBO [Edkins] 1894:I:148). Chinese formulas and recipes that date from the 1500s and 1600s attest to its medicinal value for these people (GBO [Batten] 1894:I:136–37). And under no circumstances did the British impose the drug upon the Chinese. The Asians wanted it for various medical and nonmedical reasons before the beginning of the India trade in the mid-1700s. Other Europeans, not the English, introduced them to the custom of smoking the substance. The practice began on Formosa (Taiwan) and spread to China (GBO [Edkins] 1894:I:148; GBO [Batten] 1894:I:136–37). The only thing the British had ever done was to make more of a safe, high-quality product available to Asian customers.[9] Batten supported this account of British involvement with Sir Robert Hart's statement of 1881. Hart, also affiliated with the Chinese Customs Service, documented the drug being known, produced, and used long before Europeans established trading stations on the Chinese coast. Hart also provided statistics proving that the increase in native production when he wrote the report was due to Government of India's unwise taxation of its exported product. The policy raised prices of the Indian commodity in China. This in turn encouraged Chinese people to produce their own, less expensive drug within the Empire (GBO [Batten] 1894:I:138). Batten used Hart's 1881 assessment to castigate the SSOT in the early 1890s. The moralists' success in forcing the Government of India to increase price as a technique to discourage Chinese consumption was silly. The Chinese would manufacture even more of their own drug in this new decade if the foreign substance became too expensive. In other words, the anti-opiumists were oblivious to what they were advocating.

Batten also used the experience of a missionary in China to refute charges of British unethical behavior. Sometime around 1881, the Reverend F. Galpin of the English Methodist Free Church, whom Batten described as a "respected missionary at Ningpo, an important port on the east coast of China," vigorously refused to sign a petition opposing opium imports. Anti-opiumists eventually sent the petition to the House of Commons. Galpin disagreed with their claim that the people and Government of China were eager to end opium abuse (GBO [Batten], 1894:I:138). Galpin retorted that the citizenry always had many opportunities to do so but they chose otherwise. Batten then elaborated. He suggested the Chinese could not stop using the drug even if they desired; predilection to smoking opium was a consequence of biology as much as it was a result of politics. Batten was not acknowledging the reality of addiction; he was implying that many Chinese were genetically programmed to engage in excessive indulgence. They were born to be chronically habituated.

Genetic heritage and innate predisposition also determined drug consumption in South Asia. According to Batten, Samuel Laing, the finance minister for the Government of India, provided an explanation in 1862. Laing stated that every "civilised or semi-civilised race of mankind seems to affect some peculiar form of nervous stimulant, and as the natives of Northern Europe take to alcohol, so the Chinese take to opium" (Laing, quoted in GBO [Batten] 1894:I:145). Laing then suggests that the Chinese preference for the substance is a consequence of their limited intellectual capability.

> [P]ossibly, in each case, the craving . . . for something to supply an innate want. The Englishman, the Dane, the German, and the Russian resort to that the specific effect of which is to raise the spirits and produce temporary exhilaration. The Chinese, whose greatest deficiency, as shown by the whole history, religion, and literature of the race, is in the imaginative faculties, resorts to that which stimulates the imagination, and makes his sluggish brain see visions and dream dreams. Be that as it may, the fact is certain that, under all circumstances. . . .We have . . . one of the great natural instincts of a large population. (Laing, quoted in GBO [Batten] 1894:I:145)

Calling the Chinese dimwitted is part of the vocabulary associated with the "racialist" hypothesis to explain cultural traits and physical traits. It relegates history, economics, and politics to irrelevancy in comprehending patterns of opium consumption. People indulge, or refrain from doing so, because of their genetic heritage. For Batten and fellow pro-trade advocates, biology elevated British behavior beyond reproach. They failed to realize, or chose to ignore that in 1862, and most definitely by 1891, simplistic variants of the hypothesis had diminished credibility among Anglo-European medical researchers and addiction specialists.

THE FALSE ANALOGY BETWEEN OPIUM AND ALCOHOL CONSUMPTION

Laing, much to Batten's delight, also pontificated about the anti-opiumists' opium and alcohol analogy. Laing conceded he was not a medical doctor. But extensive reading and experience permitted him to state unequivocally that little or no comparison was justified regarding the effects of alcohol and opium upon the human constitution. For Laing, the "excess of alcohol is far more destructive to the human frame than that of opium, for one attacks the tissues and the other produces only functional derangement." He also cautioned against ending Indian natives' easy procurement of the drug. Deprivation would force them to use the far more dangerous alcohol, and also the hemp "which grows wild in many parts of the country, and the effects of which are, when taken in excess, maddening" (Laing, quoted in GBO [Batten] 1894:I:145).

Batten also cautioned his audience not to make wrong judgments about opium indulgence based upon the experience of celebrated consumers. He was referring to Thomas DeQuincey. Less well known, according to Batten, was that DeQuincey and other habituates never descended into torpor. Just the opposite occurred. DeQuincey consumed the drug before going to the Italian opera because "he found it greatly increased his mental activity and appreciation of the entertainment." The experiences of DeQuincey and fellow consumers enabled Batten to affirm his belief that moderate use of opium by a person in good health had "absolute benefits" (GBO [Batten] 1894:I:139).

Batten thus far had "proven" opium was no problem in India and the British were not responsible for alleged habituation among the Chinese (GBO [Batten] 1894:I:136). Indeed, if the Chinese failed to obtain the highest quality opium due to cessation of Indian exports, an inferior drug from locales other than South Asia would satisfy their demand (GBO [Batten] 1894:I:134). A worse scenario was that stopping Indian imports might stimulate, not discourage, indigenous and surreptitious production of the drug (GBO [Batten] 1894:I:138). In either case, the SSOT was not acting in its best interest by pursuing an end to poppy cultivation and opium production anywhere in Asia.

THE SSOT PENCHANT FOR SELECTING ATYPICAL AND RARE EXAMPLES OF OPIUM ABUSE

Batten then chastised anti-opiumists who claimed that "except for medical purposes," the "use of opium is wholly pernicious, that it demoralizes and ruins, body and soul, the consumer, and that it produces no countervailing benefits which for a moment can be compared with the evils it causes" (GBO [Batten] 1894:I:136). Batten said this was an outrageous conclusion, the result of using only atypical and very rare cases to make a point. The search for accuracy and truth mandate a focus upon the typical consumer. It is deceitful to emphasize only the extreme types that are always found among the eaters of crude opium in India, the drinkers of laudanum in England, and the opium smokers of China. Examples of excess exist everywhere. It was misleading to make generalizations and to utter silly contentions based upon exceptional incidents.

The anti-opiumist proclivity for using only cases of serious abuse ostensibly found in opium dens was just as misleading. Conclusions derived from these examples were as erroneous as those of a person

> who derived his knowledge of the effects of alcohol solely from the gin palaces, or lower drinking shops in London, should conclude that habits of intoxication, brutality, and social and physical degradation there to be seen, were typical of the mass of alcohol consumers in England; in short that everyone who was not a total abstainer was a confirmed drunkard. We know this is untrue, and that the great body of Englishmen, whether the upper or the working classes, take their liquor in

moderation, and with positive benefit to themselves. So, too, with the consumers of opium in China and India. (GBO [Batten], 1894:I:138)

The anti-opiumists also refused to tell the public that in many cases even the most serious abuser began the habit in an attempt to escape suffering caused by a disease (GBO [Batten] 1894:I:138). For Batten, the rationale for initiating and continuing indulgence was, therefore, understandable and common to many human beings.

THE OPINIONS OF REPUTABLE MEDICAL PROFESSIONALS IN INDIA CONTRADICT SSOT CLAIMS ABOUT THE DANGERS OF OPIUM CONSUMPTION

Batten also asserted that eminent medical professionals rejected notions about the negative consequences of opium use as forcefully as did administrators in British India. And the former would most certainly agree with his criticism about the anti-opiumists constructing an argument using atypical cases. The thoughts of some of the medical professionals that Batten cited are mentioned earlier in this chapter. For India, there was Dr. W. B. O'Shaugnessy's 1841 observation about habitual opium eaters in Bengal living to a very old age. This discredited the anti-opiumists claim concerning premature death, and for Batten, O'Shaughnessy's statement proved that moderate opium indulgence was no more deleterious than imbibing moderate amounts of liquor (GBO [Batten] 1894:I:145). There also was Dr. D. MacPherson's 1843 depiction of the opium habit in China. He found that indulgence did not produce a "shrivelled [sic], and emaciated, and idiotic race. . . [but instead] a powerful, muscular, and athletic people, and the lower orders more intelligent and far superior in mental acquirements to those of corresponding rank in our own country" (MacPherson, quoted in GBO [Batten] 1894:I:145). A more recent study by a physician in India provided evidence that Batten found sufficiently convincing to discredit the SSOT claim about the drug inducing antisocial behavior. In 1877, a Dr. Vincent Richards published his conclusions from data collected in Balasor, located in Orissa province. The purpose of the study was to determine if opium eating predisposed an individual to crime and insanity. Richards found that people began to consume opium during an 1868 famine and continue doing so after the famine ended. Edwards did not discuss why or how nutrition was related to starting the habit, but he did conclude that opium eating

> does not conduce to either crime or insanity, since the inhabitants are a particularly law-abiding race, and the insanes are only .0069 percent of the population. (Edwards, quoted in GBO [Batten] 1894:I:145)

In Batten's mind, Balasor was not a unique situation. No correlation existed between opium consumption, crime, and insanity anywhere in India.[10] The anti-opiumists were wrong.

TERMINATING OR RESTRICTING POPPY CULTIVATION AND OPIUM PRODUCTION ANYWHERE IN SOUTH ASIA IS UNREALISTIC AND RIDICULOUS

Batten condemned anti-opiumists for making broad generalizations about China and India based upon a limited number of cases and a few experts. But he did the same thing, and his conclusions were also questionable. The man's critique of the SSOT's procedures to end production and consumption in South Asia was more credible. The organization demanded that the Government of India prevent any increase in poppy cultivation in the quasi-independent native states of Central India. This was Malwa opium. The SSOT did not want an increase in the Malwa product sold to compensate for the reduced amount of poppy grown in British India's territories. Batten said this demand was unrealistic. He claimed the opium poppy was abundantly cultivated in many districts of the country. These locales had very fluid borders. This made any attempt to curtail clandestine importation and consumption utterly futile. Equally ineffectual was the anti-opiumists' insistence that the British request the Chinese government to stop importing Malwa opium (GBO [Batten] 1894:I:143). Great Britain had no right, according to Batten, to interfere in the internal affairs of that country. And in response to the SSOT demand that the British ask the Chinese government to halt opium production in their own country, Batten barely concealed his contempt.

> I do not wish to use disrespectful language, but I can hardly believe of such a proposal with gravity. The Chinese government, who have for centuries fulminated futile edicts, threatening the heaviest pains and penalties against the growth of the poppy and the use of opium, but whose officials have never had the will or the power to enforce them, and who are known to connive at the open and unconcealed infringement of the law, are to be 'approached' by the British Government. . . . How would such a request be met? If the solemn and self-possessed Chinaman has any sense of humour, by inextinguishable laughter. (GBO [Batten] 1894:I:143–44)

Batten illustrated the proposal's foolishness by asking readers and listeners to imagine a similar event occurring in England. Before China was requested to do such a thing, he suggested, Parliament should set an example and prohibit the use of alcoholic drinks in Great Britain except for medicinal purposes. It was easy, he continued, to imagine the ensuing uproar from any attempt to "forbid by law the cultivation of the hop plant, and the growth of barley for distillation or malting; . . . [to] forbid the import of wine and spirits from the Continent of Europe and elsewhere, and then they will be in a position to 'approach' China with a prayer for the destruction of the poppy cultivation and the trade in opium" (GBO [Batten] 1894:I:144).

Just as nonsensical was the SSOT plan to implement a program similar to the 1868 Pharmacy Act, which purportedly would ensure that the drug was sold only for "legitimate medical use." Batten asked what "legitimate medical use" means. Did the phrase apply to "whole tribes of people, living in malarious and fever-stricken tracts, using the opium daily as a prophylactic?" How, in a country such as India, could one even contemplate ending public accessibility to a substance such as opium except for legitimate medical use? The idea is truly ridiculous if it meant that "no one shall be permitted to purchase opium except under the written authority of a duly certified member of the medical profession" (GBO [Batten] 1894:I:143). He asked how many doctors existed in India for opium consumers to consult? And, could anyone

> trust the Baids, [Sic] Hakims, and Pansáris, the doctors and druggists of the country, with this power? Anybody with any knowledge of India would laugh at such an idea. How then are you to meet this great practical difficulty? (GBO [Batten] 1894:I:143)

Batten believed everything the SSOT proposed in its 1890 memorial to Viscount Cross would have no effect upon ending opium smoking in China. Accepting the anti-opiumists' demands would also hinder the Government of India's ability to rule wisely and benevolently, and it would result in irrevocable harm for millions of innocent people in the country (GBO [Batten] 1894:I:146). Their health, and most of all, their pocketbook would suffer; the Indian government would lose 13 million pounds sterling in annual revenues if opium exports to Asia ended.

Batten's 24 March 1891 Society of the Arts critique of the SSOT's program for the trade's immediate end was more convincing than his attack upon their beliefs about the alleged physiological and psychological consequences of opium ingestion among Asian natives. 'Proof' obtained primarily from testimonials and opinions of British India bureaucrats and several medical professionals from earlier decades was dubious verification.

Defenders of the trade after Batten attempted to do what he started: attack the anti-opiumist medical arguments and use health professionals with much India experience to do it. In the interim, Batten's tirade did not dissuade the SSOT from pushing on, and doing so successfully barely two and a half weeks later.

The SSOT Resolution of 10 April 1891:
The Anti-Opiumist Response to Batten's Critique

On 10 April 1891, Alfred Webb, newly elected to Parliament, introduced a resolution. Sir Joseph Pease, a fellow member and now the SSOT president, seconded it. Similar to the 1890 memorial Viscount Cross, the document called upon Parliament to terminate the morally indefensible opium trade, to cease issuing licenses for poppy cultivation, to stop transporting the Malwa drug, and to manufacture sufficient opium for a legitimate medical purpose and nothing more (GBO [Anti-Opium Society] 1894:I:162; Johnson 1975:311; Lowes 1966:67; Owen [1934] 1968:312, 314; Berridge & Edwards 1981:185; Scott, James Maurice 1969:107; Crafts & Leitch 1911:92).

To press the point, Pease repeatedly referred to numerous petitions he had received supporting the motion. These included "the convocations of Canterbury and York, the Wesleyan conference, the Roman Catholic Bishops, and from virtually every other important church body in the British Isles" (Owen [1934] 1968:312).

Their collective effort to mobilize the masses was indeed impressive. Lowes (1966:67) and Owen ([1934] 1968:314) say at least 2,500 petitions were circulated and 205,000 signatures collected. Another source says that Pease and other Parliamentarians received 3,352 petitions (with 192,106 signatures) demanding an immediate end of the trade (GBO [Anti-Opium Society] 1894:I:162). In either case, the Government of India took notice.

Sir James Fergusson, undersecretary for Foreign Affairs, and W. H. Smith, two spokespersons in attendance for the Government of India that day, then spoke. Anti-opiumists' were delighted when Fergusson said

> "I freely admit that the Government of India have [sic] never denied that it would be very desirable that this source of revenue should be altered. They have taken means to reduce it, and they have diminished the area on which the poppy is grown." (Quoted in Owen [1934] 1968:295)

Smith then persuaded hesitant anti-opiumists to agree that "deficiencies in the Indian budget might be made good by grants from the imperial treasury, stating that the government would oppose the [SSOT] motion unless such a provision were added" (Owen [1934] 1968:313). To placate the Government of India, Sir Robert Fowler suggested that such a provision be added to the Webb and Pease resolution. The House proceeded to debate the merits of the original resolution. After nearly four hours of discussion, the amendment that forced the British treasury to compensate the Government of India for forfeited income was introduced (Johnson 1975:311). However, the late hour forced Parliament to adjourn before a vote on the reimbursement issue could be taken (Owen [1934] 1968:313).

Pease was pleased with the Government of India's declaration and decided to forgo calling for a vote. He had reason to be elated. Only two liberal members of Parliament had voted against the resolution, and there was a good chance the resolution would pass if the Liberal Party dominated the next election (Johnson 1975:311). Pease also realized pro-trade activists might use Fowler's amendment to persuade British citizens that they had to pay for the lost Indian revenue. English taxpayers would object and not reelect any representative voting for the amended resolution. This, he reasoned, would threaten members of Parliament who harbored anti-opiumist sentiments (GBO [Baines] 1895a:VI:168, Johnson 1975:311).

Pease's decision not to force a vote on the revenue reimbursement provision was a mistake. Two weeks later the Undersecretary of State for India announced that Fergusson had either been instructed to mislead anti-opiumists in Parliament or had spoken only for himself. Henceforth, the Government of India rejected SSOT claims about the 1891 resolution reflecting its intent to reduce poppy cultivation. Gladstone, the foremost liberal party member of Parliament, said the Fergusson and Smith comments indicated an opinion and nothing else.

The SSOT insisted otherwise. It interpreted the "no vote" of 10 April 1891 as Parliament's acknowledgment that the trade was ethically indefensible. The anti-opiumists then declared a "moral victory" (Johnson 1975:311).

It was a hollow triumph. The Government of India had no intention of reducing poppy acreage. And if forced to do so, the amended resolution required reimbursement from the Imperial treasury. Supporters of the trade added insult to injury several months later. On 27 July, Mr. A. Godley, undersecretary of state for the India Office, submitted to the House of Commons a monograph written by a Dr. Watt. The author of several monographs about Indian opium, Watt's credentials as an authority were impressive, and he undoubtedly influenced some undecided Parliamentarians perusing the document. His argument was a pro-trade political and economic commentary about anti-opiumists' depiction of physiological and psychological processes. Although acknowledging the existence of much material about the chemistry of opium and its alkaloids, Watt used none of it in critiquing the anti-opiumists. It apparently was not necessary. He "disproved" the SSOT's portrayal of bad things happening to people by simply dismissing the scenario as unrealistic. The anti-opiumists' argument for the Indian government desisting from *all* involvement in poppy cultivation and drug production was predicated on faulty theory and guaranteed much harm for India's population (GBS [Watt] 1891:25). The British administration would be immoral if it merely grew the poppy and left drug manufacturing and sale to others. The SSOT also incorrectly assumed the Chinese government really wanted to curtail consumption within their country, whereas nothing happened when it had a chance to do after the 1857 Chefoo Convention. Pease's efforts in Parliament were, therefore, a waste of time. Watt proceeded to reject the man's allegations about the analogy between the slave trade and commerce in opium (GBS [Watt] 1891:25–8).

Watt's critique did not deter the SSOT, because in March 1892 it sent another memorial to the Secretary of State. The document expressed continued dissatisfaction with the Government of India's opium policy in Burma. The SSOT balanced its accusation by recognizing the beneficial changes produced by the government since the last memorial. It, however, warned that additional measures were required to further reduce consumption. Moreover, nobody had yet articulated a convincing argument that regulations for selling opium in Great Britain were inappropriate for India (GBO [Baines] 1895a:VI:168). The Secretary of State did not respond to the memorial. Another official did react.

The person was Dr. F. J. Mouat, a retired government medical inspector in India. His experience with opium began in 1840 when given the responsibility for estimating morphine content in opium cakes exported to China. Mouat claimed this work qualified him for critiquing the anti-opiumist argument, a line of reasoning he chastised as being prompted by passion and invalidated by erroneous facts. Both traits had no place in scientific discourse (Mouat 1892:959–60). Opium eating in India, he asserted, was far less detrimental than drinking alcohol. Opium eaters did not beat their wives, and they were not guilty of other antisocial acts as was frequently the case with alcohol consumers. Mouat warned that preventing Indians from obtaining opium would result in increased use of the much more harmful alcohol or ganja (Mouat 1892:960–61; Parssinen 1983:90–1).[11]

Mouat also derided the SSOT's distinction between medical and nonmedical use as a useless dichotomy in South Asia. The drug had positive benefits regardless of how it was ingested and the reason given for its consumption. Although Mouat admitted this was

> not the place to discuss the physiological and therapeutic action of opium in the treatment of disease, . . . I believe it to be undoubted that it is a valuable febrifuge and pick-me-up in the fevers of all alluvial and marshy soils. . . . The older, and some of them are among the best, writers on tropical disease placed great and well-founded reliance upon it. I have myself used it in my hospital practice in cases of pernicious remittent fevers, where there was an intolerance to quinine, and I had no reason to be disappointed with it. (Mouat 1892:960)

He provided statistical data from 1843 about people who had been admitted for 'fever' and other maladies. This material indicated that opium eaters fared neither better nor worse regarding prolonged illness or mortality (Mouat 1892:960). The absence of a correlation, for Mouat, sufficed to prove that opium was not dangerous. The data obtained from marshy areas clearly corroborated the Government of India's position about the drug doing much good. Mouat most likely was appalled by what happened in Parliament soon after publication of his comments.

August, 1892: Gladstone as Prime Minister and Liberals in Power

Pease's 10 April 1891 optimism was prescient. The Liberal Party was elected to power in August 1892. Gladstone, now eighty-two years old, became prime minister. Three members of Gladstone's cabinet were SSOT members and there were approximately 240 anti-opiumists in the new House of Commons (Johnson 1975:311; GBO [Baines] 1895a:VI:168–69; Owen [1934] 1968:313; Berridge & Edwards 1981:186). Sympathizers also held many government positions. George Russell, parliamentary secretary at the India Office, was one of them (Berridge & Edwards 1981:185). The pivotal official was, however, the Secretary of State for India. The Earl of Kimberley, a pro-trade advocate, still held the position. An SSOT delegation visited Russell, Kimberley's undersecretary. Members of the group implored their fellow anti-opiumist to persuade Kimberley to accept SSOT demands.

The SSOT executive board waited in vain for two months. Then, in November 1892, eighty-five SSOT officers signed still another memorial and sent it to Kimberley. The document, written to appeal to Kimberley's moral sensitivity and pragmatism, was the clearest exposition to date of the anti-opiumists' sense of mission, their belief in the prospect of unrecognized benefits for all parties involved, and how to fulfill this mission. Kimberley's response to this seminal document was a forecast of things to come regarding Parliamentary discourse about the purpose of the future Royal Commission on Opium.

The memorial begins by reiterating the controversial interpretation of the events of 10 April 1891. It stipulates that adoption of the resolution by a majority of thirty-one votes was tantamount to a confession; the House of Commons viewed the opium monopoly as morally indefensible (GBO [Anti-Opium Society] 1894:I:162–63). The SSOT then proposed steps to eliminate this blight. Details differed slightly from previous provisions in order to refute the most recent pro-trade objections.

The SSOT wanted an immediate prohibition of licensing for poppy cultivation in areas of India under direct British control. No opium was to be manufactured in India other than that required for legitimate medical purposes (GBO [Anti-Opium Society] 1894:I:162–63). The principle also determined who could obtain the drug. The SSOT continued to believe that a system patterned after the 1868 British Pharmacy Act would control domestic consumption in India. The anti-opiumists stipulated that "sale of poisonous drugs is to be restricted to medical and scientific use, and that the discretionary powers for such sale should be entrusted only to responsible and carefully-selected persons, who possess adequate knowledge of the deleterious properties of these drugs, who can readily be called upon to account for any improper use of the discretion conferred upon them, and whose remuneration in no degree depends on the amount of their sales" (GBO [Anti-Opium Society] 1894:I:163). The SSOT qualified its previous declarations about the central India [Malwa] transit trade. It now called for reduction, not termination. However, the commerce should stop altogether if opium from these native states was destined for nonmedical purposes (GBO [Anti-Opium Society] 1894:I:162–63).

The memorial also warned members of the House of Commons who were wedded to the status quo. They should realize there is widespread hostility to the trade's continuance "amongst the thoughtful people of this country, and especially amongst the Christian Churches." The British people are upset "by trading in an article which is prepared for vicious uses, which brings misery to countless myriads [sic] in China and other Eastern lands, and the sale of which, in our own country, is subject to restrictions based on its recognition by the entire medical profession as a dangerous poison" (GBO [Anti-Opium Society] 1894:I:162).

Furthermore, the politicians who were hostile to the steps adumbrated above should remember that the several thousand petitions during the 1891 session of Parliament had become outdated. This material contained approximately 200,000 signatures. The number had now increased to 271,680. The SSOT message was obvious: recalcitrant Parliamentarians in future elections would experience the public's wrath.

To encourage compliance, the SSOT gave credit to the Government of India where it was due. They congratulated Sir Alexander MacKenzie, chief commissioner for Burma, for his endorsement of its 1890 plea that opium sales in that province be severely curtailed. The memorial also credited him for recommending that Chinese opium smokers in Burma not be exempt from these restrictions. MacKenzie's courage was an example for other officials because additional measures to reduce opium sales were necessary in Burma and in other locales. There has to be, for example, an immediate halt to the licensing of poppy cultivators in the Punjab province (GBO [Baines] 1895a:VI:168; Spangenberg 1976:241–42). The Government of India effort to reduce the number of opium chests offered for sale thus far was encouraging, but

> we are unable to recognize them as satisfying the conscientious objections of the Christian and thoughtful people of this country to the existing system. The scope of these measures obviously falls short of carrying out the resolution which the House of Commons has approved. (GBO [Anti-Opium Society] 1894:I:162)

The SSOT again attempted to end administrators' reluctance to what it assumed was the sentiments of the public and Parliament. The anti-opiumists claimed the English people would be very willing to compensate the Government of India for any revenue loss that might result from the trade's termination. The English taxpayer would have to compensate nobody if administrators in South Asia were truly efficient in governing their part of the British Empire. The key was to implement cost-saving measures.

The SSOT then enumerated the long-term economic and social effects of its resolution. It was euphoric about the consequences of terminating the sale of British India's Provision opium in Calcutta. Money that Chinese citizens wasted on opium would be used to purchase products manufactured in Great Britain and on non-opium related goods from India. This in turn would persuade other European nations to stop distributing the drug throughout Asia (GBO [Anti-Opium Society] 1894:I:164). The end result was goodwill and prosperity for all parties involved and all of it was drug-free (GBO [Baines] 1895a:168–69). The Reverend Griffith John of the London Missionary Society, a veteran of thirty-five years of proselytizing in the city of Hankow, stated it well. China, he proclaimed, "may begin to glorify God in us" and would rid itself of the centuries' old hostility to the west and all nations, east and west, would commence friendly, trusting trade with each other (John, quoted by the Anti-Opium Society, in (GBO [Anti-Opium Society] 1894:I:164). And most important, the

> message of salvation will once again resume its westward course. America will be stirred up to a holy and generous emulation. From the western shores of that continent and by railway access to its northern hills and plains, thousands of ardent evangelists from the British Isles, from the United States, from the Canadian Dominion, with the Gospel in their hearts and on the lips, will speed forward, with the sun, to the abodes of this ancient but still vigorous nation, will supply the lamentable defects of the noble but mournful teaching of Confucius, and will sow seeds of Divine Truth, that may grow up in a soil still strange to it, and yield at length some new proof of its transforming power, to the glory of Him who is Truth and who is Love. 'Glory be to God in the highest; on earth peace, goodwill towards men.' (GBO [Anti-Opium Society] 1894:I:165)

The SSOT ended this dithyrambic proclamation with an equally emotional plea specifically addressed to Lord Kimberley. The anti-opiumists "desire no greater honour for your Lordship and for the Government of which you are a member, than that you may be the instrument in the Divine hands of bringing about so blessed a consummation" (GBO [Anti-Opium Society] 1894:I:165).

Lord Kimberley's Response to the November 1892 SSOT Memorial

Kimberley had no desire to be an instrument for any kind of consummation envisaged by anti-opiumists. His response to the memorial was negative. He first said many members of Parliament still had serious reservations about assumptions implicit in the March 1892 SSOT document. Anti-opiumists' correspondence and activities since then continued to misconstrue Chinese intentions. The Chinese had demonstrated no desire to stop the trade and there was no indication they would do so in the future. Despite SSOT optimism about cost-cutting measures in India, and despite the Chinese purchasing non-opium western goods to offset loss of opium revenue, it was unfair and unrealistic to force taxpayers in the United Kingdom to assume such a debt if the scenario was wrong. Furthermore, while most members of Parliament now conceded some restriction upon opium sales and consumption was beneficial, few saw any sense in supporting the SSOT demand for excessive regulation of opium, especially in a distant country. As for the Burma question, the authorities were unanimous.

> [T]he Burman race was affected by the drug in a manner very different from that in which the Indian population was affected, and, whilst it had been found practicable to restrict the use of the drug to Chinese, Shans, and hill tribes in the Upper division of the Province, it had not been then decided whether the necessary machinery was available in the Lower division to enable the authorities to enforce the same system there, and the inquiries on this point alone delayed the introduction of uniformity in practice throughout. (GBO [Baines] 1895a:VI:169)

Lord Kimberley said he was speaking for all members of Parliament in rejecting one of the SSOT's key medical arguments. The opium–alcohol analogy had no scientific merit and any program based upon its veracity was impractical. Regulations governing alcohol use in Great Britain are not a model for any program to reduce opium consumption in India. The two countries were too different and so were the two products. There also were far more pernicious drugs in the subcontinent causing much greater damage than opium, and any attempt to stop Indians from using the latter would only increase clandestine sales (GBO [Baines] 1895a:VI:169).

Kimberley also did not tolerate indiscretions from subordinates in the battle against anti-opiumists. Neither did the Government of India. An illustration was the aforementioned Sir Alexander MacKenzie. Upon leaving the position of chief commissioner of Burma on 30 April 1892, he expressed agreement with the anti-opiumist position. The unfortunate MacKenzie "had helped [to] create an embarrassing financial crisis for the Government of India, and had inadvertently committed the greatest faux pas of his career . . . [when he] failed to consider the financial consequence of such a policy for the Government of India"

(Spangenberg 1976:240). MacKenzie had said the wrong thing at the wrong time. British India's administration believed that "any campaign to limit opium in Burma, especially the total prohibition proposed by the Chief Commissioner, might well become an opening wedge for an attempt to stop the sale of opium elsewhere" (Spangenberg 1976:241). MacKenzie also suffered from being cited in the SSOT November memorial as favoring almost total prohibition of opium throughout the province. He allegedly recommended complete prohibition in the northern tract and selling the drug only through licensed brokers in lower Burma. MacKenzie's superior chastised him for poor judgment and gave no assurance about future advancement. Despite the indiscretion, he was appointed Lieutenant Governor of Bengal in 1895. His resignation twenty-eight months later ended a long career in India (Spangenberg 1976:239, 242–43).

In contrast to the SSOT, pro-trade activists had infrequently solicited support from the Anglo-European medical community. The Government of India and its supporters now recognized the importance of physicians' testimony in refuting their opponents' arguments. Opinions from Sir George Birdwood, Dr. William James Moore, and several others had been welcomed, but additional confirmation from medical personnel with experience in India was needed. The administration got it on 11 May 1892.

The Calcutta Medical Society

Speakers at the fifth meeting of the Calcutta Medical Society (May 1892) were alarmed about the SSOT's affiliation with Norman Kerr's Society for the Study of Inebriation. The fear prompted them to send excerpts of the convention's proceedings to Parliament in the form of a memorial.[12] The document is important. It is the first time that an indigenous organization composed of physicians had attacked the SSOT. Conference attendees had many years of experience in the country. And some of them had had prolonged contact with opium consumers in East India, especially in the city of Calcutta.

The document is also important because it shows how much these physicians knew about opium. They evince no awareness about the numerous analyses of the mother drug and its alkaloids. For them, opium remained an undifferentiated whole. They were oblivious to, or chose to ignore, that the proportions of active ingredients produced the varied physiological and psychological reactions long noted in human beings. They also said nothing about the role of environmental factors in determining the quantity and potency of alkaloids. The conference attendees apparently assumed that all opium was the same regardless of the variables that affected its actual contents from year to year, from field to field, and from region to region.

The comments of Surgeon–Lieutenant–Colonel A. Crombie, who read the first paper, comprise most of the document. Crombie, a member of the Indian Medical Service, was not a neutral observer.

Crombie said there were no evil consequences associated with the drug because excessive consumption was rare among all castes and occupational strata in the country. Hindus, Muslims, Sikhs, and other religious communities also used opium sparingly. He claims that numerous medical practitioners and western people having much experience in India agree (GBO [Calcutta Medical Society] 1894:II:411–20).

Crombie acknowledged that medical men in every part of the world were familiar with the negative effects of alcohol. But he rejected SSOT allegations about the detrimental consequences of eating opium (GBO [Calcutta Medical Society] 1894:II:407). And he was especially upset about a petition supposedly signed by 5,000 medical men in Great Britain. The misguided souls had declared the drug and spirits were equally harmful to human health. No evidence from India supported this contention. The only thing the two substances had in common, which he called an example of "perfect parallelism," was that opium in India and alcohol in Great Britain were offered to friends and guests as expressions of hospitality.

Crombie did classify alcohol and opium as stimulants affecting mental capabilities and he believed the initial effect of each substance was "excitation of the mental functions" (GBO [Calcutta Medical Society] 1894:II:408). No similarity between the two existed beyond this, so postulating an analogy was spurious.

For Crombie, DeQuincey's early nineteenth-century opium experiences, and Addison's observations about spirits, proved that a person who consumed alcohol over a period of time experienced a "blunting of the highest cerebral functions." A man's intoxication from liquor also produced situations in which "emotions are let go." This resulted in expressions of "eternal friendship, he weeps and blubbers, or he is furious and aggressive, staggers home, and assaults his wife in a brutal fashion before he sinks into the vomit and bestiality of a drunken sleep" (GBO [Calcutta Medical Society] 1894:II:408).

The opium eater's experience was much different. Any amount of the drug affected muscular coordination far less than the same quantity of alcohol. Furthermore, all reputable authorities indicated "that under the primary influence of small doses there is increased mental keenness; the individual has the power of directing his energies with greater force to any particular object, and he is enabled to do well whatever he wishes." For Crombie, even massive doses were relatively benign. They engendered a "state of calmness, and sometimes lassitude," not the revolting characteristics common to people drunk on alcohol (GBO [Calcutta Medical Society] 1894:II:408).

Crombie also rejected the SSOT argument about opium eating damaging internal organs and shortening life spans. They were correct about alcohol but nothing bad happens when people ingest moderate amounts of the drug. And moderation, he proclaimed, was the norm in India. SSOT agitators only use the atypical abuser of opium—the consumer of excessively large amounts—to generalize, and it was not too difficult to find examples of premature death ostensibly resulting from massive internal organ damage.

Crombie cited scientists and data from different places in the world to support his critique. Christison, for example, found no emaciated and shriveled opium smokers in China and no evidence indicating damage to tissues and organs. Crombie also alluded to data from England and the British Isles that cast doubt on the opium habit being dangerous to health and longevity. He did not, however, identify references (GBO [Calcutta Medical Society] 1894:II:409).

Opium is not, as the SSOT proclaimed, a dangerous poison because most substances are toxic if consumed in sufficient quantity. The organizations also erred about opium consumption causing insanity. There are no data from India to support either allegation. Crombie then compares statistics from lunatic asylums, prisons, and other locales in Burma and Bombay Presidency with alcohol-induced insanity data from Europe. The two substances are simply not comparable (GBO [Calcutta Medical Society] 1894:II:410–11). The tone of Crombie's comments suggests that the SSOT's hyperbole might be the only form of mental illness associated with the drug. The organization, he recommends, might perform a public service for India if its members recognized "that the prematurely senile and decrepit opium-eater is the exception and not the rule, and that the rule is rather a godly, righteous and sober life, and a hale, hearty, and respected old age" (GBO [Calcutta Medical Society] 1894:II:410).

The eight Indian physicians presenting papers at the meeting agreed with Crombie. Drs. Koylash Chunder Sen, Jaganath Ghosh, Debendra Nath Roy, D. Chuckravarti, D. M. Moir, Ram Moy Roy, and Amrita Lal also concluded that restricted availability to opium would prompt people to increase their consumption of the much more onerous alcohol and ganja. Furthermore, the vast majority of law-abiding Indian citizens preferred opium to either of the aforementioned because it was inexpensive, and

> . . . it is little harmful and seems to offer them some protection against malaria . . . [and] [t]he peasantry of Bengal take to these intoxicants, not from vice, but because of the miseries of their lives, their ague, their rheumatism and the hardness of their lot, and they will probably do so 'as long as the heart has passions, as long as life has woes.' And if it is so, if it is to be a question of alcohol, or ganja, a thousand times let it be opium. (GBO [Calcutta Medical Society] 1894:II:420)

The eighth person, and the only Indian physician to voice pessimism about opium use, was Dr. Boyle Chunder Sen, whose "more gloomy view . . . cannot . . . be accepted without considerable qualification" since his colleagues provide documentation to the contrary (GBO [Calcutta Medical Society] 1894:II:419). The leaders of the Calcutta Medical Society wanted no negative comments to sully their memorial.

Parliamentary Debate of 30 June 1893

The SSOT, sensing that momentum was swinging in its favor, wanted no change in the 1892 memorial. Parliament must acknowledge the opium trade as morally indefensible. Issuing licenses for poppy cultivation without just cause must be stopped immediately. And there must be an end to drug shipments from the landlocked native states of Central India. This provision denied these enclaves of poppy cultivation access to the coast, thereby terminating the export of their pernicious product.

Pease had no quarrel with these goals. It was the economic ramifications of the fourth document that bothered him. He knew that no politician would vote for a bill that forced English taxpayers to compensate the Government of India for revenue loss if cost-saving measures were insufficient. To condone such a thing was political suicide. The next SSOT resolution had to be modified and the change had to accomplish two things: (1) compel the Government of India to comply with Christian moral precepts in reformulating its drug policy, and (2) enable sympathetic Parliamentarians to implement the SSOT resolution without jeopardizing their political careers.

Pease prevailed. On 30 June 1893, Alfred Webb introduced a modified version of the resolution. The four demands remained the same. The change was a proposal that called for the creation of a special body, a neutral entity to address the fourth demand. This commission would identify what could be done to reduce the civil and military expenses incurred in ruling India. It also would determine what kind of help or money Great Britain would have to provide to offset revenue loss created by the suppression of the opium trade (GBO [Baines] 1895a:VI:169–70).

Prime Minister Gladstone and other liberals now in power seized upon SSOT willingness to accept an investigative body as an opportunity to resolve a controversial domestic problem unrelated to opium. Gladstone's bill for Irish Home Rule was doomed in Parliament unless he could get pro-opiumist votes (Owen [1934] 1968:314, 316; Scott, James Maurice 1969:107). Long sympathetic to the anti-opiumist cause, this consummate politician also was pragmatic.

The SSOT wanted the Commission to investigate, in England and in India, *how* the trade between China and India *was* to be terminated, *how* the English opium monopoly in India *could* be suppressed, and *how* the Indian government *might* be reimbursed for the loss of revenue. But Lord Kimberley, the secretary of state for India, threatened to resign from office before consenting to a surrender of the opium revenue. He pressured Gladstone to accept an alternative wording. Kimberley's resignation would strengthen pro-trade hostility to the SSOT and a loss of votes for the Irish Home Rule bill. Much to the chagrin of many SSOT members, the prime minister capitulated to Kimberley's demands (Lowes 1966:68).

The Commission's mission statement was reworded. It was to investigate *if* opium should be prohibited except for medical purposes, to inquire *if* opium consumption had negative physical and moral consequences. It also was to determine what measures *could be taken if* anti-opiumists' proposals were not followed, and what did the citizens of India think about prohibiting the trade? Anti-opiumists were unable to organize a united front to oppose the rewording. Parliament then accepted Gladstone's amendment by a vote of 185 to 108 (Johnson 1975:312; Lowes 1966:59; Owen [1934] 1968:315–16; Scott, James Maurice 1969:107; Berridge & Edwards 1981:186).

The creation of a special investigative body was a hollow victory for anti-opiumists. A resolution establishing a timetable for quickly ending the onerous trade first in India and then throughout Asia had been transformed into a debate as to whether there was going to be anything done at all (Lowes 1966:68; Johnson 1975:312; Brown, J. B. 1973:107–08; also see Owen [1934] 1968:315–17). Gladstone had diverted the forthcoming inquiry away from *any* consideration of opium smoking in China, the anti-opiumists' major issue for many years, to opium eating in India. This was bad news for the SSOT; it had much less data about the practice compared to the material for China (Lowes 1966:68). Nonetheless, the organization's leadership tried to portray Gladstone's perfidy as progress in eliminating evil from the world. It was not.[13]

The Government of India now had time to organize a potent defense in India, a region they controlled. British administrators and pro-trade supporters could influence, much more so than in China, the kind of data to be placed before the Commission and the type of witness to be interviewed. In short, the investigation was amenable to management. Anti-opiumists were not blind to this possibility. Nonetheless, optimistic members remained confident their views would prevail, and that the Commission's revelations would vindicate their stance. The absolute correctness of their goal, consequently, would eventually triumph regardless of what pro-trade advocates proffered (Berridge & Edwards 1981:186).

Other anti-opiumists disagreed. The National Righteousness felt the Commission now had the opportunity to "whitewash the problem, delay effective decisions, and give the treacherous Indian government considerable power in influencing the findings" (Johnson 1975:312). The periodical's warning was justified.

The British Indian Association's Condemnation of the SSOT and the Royal Commission Mission

Calcutta's business community quickly expressed its discontent. Messieurs Narendra Krishna and Rajkumar Sarvadhikari, vice president and secretary, respectively, of the Committee of the British Indian Association, sent a memorial to the Honorable Sir Anthony Patrick MacDonnell, the Lieutenant Governor of Bengal on 23 August 1893. They objected to a minority of English Parliamentarians acting contrary to the wishes of the majority. They also decried the SSOT goal to restrict or eliminate opium use as utopian because narcotic consumption had existed everywhere from time immemorial and "a divine origin is claimed for its introduction." The document provides no more details about this spiritual source (GBO [British Indian Association] 1894:II:313).

Krishna and Sarvadhikari and the people they speak for also reject the opium and alcohol analogy. Opium, they assert, is less harmful than alcohol even when the drug is used in excess. It also causes no crime anywhere in the world. And for some people *Papaver somniferum Linn* was necessary for survival. Evidence for this claim was the "very large number of the poorer portion of the population . . . particularly . . . the cultivators of the soil in the swamps, marshes and inundated lands of Lower Bengal, as also for night watchmen, palki-bearers and fishermen in such parts." Prohibition would result in the death of many poor people. Another consequence was the possibility of large-scale unrest and rebellion in the countryside. It also was inevitable that people whose desire for opium remained unfulfilled would turn to liquor "which . . . memorialists cannot but believe would be socially and morally a great curse to the people" (GBO [British Indian Association] 1894:II:313).

Krishna and Sarvadhikari concluded with a plea to the Lieutenant Governor to convey their objections to His Excellency the Governor-General of India. The creation of the Royal Commission was a travesty and India's citizens should not be forced to pay its expenses during its stay in the subcontinent. The "promotion of the scheme," according to the authors, "is due more to misguided philanthropy than to sound statesmanship" (GBO [British Indian Association] 1894:II:313).

The Calcutta Missionary Conference Response: Critique of the Pro-Trade Scenario and Its Castigation of Unethical Attempts to Influence the Forthcoming Royal Commission Investigation

Less than a month later, on 21 September 1893, a missionary organization castigated the behavior of groups such as the British Indian Association. The missionaries said the conduct was a violation of parliamentary rules. The Reverend J. Brown, chairperson of the Calcutta Missionary Conference, presented a memorial to His Excellency the Viceroy and Governor-General of India in Council and requested that the document be brought to the attention of the appropriate authorities in London. Brown protested the sudden appearance of pro-trade arguments by "public bodies" as an unethical attempt to prejudice the forthcoming Royal Commission investigation in India. He wanted to make clear that positions espoused by organizations such as the British Indian Association do not represent everyone's opinion in India (GBO [Calcutta Missionary Association] 1894:II:314). People belonging to these kinds of organizations are nonphysicians. They are pontificating about topics beyond their expertise and their statements lack credibility.

Brown first challenged the pro-traders' hostility to using Great Britain's opium policy as a model for India. He claimed that all standard works on drugs that were recognized as authoritative textbooks in Indian and British Colleges, as well as in courts of law, concur about a principle issue. All of them abundantly affirm opium's classification as a poison, and that the drug should be available only with a medical prescription. Brown cited the opium research of Sir Benjamin Brodie, Drs. Brunton, Ringer, Pereira, Garrod, and many others. He believed their cautionary observations about the drug justified "dealing with it in India as it has been dealt with by law in Britain" (GBO [Calcutta Missionary Association] 1894:II:314).

The Government of India harmed the country by allowing easy accessibility to the drug and encouraging consumption. The administration's behavior was immoral when, in some cases, officials created a desire for the product where none existed before. And it was loathsome for British India to manufacture vast quantities for export to other countries. Brown asked how could the British, who now restricted distribution of the drug in their own country, tolerate such a different situation in a nation over which they were attempting to rule wisely and fairly? He said that the public press deepens this conviction because it reports numerous deaths from opium poisoning. These are cases of homicide and suicide. It was indeed very peculiar, Brown lamented. Officials claim opium to be a dangerous substance in one sentence. Then, in the next utterance, they defend its continued production and distribution in the next utterance (GBO [Calcutta Missionary Association] 1894:II:314).

Ignorance, according to Brown, compounded the contradiction. He categorized pro-opiumists' assertion that drug restriction would lead to increased abuse of alcohol as a "mere assumption, equally difficult to prove or disprove, because it is based on no authenticated experience or known scientific or historical analogy" (GBO [Calcutta Missionary Association] 1894:II:314). Even esteemed members of the British establishment supported the anti-opiumist position. For example, Sir Thomas Wade, the deceased British minister in China, declared in one of his publications that the drug in China was

> a habit many times more pernicious, nationally speaking, than the gin and whisky drinking, which we deplore at home. It takes possession more insidiously, and keeps its hold to the full as tenaciously . . . [and the result is] steady descent, moral and physical, of the smoker. (Quoted in GBO [Calcutta Missionary Association] 1894:II:313)

Then there was the testimony of Sir Dennis Fitzpatrick, whom Brown referred to as an "expert." In a Government of India dispatch dated 4 October 1891, Fitzpatrick said "that there are places in India, where, owing to a want of proper supervision or control, abuses have prevailed, which at least strike one with greater horror than any corresponding abuse in countries which are demoralized by drink" (Fitzpatrick, quoted in GBO [Calcutta Missionary Association] 1894:II:314). This kind of evidence prompted Brown and his fellow missionaries to declare that "if drink is quantitatively, opium is qualitatively, the more demoralizing evil" (GBO [Calcutta Missionary Association] 1894:II:314).

Brown continued his attack. The experts cited above, and firsthand observers in India such as Dr. Valentine of Jeypore, had discredited sentiments about opium being both necessary and "most beneficial" to Rajputs and "other warlike races" in India. There also was no possibility that cessation of China's opium imports would force its citizens to procure the drug elsewhere.

Brown provided no evidence to support the declaration, but did say that the Government of India would benefit by doing the right thing. Past "[e]xperience," he continued, "has proved that the abandonment of evil habits has always brought material as well as moral prosperity" (GBO [Calcutta Missionary Association] 1894:II:314). The experience being referred to is not specified. Brown also critiqued other pro-opium arguments and remained confident that the British administration would follow the moral path. This meant embracing a policy guaranteeing India's people that the amount necessary for legitimate medical use would determine the number of acres cultivated in poppy and the quantity of opium manufactured (GBO [Calcutta Missionary Association] 1894:II:315).

Lyall's Outrage and the Government of India

Mr. D. R. Lyall, a Government of India official, read the Calcutta Missionary Conference memorial on the day it was submitted to the Governor-General. Lyall was infuriated by the missionaries' insinuation that the Government of India condoned behavior contrary to the instructions of Parliament. He immediately wrote a stinging denial in which Brown and his colleagues were accused of inventing data, misquoting sources, and taking statements out of context. The "scientific" data that made the SSOT and moral arguments of other antiopiumists more palatable to observers was, consequently, suspect. Lyall first questioned the accuracy of the authorities Brown cited when classifying opium as a poison. He claimed Sir Benjamin Brodie's statements about opium being a poison could not be located for verification. Therefore, Brodie's view about the topic carried no weight (GBO [Lyall] 1894:II:315). Lyall attacked Brown's other experts; Brunton was qualified to speak about therapeutics, but he never investigated opium eating. This made him an opium nonexpert engaged in perpetuating popular misconceptions. The Missionary Conference memorial also performed a disservice for Dr. Ringer because the people who wrote it used only partial statements beneficial to their cause. They ignored everything else. Ringer's comments about toxicity applied only to excessive use of the drug. Brown, however, failed to mention that Ringer found moderate use of the opiate no more detrimental to health than tobacco smoking. Ringer said the same thing about alcohol; moderate use did no harm but this might not be true for excessive consumption. Brown's use of the esteemed Dr. Pereira's ideas also was suspect. Pereira, according to Lyall, was decrying the condition of "an opium wreck" and not the typical user who consumed opium in moderate amounts.

Dr. Eatwell, Lyall asserted, provided accurate information about the effects of opium smoking. The missionaries would do everybody a favor if they read what he wrote. Eatwell did acknowledge negative consequences of excessive consumption. He also recognized that "morbid impulses" did explain some cases of abuse just as they did in England for alcohol, but the primary cause regarding opium was a desire to find relief from a painful disease. Eatwell unequivocally rejected any claim that habitual use of opium by the masses in India or in China was injurious to their mental, moral, or physical health. Indeed, there was no proof that the moderate consumption of alcohol or opium was harmful to anyone. Alcohol abuse was another matter; it was far more disastrous for society than excessive opium consumption. Eatwell, with Lyall's blessing, asked the reader to "[c]ompare the furious madman, the subject of delirium tremens with the prostrate debauchee, the victim of opium; the violent drunkard with the dreaming sensualist intoxicated with opium; the latter is at least harmful to all except his wretched self, whilst the former is but too frequently a dangerous nuisance, and an openly bad example to the community at large" (Eatwell, quoted in GBO [Lyall] 1894:II:316).

Lyall thought Brown and his sympathizers continued to wallow in sloppy thinking. The missionary's use of a quotation from Dr. Garrod, for example, was unacceptably selective. Garrod was describing one case of opium poisoning from a single overdose. Lyall said the incident "has nothing to do with the habitual use or abuse of opium" (GBO [Lyall] 1894:II:316). The anti-opiumist demand for prohibition of opium use in India except for medical use also has no scientific justification. Nowhere in Brown's references is there any discussion "that opium should be used only under medical prescription and treated as a poison, or that any of them touched on the question of dealing with opium in India as it is dealt with in Britain" (GBO [Lyall] 1894:II:316–17). The Calcutta missionaries also said that opium consumption in India was increasing. Lyall claimed they had no proof for such a statement, and a lack of substantiation meant they simply had no credible argument for prohibiting Indian citizens' use of anything, especially a substance with obvious benefits. Opium, for Lyall, was "the medicine of Bengal," and it qualified as the "safest and least harmful of all habitual stimulants" when used in moderation (GBO [Lyall] 1894:II:316).

Reverend Brown's Rebuttal

On 27 November 1893, Reverend Brown responded to Lyall's attack. The sole purpose of the Calcutta Missionary document, he contended, was to ensure that British officials were provided with medical evidence demonstrating that every respected authority classified opium as a dangerous poison. Brown rejected Lyall's criticism about citing only favorable quotations. There was enough material from Brunton, for example, to infer that the man was issuing a warning about the drug's addictive potential (GBO [Brown] 1894:II:318).

Brown then mimicked his antagonist. He accused Lyall of inventing statements that Ringer had never written and then using these nonexistent utterances to rebuke the missionaries. The veracity of everything else Lyall alleged about Ringer's actual statements was equally suspect. For Brown, Lyall was no better than the people he criticized; Lyall was dangerously close to committing the sin of using self-serving quotations from Pereira (GBO [Brown] 1894:II:318). The missionary concluded his rebuttal by saying the remainder of Lyall's critique was "purely controversial, which implies defects of intelligence rather than defects of integrity" (GBO [Brown] 1894:II:319). Lyall's reaction to a missionary calling him stupid is unknown.

W. B. Phillips' Attempt to Mediate

On 30 November 1893, British government officials asked a Mr. W. B. Phillips to resolve the vitriolic dispute between Lyall and Brown. Phillips said the Calcutta Missionary organization wanted to make no public comment about its views concerning opium consumption in India before the Royal Commission's arrival in India. When the British Indian Association attempted to "prejudice the public mind, at a critical time, upon a great question," the Calcutta missionaries knew they had to show clearly that the businessmen were not speaking for a wider public. The Conference memorial was not intended to be an "exhaustive document" but only a "brief counterblast to the unexpected Memorial of the British Indian Association of August 23" (GBO [Phillips] 1894:II:319).

Phillips defended the document's accuracy. He said the people who selected the data did not believe that members of the Royal Commission on Opium would accept fictitious and erroneous statements. The missionaries also were distressed because Mr. Lyall worked for the Government of India. They believed this would unfairly increase the influence of Lyall's critique among the commission's members. The Government of India, after all, was supposed to be the entity being investigated, not the institution that evaluated what was accurate or inaccurate (GBO [Phillips] 1894:II:319).

MORALITY, SCIENCE, AND INDIA'S OPIUM DURING THE NINETEENTH CENTURY

The creation of the Royal Commission on Opium in 1893 should have delighted all of the trade's opponents. The event seemed to signify the beginning of imperial rule imbued with Christian principles of right and wrong as defined by the anti-opiumists. This was not to be.

Gladstone's reinterpretation of the controversy and Parliament's subsequent passage of the resolution ensured that each issue associated with anti-opium agitation during the preceding decades would be debated again. This time there would be no data from China. The anti-opiumist victory was, in reality, a treadmill in which the arduous process of education and persuasion had to be repeated. The argument seemed destined to go around, and around, and around once more. Pessimists admitted defeat. Optimists in the SSOT did not.

Parliament ordered the Government of India to plan the Royal Commission's itinerary and to select witnesses to testify. The administration also was instructed to assemble documents that would, ostensibly, permit an unbiased study of the question. Anti-opiumists were told to find their own witnesses in India. This was an exceptionally difficult undertaking given the meager resources at their disposal and the little time to arrange anything.

The trade's defenders expected no diminution in anti-opiumist dedication. They knew that each point presented to justify continued noninterference would be attacked with moral and "scientific" evidence to the contrary. Opponents of prohibition needed some evidence capable of persuading skeptics and neutral observers about the rashness of interfering in poppy cultivation, opium production, and distribution in India. The Government of India officials needed a thesis so convincing, a 'mission' so worthy that it would discredit rumblings about their ability to manipulate contents of the forthcoming proceedings, hence the outcome. The possibility of formulating an argument to continue the status quo capable of persuading members of Parliament, the Queen, and international opinion might be enhanced if it incorporated 'scientific' data and if it was inextricably related to the welfare of people in India. In other words, the Government of India needed an unimpeachable, empirically verifiable issue to invalidate the imminent anti-opiumist attack. It had to be a topic that the most fanatical missionary could not condemn as immoral. The anti-opiumists provided an opportunity to find one.

Common sense and science had already modified the anti-opiumists' abhorrence of opium use. The SSOT position during the last quarter of the century consistently stated that the Government of India's involvement in poppy cultivation and opium production for "legitimate medical use" was acceptable. The

SSOT's cognizance of data illuminating the utility of opium and its alkaloids for human maladies, however, provided defenders of the trade with a counterargument so impressive that few anti-opiumists challenged it. Those moralists who did so were ineffective and too late. It was in this milieu that the South Asian folk belief about eating opium to prevent and cure 'malaria' became a vehicle to invalidate many of the anti-opiumist assertions about the drug. Protecting peoples' right to consume the drug became an expression of imperial benevolence. It was conduct that befitted India's rulers from a Christian nation.

NOTES

1. Sir George Birdwood's views are discussed in the next chapter.
2. Peters says that Kerr had no pathological evidence at the time to justify the terminology and that his interpretation of addiction lacked a clear distinction between disease and vice (1981:475–76). She then describes how Francis Anstie's confirmation of aspects of Kerr's interpretation ultimately contributed to the merging of secular and religious perspectives in theories of addiction. The result was that Kerr and Anstie slid "smoothly from the physical to the moral . . . [and illustrated] the ease with which the disease model could in later years be characterized somewhat condescendingly as a 'hybrid 'disease of the will concept'" (Peters 1981:478). Berridge alludes to the same thing. She claims Kerr proves her contention that the "British version of the disease model had close links with temperance and anti-opium ideology through the concept of inebriety which linked both alcohol and opium" (1978:457). Also see Parssinen (1983:86–90) for comments about the contributions of Dr. Norman Kerr and the Society for the Study and Cure of Inebriety to the SSOT, and for Edward Levinstein's inadvertent contributions to the anti-opiumist cause.
3. The pro-traders had a point regarding opium and the sex drive. As Kathleen Lodwick explains in her description of addiction among the Chinese, "[m]any foreign doctors in China noted that opium addicts had few children and tended to blame the fact that they were interested in little but smoking. Only in the late nineteenth century did some doctors realize that opium addiction diminished sexual desires and long-time addicts had lost the ability to procreate. Even the importance of continuing the family line was of no interest to the addict. If two generations of a family were addicted, it was generally assumed that they would be the last of their line" (1976:33).

Opium consumption and diminished sex drive was one of the few pro-trade arguments that had scientific credibility.

4. Lowes says the "attack was no longer directed against China, but against its subsidiary, the Indian Government, for its control over the sources of the trade" (1966:65). This posed problems for the SSOT. Owen suggests that with passage of the Chefoo Conference provisions, "the anti-opium movement waned palpably. Coercion of the Chinese had now ceased and internal dissension, lack of funds, and above all the absence of any clear-cut purpose nearly ended its usefulness" (Owen [1934] 1968:311). Also see Berridge & Edwards (1981:180, 183) for comments regarding the effects of the Chefoo Convention upon the Society. Some SSOT members continued to disagree with the July

1885 decision to focus upon India. In 1888, the debate led to the creation of the Christian Union for the Severance of the Connection of the British Empire with the Opium Traffic. The organization published the periodical *National Righteousness*. Its editor was Benjamin Broomhall, the secretary of the China Inland Mission from 1888 until his death in 1911. The group's ideology, was "closely identified with the missionary view of things, and missionary influence among its leadership and supporters was strong" (Berridge & Edwards 1981:183–84).

5. Inglis agrees. He describes Batten's paper as a very "impressive display of its [i.e., opium trade's] supporters" (1975:92).

6. Copies of many of the regional replies are found in GBO [Appendices I–L] 1894:II:313–664. The views of people whom Batten cites are found on pages 13–64 in GBC [Consumption] 1892:1–109. This report, compiled soon after the SSOT sent its 1890 memorial to Viscount Cross, was not formally submitted to Parliament until 1892. Government of India officials were able to cite its contents in the interim (GBO [Baines] 1895a:VI:168).

7. A skeptic might conclude consumption is so great and abuse so prevalent that a brief report is inadequate to convey the problem's severity.

8. Batten provided no reference for the assertion and this author can find none. A more accurate assessment of the past and present anti-opium stance is that they either said nothing about the relationship or only referred to inhabitants of 'malarial zones' who considered opium useful as a prophylactic. Anti-opiumists' were preoccupied with the immorality stemming from opium use. The relationship between the drug and the disease was not a paramount issue in their agenda.

9. Batten selected a work specifically written to refute earlier accusations of British immorality. Edkins' list of facts is not inaccurate. The data, however, are amenable to various interpretations depending upon the commentator's ideological leaning. This characterized Edkins' statements. Other analyses of the time disagreed with his view of English motivations and about his employer engaging in nothing other than normal commercial trade. The title of Edkins' manuscript is "Historical Note on Opium and the Poppy in China." A copy of Edkins' manuscript is found in GBO [Edkins] 1894:I:146–61. Edkins mentioned several of the sources that Batten used in his argument.

10. Batten also mentioned Sir William J. Moore as providing medical information that illuminated the SSOT's facetious allegations. But Batten merely said that Moore's ideas were so well known they did not have to be repeated here (GBO [Batten] 1894:I:146). The Anglo-European medical literature of the era indicates that Moore's ideas were not as widely known as Batten implied. His prominence was restricted to a theoretically conservative segment of the British medical community in India. The explanation of disease and cure envisaged by this surgeon general of Bombay Presidency emerged as an important part of the pro-trade defense as the decade progressed. See the next chapter for a discussion of Moore's ideas.

11. Ganja [Gánja, or Gánjha] most often refers to a preparation made from hemp (Cannabis sativa). There are regional variations in India. In the "northwest provinces the term also designates an intoxicating liquor, an infusion of young flowers and leaves in water. In Bengal, the same are dried and pounded, and then used in smoking. The intoxicating property depends in either case upon the resinous exudation of the plant adhering to the vegetable substance" (Wilson, H. H. [1855] 1968:165).

12. A note in the Royal Commission document indicates the memorial also appears as a supplement to the August 1892 issue of *The Medical Gazette* under the title: "The Ef-

fects of the Habitual Use of Opium on the Human Constitution" (GBO [Calcutta Medical Society] 1894:II:407–20).

13. Anti-opiumists expressed their true feelings after Gladstone's death in 1898. According to J. F. Brown, "*The Friend of India*" politely accused the dead Liberal statesman of moral bankruptcy: 'In office, however, the man who had thus spoken out against this national inequity was again and again its defender'" (1973: 108).

4

The Serendipitous Nature of "Except for Medical Use" and Participants in the Royal Commission Hearings

INTRODUCTION

References to opium preventing and curing 'malaria' appear infrequently in the pro-trade polemic before 1879. This changed in the next decade. Anti-opiumists' use of medical evidence to support their moral argument meant that opponents could no longer dismiss SSOT accusations as hysterical foolishness. It was in this milieu of growing ethical and medical disquietude about drug consumption that the opium and 'malaria' connection emerged in official British documents and the English press. What had been a rare observation in western society about an insignificant folk belief held by some natives in India began to emerge as part of a medical justification for noninterference in any aspect of the trade.

SURGEON-GENERAL SIR WILLIAM JAMES MOORE AND SIR GEORGE BIRDWOOD

The opinions of several opium–malaria proponents appear in the public media during the 1880s. These people also are cited in memorials and testimonials presented to Parliament and in various British and Indian government department documents. The most frequently mentioned individuals are Sir William James Moore (1828–1896) and Sir George Birdwood (1834–1917). Defenders of the trade did not question the two men's assumption about composition of the drug and its effect upon human physiology and psychology. The data that Moore and Birdwood portrayed as demonstrating the preventive and curative power of opium for 'malaria' was then used to invalidate the anti-opiumist scenario.

Sir William James Moore provided them with a coherent 'medical' argument for the veracity of the folk belief based upon his long experience in Rajputana, then as the deputy surgeon-general of Bombay Presidency, and later its surgeon-general.[1] Moore's orientation is best described as "chill" theory. It was a dominant explanation of disease causation (and therapy) among influential members of the British medical establishment in India during the latter part of the nineteenth century.

Sir George Birdwood also had impressive credentials. As of 1882, he had been a professor of *materia medica*, botany, anatomy, and physiology at Grant Medical College in Bombay, and curator of the city's Government Central Economic Museum (Birdwood 1882b:230).[2] Although far better known in Great Britain than Moore, a combative style of writing did nothing to enhance the credibility of Birdwood's argument among discerning physicians. One influential English medical periodical called it farfetched.[3]

SIR WILLIAM JAMES MOORE

Surgeon-General Sir William James Moore's Work between 1880 and 1894

Moore's discussions about the relationship between 'malaria' and opium occupy two categories.[4] Items in the first category are apolitical endeavors to educate medical practitioners about maladies common in South Asia. These publications critiqued current trends in medical theory. They also presented his perspective about the cause, diagnosis, and treatment of fever and disease in India. The creations of William James Moore the scientist-cum-politician comprise the second category. These were responses to anti-opiumists' accusations. They were designed to influence the British Parliament's formulation of opium policy and to protect the Government of India's reputation among the reading public.

Moore's Apolitical Writings:
The Man as a Medical Practitioner and Scientist (1886)

One of the most informative examples of Moore's apolitical publications was the second edition of his 1886 *Manual of Diseases in India; with a Compendium of Disease Generally*.[5] Moore was dissatisfied with contemporary theories of health and sickness. He rejected observations that presented the old miasmic explanation in the guise of varieties of contagion theory. He also dismissed the role of germs. Colleagues were remiss, he tells us, for accepting notions of disease causation that Pasteur, Koch, and others had articulated several decades before 1880. The term 'germ' indicated the existence of a tangible entity. This entity could be isolated and then studied independent of its surroundings if the appropriate technology was available. Moore knew the technology for doing this did exist. However, impartial observers had not yet demonstrated that germs "long reputed to be the cause of paroxysmal fever . . . [and] credited with the excitation of a vast number of other maladies . . ." were present in water, soil, or air (Moore 1886b:258–59). For Moore, it was conjecture, not science, to say that malarious microbes caused many afflictions. The idea was as fallacious as an elusive poison in the atmosphere creating sickness. The presence of germs was, at best, a subjective assumption. Indeed, "[a]ll that we are taught regarding the characteristics and habitat of malaria has been deduced by inference from presumed consequences; . . . [from] 'its pathological action' (Moore 1886b:259).

Moore attacked other variations of the microbial theory. Equally invalid was a claim about the "bacillus formed in typhoid fever" being "the germ causing the disease [because] inoculation has not proved such to be the case" (Moore 1886b:253). The Klebs and Crudeli "discovery" of malarial bacilli in water and soil also was a mirage. So was the Marchiafava and Cuboni "confirmation" of the Klebs–Crudeli breakthrough. Moore was referring to Marchiafava and Cuboni's isolation of "spherical mobile microorganisms in the white blood-corpuscles, which, [Marchiafava and Cuboni] theorized, might be the spores of the bacilli" (Moore 1886b:268). These scientists were wrong because the so-called malarious disease

> has been found in many kinds of surfaces, so it cannot be linked to a certain kind of geological formation . . . [or to] one form of low vegetable organism. . . . It is scarcely reasonable to presume that alluvial soils, ferruginous earths, decaying granite, limestone rock, marshes, dry sand, all produce the same rather poisonous emanation, or of vegetable organism. If malarious poison is really evolved from the earth, it seems reasonable to suppose various geological structures would produce different results, and that therefore the characteristics of malarious disease would differ. Yet malarious disease prevails on all the structures named, and when typical it presents very similar characteristics everywhere. (Moore 1886b:268–69)

Moore also dismissed "periodicity," a phenomenon that Patrick Manson had detected while conducting elephantiasis research in China. Numerous other researchers subsequently verified its existence. For Moore, people are wrong if they believe periodicity is a defining characteristic of 'malaria.' Periodicity is the appearance and abatement of fever episodes. These people do not realize the "event" is "an ever-present and essential condition of all disease, but more marked in tropical climates, where atmospheric periodicity, or change, or vicissitude, is most powerfully felt by the human frame, in consequence of the debility of the skin caused by heat" (Moore 1886b:269). This ubiquity in nature meant there was nothing special about the presence of periodicity in so-called malaria, in other tropical diseases, or anywhere else it was detected. There also was no justification for associating microscopic living creatures with the phenomenon. The Anglo-European medical community's acclaim given to Manson and his supporters, Moore implied, was unjustified. Furthermore, researchers in the post-1886 era who accepted the idea of minuscule villains would discover nothing.

Moore's Rejection of the "Malarial Poison" Hypothesis (1886)

Moore credited Lancisi's 1745 belief about decaying vegetation and swamp gas with having spawned contemporary "malarial poison" explanations. But

Moore thought variations of the atmospheric miasmic theory of disease were just as unproductive as ideas about germs. None of these theories of contagion resolved the contradictions he had noted during many years in India. And the errors made by relying upon permutations of miasma theory were as serious as the fallacies preventing an accurate classification of fevers (Moore 1886b:260–66).[6]

Moore declared contemporary fever diagnosis to be a mess. Medical practitioners had, by the mid-1880s, identified more than sixty kinds of "remittent fevers" and eighty types of "typhoid fevers." Furthermore, they construed each one as a separate and distinct disease. Moore criticized this as confusing and speculative (1886b:249, 251). He also thought the mistake was understandable. Similar to his comments about "periodicity," conditions unique to the tropics caused the error. Fevers tended to "shade off into one another" in southern locales. Hence one "fever disease" that displayed distinctive characteristics in its initial stage might soon deviate from the expected scenario. An observer then confronted a confusing situation in which a fever appearing to be typhoid ended up as remittent and vice versa. Difficulties in explaining why this happens were exacerbated if the transformation occurred, as it often did in the tropics, during a brief period (Moore 1886b:249, 251–53).[7] Moore asserted that most of these fevers were deviations from "some well-recognized typical disease." They were not, contrary to his contemporaries' statements, unrelated maladies (Moore 1886b:249). Moore said he was not alone in postulating a single source of virtually all instances of elevated temperatures. Even contagion theorists believed cholera was not a separate disease. It was the "'ultimate' result of the highest intensity of that malarial poison which under other circumstances excites the mildest form of ague" (1886b:252).

Moore also concurred with these "malarial poison" theoreticians in rejecting the plethora of 'separate fevers are separate diseases' interpretation. However, his agreement with these people ended here. They had failed to isolate their villain from other variables; it still was "invisible, imponderable, and not recognizable by any chemical or other test" (1886b:259; see also pages 252–53, 259, 266–67). Malarial poison, for Moore, remained a mirage. And all people believing in the existence of a distinct entity made a questionable "inference . . . [that is] admitted by the supporters of the malaria theory" (Moore 1886b:272).

Malarial poison theoreticians also avoided explaining the significance of diurnal variations in "continual fevers." They compounded the error by refusing to realize that a "continual fever" often was virtually identical to a remittent paroxysm and an intermittent fever. In other words, they were seeing distinctions where there were none (Moore 1886b:252).

Moore condemned the "malarial poison" interpretation as simplistic and inadequate to account for the idiosyncrasies he recorded in South Asia. This prompted him to suggest that cases involving one kind of tropical fever evolving into another type were more accurately portrayed as falling along a continuum. He inclined "to the view that fevers in their several forms are further developments of the mildest form, and are due to the same causes; just as I regard a catarrh, a tonsillitis, a bronchial affection, and a pneumonia, as further developments of cold or chill, acting on the mucous membrane of the parts implicated" (Moore 1886b:253).

Proponents of "malaria poison" theory made still another mistake when they envisaged it as a substance ascending from the ground into the air during the night. They also were wrong for blaming trees for its appearance (Moore 1886b:260–66). India furnished no support for a relationship between sickness and darkness or trees. Many places remain free from fever and malaria after sunset. The malady also appeared in locales void of trees. Moore also said impure water did not "excite malarial fever" (Moore 1886:267). People forced to use dirty water in India and elsewhere suffered no more than those using clean water. While he admitted there were "numerous poisons and diseases which may be introduced into the system by water, . . . there is no necessity to add malaria to the list, in order that the importance of pure water may be demonstrated" (Moore 1886b:267). Another false lead in explaining the presence of the diseases was various environmental factors portrayed in popular and scientific literature. Moore cited nightfall, trees, and contaminated water as examples of misconceptions.[8]

Moore's Theory of the Etiology of Disease and Febrile Diseases

Moore's refutation of another observation that ostensibly proved the existence of malarial poison further illustrates his interpretation of disease etiology, fever diagnosis, and therapy. He said that miasma theoreticians postulate the clearing of land for crop planting as dangerous because "malaria" was "released" to infect a human population. Moore condemned the idea as nonsense. Removing vegetation for cultivation was arduous work, and it was

> undertaken under difficulty and discomfort. Without sufficient shelter and adequate food, and with great physical exertion, sickness would prevail whether the ground was disturbed or not. As countries become cultivated, damp is lessened, and the inhabitants are proportionately better fed and housed. Sir R. Christison attributed the cessation of ague in Scotland not to diminution of malaria, but to the people being better fed. (Moore 1886b:266–67)

Moore was suggesting that mundane social, political, and economic factors over which individuals had some control were the source of most human afflictions. This included all the examples mistakenly attributed to the mysterious, invisible entity called "malaria" and the equally nonexistent microscopic germs. The explanation of sickness was found in "exposure, in working in water, in bad food, or in the class of people employed (perhaps prisoners)" (Moore 1886b:267). The liberation of a hypothetical poison that caused sickness was irrelevant. Human misery was primarily a product of society itself, and in "any report of malarious epidemics . . . it will be found that the persons so suffering were exposed to other and recognizable causes of disease" (Moore 1886b:270).

Moore reprimanded his contemporaries for their inability to comprehend this fact. They added to the nonsense pervading medical science by failing to recognize two things: that "paroxysmal febrile diseases" were not all discrete, unrelated entities, and they also were not an undifferentiated mass. Moore eliminated the confusion in classification by postulating the existence of only two categories of fever found in the tropics and elsewhere.

Moore's Revised Fever Classification and the Nature of Disease and "Malaria" (1886)

The first category contained the "eruptive fevers" generated by a very small number of separate maladies (Moore 1886b:252, 258–59). One example was pustules associated with smallpox. He also placed skin eruptions that produced unusual disfigurement in the same category.

Comprising the second category were the remaining fevers that Moore claimed his contemporaries mistakenly recognized as different diseases. In 1874, and again in 1886, Moore said the most common type of elevated temperature in South Asia was a "mixed form of fever." He said it should be labeled "undefined climatic fevers" (1886b:274–75). Other fevers present in India were "continued fever," "enteric fever" (a term he preferred to typhoid), "typhus fever," "relapsing fever," and "cerebro-spinal fever" (Moore 1886b:275–330).

Moore's comments about the remaining fevers in this category identify them as the product of malarial plasmodia. Moore placed the varieties of tertian fevers he found in the rejected typologies in the "intermittent fever" category. All "intermittent" entries had a "cold" stage. His "typical ague" had both a "cold" and a "hot" stage. And another hint this was malaria as it is now understood was his recommendation of quinine to treat sufferers. "Remittent fever," another type, also had a "cold" stage. It was so similar to "ague" that Moore called it "exaggerated ague" (1886b:278–81).[9] The last member was a peculiar consequence of the "operation of various conditions of climate and circumstances" and he called it "masked malarial fever" (Moore 1886:333). "Masked malarial fever" was not always accompanied by a rise in the patient's pulse. The most reliable trait indicating its presence was increased excreta (Moore 1886b:330–34).[10]

Moore stated that the combined effect of diet, stress, and fatigue was the underlying cause of paroxysms in both categories. Scientists had ignored these factors simply because they were so obvious and "sensible." But Moore contended that a deficiency or excess of these items determined both the appearance and the clinical course of any "fever" malady. Poor food, excessive fatigue, and too much stress quickly disrupted a person's nervous system. Factors unique to the sufferer, to his family, to her race, and to all people in that society created the slight variations in elevated temperature. These variations were responsible for most of the confusion among medical practitioners. Moore thought his interpretation of the clinical consequences of a damaged nervous system ended the problem of inaccurate fever classification.

Continued malfunctioning of the nervous system could lead to organic damage as well as sickness with fever. The latter produced a diagnostic nightmare; elevated temperatures manifested so much diversity that observers mistakenly construed them as distinct diseases. Moore, however, maintained that an elevated temperature was neither proof nor a symptom of a separate malady; it was a "clue" to the existence of something more fundamental. People citing the hypothetical existence of "malarial poison" to explain the presence of fever were wrong. They were actually observing one gradation of "chill" or the body's external expression of a dysfunctional, disturbed nervous system. These people simply failed to realize that "all febrile disturbances . . . from a common cold, . . . affecting the Schneiderian mucous membrane, to severe typhoid affecting the intestinal mucous membrane, are characterized by . . . more or less chill, succeeded by more or less pyrexia; or in other words, the first apparent event in the chain of sequences constituting any kind of fever is functional injury of the nervous system, followed by functional inactivity of the most important organs of the body, proceeding in some instances to organic disease" (Moore 1886b:252).[11]

The medical community's preoccupation with hypothetical, contagious swamp emanations and imaginary tiny bugs, Moore suggested, also had precluded them from realizing the consequence of lowered climatic temperature upon human skin. A sudden decrease produced "excitement and debility" of the "cutaneous system" (Moore 1886b:256–58). Moore claimed these conditions contributed to the development of fever. The primary reason for the unacceptable state of fever classification and low level of sophistication regarding disease therapy was, for Moore, a lack of common sense among people who should have had much of the trait.

All fevers, for Moore, were ultimately manifestations of a damaged nervous system. Distinct fevers indicated the severity of harm to the nervous system. This in turn affected the functioning of separate organs and processes in the human body. These became "types" or "classes" of fever. Characteristics idiosyncratic to the person who experienced fever, to his or her family, caste, religion, race, and so forth, were responsible for the subtle differences within the "types" or "classes" of fevers that the observer detected.

Moore's Theory and Evidence from India and the Tropics

Moore believed his knowledge about the tropics enabled him to expose the fallacies of contemporary Western medicine and therapeutics. He was convinced "writers confound climatic and other influences with malaria." This error led to a situation in which the many cases of elevated temperature blamed on some "malarial poison" were degrees of "climatic fevers" or "undefined climatic fevers" (1886b:272). South Asian data, in particular, permitted Moore to conclude "that there is no such thing as a specific fever, each variety being a phase of the general state fever, modified into different types by the influence of attendant circumstances . . . in other words, by regarding them as typhoid, modified by malarious influences, or as malarious, modified by typhoid influences" (Moore 1886b:253).

The maladies that some people claimed to be distinct were actually points along a continuum in which the "least severe form of fever is . . . an ordinary cold, the more severe phases being ague, continued fever, remittent, relapsing, typhoid, typhus, cerebro-spinal fever, and undefined climatic fever, all of which are observed in India, the last mentioned being the most common" (Moore 1886b:274–75). Moore also thought that all variations of fever had a common origin. In India, for example, people existing on a vegetarian diet had only two small meals of rice. This produced an insufficient amount of body heat required for the kind of labor most natives performed and for coping with the climatic conditions they confronted. A person who worked under an intense sun and in severe heat during the day, followed by coolness at night, experienced "chill." This occurred because the human "system must be compensated by a supply of heat from its own inadequate carbonaceous store" (Moore 1886b:271). The amount of internal warmth generated by digested food was inadequate to ameliorate the sudden and profound effect of the temperature contrast.

According to Moore, the negative effects of a poor diet were akin to shock. And the kinds and amount of vegetarian food consumed exacerbated the condition. Other factors contributing to sickness were the effect of too much exertion, unrelieved stress, and continued fatigue. Also involved were the aforementioned many variables that are idiosyncratic to the individual, her subcaste, his caste, and so on. All these factors were responsible for the "chill" that people experience in varying degrees of intensity. And each instance of "chill" was a prelude to the development of sickness.[12]

Prolonged exposure to intense sun and heat followed by dampness after sunset had insidious consequences throughout the tropics. Moore also believed that the absence of these variables also affected people. In other words, he claimed his theory about the relationship between environment and disease had worldwide applicability. The variables responsible for the gradations of fevers found in the tropics were not present in northern countries. In Scandinavia, for example, the climatic contrast between day and night was moderate. Inhabitants also ate other kinds of food, and heat-producing meat was a staple in their diet. Only a mild "impression on the human system" was generated. This, in turn, rendered Scandinavians much less susceptible to the "chill" experienced by natives in such places as India (Moore 1886b:271).

Moore's Concepts of Therapy, "Malarious Zones," and "Malarious Influences"

Moore's solution to prevent and cure fever diseases was easy to understand, it was optimistic, and it was simplistic. Germs and "malarial poison" were absent from his list of culprits because they did not exist. A healthy region was created by diminishing "malarious influences" found in a "malarious zone." The former alluded to the general environment of people, the way of life encouraging the evolution of detrimental social, economic, and political characteristics of a population. A "malarious zone" existed when the negative consequences of these factors in a particular locale were severe. These locations, Moore tells us, were "too low and damp, or the accommodation or food or general hygienic arrangements will be found defective" (Moore 1886b:271–72).

Eliminating a "malarious zone" and freeing its people from "malarious influences" was a simple procedure. Consumption of "nutritious food," avoiding work patterns requiring prolonged exposure to the sun, and other procedures, was central to Moore's therapeutic method. These steps prevented or cured disruption of the human body's nervous system, which in turn inhibited conditions conducive to the appearance of "chill" and subsequent evolution into varieties of fever. It therefore was of paramount importance that leaders of the society maintain "good sanitary surroundings." This included "good drainage, with consequent freedom from damp and its effect, chill." Equally important was "[g]ood personal hygiene" because "[g]ood conservancy and cleanliness generally prevent that vitiation of the atmosphere which leads to contamination of the blood, and consequent further susceptibility to changes of temperature" (Moore 1886b:334).[13]

Moore's ultimate cause of fever was the "general environment." There were many possible elements in this single category. Prescribing therapy in detail for a particular fever, therefore, was exceptionally difficult. He said a change in the climate was the only certain cure for "masked malarial fever." The patient should be given meat, "strong ale, [but] not wine," . . . [and] "liquor potassœ arsenitis" if a change in climate was impossible to experience (Moore 1886b:333).

Other than suggesting that mental and physical inactivity combined with a proper diet was the best "cure" when a fever appeared, Moore was either vague or said nothing about specific steps needed for any of the remaining fevers. The minor distinctions between them did not warrant special therapeutic measures. What remained was an attractive albeit generic scenario involving proper food (including the "juice of a lemon twice a day"), clothing (especially flannel), relaxation, housing, and protection from the sun. These items eliminate, or at least moderate, the severity of "fever" diseases; they rectified imbalances in caloric intake, levels of stress, and amounts of fatigue (Moore 1886b:38, 329, 334). The nervous system of a human being then functioned properly, and this prevented a "chill" from developing.

Moore also believed minor reliance upon chemicals could restore health. For example, he recognized quinine's "tonic and stimulating effects on the nerves, whereby the system is braced against changes of temperature" (Moore 1886b:334).[14] Quinine, however, should always be given in small doses. Moore also was unenthusiastic about prescribing *Papaver somniferum Linn* or its alkaloids. In this 1886 document, he declared both opium and narcotine were useless for the prevention or cure of the paroxysms that "malarial poison" theoreticians had observed. He rejected the drug and the alkaloid because there was reason for "doubting the very existence of malaria, and if there is no poison there can be no specific action on it. . . . [Hence the] various remedies from time to time brought forward as anti-periodics have in reality the slightest power over fever" (Moore 1886b:322). In other words, Moore is saying that these assertions about opium and narcotine being efficacious agents were erroneous because the "thing" they purportedly attacked did not exist.

Moore's reservation about the significance of opium in the fallacious "malarial poison" theory is also found in his own typology of fever. The drug could be used for some complications associated with "cerebro-spinal fever," but it should always be administered in combination with other ingredients such as quinine or belladonna liniment (Moore 1886b:328). Furthermore, his discussion of "intermittent," "typical ague," "remittent" or "exaggerated ague," and "masked malarial fever" identified characteristics peculiar to malaria plasmodia. But he did not recommend opium for treating any of these four gradations of a human being's disturbed nervous system in the 1886 *Manual of Diseases in India* publication. The drug was unimportant in the therapy he recommended to medical practitioners laboring in South Asia.

Although Moore's apolitical treatise did not prescribe opium to prevent "chill," the man's responses to anti-opiumists' increasing influence in Parliament indicate a very different attitude about the drug's status. Moore's theory of human physiology, psychology, plus his perception of fever and curing, provide a clue to understanding the very different tack he followed in refuting anti-opiumists' assertions. They also clarify why defenders of the trade embraced his ideas.

Human Physiology and the Status of Opium in Moore's 1886 Apolitical Treatise

Moore could not eliminate all factors that prevented sufferers in India from obtaining more restful, less stressful working conditions, adequate clothing, and proper shelter. But his theoretical framework permitted more than one interpretation of the effects of opium. This trait enabled supporters of the trade to proclaim their program helped to reduce "malarious influences" and eliminate "malarious zones."

Moore's ideas enabled opium to be construed as a dietary supplement. Consuming this "food" prevented the appearance of 'fever' or stopped a paroxysm once it had developed. Opium was able to eliminate conditions conducive to the generation of "chill" by sedating internal organs and "calming" human skin. This precluded "excitation" which in turn conserved internal warmth. *Papaver somniferum Linn*, in this variation, ameliorated the problem of insufficient body heat that contributed to the development of fever (Moore 1886b:323, 328).

Moore's understanding of human physiology also contained a tacit justification for eating opium in India, although he mentions this nowhere in the 1886 manuscript. Opium functioned as a thermostat because daily consumption of the sedative reduced the amount of excessive heat accumulated in the body. For Moore, this "cooling" lessened the difference between what a person experienced during the day and what the individual felt after sunset; the great contrast between daytime and night caused a chill. Opium ingestion reduced the degree of severity. One can infer that Moore believed opium cured nothing; the drug merely ameliorated the intensity of a factor responsible for the appearance of the disease called 'fever.'

Moore's Medical-Cum-Political Opium Publications between 1880 and 1894

There was nothing ambiguous or implied about the status of opium in Moore's medical-cum-political pronouncements between 1880 and 1894. The drug was indeed a form of nutrition. It enabled consumers to perform hard work by replacing dissipated heat that a meager and unhealthy diet did not replenish. And in very hot weather the drug sedated or quieted overheated internal organs. *Papaver somniferum Linn* retained this dual status regardless of how it was prepared, how it was ingested, or the reason given for its consumption. For Moore, opium was simply good for Asians. They should use it in any way, in any place, at any time, and in any quantity vaguely defined as less than excessive. For Moore and others of similar mind, there was no need for further discussion.

These writings also reveal a much more tolerant attitude about the 'malaria is a poison' explanation he vigorously criticized in the 1886 treatise. Two of these documents are illustrative.

As mentioned in the opening chapter, Western scientists discovered nothing between the early 1880s and mid-1890s that enhanced the credibility of the 'malarial poison' scenario. But much data also had been accumulated that indicated one of Moore's contentions was not erroneous. This was his identification of variables in the general environment being linked to disease. The level of sophistication characterizing late-nineteenth century science did not exclude the possibility that one component of therapy might indeed be proper food, clothing, and shelter. Nonetheless, relying exclusively upon them did not guarantee the restoration and preservation of health. Furthermore, nobody had validated Moore's contention about opium functioning in the human body exactly as he said it did. And there was abundant evidence that under no circumstances could the drug be considered a simple, undifferentiated whole. Moore revealed ignorance about pharmaceutical achievements, and to a lesser extent about progress in unraveling the complexities of human physiology. This intellectual lapse was not the consequence of being isolated in distant India. He returned to England in 1878 and worked in the Revenue and Statistics Department of the India Office in London until 1899.

In 1892, Moore adamantly proclaimed that opium was "not the destructive agent which anti-opiumists have declared it to be." He accused them of being as "noisy as the Salvation Army," and "if their statements are not actually untrue, they are often sensational exaggeration." Moore had a point. Anti-opiumists were vociferous but the man was as noisy and prone to hyperbole as the people he attacked. The Chinese, he tells us, had been a civilized nation from time immemorial. They could take care of themselves, which means the Christian moralists should not interfere in the internal affairs of this foreign country. These loud people attracted quack doctors in England and together they have pontificated about the evils of opium consumption. Hence, both groups contributed to the misguided notion of abolishing availability of a valuable, indispensable substance in the Orient. This, for Moore, was not only stupid; it was a crime. Thousands of poor people in India who suffered "from want of food would not be able to appease the hungry edge of appetite by the customary dose of opium; and when scarcity or famine occurs, thousands more would die than before." The situation was not much better for survivors of starvation because a "person having to undergo great physical fatigue would not be able to render himself proof against it by opium . . . " (Moore 1892c:224).

Moore said the anti-opiumists' aberrant morality derived from incorrect assumptions about the drug. Consumption hurt no Indian. The smoke from opium, for example, was rendered totally benign because the substance in crude form was boiled to produce the extraction called "chandul" or "chandoo," whereby "much of the narcotic principle of the opium is dissipated" (Moore 1892c:224). Moore did not reveal what narcotic principle he was talking about. He also did not indicate if this pertained to one, several, or all members of the two families of opium alkaloids known to exist at the time. He agreed with Sir George Birdwood's opinions (published in the early 1880s and discussed below) about an opium smoker's absorption of only the harmless "volatile resinous constituents of the opium" (Moore 1892c:225). Moore was referring to the physiologically inert, nonaddictive components described in chapter 1. The moralists, Moore lamented, castigated in ignorance "and without the grace of that best of virtues, charity" when they blamed patronization of chandoo shops as the cause of people's maladies (Moore 1892c:225). These customers were poor souls who indulged in this "harmless enjoyment" because of the comfort it brought. A phony righteousness held by individuals who did not know what they were talking about would prolong the misery of those "suffering from some malady . . . [who have] a bad cough, . . . [or are] evidently asthmatic or consumptive, . . . [or] weakened by rheumatism, . . . [or] shivering in the cold stage of ague, . . . [or have] some painful skin disease" (Moore 1892c:224). Only the heartless could conclude otherwise. They should do everyone a favor by keeping their mouths shut.

Moore further strengthened the case for Indian citizens' unfettered use of opium by presenting evidence that frequent use was "a safeguard against malarious fevers, which could not be done if a physician's prescription were required." His elaboration of the components of a "malarious fever" indicates he was referring to some of the numerous paroxysms whose existence he rejected in the 1886 *A Manual of the Diseases in India*. Moore also acknowledged that the anti-opiumists challenging his contention about the prophylactic capability of the drug had a valid point. One critic, for example, said he never met a native rationalizing indulgence because of the antiperiodic virtues of *Papaver somniferum Linn*. Moore also admitted to never having met anyone who said it, but he had heard about many Indians living in "malarious seasons and localities" who consumed the drug.[15] Moore supported this statement by presenting "evidence" gathered by British observers. One was the previously mentioned Dr. Vincent Edwards. This is the individual whom Batten cited in his 1891 Society of the Arts presentation. Edwards, according to Moore, found that opium consumption was "much more common in malarious than in healthy localities." Moore then mentions a Mr. Foster. This commentator said that in Godavery district of India, "all classes use it, not as an indulgence, but because it is considered as an admirable febrifuge, preventing cold, rheumatism and ague" (Moore 1892c:225). Foster also believed that opium use would cease only if fever was eliminated. The correlation of opium consumption with prevalence of fever also was observed in China, this time by a Dr. Winchester. This evidence led Moore to conclude that

> [t]here is no doubt that a poorly fed people, living in a malarious country, would be much worse in health without opium. In my own experience during feverish seasons, those who escaped of a large establishment were the opium users. Since the days of Pliny and Paracelsus, opium has been regarded as a preventive of malarious fevers. We need not, however, go to ancient times, nor to the East for evidence. Opium has always been the favorite prophylactic against ague in the English fen country. (Moore 1892c:225)[16]

In 1892, Moore said opium had been a dietary supplement since antiquity despite consumers proffering other explanations for its functions and effects. He still believed the most accurate depiction of opium was that it was a kind of "food." He was in a minority. Nineteenth-century scientists' discoveries had already demonstrated the nutrition idea was a simplistic explanation. The drug was a complex entity and its effects upon animals, including humans, were just as complex.

One year later, Moore was indignant, and even more insistent. He said the "several occasions when I have mentioned that opium is preventive as well as curative of so-called malarious fever the statement has been doubted or even contradicted" (Moore 1893:1196). He now introduced additional evidence from India to support his contention. This time it consisted of Dr. O'Shaughnessy's statements earlier in the century. Moore also included an apparently recent declaration by Surgeon-General Rice in Calcutta about some natives in parts of India who believed that opium prevented 'fever.' Rice also said the drug increased human life spans even if a disease or a paroxysm was absent.[17] The only other proof Moore presented was a few people's opinions about opium consumption. These utterances were inferences. They were no different from the statements he had labeled as subjective in the 1886 *Manual of Diseases in India*. Moore's experiences in south Asia enabled him to also make inferences that, for him, constituted proof.

> In my own experience I have known opium consumers alone remain free from fever when most others suffered during extraordinary malarious seasons. And as servants in India I preferred opium users, they being less liable to get sick from exposure on the march or when taken into the colder climates of the hills. (Moore 1893:1196)

Moore also used narcotine to enhance the argument for opium. This alkaloid, we are told, had "been proved to be an antiperiodic" but Moore provided no citation (Moore 1893:1196).[18] The evidence furnished about narcotine, no less than opium itself, apparently consisted of individuals who believed the drug did many good things. If not, then they were informants paraphrasing the beliefs of other people about the alkaloid's medical efficacy. The data available to Moore and upon which he based his argument was as moot as any of the material he rejected between 1880 and 1893. And the western allopathic medical community during the period did not classify narcotine as an antiperiodic.

Moore avoided discussing how narcotine performs its function. He apparently thought the clinical course of the alkaloid in the human body was identical to opium, the mother drug. He then equated the consequences of smoking the drug with the results produced by eating the crude or semi-processed substance. Similar to the 1886 apolitical statements, opium used in small quantities does things to the human body. But now he now includes beneficial stimulation as a complementary trait. The drug

> excites the circulation, and produces a glow throughout the whole system. In large quantities, it soothes the system and blunts nervous sensibility. Both actions are antagonistic to chill . . . (Moore 1893:1196)

Consumption of the drug in any amount, consequently, was not invariably detrimental to human health. The scenario Moore articulated in this 1893 publication was identical to the process proposed in the apolitical 1886 treatise. An Indian peasant who lacked adequate clothing and diet ate opium. Then "instead of feeling cold and shivering, he remains warm and glowing, and so escapes chill, which, if not the real and only cause of malarious fever, is certainly the cause of so many repetitions of the attack" (Moore 1893:1196).

Moore's admission that "malarious fever" might be explained by variables different from those that he espoused indicated some cognizance of progress. The awareness refers to discoveries by physiologists, bacteriologists, and scientists in related disciplines circa 1893. Moore, however, refused to admit his ideas were outdated. The recent "great increase of malarious fever in certain parts of India" he suggested, was probably due to the elimination of opium shops and from prohibiting a person from buying no more than "one tolas weight, rather less than half an ounce" (Moore 1893:1196). With nothing to protect the poor person from a disadvantageous environment, fever was the inevitable result. Ignorant, misguided Christian moralists were the human cause of misery for millions of Indian peasants.

In an 1892 article entitled "The Errors of the Anti-Opiumists," Moore paraphrased the comments of a prominent pro-trade activist. This individual, according to Moore, portrayed "the history of the Anti-Opium Society [as] a dreary record of energies wasted, talent misapplied, wealth uselessly squandered, charity perverted, and philanthropy run mad" (1892a:62). Moore fully shared these sentiments in 1892 and 1893. His assessment would not change in the coming years.

Details of Moore's depiction of the physiological effects of opium in the human body first appeared in the early 1880s. At the same time, Sir George Birdwood published his interpretation. For the remainder of the century, the pair attacked anti-opiumists' contentions. Both men testified before the Royal Commission on Opium during the first week of hearings. Birdwood's influential article, "The Opium Question," was published in the 20 January 1882 issue of *The Times (London)*. Pro-opium supporters immediately proclaimed his opinions about all aspects of the drug to be authoritative. They continued to do so for the next two decades. Other people were unenthusiastic; some said his explanation about how opium prevented and eliminated sickness, including malaria and its fevers, was nonsense. Even George Batten decided not to include Birdwood's most unconventional ideas in the 1891 Society of Arts address. Ardent anti-opiumists, preoccupied with petitioning members of Parliament and building a case proving the evils of inevitable addiction upon consuming the substance, ignored Birdwood's orientation before the Royal Commission began its deliberations.

SIR GEORGE BIRDWOOD

Sir George Birdwood's 1882 Perspective about Opium

Birdwood's ideas about opium had not changed since first expressing them while a university student. He restated them in an 1865 publication entitled *Catalogue of the Vegetable Products of the Presidency of Bombay; including a List of the Drugs Sold in the Bazaars of Western India*. Birdwood contended the critics who attacked his past scenario had been wrong. He repeated the same warning in 1882. Contrary to what these skeptics implied, his perspective was based on "facts from every region of the globe" and he took no side in the current, volatile opium controversy (Birdwood 1882a:3). Like Moore, Birdwood viewed opium as a dietary supplement useful in the prevention and cure of disease.

> To me the whole weight of trustworthy evidence, and particularly of professional evidence, which probably is alone trustworthy evidence in such a matter, seems to be in favour of the use of such a contra-stimulant as opium by the inhabitants of tropical countries, more particularly by those who live in malarious regions and feed chiefly on a vegetarian diet. (Birdwood 1882a:3)

Birdwood said he was aware of only two eminent authorities on India and elsewhere in Asia who mentioned the detrimental effects of eating and drinking opium among natives. He rejected their opinions. James Tod was the sole India expert who, in his *Annals and Antiquities of Rajast'han or the Central and Western Rajpoot* [sic] *States of India*, discussed the pernicious effects of Rajputs' eating excessive amounts of the drug. But Tod wrote very early in the century, hence his observations, Birdwood argued, applied only to the past. Tod also discussed only one group claiming Rajput status in one region of India. There were, however, many Rajput clans throughout the country. Rajputs, furthermore, comprised only one of the five Varnas or ritual categories of Hindus in the society (i.e., they were Kshatriyas), and not everyone in India was a Hindu.[19] Tod's observations, consequently, were not only outdated, they applied, if valid at all, to only a small percentage of India's population. The other negative comment concerning the drug, according to Birdwood, had nothing to do with physiology, psychology, or any other physical science. It was the result of "commercial jealousy"; Sir Stamford Raffle's "emphatic condemnation of opium obviously . . . [being] . . . but a reflection of Dutch prejudice against it" (Birdwood 1882a:3). Birdwood ignored every individual, and all arguments, against unrestricted accessibility to the drug in Great Britain. Nothing articulated since the 1830s had validity. This was true for India as well. He also ignored all laboratory research relevant to opium alkaloids since the 1820s.

Birdwood instead asserted that few trustworthy observers were hesitant about using the drug. Many people hailed its utility in India and they were not even trained medical professionals. In other words, the benefits of consumption were so obvious that even a layperson could easily recognize them. Birdwood cited such well-known authorities as Sir John Malcolm whom, in his *Memoir of Central India*, condoned the habit in that part of the country. James Burnes said the same thing for the Sindh Province in his *Narrative of a Visit to the Court of Sinde, and a Sketch of the History of Cutch*. An unequivocally favorable attitude toward consumption of the drug, according to Birdwood, was W. C. B. Eatwell's often-cited 1851–1852 publication about opium preparation in British India. Birdwood also mentions the positive comments found in Dr. Elijah Impey's 1848 *Report on the Cultivation, Preparation, and Adulteration of Malwa Opium*. The East India Company or its successor, the Government of India, employed for some time or for their entire career Malcolm, Eatwell, Impey, and Burnes. Birdwood also agreed wholeheartedly with the ideas that Sir William James Moore articulated in 1882. He also noted John Crawfurd's strong preference for using opium instead of alcohol as the preferred stimulant. The idea is found in the latter's *Dictionary of the Malay Archipelago* (Birdwood 1882:3).

Lest anyone question the medical veracity of these esteemed Asian specialists, Birdwood selected statements from famous nineteenth-century medical experts as well. He briefly mentions Sir Robert Christison's abstract of eleven cases in the latter's volume *Poisons*, and cites Pereira's speculation about the drug not shortening the human life span.

Birdwood presented other material to refute well-known anti-opium allegations concerning degraded morality, the drug's nefarious dubious reputation as an aphrodisiac, and so forth. Most germane, however, were his comments about the beneficial aspects of opium eating and the totally innocuous custom of smoking the opiate. Oral consumption of the drug was a suitable, if not superb, method of treating or eradicating what he was calling 'fever,' and 'malarial' and 'non-malarial' fever.

Birdwood's Proclamations Regarding Opium Smoking

Birdwood said that condemning the Government of India for encouraging Asian natives' opium smoking was silly because the habit was "an infinitely milder indulgence" than smoking tobacco. In fact, smoking the opiate was so "absolutely harmless" it could not even be compared to tobacco. The latter "may, in itself, if carried to excess, be injurious, particularly to young people under twenty-five; but I mean that opium smoking in itself is as harmless as smoking willow bark or inhaling the smoke of a peat fire or vapour of boiling water." Although Birdwood cited several people challenging his assertions, he offered opinions of many others who wrote about the innocuous or beneficial consequences of using the smoking extract. Prominent among these was Sir William James Moore's observation that "the freedom of opium smokers from bronchial and thoracic disease is deserving of deepest consideration" (Birdwood 1882a:3).

Birdwood also believed the method of preparation partially explained the benign consequence of smoking opium. Various items already added to the drug had diminished its "narcotic power." The reduction continued during the substance's manufacture into an "extract." He provided no information about what was added and how this reduced narcotic capability. Nonetheless, the result was an opium pill that could be

> placed in a flame, where it is instantly set ablaze. It blazes furiously, and its vapour is at the same instant inhaled into the throat and lungs in one inspiration. . . . But none of the active principles of opium are volatizable! [sic] (Birdwood 1882a:3)

If the consumer was getting none of the active drugs found in the crude drug, then what was the sense of smoking the product and what good did it do anybody? Birdwood answered this question using his knowledge of chemistry circa 1850–1854. He admitted this information was "quite out of date" but continued nonetheless, and asserted that if anyone bought

> Indian opium, as retailed in the bazaars, and prepares pure chandoo from it, and smokes as many pills of it as he pleases . . . he will find that they will not produce the slightest effect on him, or any one else, one way or the other, beyond causing that pleasant and peaceful warmth throughout the body which comes of sitting over a peat fire on a chilly day, or inhaling the fragrant vapour from a bowl of whisky toddy as you stir the boiling water into it, or, for that, from the simple steam issuing from a jug of boiling water. I conclude myself that nothing passes from the deflagrating chandoo pill into the lungs but the volatile resinous constituents of opium . . . if this be the fact, it explains the antiseptic and prophylactic action of opium-smoking in the pulmonary affections of the Chinese. (Birdwood 1882a:3)

Birdwood's reliance upon mid-nineteenth century chemistry in the context of 1882 permitted him to explain the process. He claims the inert components of opium coat, and therefore protect, the bronchial passages and lungs from "outer air." This helps to reduce infection. Furthermore, the drug was so completely incinerated that only "harmless smoke [entered] the lungs." The lamentable effects that anti-opiumists dramatically and consistently reported from China were indeed real. But the cause of this deterioration was the "general debauched habits of the lower outcast populations of the cities of China" and "not the accidental circumstances that some of them indulge in opium smoking" (Birdwood 1882a:3). Addicts in China, for Birdwood, had no one to blame but themselves for the misery observed so keenly, and for so long, by misguided Christians and people of similar inclination. The people responsible for the anti-opiumists' lament were moral degenerates. They would be reprobates regardless of the presence or absence of the drug.

Birdwood's General Conclusions about
Opium Smoking Among Asian Natives

Smoking opium did nothing to reduce or destroy the morality of the Chinese. It also was not the source of the alleged physical misery that these people experienced daily. Those who believed otherwise had no idea about "what morality means in Eastern Asia—much less immorality." Furthermore, the custom did not cause the daily misfortunes so often reported. Just the opposite was true; opium smoking might prevent their occurrence. Indeed, the custom was

> in short, . . . a strictly harmless indulgence, like any other smoking, and the essences of its pleasure to be, not in the opium itself so much as in the smoking of it. If something else were put in the pipe instead of opium, that something else would gradually become just as popular as opium, although it might not incidentally prove so beneficial. (Birdwood 1882a:3)

Birdwood never considered how to answer an obvious question; if opium was no different from other substances that were capable of being consumed in this manner, then why did the English for decades go to so much trouble to export an essentially vapid product to China? It would have been just as lucrative and much easier to have avoided the previous eighty years of controversy by selling pipes to the Chinese instead of *Papaver somniferum Linn*.

Birdwood's Conclusions about
Eating and Drinking Opium in South Asia

Birdwood also had a favorable attitude about people in India eating the drug, and drinking it when dissolved in solution. He claimed that a native asked about the dangers of opium eating would be rendered incredulous by such a question. The only response would be "if you take away our opium, what shall we do against fever?" (Birdwood 1882a:3). Even Englishmen in India consumed the drug for this purpose. He cites the deceased Consul Margary who ate one pill per day to ward off fever as he journeyed to a location identified as Bhamoo. For Birdwood, this one example sufficed to refute any claim about the negative effects of opium eating among non-Indians or Europeans in the subcontinent.

Birdwood also asserted that awareness of opium's healing capability was not restricted to the natives of India and their English sympathizers. History, he opined, condoned consumption of the opiate. Pliny and other famous people from the distant past advocated its use. And Birdwood echoed Moore in alluding to opium being a kind of food because it was "probably absolutely beneficial to the nutrition of a vegetarian population like India." It also functioned as an aid in digestion. He used some of Sir Benjamin Brodie's ideas to describe the physiological process. Brodie, whom Birdwood describes as "the most distinguished opponent of the dietetical use of opium," was important because even this skeptic admitted that consumption did not incite the emotions as did alcohol; it pacified them. This meant that the two substances were not in the "same category as dietetical corroborants" (Birdwood 1882a:3). Brodie provided substantiation for the soothing, hence very positive, powers of the drug.

> The effect of opium when taken into the stomach is not to stimulate, but to soothe the nervous system. . . . The opium eater is in a passive state, satisfied with his own dreamy condition while under the influence of the drug. He is useless, but not mischievous. It is quite otherwise with alcoholic liquors. (Quoted in Birdwood 1882a:3)

The drug also affects the intestines of a human being. It calms, soothes, and prolongs food retention by rendering the digestive tract lethargic. Any discomfort that the vegetarian experienced was more than offset because all nutrients were extracted from the material undergoing digestion. This longer period of time resulted in a life being saved.

Birdwood provided anatomical reasons to support this contention. "Carnivorous animals," he declares, "have proportionately shorter intestines than graminvorous, while man, being by nature both carnivorous and graminvorous, has intestines of intermediate length between the extremes adapted to an exclusively animal and an exclusively vegetable diet" (Birdwood 1882a:3). Influenced by Buddhists, the Hindus in India had become strict vegetarians, and vegetarianism is woefully "unsuited to the human constitution." The result was that "after weaning they [Indians] all suffer more or less from inordinate indigestion, which continues to the end of their lives, except among those who moderately indulge in the habitual use of opium." Opium, Birdwood contended, now functioned to ensure proper digestion of whatever entered the human body. In a profound way, it helped the internal organs to obtain as much nutrition as possible from a diet fundamentally inadequate for satisfying human needs, or at least detrimental to ensuring a long and healthy life span. Opium, therefore, alleviated damage wrought by a defective food custom because it "delays the process of digestion, and has, in fact, the effect, as it were, artificially prolonging the human intestine, and thus promoting the more complete digestion, and assimilation of vegetable food" (Birdwood 1882a:3). Food retention in the intestines or an inability to evacuate was a very beneficial consequence for those who did not eat meat. For Birdwood, constipated vegetarians were lucky people. They all enjoyed longer, healthier lives despite a diet void of animal flesh. Taking away opium increased the possibility of their premature demise.

Birdwood's choice of medical experts in this 1882 document was selective. He ignored the growing cadre of scientists and lay people voicing increasing concern about the drug's potency no matter how it was consumed. Birdwood also was conveniently unaware of data available during the 1880s concerning the potential toxicity of opium and some of its alkaloids.

THE 1882 *LANCET* CRITIQUE OF BIRDWOOD AND MOORE

Birdwood's declaration about opium and the digestive process was immediately attacked, as were the ideas of Moore found in a volume of articles published before 1882. Moore's book is entitled *The Other Side of the Opium Question*. The challenge came not from moralistic Christians but from the editors of the medical journal *Lancet*. They reject the two men's bold assertions about habitual, albeit moderate, consumption of the drug being "positively beneficial to the Eastern races." The logic, especially Birdwood's reasoning, was suspect. Birdwood was criticized for relying upon outdated medical knowledge from his college years and arriving at conclusions before even setting foot in India. Current research did not support his contention that opium smoking exerted no narcotic influence upon the consumer. And anyone witnessing what occurs among opium smokers in London's East End realizes that Birdwood is completely wrong. This kind of evidence, the editors continued, was "scarcely disproved by being dismissed as the product of sensational writers, and is abundantly confirmed by Mr. Moore" (*LAN* 1882:233).

Birdwood's contention about the effect of opium being a "lessening of the peristaltic action of the intestinal canal is of distinct value to those whose diet is chiefly vegetarian, assimilating their digestive tract to the longer canal of the herbivore . . . is certainly farfetched." A diet of rice was not comparable to the food ingested by a herbivore and Birdwood was confused about physiology. The effect of opium was "exerted chiefly on the lower part of the intestinal canal, where the digestion and absorption of starchy food do not take place." Birdwood also said the constipation experienced after consuming opium was a benefit whereas Moore admitted it was one of the "evils of its use" (*LAN* 1882:234).

The periodical's editors rejected any notion that moderate use of the drug was innocuous or beneficial. Opium was a stimulant leading to addiction with tragic results. The innocent individual "after a very brief habituation, is wretched and feeble without his artificial strength." Even the "minimum opium-eater is a slave [whereas] the moderate alcohol-drinker is not . . . [and] the testimony on this point is overwhelming, and so also is the evidence of the rapidity with which the opium-eater becomes enslaved, and the extreme difficulty and rarity of rescue" (*LAN* 1882:234).

Moore fared little better. Both men ignored the mass of evidence that unequivocally proved the unfortunate consequence of opium indulgence. The *Lancet* editors said one example was the depressing contents of recent Chinese consular reports concerning voluminous drug importation into the country. Furthermore, how could anyone accord much credibility to an observer who used a "racialist" argument to defend contemporary British and Government of India opium policy. Birdwood, the *Lancet* tells us, merely paraphrased Moore's statements. The result was a vindication of the trade by engaging in a "violent tirade against the Chinese as the most drunken, debauched, and dissolute people on the face of the earth, and we are therefore justified in forcing upon them an additional intoxicant suited to their venery in its aphrodisiac properties (denied by Birdwood, but admitted by Moore), on the chance that we may thereby lessen their drunkenness" (*LAN* 1882:234). The medical journal's dismissal of Birdwood's digestive tract scenario and its castigation of Moore's racial argument were stinging. Nonetheless, some people ignored the criticism.

DEFENDING OPIUM: PRO-TRADERS' APPROPRIATION OF THE BIRDWOOD AND MOORE ARGUMENTS

Moore's theory of disease and its cure and Birdwood's interpretation of opium and 'malaria' provided defenders of the status quo with a medical justification for no additional regulation of the trade. Each man accorded paramount status to opium. Keeping the drug inexpensive and available for all people reduced their susceptibility to 'fever' maladies. Most people in India could not change their diet or the conditions under which they worked. Too often a person's life depended upon the ebb and flow of invisible, intangible emanations from swamps, trees, soil, and so forth. Opium provided a helpless person with a sense of mastery over one's fate: eating the substance reduced excessive heat in the hot season or increased its quantity during cold periods. In both cases, *Papaver somniferum Linn* made a person less prone to chill; the precursor of 'fever,' 'malaria,' and possible death.

The SSOT demanded that opium production and consumption be restricted to legitimate medical purposes. Moore and Birdwood 'proved' that all consumption was medicinal. Pro-traders welcomed the evidence. But few of them were qualified medical practitioners. Still fewer defenders of the trade had the expertise or the inclination to conduct laboratory tests to confirm what Moore and Birdwood said about the drug. Who was appointed to the Royal Commission on Opium and the format for selecting witnesses was therefore crucial. The SSOT and its opposition needed people to demonstrate the veracity of their respective positions to Commission appointees. Pro-traders had reason for optimism.

COMPOSITION OF THE ROYAL COMMISSION ON OPIUM

Queen Victoria announced the composition of the Royal Commission on Opium on 2 September 1893, in the fifty-seventh year of her reign. Sir Thomas Brassey was the chairperson. Three other appointees were knights and one of them was an Indian. He was Sir Laksmiswar Singh Bahadur, maharajah of Darbhanga. Darbhanga was a native state located northeast of Bombay Presidency. Sir James Broadwood Lyall, a Government of India nominee, was a member of the "Most Eminent Order of India," and a "Knight of our Most Exalted Order of the Star of India." Lyall and the maharajah provided "India experience." Sir William Roberts would be the Commission's source of "medical expertise" (GBO [Court of St. James/Lord Kimberley] 1894:I:v–vi).

Other Members of the Royal Commission on Opium

Mr. Haridas Viharidas, a former high ranking official of the native state of Junargarh, was the Commission's second Indian national. The remaining appointees were four British commoners. Two of them, Robert Gray Cornish Mowbray and Henry Joseph Wilson, were members of Parliament.

Mowbray, a conservative and unionist, had been secretary to the chancellor of the exchequer from 1887 to 1892. After his stint with the Royal Commission on Opium, he was a member of the Royal Commission on Indian Expenditure. This assignment lasted from 1896 to 1900. Henry Joseph Wilson had replaced W. P. Caine. Caine, an anti-opiumist appointee to the Commission and knowledgeable about India, could not accept the assignment. Prior to his appointment, Wilson had not been a "conspicuous anti-opium leader" in Parliament (Johnson 1975:312).

Arthur Upton Fanshawe was the second person nominated by the Government of India and the seventh member of the Commission. Born in 1848 and educated at Repton, he entered the Bengal Civil Service in 1871 and worked in the Central Provinces. Fanshawe was the postmaster general of Bombay in 1882 and later held the position of secretary in the Finance and Commerce Department to the Government of India. He then became director-general of India's post office in 1889 and held this position when appointed to the Royal Commission on Opium. Completing the eight-person board was Sir Joseph Pease's brother Arthur, a Quaker and the SSOT's second representative (Buckland [1906] 1969b:143); Johnson 1975:312; GBO [Court of St. James/Lord Kimberley] 1894:I:v–vi).

Biographical Comments about Principal Questioners

Sir William Roberts, Lord Brassey, and Sir James Lyall, in that order, asked witnesses most of the questions pertaining to medical aspects of the opium habit in India. They were followed by Henry Wilson and then in equal, albeit minor, frequency Arthur Fanshawe, Robert Mowbray, Haridas Viharidas, and Arthur Pease. Sir Laksmiswar Singh, the maharajah of Darbhanga, asked nothing germane about the topic.

In a Minority Report submitted to Brassey as the Royal Commission completed deliberations, Henry Wilson condemned the format for collecting evidence and rejected almost all recommendations made by its members. The behavior of Roberts, Brassey, and Lyall, according to Wilson, affected the nature of the hearings, and the contents of opium and malaria questions posed to witnesses. Since their conduct was partially responsible for Wilson's negative reactions (and for the anger of many other people), some comments about the backgrounds of these principal questioners, as well as Wilson, are in order.

Sir James Broadwood Lyall was born in 1838 and died on 4 December 1916. He was educated at Eton and Haileybury College. Appointed to the Bengal Civil Service in 1857, he arrived in India during 1858 and became a member of the Punjab Commission until the end of 1859. Lyall was the financial commissioner of this northwestern province before being sent to southern India. Here he served as British resident in Mysore and chief commissioner of Coorg (south India) from 1883 to 1887. Lyall then returned to the Punjab as its lieutenant governor and governor-general until 1892. The Government of India then appointed him to the Opium Commission. Lyall was president of the Indian Famine Commission in 1898 and during his long career he visited China, Japan,

Canada, and the United States (Buckland [1906] 1969c:257; *WWW 1916–1928* 1929b:II:63; Berridge & Edwards 1981:186).

Sir James Lyall's long career with the Government of India made him no friend to the SSOT. According to Berridge and Edwards, he thought the purpose of the Royal Commission inquiry was "silencing of the anti-opium agitation." And in a letter sent to Viceroy of India when the Commission was beginning its work, bias is obvious when he declares that "'[t]he facts of the case are all really well known enough, and the object appears to be to get an expression of opinion, of native opinion in particular, which will carry sufficient weight to enable the question to be shelved'" (Lyall, quoted in Berridge & Edwards 1981:186).

During the forthcoming Commission hearings, Lyall did not desist from voicing his belief about the harmlessness of moderate amounts of opium. Berridge says the opinion of a single Englishman from the Fens region was, for Lyall, sufficient to illustrate the consequences for Indians using the drug. Lyall produced a letter from Thomas Stiles, a ninety-six year old doctor who began practicing medicine in the Fens in 1813. The physician retired sixty-two years later. Stiles claimed that he had never been exposed to any case in which use of the opiate shortened the life span of the consumer, or was the cause of any disease (Berridge 1977:281). Brassey and Roberts were more circumspect in indicating their feelings about anti-opiumists' protestations.

Thomas Allnut Brassey, the "first Earl Brassey, of Bulkeley, Chesire," was born in Stafford, 11 February 1836. Other than a publication entitled *Problems of Empire; the Case for Devolution*, there was little about India or any subject related to opium production and consumption or to disease and drugs in Brassey's background that made him especially qualified to be Assistant Secretary to the Royal Commission on Opium (WWW 1916–1928 1929a:II:120–21; V. W. B. 1927:62).[20] The 1927 edition of *The Dictionary of National Biography* describes him as a "rich man, of no outstanding ability" but very conscientious, highly patriotic, kind, pleasant, and even-tempered (V. W. B. 1927:62). His brief career in Parliament (1880–1886) was undistinguished. The man's most enduring contribution to British society was *Brassey's Naval Annual*. First published in 1886, it was recognized for many years as the "most authoritative survey of naval affairs throughout the world" (V. W. B. 1927:62–3).

Henry Joseph Wilson was born in Nottingham in 1833 and educated at University College, London. He was a businessman who, upon election to Parliament in 1885, represented Holmfirth division of Yorkshire when he replaced W. P. Caine on the Royal Commission (*WWW 1897–1915* 1935:771; Stenton & Lee 1978b:377). Besides the opium assignment, Wilson's South Asia experience included membership on the India Office Committee on Regulation of Prostitution during 1893 (Stenton & Lee 1978b:377; *WWW 1897–1915*:771). Wilson's "progressive" inclinations earned him posthumous portrayals as being "[a]ctively connected with Liberal organisation in Sheffield; temperance, abolition of State regulation of vice; a Radical, strongly opposed to Militarism and Protection" (WWW 1897–1915 1935:771). Another citation describes him as a "[r]adical, opposed to Aggressive Foreign Policy, Militarism, Protection, etc . . ." (Stenton & Lee 1978b:377).

Added to this mix of Lyall, a Government of India loyalist; Wilson, a liberal unenthusiastic about what the British presence in South Asia symbolized; and Brassey, the epitome of patriotism and privilege with no India experience, was the apolitical Sir William Roberts. Roberts was appointed to evaluate the oral and written medical evidence. Since the Royal Commission was deliberating the future of opium in the British Indian Empire and Roberts was central to the discussion, a few comments about what the man had done to earn his appointment are indispensable. The material also shows why defenders of opium welcomed his appointment.

SIR WILLIAM ROBERTS' QUALIFICATIONS

In 1885, William Roberts was knighted for a career marked by valuable contributions to physiology, nutrition, and disease prevention.[21] His brilliance and analytical thoroughness earned him many honors prior to this consummate honor. Soon after graduating with distinction from University College in London in 1851, he became a member of the Royal College of Surgeons, and received a licentiate from the Society of Apothecaries. Roberts then excelled at the University of London, and the institution awarded him the M.D. in 1854. He was immediately appointed to the faculty of the Manchester Royal School of Medicine, and would spend nearly thirty years at the institution. His affiliation was replete with additional honors. One of many came in 1877, when the Royal Society awarded him the title of Fellow for contributions to histology, pathological chemistry, and physiology (*BMJ* 1899:1063–64).

The Early Years of Sir William Roberts' Research

Part of Roberts' career suggests he was capable of providing the SSOT with an incisive critique of the oral and written evidence offered to the Royal Commission. Another phase illustrates why the Government of India and pro-traders wanted him to be the Commission's only medical expert. The two periods overlap although Robert's early research interests and observations indicate his cognizance of current arguments in physiology.

Roberts' Skepticism of Alternatives to Traditional Allopathic Medicine

Interested in many subjects, Roberts investigated several at the same time and made significant contributions to each one. One of the earliest was a critique of homeopathy. This new, unorthodox approach to disease causation and cure was very popular in Great Britain at the time. Roberts doubted its veracity. The suspicion was confirmed when he found that some concoctions contained large doses of potent drugs, not the infinitesimal amounts a person was supposed to find. He then concluded that many homeopathic practitioners were frauds and published a "crushing indictment" about the doctrine's absurdities (Leach 1899:159, 162–3).

Roberts' investigations qualify him as being part of the reform movement in Great Britain. It included the chemists, pharmacists, and physicians who were challenging the alleged capabilities of traditional opium concoctions.

The Human Kidney and Its Malfunctioning

Roberts' investigation of kidney functions and secretions resulted in the 1865 publication of *A Practical Treatise on Urinary and Renal Disease including Urinary Deposits*. For more than twenty years thereafter, the volume was hailed as the "most important contribution to practical medicine" and of "equal importance to the physiologist." His research into the cause and cure of gout received similar praise (*BMJ* 1899:1064; see also Stephen & Lee 1921–22:22–Supplement:1171). An important corollary of this interest is that Roberts not only identified what caused these problems, he proposed methods to both prevent and avoid their malfunctioning. The man was a pioneer in what his admirers called practical therapeutics.

The Etiology of Misery: Roberts and the Germ Theory of Disease

Roberts also favored germ theory over old notions of disease causation early in this era of paradigmatic change. He was, after 1865 and through 1877, active in a debate spawned by the Pasteur and Lister discoveries about microorganisms in disease. The scientific community disagreed about how the entities were produced and what function they performed. Some people believed germs "might arise de novo, from the media in which they grow." This was an argument for spontaneous generation. Other scientists said this was impossible; pathogenic organisms must "always spring from organisms like themselves" (Leach 1899:167; see also Stephen & Lee 1921–22:22–Supplement:1171).

Over a period of four years, Roberts conducted experiments to test each explanation. The results were published in 1877. Roberts concluded that normal tissues and fluids had no inherent capability to spawn pathogenic organisms. Germs imported from outside were responsible for their appearance in media. Typical of Roberts' cautiousness, he suggested the findings did not completely invalidate the possibility of spontaneous generation, but it was highly unlikely (Leach 1899:168). This research also provides information about his understanding of the origin and cure of 'fever.'

Roberts' Research Interests and Explanation of 'Fever'

Roberts was very aware that slightly elevated temperatures and serious paroxysms were a symptom of infection. And he was equally convinced that microbes were the common underlying cause of these fevers. In 1877, for example, he discussed the different kinds of paroxysms associated with "relapsing fever," septicæmia, "splenic fever," anthrax, diptheria, scarlet fever, cholera, and typhoid fever. Although he mistakenly suggested that some of these microbes might ultimately be linked to one harmless organism that had undergone morphological change, he was correct in associating different patterns of fever with specific microorganisms.

Roberts also accepted the notion of periodicity, the recurrence of identical paroxysms in a patient over a period of time. His discussion of "relapsing fever" explained the phenomenon. And the animal experiments he conducted demonstrated that pathogenic organisms, created by decaying tissues, could be injected into healthy creatures. The result was animals suffering from the malady. Last but not least, he proposed that microorganisms could survive outside of a host in very adverse conditions. Given appropriate conditions, these microbes could emerge from dormancy to infect new subjects with devastating consequences (Roberts 1877:168–73).

Another event demonstrates Roberts' perspicacity. Early in his career he tested, for many kinds of ailments, the usefulness of Wunderlich's newly introduced clinical thermometer. Roberts, aware of the confusion characterizing fever classification, spent most of 1864 using the instrument, refining diagnostics and prognostication. He almost died from typhus contracted in the Royal infirmary while doing so (Stephen & Lee 1921–22:22–Supplement:1171; Leach 1899:163).

In short, Roberts rejected paradigms of sickness that ignored small bugs and the complications these microbes created. He also was fully conscious of the confusion generated by faulty systems of fever classification. He demanded precision and proof—not conjecture—from anyone pontificating about the cause and cure of disease.

The Later Years: Sir William Roberts' Perspective on Nutrition, Disease, Progress, and 'Race'

Nutrition, Disease, and Practical Therapeutics

Sir William Roberts' principal interest during the sixteen-year period before 1893 was the link between nutrition, physiology, and sickness. Sometime during 1877, he resumed studying facets of human digestion and emphasized its implications for the treatment of disease. This contribution to "practical therapeutics" earned him the Cameron Prize in 1879 (*BMJ* 1899:1065; Stephen & Lee 1921–22:22–Supplement:1171). The honor was followed by an invitation from the Royal College of Physicians to be the Lumleian Lecturer for 1880. Roberts selected "digestive ferments" and "artificially digested foods" as his presentations. Many years of studying pancreatic extracts enabled him to demonstrate how ferments broke down starch and other food constituents. He was able to calculate the dietetic utility of "artificially digested foods" and how they could be prepared to maximize nutritive value for human consumers (Leach 1899:169–70). The lectures were applauded for their theoretical significance and importance for practical medicine. A compilation of addresses and articles responsible for the 1879 Cameron Prize was published six years later under the title *Lectures on Dietetics and Dyspepsia, delivered at the Owens College School of Medicine in February and March, 1885.* (*BMJ* 1899:1063–64; Stephen & Lee

1921–22:22–Supplement:1171). Roberts kept active between 1879 and 1885 refining earlier observations, making new ones, and experimenting. He also recognized the wider implications of his then current research. What he said about this work affected his conduct in India.

Two 1885 and 1890 public addresses published in the *British Medical Journal* present the man's perspective about nutrition, disease, and practical therapeutics before the Royal Commission on Opium appointment.[22] Roberts discussed the tack that observers should take when confronting dietary customs of people around the world, the origins of such habits, and what physiological and psychological functions these foodstuffs performed for the human animal. He also discussed the appropriate role of secular and religious institutions in telling people what to consume, and he described the consequences for a technologically advanced nation in relying upon "prepared foods" as sources of nutrition. Roberts' previous accomplishments were impressive. Nonetheless, his perspective about "practical therapeutics" between 1885 and 1891 most likely was the paramount factor that convinced Queen Victoria and her advisors to accept Roberts as the source of "medical expertise" for the Royal Commission on Opium.

Food Preferences in a Society Are the Result of Biological Heritage

Roberts opened his 1885 address to the British Medical Association at Cardiff by declaring that dietetics was a "somewhat neglected" science which would be beneficial to humankind only if practitioners avoided exclusive reliance upon "a priori data supplied by physiology" (Roberts 1885a:188). The discipline must instead be based upon observing and studying the eating and drinking customs of people around the world. These practices, he asserted, were not

> random practices adopted to please a palate, or to gratify an idle or vicious appetite. . . . [They] must be regarded as the outcome of profound instincts, which correspond to important wants of the human economy. They are the fruit of a colossal experience accumulated by countless millions of men in successive generations. (Roberts 1885a:188)

The instinctive origin of dietary preference was reiterated in the 1890 address to the Manchester Medical Society and the *British Medical Journal* article when he declared these preferences were

> as much sober, unsophisticated facts of natural history as are the food habits of wild animals. They have grown up by the free play of natural instincts, under the regulating force of universally acting biological laws, under the pressure of the sleepless vigilance of the law of the survival of the fittest and the sure incidence of the laws of heredity. (Roberts 1890:883)

Roberts' insistence upon the necessity for careful study of "national diets" reflected pragmatism as much as it did a respect for cultural differences. He declared it was impossible to compel people through legal or religious mandate to change their food habits and expect any change to be permanent. The probability of failure was multiplied if this coercion came from nonindigenous institutions or people. Roberts implored readers to beware of the harm caused by ignorant meddling (Roberts 1885a:188).

Roberts realized that some individuals might not follow societal norms about what was good to ingest and that "personal idiosyncrasies" or differences in "constitution" accounted for these exceptions. Some people might be "natural born vegetarians who have a life long distaste for meat" while others might be "intolerant" of such items as coffee and tea (Roberts 1885a:189). There also were individuals in any society with "altogether perverse and depraved" nutritional preferences (Roberts 1890:884). These exceptions should not be condemned; their occurrence should be anticipated and understood.

Roberts' comment about what tasted "good" was another expression of his eclectic cultural relativity. What was delicious or unpleasant depended upon the kind of creature being discussed. There was, for him "no such thing as an absolutely bad flavour . . . [because] [e]ach animal has its own gustatory standard, which is accurately adjusted to the wants of its particular economy" (Roberts 1890:884). The animal palate functioned as a

> dietetic conscience at the entrance gate of food, and its appointed function is to pass summary judgment on the wholesomeness or unwholesomeness of the articles presented to it. It acts under the influence of a natural instinct, which is rarely at fault. This instinct represents an immense accumulation of experience, partly acquired and partly inherited. (Roberts 1890:884)

Roberts' tolerance for dietary differences around the world did not preclude him from linking these habits to the intellectual, moral, and technical progress of a nation. The stage of "civilization" attained by a particular "race" and what its members ate was neither accidental nor unrelated. The "British races and other races of Western Europe, together with their kindred and descendants in different parts of the globe . . . are [in] every way, but especially in intellectual power, and in their productiveness of men of originality and eminence, far in advance of all others . . ." (Roberts 1885a:188). Domination in international commerce had introduced the English and their kin to foodstuffs from diverse parts of the globe. Some items had been assimilated into the national diet. Other things were ignored. The choice, however, had resulted in the customs of occidental people such as the English becoming a "beneficial model" for less civilized people to emulate (Roberts 1885a:188).

Composition of the Occidental or Western Diet

This "beneficial model" consisted of fruit and green vegetables as well as cereals, legumes, and other "farinaceous articles." An equally important ingredient was "the various forms of animal flesh" as well as much consumption of coffee, tea, or cocoa, or all three. And universal to all people adhering to this "beneficial model" was a "systematic use of alcoholic beverages . . ." (Roberts 1885a:188).

Roberts defended his model by declaring that a human diet must perform two functions in the struggle for survival. A diet had to provide "general nutrition." Bread and related cereal items, seeds of legumes, fruits, vegetables, dairy products, fish, and meat satisfied this need. The second function was nutrition for the "higher faculties" which, for Roberts, were the brain and nervous system. The "brain foods" were coffee, tea, and the numerous kinds of alcoholic drinks and tobacco. Alcohol, tea, and coffee were not "luxuries" as some misinformed people believed. They were very important for human survival because the "struggle for existence—or rather, for a higher and better existence—among civilised men is almost exclusively a brain struggle." Hence, these three items were tools enhancing the quality of life in the world whereas tobacco, "although [it] cannot be strictly classified as a food . . . [still] must be ranked with our dietetic customs" (Roberts 1890:883).

Meat had a dual status. It qualified as "general nutrition." It also satisfied the needs of the brain and nervous system because it possessed "certain stimulating properties" that distinguished it from vegetable and dairy products (Roberts 1890:883; see also Roberts 1885a:189). Eaters of animal flesh, drinkers of coffee, tea, and alcoholic beverages as well as people avoiding these things, however, were all reflecting the "spontaneous outcrop of natural instincts, and the fruit of an immense experience, and the sanction they derive therefrom constitutes an incomparably higher authority than the opinion of the wisest amongst us" (Roberts 1885a:189).

Effect of Gender and Age upon a "National" Diet

Roberts realized that dietary variation could exist in the population of any society. The cause of this divergence was most often sex and age, or differences in "constitution." Women ate much less meat than men did among people who adhered to the "beneficial model." The English were illustrative. The contrast was even more marked regarding alcohol consumption. "My impression," he asserted, "is that, in this country, three-fourths, if not four-fifths, of the alcohol consumed is consumed by men, and only one-fourth or one-fifth by women . . . [because] women are more sensitive to the effects of alcohol than men, and are more easily injured by the excessive use of it." English females satisfy their need for "brain food" by ingesting "much more tea and coffee . . . especially tea . . . [and] women consume, in proportion to the totality of their food, more milk and more bread than men do" (Roberts 1885a:189).

Growing old affected dietary consumption in every society on earth. Peoples' "nutritive processes decline in elasticity and power" the longer they live. Proof of the change is their inability to "absorb a quantity of stimulant" such as alcohol. This had not been a problem earlier in life (Roberts 1885a:189).

Roberts' Beliefs about Alcohol Consumption

Roberts disagreed with the temperance movement extremists who wanted complete prohibition of alcohol in Great Britain. He said liquor was not harmful to a "race" as long as people did not imbibe excessively, a situation he admitted did occur. Excessive consumption indeed harmed some individuals, but alcohol was still a useful article of diet and posed no threat to society as a whole. Roberts also acknowledged that drinking in his country had inflicted more "physical, moral and intellectual ruin on individuals" compared to all other "civilized communities" but the nation still had a low death rate, and the "moral and intellectual vigour of the race is high" (Leach 1899:171–72). England was not the only country benefiting from the positive relationship.

Roberts correlated alcohol consumption with levels of civilization around the world. All "advanced" western societies consumed alcohol, but

> the nations abstaining from the use of alcohol are, upon the whole far inferior to the alcohol-bred races of the West. The Japanese are the only Asiatic people who have for centuries consumed alcohol largely, and they display a mental receptivity and love of progress, which are in marked contrast to the stagnation around them. (Leach 1899:171–72)

Alcohol use among people in a society, therefore, was not a sign of inevitable moral and physical degeneracy. If consumption was modest, it performed "some real service to man" as a beneficial stimulant. A society that prohibits all use of "spirits" jeopardized its chance to ascend the ladder of "civilization." Roberts knew that viewing liquor as a "civilizing" force was an unusual perspective, and rarely did he "allude in his writing to the advantages of alcohol, fearing lest he might create a wrong impression on the subject" (Leach 1899:172). Leach does not identify the source of Roberts' concern.

Roberts' stance undoubtedly offended participants in the influential Temperance Movement, but it probably delighted the Government of India administrators and pro-trade individuals who were familiar with his writings. Roberts' assertion about alcoholic beverages nourishing the brain explained why Asian nations, Japan being the exception, were poor and backward. He was rejecting a portrayal of liquor use as intellectually, morally, and physically degenerating. Central to the SSOT strategy for India, however, was persuading Commission members that opium consumption was as bad as imbibing liquor or more so. Roberts did them no favor by declaring alcohol was cerebral nutrition in the struggle for survival and using Japan as an example. If liquor was good for people and contributed to a "better" society, then what was the status of opium when it was construed as being in the same category as alcohol?

Laboratory work started during 1885 was one factor that prompted Roberts' declaration of a positive role for alcohol in society. He analyzed how wine, tea, coffee, and cocoa affected pancreatic digestion, and salivary and peptic activity. He chose these "food accessories" because they were "used more or less by all nations, and seem to be essential to the comfort of mankind" (Leach 1899:169–70; Roberts 1885a:189). Roberts concluded their common effect was to slow down the digestive process and that retardation was not a wholly negative consequence. The "advance of civilization" was characterized by food being "constantly rendered more digestible" which resulted in "too rapid digestion and a waste of material" (Leach 1899:171). It was desirable, therefore, that "the digestive fires should be damped down in order to ensure the economical use of food" (Roberts, quoted in Leach 1899:171). For Roberts, infrequent bowel movements might contribute to good health, a conclusion that Sir William Moore and Sir George Birdwood probably read with pleasure.

Roberts' Perspective about Diets for the Sick

Roberts distinguished between completely debilitated people and the "walking" sick, or those people still able to perform normal activities (1890:883). When a person was struck down with fever or had some "organic disease," a physician should not be concerned with what was "the best fitted to bring out his physical and mental powers; the business at hand is to advise what is best to keep body and soul together until the fever storm be passed, or what is best to minimize the incidence of organic trouble, and to lengthen out existence to the utmost possible span" (Roberts 1890:883). Caregivers performed a disservice if their therapy violated the dietary customs of the ambulatory patient and the completely debilitated. This mistake was the result of ignorance, not maliciousness.

Roberts preferred not to alter diets for anyone, including the sick. He believed that eating a familiar food was part of the healing process unless the item was undeniably negative. Taking away what people were accustomed to consuming heightened their sense of insecurity. The psychological consequences might be detrimental to health. In situations where physiological liabilities negated psychological benefits, Roberts advised practitioners to proceed slowly and cautiously. Although he believed benefits resulted from changing a diet, one should only suggest change, not insist upon it. A caregiver should not forget that it was "better to lessen the quantity than to forbid" (Roberts 1890:884). They also should be tolerant of custom unless there was sufficient proof to the contrary. In situations where the cause of sickness was in doubt, there were two questions to ask: did people like the food they were told to eat; and did the food agree with them? "Do not interfere with a patient's customary preferences if the answer to both queries is yes" (Roberts 1890:884). Roberts honored a central tenet in the applied phase of his career. He said that insisting upon changing a sick person's dietetic habits for no "clear reason" was nothing more than the imposition of "irksome and needless restrictions" (Roberts 1885a:189). He would not forget it during his association with the Royal Commission on Opium.

Roberts believed liquid foods helped sick people. He recommended milk, "[b]eef-tea and other [m]eat concoctions," "[c]old-made [m]eat infusions," "[b]eaten-up eggs," and "[f]ortified [g]ruels (Roberts 1885a:190–92). Biological endowment, however, prevented vegetarians from ingesting these items with beneficial results. Substitutes might be found in the native diet, and a medical practitioner should not discourage consumption of these items regardless of what they were. Caregivers also must realize that the aging process could necessitate a revised diet (Roberts 1890:885). This phenomenon was found in societies classified as vegetarian and meat eating, as well as among people who consumed alcohol, tobacco, and other stimulants. It also was present in cultures whose population abstained from some or all the aforementioned. The detail of appetite adjustment during the aging process varies from society to society, and the change might include items objectionable or unconventional to members of another cultural tradition.

A "hands-off" attitude toward indigenous culinary preferences was particularly important if the health-care giver was not native to that population. Again, Roberts admonished, be tolerant of a diet different from your own merely because it lacked similar "brain foods" or substances "nourishing" the nervous system. People who desired these items, be they vegetarians or abstainers from coffee, tea, cocoa, and other "food accessories," might be ingesting another, unfamiliar, form of "brain food" or mental nutrition that the observer incorrectly labeled as a nonfood, or as unsavory. Tolerance, however, did not alter reality: vegetarians and people who abstained from modest amounts of alcohol, tobacco, and other substances stimulating the "higher faculties" were at a disadvantage. Their diet prevented them from reaching the level of civilization enjoyed by people in the meat-eating, alcohol-consuming nations of the western world.

In 1891, Roberts' most recent thoughts about the theory and practice of physiology, medicine, diet, and disease appeared in *Collected Contributions on Digestion and Diet* (*BMJ* 1899:1064; Stephen & Lee 1921–22:22–Supplement:1171). The book's contents indicate his ideas about the relationship between dietary preference and biological inheritance, and about how to feed the sick, had not changed. A second edition of the 1891 book was published in 1897.

Intimations of Roberts' Response to Witnesses' Testimony

Roberts' appointment ostensibly ensured that the Royal Commission included at least one person who would insist upon stringent standards of proof being met before accepting any claim about what opium could do or did not do. Roberts' participation bestowed scientific credibility upon the entire enterprise. The SSOT, as well as their opponents, would have to convince him of the veracity of their respective positions. The man's mind, however, was not a tabula rasa to be filled only by witnesses' recitations; it had been shaped by decades of immersion in physiology. His views about some topics would undoubtedly influence responses to what he was about to hear during the Royal Commission sessions. Roberts' reputation as a careful researcher at least suggested a degree of impartiality would inform his evaluation. Nonetheless, some of the man's preconceptions did not bode well for the SSOT members or sympathizers attempting to discredit the drug and disease connection at the hearings.

Roberts' investigation of homeopathy indicated that he questioned a new or unorthodox way of healing until he was convinced that its practitioners were honest and accurate. Merely proclaiming that a technique was either efficacious or worthless was an opinion, not a fact, and Roberts was predisposed to demand convincing proof before it, or any drug or substance, received his stamp of approval or disparagement. The preferred form of validation for this careful researcher was a controlled experiment conducted in a laboratory setting over a long time before making any proclamation. And if this were not possible, the rigor and scrupulous accuracy he insisted upon would have to be attained in some other manner. The importance he attached to curing the sick demanded nothing less.

Roberts' exposure to homeopathy also made him aware of inaccurate claims about amounts of chemicals in a prescription. The real contents of a medicine often differed from stated quantities. In other words, the importance of quality control was not a foreign idea to the man. And in his evaluation of the unorthodox or the new, be it a therapeutic technique, a chemical substance, or anything else, Roberts' skepticism did not preclude him from announcing any merits that the unconventional possessed. If Roberts' experience was any indication, people proclaiming that opium prevented or cured malaria or both, as well as those who belatedly tried to disparage such a notion, would not have an easy time convincing the man that what they said was accurate.

Roberts' participation in the spontaneous generation debate spawned by Lister and Pasteur indicated he was aware of new explanations of disease and living microscopic creatures as causative agents and possibly as vectors. His acceptance of germs as an etiological variable in sickness evolved from a skepticism about monocausal scenarios inherited from the distant past. These included humoral theory, dogmatic interpretations of miasmatic influences, and so forth. But a skeptical mind was not synonymous with complete denial of the utility of old ideas. Roberts, therefore, would insist that contemporary interpretations of old notions had to satisfy the same criterion he expected from unorthodox approaches to healing. Merely being ancient, commonplace, familiar, widespread, and popular was neither proof nor invalidation of scientific merit.

Roberts' acceptance of a link between microscopic organisms and noncontagious sickness, infection and infectious diseases included a realization that there also was a correlation between these tiny creatures and fevers. It also made him aware of the phenomenon of periodicity and its link to recurrent paroxysms and dreaded epidemics.

Roberts at times implied, and at other times explicitly suggested, that a society is what its people ate and that dietary custom was a reflection of biological destiny. Genetic makeup mandates a preference for certain foodstuffs and avoidance of others. This applied to individuals and to entire populations. Roberts acknowledged the existence of acquired tastes and that preference for items might entail something more than only genetic determination. Changing food habits among individuals, even more so for an entire population, was a slow process, a perhaps impossible task; a futile struggle against nature to instill a permanent change among people who could not change. This biological trait suggested that, in Roberts' view of the world, some nations were destined to remain less than fully "civilized."

Meat eaters and alcohol consumers were salient contributors to worldwide societal progress. And for Roberts, alcohol and tobacco were the opposite of what fervent anti-opiumists proclaimed them to be. He associated alcohol and tobacco use with a better life on earth, whereas the moral reformers lumped them in a category of items negating any decent existence whatsoever. Japan, the only Asian nation occupying a level of civilization approximating Anglo-European societies, was proof of the benefit of alcoholic beverages. And he implied that other "stimulants" had similar consequences for the human brain and nervous system. Roberts' pronouncements indicate that he was intellectually at odds with anti-opiumists even before commencement of the Royal Commission hearings. He also was predisposed to be more sympathetic to pro-traders' claims about the positive, or at least the benign consequences of opium use, in moderation or otherwise.

Roberts was also inclined to accept sex and age differences in food preferences as virtually immutable, hence acceptable and to be expected wherever they occur. Therapeutic specialists should not condemn the elderly because they ingested a substance or substances which younger generations did not consume. There should be no disparagement of anything that the old prefer because it was suitable for biological requirements at that time in their lives. And there was a high probability that no one single thing could satisfy the needs of the elderly in every society around the world: old folks were different from younger people, but old people were not clones of each other. What they needed to combat the physical and mental deterioration of aging depended upon the society in which they lived and their genetic inheritance. Sex as well as age differences in "brain food" substances did not invalidate the "truth" of meat, alcohol, and tobacco being good for mental prowess or powers. They indicated the role of genetics and the inevitable life cycle in humans for influencing what kinds of "brain food" one was attracted to, and at what age.

Roberts' skepticism about the proliferation of processed foods available to citizens of modern society was the product of his physiological experiments and study of nutrient absorption. His research led him to believe that food passing too quickly through the digestive system precluded complete extraction of its nutritive value. He might not be shocked or hostile, therefore, to someone advocating or condoning the consumption of substances that prolonged food retention in organs responsible for digestion. He also appears to have been predisposed not to summarily reject the testimony of witnesses who commented favorably upon William James Moore's idea of opium being a food because it was a mechanism preventing dysentery or rapid propulsion of material through the body. If Moore's proponents furnished sufficient and convincing proof during the hearings, Roberts just might accept the "unconventional" interpretation of the drug being nutritious due to its ability to impede evacuation, thereby helping to prevent and to cure 'malaria'. The number and kind of witnesses plus the quality of their testimony would be crucial in the man's decisions. Also important were the locations Roberts and his colleagues would visit in South Asia to gather evidence for their recommendations to Queen Victoria and Parliament. In both respects the Government of India and supporters of the opium status quo had a dismaying advantage.

THE ROYAL COMMISSION ITINERARY
IN INDIA AND SELECTION OF WITNESSES

Anti-opiumists had problems even before the Commission's first hearing on 8 September 1893. Lord Brassey invited the Government of India to select witnesses. One unidentified Commission member, most likely Henry Wilson, objected. This dissenter claimed the British India administration would choose only people who supported its position. The Commission thereafter performed this task to avoid the appearance of bias (GBO [Final Report] 1895:VI:4). The Government of India, however, refused to search for any anti-opium witnesses in the country (Owen [1934] 1968:320; Johnson 1975:313). The SSOT had to find its own people.

Having the Royal Commission select witnesses did not allay SSOT suspicion. The Commission's mission was to evaluate the medical utility of opium only in India. Lord Brassey disagreed. He thought the review should include responses from opium-consuming regions beyond South Asia. Brassey then had questionnaires sent to British Governors of Hong Kong and the "Straits Settlements," i.e., Singapore, Penang, and so forth, and to Her Majesty's Minister in China. These officials in turn would request responses from "competent witnesses" (GBO [Final Report] 1895:VI:1–2). Anti-opiumists had neither the time nor finances to follow suit. Their evidence would be colleagues' previous comments about the drug's status in China and other Asian locales and Anglo-European opiate research findings; they hoped that Brassey's supplementary information would be unbiased.

The SSOT faced another problem. Lord Brassey had also instructed the Indian government to choose the locations to visit in the subcontinent. It did so. Members of the Commission, however, had neither the time nor the endurance to travel throughout the entire country listening to testimony. The strain was not relieved despite some witnesses journeying to selected locations to testify.

India's administrators then proposed a revised itinerary and Lord Brassey accepted the change. Travel was limited to places in the northern part of the subcontinent where opium consumption was prevalent. The locations formed a wide belt from the Northwest Provinces to the eastern borders of Burma and Assam and extending south to Rajputana, Bombay Presidency, Central India, and Orissa.

Witnesses from "Lower" or south (peninsular) India, consequently, were underrepresented in the oral testimony. The Government of India claimed the omission was unimportant because opium was less significant in the life of south Indians. Supplementary evidence could be obtained by questionnaires sent to responsible individuals if this information was deemed necessary (GBO [Final Report] 1895:VI:2).

Relegating south India to secondary importance was a setback for the SSOT. The Government of India was correct; people in this part of the country consumed much less opium but they were not immune from the diseases that harmed fellow citizens in the north. The probable dearth of oral evidence extolling the drug among the inhabitants in peninsular India would have enabled the SSOT to challenge pro-traders' proclamations about opium's alleged indispensability or utility. The reason for minimal consumption in the south was that most of these people might not view the drug as a prophylactic or cure for malaria, 'malaria', or any other disease.

SSOT naivete now became painfully obvious. As discussed earlier, its leaders had assumed that taxpayers in India and Great Britain would gladly reimburse the Government of India for lost revenue. One consequence of the incorrect assumption was soon evident after the government announced its refusal to locate witnesses that were sympathetic to the SSOT position. The responsibility fell to Henry Wilson and Joseph G. Alexander. The Commission first questioned thirty-nine witnesses in London. Seventeen were Protestant evangelists from China (Beattie 1969:122). Wilson and Alexander then departed for India to organize the anti-opiumist defense. This work had to be completed before the Commission reconvened in Calcutta on 18 November. The response in India dismayed the two men. Groups that were assumed to support the SSOT offered little or no help. Indian doctors who had signed an 1892 anti-opium memorial now refused to testify for the organization. Other physicians recanted their signatures on the document during their appearance before the Commission. Anti-opiumists' disappointment was exacerbated when Indian political associations, including the forerunner of the Congress Party, announced opposition to prohibition. The refusals were understandable. An SSOT success meant that people in these organizations would have to compensate the Government of India for lost revenue. And it is difficult to imagine why any indigenous politician or political party would want to be identified with a policy that guaranteed increased taxes for Indian citizens.

The SSOT cause was further damaged by the behavior of Commission appointees when they were in India. All of them except Henry Wilson stayed in the British compounds during the hearings. This meant they avoided contact with natives, and the possibility of hearing informal, unsolicited evidence that might influence their opinions in the final deliberations was negligible. Wilson, however, was amenable to listening to all people. This receptiveness was not much help. He and Alexander "worked hard to find evidence and witnesses against opium, [but] they seldom encountered any" (Johnson 1975:313).

Lord Brassey announced completion of the Commission's interviewing phase on 11 February 1894. Hearings had been held on seventy of the eighty-three working days spent in India. Commission appointees had interrogated 723 people, of whom 257 were Europeans and 466 were natives of China or India (GBO [Final Report] 1895:VI:5). The SSOT, however, nominated only a fraction of the total: 152 witnesses with ninety-two being either Indian or Chinese. The remaining sixty witnesses were American or European. English nationals are classified as "European" in Commission documents.

The majority of anti-opium witnesses were "missionaries," a total of thirty-nine people. With the exception of five Chinese and Indians, all missionaries were European and American. Other church-affiliated individuals included five Indians and Chinese described as "catechists and mission teachers." There also were two Chinese and Indian non-Christian "Preachers." The last entry in the

"Missionaries" category was thirteen European and American "medical missionaries." The Royal Commission report states that all these witnesses admitted their testimonies were based upon religious convictions. Furthermore, their work experience and observations had confirmed these moral sentiments.

The Royal Commission's comment can be construed as a criticism of the SSOT witnesses' lack of objectivity. If this was the Commission's intention, the same comment regarding the influence of ideology upon judgment is applicable to the numerous people the Government of India successfully nominated as witnesses.

The second largest anti-opium contingent was twenty-six "Representatives of Associations." This category had twenty-three Indians and Chinese, three Europeans and Americans. One person belonged to

> a political association in Calcutta, and addressed the Commission on the system of poppy cultivation in Behar. Of the others, three appeared on behalf of the English Anti-Opium Society, eight represented the Brahmo Samaj of Bengal, and the rest, societies for the promotion of abstinence from stimulants in upper Indian and Bombay. (GBO [Final Report] 1895:VI:15)

Fourteen "medical practitioners" presented their views supporting facets of the SSOT cause. Ten were native to China or India and four were European or American. There were also three Europeans or Americans plus eight Chinese and Indians designated as "Merchants and Shopkeepers" testifying on behalf of the anti-opiumists. Eleven other individuals (three Europeans and Americans, eight Indians and Chinese) were classified as "Miscellaneous." All people in each of the remaining occupational categories were Indians and Chinese: eight former government officials, four people then currently employed as "government officials," seven "lawyers," six "landlords and tenants," four "journalists," and two people classified as "Professors and masters" (GBO [Final Report] 1895:VI:15).

The one potential bright spot for the SSOT in this underrepresentation was that "volunteer" witnesses unaffiliated with the anti-opiumist cause—even those selected by the Government of India—might not offer unqualified support for the present pattern of opium consumption in South Asia. Some of these people might be sympathetic to the SSOT's moral argument or they might give evidence challenging the use of opium except for medical purposes.

The chance of that happening was slim. The Government of India selected members of three groups to speak on its behalf. "Official" witnesses comprised the first category. They were qualified to provide information regarding the extent of poppy cultivation as well as the processing of opium and its sale in India. The group also included people familiar with systems of taxation in British India plus the native states and individuals having information about general financial and administrative aspects of the opium trade.

The second group consisted of civil and military officers knowledgeable about opium consumption among the "different races" in various parts of the country. Here were the police officers and individuals involved in the administration of criminal law, and "gentlemen of the medical profession" in government service as well as those in private practice. All of them purportedly had "opportunities of observing the moral and physical effects of the consumption of opium."

The last category were the "European" and "'Native' non-official gentlemen of recognized standing" (GBO [Final Report] 1895:VI:3). They were competent in discussing the opium question from a different perspective. This meant the witnesses would express personal opinions or the position of the organizations they represented.

The Royal Commission's Final Report indicates that many Government of India witnesses who testified about the consequences of opiate indulgence were members of the Indian Medical Service (IMS). The institution is portrayed as being beyond reproach. It accepted only individuals "qualified as medical men in the United Kingdom" who had survived "severe competition" during the selection process. After completing contracts, many of these physicians remained in India to serve as "civil surgeons." Therefore, all past and present IMS personnel were qualified to "speak with authority" about the effects of opium upon the health and morality of the Indian population. Equally important, their "professional standing is a guarantee of their independence of character," which meant that Royal Commission appointees could assume the testimonies of these witnesses were untainted by nonmedical issues relating to opium (GBO [Final Report] 1895:VI:16). These pronouncements are moot.

NOTES

1. Moore entered the Bombay Medical Service in 1852. After serving in the Persian War during 1856–1857, he was the residency surgeon at several locations in Rajputana from 1862 to 1877. Appointed deputy surgeon-general of Bombay in 1877, he was promoted to surgeon-general in 1885 and retired in 1888. He received the K.C.I.E. in the same year and was appointed an honorary physician to Queen Victoria. Moore died 9 September 1896 (Buckland [1906] 1969d:298).

2. Birdwood was born in India to a family with long residency in South Asia. He entered the Bombay Medical Service in 1854, served in the Persian War during 1856–1857, and became a well-known philanthropist in Bombay after his return. Birdwood held many official positions in the city. Some of these were cited in this chapter. Poor health forced him to return to England whereupon he joined the India Office. He served as special assistant in the Revenue and Statistical Department from 1878 to 1899. Birdwood wrote many articles and longer publications in the arts and sciences before and after retirement. Erudition in Sanskrit, extensive knowledge about Indian art, philology, etymology, and folklore, combined with medical training and years of service in India, account for Birdwood's opinions about opium consumption. His ideas appeared in the British press during the last twenty-five years of the nineteenth century. See Buckland [1906] 1969a:43, and *DNB* 1938:46–47. Also consult Brereton 1882:230.

3. The critique is presented in this chapter. An appropriate designation for Birdwood is 'more notorious' rather than 'better known'. In his influential 1892 diatribe against the anti-opiumists, G. H. M. Batten said the "views of Sir William Moore . . . are well known

[and] they fully accord with those I have already quoted" (GBO [Batten] 1894:I:146]. The ideas of Birdwood, not Moore, strained scientific credulity at the time.

4. Material published between the early 1880s and early 1890s contains Moore's ideas. These are: *IMG* 1880:September 1 & October 1:225–30, 257–64; *Transactions of the Bombay Medical Society* 1882a:n.p.; 1882b *Other Side of the Opium Question*; *PMJ* 1892a:11:February:58–63; *PMJ* 1892b:XI: 638–40; MR 1892c:1:December 1:224–29; *BMJ* 1893:2:December 2:1196; MR 1894a:III:89–95, and his 1886b *A Manual of the Diseases of India, with a Compendium of Diseases Generally* (2nd edition), especially "Fevers," pages 249–58, and "Malaria," pages 259–82.

In the 1886b *Manual*, Moore cites his previous publications challenging aspects of fever diagnosis. These are "Famine and Fever in Rajputana" and "On the Value of Quinine." He indicates both articles are in the 1870 volume of *Indian Medical Gazette* (*IMG*). An article entitled "Malaria versus Recognisable Causes of Disease" is found in one of the *Gazette's* issues for 1876. One issue of the 1874 volume for *The Indian Annals of Medical Science* (*IAMS*) has his article entitled "Diagnosis of Indian Fevers." The IAMS published two another relevant document. The first is called "On Fever." It might be found in volume twenty-one. The other title is "Masked Malarial Fever." No more bibliographical data are available for the two articles because these issues of the IAMS were unavailable to the author. Earlier issues of the IMG also were unavailable.

The author did obtain two articles appearing in IAMS during the 1870s. They are 1878a "Marwar—The Land of Death" (20:497–530) and 1878b "Remarks on Remittent and Intermittent Fevers, and Their Complications" (20:1–95). Their contents are cited in the chapter when appropriate.

5. The second edition (London: J. A. Churchill) was not revised. This indicates that Moore's beliefs did not change after the first volume's publication. See chapter 16 for details, especially the discussion of "Fevers" (pages 249–58), and "Malaria" (pages 259–82).

6. Moore provided a prelude to his 1886 rebuttal of 'malarial poison' ideas in one section of his article "Marwar—The Land of Death." *IAMS* 1878a:20:513–17. The section evaluates variations of the explanation articulated by physicians who were working in India and elsewhere in the world. Moore presents examples from his experience in Rajputana to disprove their contentions.

7. Sir James Piaget's critique had inspired Moore. Piaget said the majority of the diseases being "discovered" were only deviations of some "well-recognized typical disease" (Moore 1886b:249).

8. By 1886, Moore had changed his mind about the role of water. In the 1878 article about Marwar (in Rajputana), he had been "inclined to believe that malarious disease more frequently arises from the use of impure water" (1878a:20:515).

9. Moore acknowledged that administering quinine was beneficial for people suffering from his "remittent fever" in 1878. See his article entitled "Marwar—The Land of Death" in *IAMS* 1878a:20:497–530) He said that when confronted with "all severe cases of fever, and I occasionally treat very violent remittents, recourse is had to quinine" (1878a:20:517). Subcutaneous injection of the alkaloid in solution produced quicker results than oral consumption. He does not mention opium as a preventive or a cure for his "malaria," "paroxysmal fevers," "malarious fevers," "severe fevers," or "very violent remittents" (1878a:20:513–18). Besides quinine, Moore cites strychnine for "long cases of continued fever," and in cases "of enlarged spleens," he used the biniodide of mercury, plus other items (1878a:20:518–19). He also describes what Indian natives ingest for enlarged spleens. *Papaver somniferum Linn* is not in the list of "antiperiodics" (1878a:20:519).

154   Chapter 4

Moore does discuss eating opium in two brief paragraphs of another 1878 article publication. The article is "Remarks on Remittent and Intermittent Fevers, and Their Complications." It also is in the *IAMS* article (20:1–95). Moore mentions "remittent" and "intermittent" fevers, and his comments about opium are cautious. He is "inclined [to suggest] that a prophylactic influence is observable," and that consumption "probably tends to prevent malarious poison taking effect in . . . several ways" (1878b:20:13).

The first "way" is that it "prevents waste of tissue, . . . [and] it also exerts its well-known direct stimulating or sedative actions on the nerves" (1878b:20:13). The second "way" is what natives believe; they claim opium "will not only preserve them from fever, but also from some other maladies" (1878b:20:13). The other supporting evidence that Moore offers for the drug is that he had frequently noticed confirmed opium eaters being able to escape "fever, when others were attacked" (1878b:20:13). For example, he mentions two opium eaters who managed to stay healthy when "every person attached to the Political Agency, suffered from one or other type of fever" (1878b:20:13). He also includes eighty patients admitted to a dispensary. All of them suffered from "one or other form of paroxysmal fever," and only twelve of them were opium eaters (1878b:20:14). The small number of consumers among the ranks of the sick was, for Moore, a clue to the drug's power.

This kind of evidence enabled him to claim that opium had long been regarded as a "remedial agent, second only to quinine, and therefore a prophylactic action might be presumed" (1878b:20:13). Except for the Indian natives cited above, Moore does not identify other people (Anglo-European physicians and observers) providing evidence for him to make this generalization.

10. See pages 330–34 for Moore's comments about "Masked Malarial Fever." Observations about continued, intermittent, typical ague, remittent, enteric, typhus, relapsing, and cerebro-spinal fevers are found on pages 278–330.

11. Pyrexia is "to be feverish . . . [or having] abnormal elevation of body temperature; Fever . . . " (*WNID* 1975:942).

12. Moore said that other India experts shared his views. Oldham "entirely rejects the theory of specific poison, and refers fevers to chill" (1886b:273). Lyons said the miasma theory was inapplicable. Bellews believed "malarious fevers are produced by chill," and Planck, Gordon, and O'Connell indicated essentially the same thing (Moore 1886b:273). The opinions of these physicians prompted Moore to declare that Dr. MacNamara's query about malaria being the result of "the sum of operations of the various conditions of climate and place by which we are surrounded may be answered in the affirmative" (1886b:274). References to other medical personnel are found throughout the volume.

13. Moore was suggesting that personal hygiene contaminated the atmosphere. But if impurities in the air cause sickness, Moore was advancing essentially the same interpretation as the malarial poison and "contagion" theoreticians whom he castigated. He was oblivious to the subtle contradiction. The difference is that Moore viewed human beings as principal creators of the pollution whereas malarial poison proponents blamed nature, such as swamp emanations.

14. Moore also recommended quinine to alleviate various symptoms associated with his cerebro-spinal fever, or spinal "affections." This was an inclusive category encompassing what fellow diagnosticians classified as enteric, undefined fever, relapsing fever, typhoid, and typhus (Moore 1886b:303–22). See pages 322–33 for Moore's other comments about quinine's power and liabilities, including its ability to reduce the body's "heat."

15. Moore was very active in 1892 attempting to provide support for the opium prophylactic argument. His publication "Malaria and Its Remedies" is one example of the ef-

fort. It is in the 1 December 1892 issue of *PMJ*: 11:638–40. Moore now disparages the idea of quinine (and cinchona) for being a "specific remedy for various forms of so-called malarious disease." There is sufficient evidence that the alkaloid has been "much over estimated as a preventive and as a curative agent." In contrast, he gives a glowing account of opium, declaring that it "is certain that . . . opium prevents malarial fevers" (1892b:11:639).

He then declares that the power of opium is probably due to narcotine. He then discusses the mother drug's ability to prevent 'fevers'. Consumption prevents "chill" among people who are "sensitive to cold and damp," it enables people to survive on a diet that most Europeans would say is "semi-starvation" and would lead to "febrile and other diseases" among non-Indians (1892b:11:639–40).

Opium also provides the same benefits that alcoholic stimulants offer to people elsewhere in the world. He admits that "[f]ear of the anathema of the 'Society for the Suppression of the Use of Opium' prevents more [discussion] on this subject" (1892b:11:640). He did not hesitate to express his contempt for the SSOT (and fellow travelers) in another 1892 publication. The title is "The Errors of the Anti-Opiumists" and it was published in *PMJ*:11:58–63). Two other articles supporting the medical benefits of opium for disease prevention and cure are his *PMJ* 1894b:13:15–21 and *PMJ* 1895:14:9.

16. Moore was wrong. As discussed earlier, massive opium consumption in the Fens had virtually ceased before 1892. Two factors responsible for the decline were disruption of supply and the better-educated population in the Fens. Availability of drugs that were capable of curing the maladies for which opium had hitherto been consumed, in addition to factors previously mentioned, also contributed to the drug's decreased popularity in the region.

17. Moore was most likely referring to the testimony that Surgeon-General Rice gave to the Royal Commission on Opium in Calcutta. Rice's perspective is discussed in following chapters.

18. It probably was the testimony of Government of India employees or officers given to the Royal Commission on Opium held in London before departure for India (Moore 1893:1196). Moore might have been aware of two obscure India documents dating from the late 1850s and 1860. This material is discussed at length in a following chapter.

19. See Tod [1829, 1832, 1914] 1971:1:553–5 and 1971:2:578–84 for details.

20. A case can be made for Brassey not being qualified if lack of bias was a criterion for appointment to the Royal Commission. The man was not free from involvement in the opium commerce. This link is discussed in another, and later, chapter.

21. Roberts was born 18 March 1830 and died 16 April 1898 (*BMJ* 1899:1063). G. H. Brown (1955:147) says Roberts was a pioneer in biochemistry.

22. The first article is 1885 "On Feeding the Sick." Address in Therapeutics Delivered Before the British Medical Association at Cardiff, 1885. *BMJ* 2:188–92. The second publication is 1890 "On Some Points in Dietetics." Address Delivered at the Opening of the Current Session of the Manchester Medical Society. *BMJ* 2:883–85. Other sources and additional material from Roberts are cited when necessary. Also see the *BMJ* 1899:1064–65, and Stephen & Lee 1921–22:22–Supplement:1171.

5

Hope for the Anti-Opiumists: Witnesses' Perspectives about Why People in India Eat Opium

INTRODUCTION

Dr. F. J. Mouat, defender of the Government of India's opium policy and occupant of the "chairs of Medicine and Medical Jurisprudence" at Calcutta Medical College Hospital, testified in London on 15 September 1893. It was the fourth day of the Royal Commission hearings. He had been an "assistant opium examiner and official chemical examiner of processed opium" during the 1840s and later became a "professor of *Materia Medica* and Chemistry." Mouat remained as convinced as he had been before creation of the Commission that the drug was a panacea about which the public was misinformed or not being told (Mouat 1892:959). The evidence offered this time, he admitted, was minimal. Nonetheless, he claimed the cases were typical (GBOW [Mouat] 1894:I:76). Mouat spoke about three individuals delivering medicine to victims of an epidemic in the Terai districts. The districts were near the city of Bareilly in the United Provinces. One person who smoked only tobacco died as soon as the group reached its destination. The second individual consumed bhang and managed to return to Bareilly with a "bad type of remittent fever."[1] The third man, a "confirmed opium eater . . . returned after the epidemic was over, much improved in health and experience" (GBOW [Mouat] 1894:I:76). Mouat did not indicate having met these people, but for him the episode was proof that eating opium guaranteed disease avoidance and survival. Mouat was a harbinger of things to come. The anecdotal evidence he presented to the Royal Commission in the early days of its inquiry was not an atypical event during the next six months.

Members of the Royal Commission asked eleven other witnesses in London specifically about the opium and malaria connection. One hundred and thirty-eight people in India were questioned about the topic. The 149 witnesses provided testimony of varying quality. Like Mouat, some offered an anecdote having limited usefulness for comprehending usage patterns and rationales throughout the country.[2] A few respondents were even less helpful; they said little more than yes or no when asked about a correlation between ingestion and disease. The Royal Commission neither requested elaboration nor did it solicit information about what these people knew about the beliefs of Indian citizens.[3] These witnesses are listed in Appendices A and B or cited in endnotes. Other individuals, however, did offer testimony providing some information about who consumed opium and why they did so. The most informative are discussed in the following pages.

Sir William Roberts drew upon these witnesses' comments about several related topics to evaluate medical aspects of the opium habit in India. This chapter presents what all people, not just the individuals who influenced Roberts, said about each of the issues. The next chapter does the same thing for related topics. Similar to Mouat, the inclusion of biographical data establishes the respondents' qualifications to speak about the subject. Excerpts from witnesses' testimonies also are used, sometimes extensively. Citing what people said and how they said it accomplishes several things. These utterances convey a sense of time and place. They also clearly document witnesses' contradictory responses about the relationship between *Papaver somniferum Linn* and the malady caused by plasmodia. The content of actual dialogue, in this case participants' comments about eating the drug and 'malaria,' also provides a clue to their acceptance or at least cognizance of more inclusive theories of disease and drugs. Some witnesses were explicit about the theoretical framework prompting their observations. Other respondents' notions were unexpressed or unrecognized. The opinions of some participants were prominent in Sir William Roberts' report to the Royal Commission. He ignored other people or accorded them marginal credibility. The testimonies that Roberts deemed to be relevant, therefore, illuminate the more inclusive ideas about sickness, health preservation and restoration he thought appropriate for South Asia.

This chapter reviews witnesses' rationalizations about why people in India ate opium. Explanations are found in their declarations about the significance of pain relief, about opium as a food, about the merits of the drug compared to quinine and other cinchona alkaloids, about exactly how opium helps or hinders a sufferer, and in their comments concerning the narcotine content of opium. The next chapter presents their comments about how sexual identity, age, religion, place of residence, caste, wealth, ethnicity, and nationality influenced opium use throughout South Asia. The material includes witnesses' explanations for nonconsumption.

Chapters 5 and 6 can be read in two ways. The summaries included for most issues discussed within each chapter are brief statements of what members of the Royal Commission were hearing about specific topics. Reading only these summaries offers a glimpse into what was transpiring. However, careful reading of the anecdotal material comprising each chapter section conveys the aforementioned sense of time and place. Performing this tedious task also helps explain why Roberts' conclusions and recommendations were so controversial at the time of their publication. In brief, the man's selective use of oral testimony translated into an evaluation favorable to the Government of India.

Chapter 1 described Anglo-European disease terminology during part of the 1800s as vague and burdened with multiple meanings. These traits characterize the statements of many witnesses queried by the Royal Commission in the mid-1890s. Since their phrases and words often lacked exactitude, the format found in previous chapters is used throughout the book. It identifies what is being referred to. Single vertical marks frequently enclose such terms as 'malarial fever,' 'malarious diseases,' 'malaria,' 'fever,' 'fever diseases,' 'malarious regions,' and so forth. These indicate, for lack of a better term, a loose use of the word or phrase. The individual's 'malarial fever,' for example, clearly refers to more than one etiologically distinct malady. A 'malarial region' described a locale plagued by two or more different afflictions.

Henceforth, these Royal Commission witnesses are called "lumpers." Lumpers are similar to theoreticians alluded to in the opening chapter who proposed one remedy for maladies subsumed under 'malaria.'

Single vertical marks also are used when the entire content of a person's testimony suggests the orientation, but brevity of the excerpt found in the chapter makes this difficult for a reader to delineate. There also are a few instances when malaria is not enclosed within single marks. This occurs when it is impossible to identify exactly what the person had in mind when using the term. It is unclear if the speaker recognized a distinction between the plasmodia-induced sickness and other interpretations of malaria. Other terms enclosed by single marks signify this author is referring to its popular meaning during the 1890s. However, no signifiers are used with the word 'paroxysm.' Today it means an intense outburst of disease symptoms. One symptom is fever. The Royal Commission on Opium volumes, however, indicate that a more restrictive definition was in vogue among many participants; it was a synonym for an episode of elevated body temperature. The author uses this definition in chapters 5 and 6. The rationale for enclosing words between quotation marks (the exception being paroxysm) also applies to the remainder of the book.

A Government of India official assigned each of the 723 witnesses (257 "European" and 466 "Native") to one of twenty-two occupational categories.[4] Although seventeen groups were represented among the 149 witnesses providing commentary about the drug and the disease, two categories of medical professionals predominated.[5] Eighty-one "medical practitioners [currently] employed by Government," most often meaning the Indian Medical Service (IMS), appeared before the Royal Commission. Forty-nine people having this classification said something about the correlation. It was the largest occupational category represented among witnesses cited in this, and the next, chapter. "Medical Practitioners (Private)" held second place; thirty-one physicians currently in private practice or retired testified before the Royal Commission. Table 1 lists the occupational categories and number of all opium and 'malaria' witnesses.

Scholars writing in the twentieth century have commented about the presence of "sometimes, well-coached pro-opium witnesses" testifying about diverse topics during the hearings (Johnson, 1975:313; see also Owen, [1934]

1968:320). In this chapter, the characterization is also appropriate for individuals whose statements supported the opium and 'malaria' correlation. It also describes a few SSOT-nominated witnesses. The interrogation style of Sir James B. Lyall, Lord Brassey, and Sir William Roberts for other witnesses occasionally made a favorable pro-opium response inevitable. The instances of Lyall "leading the witness" stemmed from his unabashed espousal of the status quo. Roberts' proclivity for the procedure most likely was a determination to extract a maximum amount of data about the medical benefits of opium use with as much precision as possible. Brassey's silence about the tactic might be due to inexperience in dealing with a controversial issue, or not wanting to interfere with colleagues' performance of duty.

This is conjecture, but what is obvious from a review of the Royal Commission hearings is that what people did for a living was not a reliable predictor of their responses. Witnesses accepting or rejecting opium as a prophylactic or febrifuge or both crossed occupational boundaries. For example, all Government of India officials, regardless of rank in the administration and department affiliation, did not provide data supporting the relationship.[6] Physicians in the Indian Medical Service did the same thing. Furthermore, the responses of these witnesses, who were all nominated by the Government of India, did not enhance the credibility of proclamations extolling opium use in India. Very few people from the small group of SSOT witnesses gave testimony that condoned aspects of official drug policy.

Equally obvious is that giving an honest opinion about the opium and 'malaria' correlation was not synonymous with articulating an accurate evaluation of disease and appropriate therapy even by the standards of that era. The testimonies reveal surprising ignorance for some people and unexpected sophistication from others. This is applicable to everybody from the occupational categories providing "evidence." This included the "Medical Experts" who claimed to be independent witnesses, those employed by the Government of India in the Indian Medical Service or otherwise, and physicians affiliated with, or sympathetic to, the SSOT.

WHY DO PEOPLE IN INDIA EAT OPIUM?

Witnesses' Awareness about Perceptions of
Disease and Curing in Anglo-European Medicine and Science

Many witnesses influenced by miasmatic and tellurian theories of sickness had something in common. They lumped etiologically distinct maladies possessing a common symptom of elevated body temperature under the term 'malaria.' Their testimonies contain numerous references to 'malarious diseases,' 'malarious fevers,' 'malarial environment,' and 'miasmatic influences.'

Other witnesses in India challenged the assumption that superficially similar symptoms were proof of a common etiology. These dissenters considered climate, topography, elevation, and so forth, to be variables in the appearance, duration and virulence of a disease, but not the only ones. Some of these witnesses were aware of current research in allopathic medicine while the rest were not, but their collective dissatisfaction with the limitations of old paradigms prompted a suggestion, often clearly stated and sometimes implied, that additional factors of equal importance were involved. For these witnesses, comprehending the nature of human sickness and how to cure it required looking beyond a simplistic portrayal of the setting in which similar overt characteristics were manifested. Henceforth, these critics are called "splitters" and the people with whom they disagreed are the "lumpers."

Splitters rejected the lumpers' penchant for placing etiologically distinct maladies in an inclusive category called 'malaria.' Splitters were aware of current western research or they had serious reservations about old explanations. For these people, idiosyncratic traits of paroxysms generated by an assortment of vaguely defined ailments labeled 'malarious diseases' indicated the presence of additional and different causative agents. This suggested that a "cure" for one disease with a fever symptom might be ineffective for a malady that generated a different pattern of paroxysm. There was, therefore, no universal cure for all diseases accompanied by elevated body temperatures. Fever-producing sicknesses were unrelated to each other for reasons other than elevation above sea level or changes in the climate and topography of a locale. These distinct afflictions required different therapeutic procedures. A drug like opium, for example, might alleviate symptoms of one kind of 'fever disease' or it might not. It might even eliminate the unknown variable responsible for the appearance of the paroxysm or it might do nothing of the sort.

Witnesses' Understanding of the Chemistry and Pharmacology of *Papaver somniferum Linn*

Witnesses demonstrated minimal awareness of western researchers' pre-1894 opium discoveries. Most lumpers and splitters, including medical doctors, viewed the drug as an undifferentiated entity. Few people in either category recognized the significance of alkaloids or thought these components were sufficiently important to mention. Some witnesses identified morphine as responsible for any possible therapeutic value opium had for preventing or curing 'malaria'. Other participants disagreed; they recognized narcotine—not morphine—as an alkaloid of importance but attributed different capabilities to it, or none whatsoever.

OPIUM AND PAIN: A RARE INSTANCE OF AGREEMENT AND THE DISPUTED COROLLARY

Witnesses' comments about virtually all arguments proclaiming or refuting opium as a prophylactic or febrifuge of malaria depended upon their acceptance of broad or narrow interpretations of the malady. One example was the difference of opinion between lumpers and splitters about inferences drawn from "pain relief." This was the only capability that everyone recognized opium as having. Some lumpers construed the power of opium to relieve pain as evidence that the drug also prevented or cured their version of 'malaria.' Other witnesses with similar inclination said the drug performed all three functions; opium was a prophylactic as well as a febrifuge for 'malaria,' and it was a general-purpose anodyne. Splitters disagreed with all of them. They were equally opposed to the frequent portrayal of quinine having limited or no value for preventing and curing any of the etiologically distinct ailments which lumpers classified as 'malaria.'

Twenty-six witnesses specifically mentioned opium and pain. All portrayed the drug as an anodyne but they disagreed about the wider significance of this trait. Some people said relief of pain proved that opium was also a prophylactic, or a febrifuge, or both, for malaria or 'malarial fevers.' The majority of witnesses indicated the correlation was spurious because pain relief, disease prevention, and cure were separate issues. Opium might comfort a person suffering from a disease but it did not prevent or cure the malady. Witnesses also had contradictory thoughts about Indian natives' beliefs regarding the status of opium as an anodyne, as a prophylactic, and as a febrifuge for 'malaria.'

Testimonies were elicited from individuals living in different parts of the country. The following responses representing both points of view are grouped according to region. The regional identification is periodically used for other topics discussed in chapters 5 and 6. The map of India (with comments) identifies these regions.

Opium Was Only a Useful Anodyne

Middle India

Reverend J. Wilkie was a fourteen-year veteran of missionary work for the Canadian Presbyterian Church in Indore, Central India. On the sixty-sixth day of the hearings, Wilkie told the Royal Commission that Indian natives realized opium neither prevented nor cured diseases. Nonetheless, they still consumed it as a "remedy" in "all cases of trouble" because it relieved pain (GBOW [Wilkie] 1894:IV:165). He also had heard opium was "used [specifically] for fever; . . . [but] so far as I know from inquiry or personal observation, the people do not value it either to ward off or cure fever, but use it to relieve the accompanying pain" of a paroxysm (GBOW [Wilkie] 1894:IV:164). The minister had firsthand experience. Although not a physician, he took medicine when visiting villages and operated a dispensary in Indore where he gave

> medicines to all those connected with me, and I know those who can get quinine prefer it to opium. I have asked people whether they would use opium for fever, and I have never had an affirmative answer. (GBOW [Wilkie] 1894:IV:165)

Another member of the clergy and two medical doctors working for the Government of India expressed similar sentiments about the population of Middle India.

Mr. Dinnonath Mazumdar, minister for the Brahmo Samaj New Dispensation Church in Bankipur testified on 5 January 1894, the eighth day of the hearings. He said that only opium addicts believed they could avoid frequent bouts of fever, and they did it by consuming the drug. They were wrong, Mazumdar continued, because they suffered from paroxysms regardless of the amount ingested. The minister also contended there was no difference between opium eaters and non-consumers in the number and severity of fever attacks. This meant the drug was ineffective (GBOW [Mazumdar] 1894:III:33).

For Mazumdar, nonaddicted Indian natives using only quinine to prevent or cure malaria refuted opium's alleged prophylactic and febrifuge status. If truly helpful, quinine users would have stopped abstaining from opium because they also wanted to avoid suffering. And having two cures was obviously better than one. Quinine also might be scarce but opium rarely was. It was reasonable, therefore, to expect people to ingest opium if quinine was unavailable, and the argument for opium lacked credibility if the public did not consume the latter. Mazumdar did say *Papaver somniferum Linn* was beneficial for dysentery and rheumatism, but he was unable to "give a definite opinion" regarding the quality of evidence supporting other consumers' assertion about the drug's usefulness in "damp, malarious districts" (GBOW [Mazumdar] 1894:III:33). He did not elaborate.

Surgeon Major-General Rice, Director of the Indian Medical Department, spoke before the Commission on the seventh day of the hearings. He agreed with the Wilkie and Mazumdar assessments about opium in Middle India. Thirty-seven years in the Indian Medical Service as a civil surgeon in the Central Provinces, medical director of a district, and superintendent of its jail, enabled this high-ranking official to declare that opium did not cure "intermittent fever" (GBOW [Rice] 1894:II:11–12). Inhabitants of malarial districts in the Central Provinces also did not believe it prevented malaria, intermittent fevers, or any other disease. They viewed the drug exclusively as a remedy for reducing pain caused by sickness. Opium was consumed only because it was inexpensive and plentiful (GBOW [Rice] 1894:II:12–13).

Surgeon-Major W. A. Quayle was the civil surgeon for Nimar district. He also had been superintendent of a jail in the Central Provinces for eight years (GBOW [Quayle] 1894:IV:339). Quayle was convinced that opium was a popular general anodyne. A few old people in every village of Nimar district used it, and consumption was almost universal among poor people. He told the Royal Commission members that the jungles of Nimar, especially the Tapti valley, were "very malarious tracts." Inhabitants of these locations were plagued by "frequent sequences of malarial fevers, and to relieve these opium is the only remedy within reach of all, and many even cannot afford to purchase it, its price being so prohibitive" (GBOW [Quayle] 1894:IV:340). A common practice among these people was to ingest opium "after ague [but] not as a prophylactic." They consumed it to relieve fever "sequences, diarrhoea, dysentery, neuralgia, and muscular pains" (GBOW [Quayle] 1894 IV:340). Quayle was alluding to rheumatism and other ailments. Although Indians said the drug was good for malarial fever because it relieved discomfort, Quayle said it was a mistake to assert that it prevented people from getting the disease. He admitted having no experience to judge if opium was an effective febrifuge for a person already suffering from the malady. Commentators working elsewhere in India voiced similar comments.

East India

Reverend M. B. Kirkpatrick spent two years in Toungoo (Burma) and then three and one half years in the Shan States. The experience enabled this medical missionary for the American Baptist Mission to discern different patterns of opium use. Responding to Sir Lyall's questions on the twenty-sixth day of the hearings about the prophylactic capabilities of opium, Kirkpatrick said malaria was rampant in rural and urban areas of the Shan States with which he was familiar (GBOW [Kirkpatrick] 1894:II:217). Two-thirds of the inhabitants of Thibau City had the malady, and it was so common elsewhere during the monsoon that everyone anticipated suffering. Despite this prevalence, Kirkpatrick had never known and had never heard of Shan natives taking opium "to relieve them of fever" (GBOW [Kirkpatrick] 1894:II:219). A closer association between the drug and the disease was found only among opium smokers who came to the hospital in Toungoo. They confessed to beginning the habit to relieve pain associated with fever. Kirkpatrick's description of the term indicates it included paroxysms caused by malarial plasmodia. These opium smokers became addicted to the drug but continued to have attacks, albeit with less pain being reported. According to Kirkpatrick, other residents of the locale and natives elsewhere in Burma never told him that fellow Burmese "used [opium] as a prophylactic: it is simply to relieve the pains when they have the fever" (GBOW [Kirkpatrick] 1894:II:219).

Two other missionaries in East India concurred with Kirkpatrick. Reverend Cushing, a medical doctor working in Burma since 1867, declared that natives in Rangoon and the Shan States rarely used the drug "directly" or "extensively" for malaria. Some local people thought it relieved the pain of 'malarious fever' and therefore assumed it prevented the malady. Cushing thought the assumption was incorrect (GBOW [Cushing] 1894:II:196). Reverend Joseph Samuel Adams, affiliated with the American Baptist Mission and a resident of "upper Burma" during 1874 through 1879, said that even in the most "feverish districts," and those in China as well, opium functioned only as a pain reliever. It never prevented the disease. His subsequent posting for thirteen years in Kinhwa city in China's Chih-kiang Province also convinced him that Chinese opium smokers got the disease quicker than nonsmokers (GBOW [Adams, J. S.] 1894:I:24).

Surgeon-Captain J. H. Tull Walsh expressed a view similar to Kirkpatrick, Cushing, and Adams. Tull Walsh, civil surgeon for the Indian Medical Service in Puri, a large district in the Orissa Province and one of East India's "Lower Provinces," said even the most healthy residents in Puri were in poor physical condition. Most natives viewed the drug as a general anodyne and consumed it "to combat various pain [sic], aches, and diseases." His description of 'fever' indicates the term included paroxysms caused by malarial plasmodia and the elevated temperatures common to other maladies. Although Tull Walsh agreed with the natives' perspective, he was unable to accept opium as a "specific" for malaria because he recognized that all fevers did not produce large spleens. He suggested many physicians and lay people either did not share this awareness, or did not think that differences in spleen size signified the existence of unrelated paroxysms. They mistakenly placed fevers stemming from different origins under the category 'malarial fevers.' Consequently, the drug might be prescribed for "two distinct diseases which have got muddled up under the head of 'malaria,' and there is a possibility that it might be useful for one disease but not the other" (GBOW [Tull Walsh] 1894:II:85–6).[7] This perceptiveness precluded Tull Walsh from proclaiming anything more remarkable about opium. It was a useful anodyne for specific maladies, and these afflictions shared only a common proclivity to induce elevated body temperature.

Dr. James Robert Wallace came from Calcutta. He had been medical doctor in India since 1872 and a private practitioner in the city for the past fourteen years. Testifying on the sixteenth day of hearings, Wallace was not reticent about expressing disdain the notion that opium prevented malaria. He asserted that none of his medical colleagues in India ever mentioned opium as a preventive for the affliction. This included Dr. Norman Chevers, renowned for his tropical disease publications, and an instructor in the medical school that Wallace attended.[8] And never during Wallace's residency in India had natives acknowledged taking opium to prevent or to cure malaria (GBOW [Wallace] 1894:II:117–18). In recognizing that the drug did "relieve the incidental symptoms of the malarial condition as an anodyne," Wallace distinguished between a disease prophylactic and a pain reliever (GBOW [Wallace] 1894:II:119). His experience in the eastern part of the country, especially Calcutta, convinced him the two capabilities were distinct; pain relief simply was not another way of referring to disease prevention.

West India

Another medical missionary working elsewhere in India was unequivocally negative about opium being a prophylactic or febrifuge for malaria. Lord Brassey's interrogation on the forty-ninth day prompted Dr. H. Martyn Clark from Amritsar, a city in Punjab Province, to declare that

> opium is . . . in no sense whatever an anti-periodic. It does not ward off attacks of malarial fever; it in no way shortens such attacks when they do occur. The city and district in which I work is notoriously malarious, even in malarial India, and I have not observed that opium-eaters enjoyed any immunity or suffered any the less. Doubtless in cases of malarial fever it soothes pain, aching of joints, and so forth, eases the malaise and general sense of wretchedness which a person has, and to that extent it is useful; but that it is in any case an antidote or specific for malarial fevers, I have not been able to observe. (GBOW [Clark] 1894:III:191–92)

A witness hailing from another locale in West India echoed Clark's sentiments during the third day of the hearings.

The Northwest Provinces (NWP) was the name for a vast territory located north of Punjab. The NWP, frequently cited in the literature as the Northwest Frontier Agency, included parts of present-day Afghanistan and Pakistan. Brigade-Surgeon R. Pringle, a NWP sanitary officer with thirty years of India experience and active in the SSOT, testified on Wednesday, 13 September 1893. This physician provided the Royal Commission with details for his rejection of the prophylactic and febrifuge argument. Eight years in Orissa (East India), two years in Central India, and twenty years in the NWP forced him to conclude opium itself prevented nothing and cured nothing. It was beneficial only if "prescribed medicinally." This meant that only qualified medical practitioners should dispense the drug to the public. Nonregulated accessibility, even taking small doses in malarial districts, was harmful because opium induced chronic habituation (GBOW [Pringle] 1894:I:54).

Pringle had distributed opium in combination with other medicines, but he never prescribed it as a febrifuge. Queried about the drug's alleged properties for 'malaria,' he replied that it was "merely a febrifuge on the principle that it is sudorific and sedative . . . [it] relieves . . . [the] system by the skin. . . . [It] gives rest and relief from pain and suffering . . . [A person] thus [has] restful sleep at night, both as regards malarial rheumatism and malarial dysentery . . . [but] opium was never suggested as a febrifuge under any condition whatever" (GBOW [Pringle] 1894:I:52–3). For Pringle, an SSOT "addiction specialist" mentioned in an earlier chapter, opium was a useful albeit potentially harmful palliative for the complications caused by malaria. It qualified as a febrifuge only if this term was loosely defined. He concluded anything more grandiose proclaimed about the benefits of consumption was unfounded.

On 1 January 1894, the forty-sixth day of the hearings, Sir William Roberts asked Surgeon-Major S. Little about opium being a "direct prophylactic" for 'malaria.' Little, a resident of India since serving in the 1879–1880 Afghan War and the current civil surgeon at Mooltan in the United Provinces, said that natives in Mooltan never consumed opium believing it has "direct anti-malarial efficacy" (GBOW [Little] 1894:III:161). He then elaborated and told members of the Commission that many maladies besieged these people. Each affliction was exacerbated by

> the malarial element [that] enters into and complicates the source of all these diseases to an enormous extent. It is also largely productive of obscure joint pains and neuralgias [sic] attributed by the sufferer to other causes; so it may be said that opium is largely used to cure or palliate many of the results of malaria, though seldom taken avowedly as a direct prophylactic against the disease itself. (GBOW [Little] 1894:III:161)

The disease, for Little, was a diffuse entity intensifying discomfort. He also rejected opium as a prophylactic for any disease, especially malaria, and so did natives whom Little knew. Similar to Pringle's contention, opium was a febrifuge only if the term was loosely defined. However, any substance capable of blunting the sensation of pain also qualified as a febrifuge, and this rendered the category meaningless. Surgeon-Major Little, as well as Brigade-Surgeon Pringle, contended that opium was, at best, a useful general anodyne.

Another medical missionary provided more details about the effect of opium upon malaria. He was responding to Lord Brassey's query during the sixty-second day of the hearings. Dr. William Huntly told Commission members about his work in the Marwar and Meywar regions of Rajputana. During this posting, he had spent most of the time in the cities of Jodhpur and Nusseerabad. Furthermore, "in all who have come before me, no native ever urged malaria as the reason for beginning or continuing the opium habit" (GBOW [Huntly] 1894:IV:60, 65). Never had he come across evidence proving that opium prevented any malady. For Huntly, no proof existed because "during the last two seasons of excessive rain when malaria was unusually severe in Marwar, the opium-eaters suffered equally with the non-eaters" (GBOW [Huntly] 1894:IV:60). He had also never heard of any native consuming opium to ward off the chills "which bring on the recurrent febrile attacks" (GBOW [Huntly] 1894:IV:61). The proverbial grain of truth that Huntly discerned in all the "talk of beneficial use of opium in malaria is its power of lessening the discomfort felt in the cold stage of the attack" (GBOW [Huntly] 1894:IV:60). For this medical missionary, opium also prevented nothing and cured nothing; the only positive function it performed regarding malaria was relief of pain during one phase of a paroxysm.[9] And Pringle seems to have been referring to the plasmodia-induced version of the disease.

Western Coast

Three witnesses from different places in this region also declared the capability of opium was limited to pain relief. Surgeon-Lieutenant Colonel T. S. Weir, an Executive Health Officer in Bombay since 1873, testified on 12 February 1894, the sixty-ninth day. Weir said that reports of people consuming the drug to prevent malaria demonstrated how little the disease was understood. Opium was useful for alleviating the pain caused by bowel disorders. One of the latter was dysentery, which he claimed was a common result of 'malarial poisoning.' Another ailment frequently found in 'malarious' locales of the Western Coast was a "congested state of the mucous membrane." Weir had "no hesitation in saying opium gives more relief in this state than any other remedy." For this physician, however, opium was useless for the prevention or cure of malaria or 'fever.' It only alleviated discomfort stemming from a malfunctioning upper and lower intestinal tract. This condition produced a "low fever" in people, and it might be the product of numerous factors. Weir admitted he experienced relief from intestinal tract pain after consuming the drug (GBOW [Weir] 1894:IV:223).

Surgeon-Lieutenant Colonel M. L. Bartholomeusz was a veteran of nineteen years of government service in the provinces of Sind and Gujerat. In Bombay, on the seventy-second day of the hearings, he told the Royal Commission that opium was indispensable. Bartholomeusz, whose current assignment was civil surgeon and superintendent of Byramji Jijibhai Medical School and "Lunatic Asylum" in the city of Ahmedabad, also declared that people living in malarious districts, meaning most of the agricultural population of Gujerat, were

> subject to various ailments accompanied by neuralgic pains . . . [for] these people living . . . far away from hospitals and dispensaries opium is a godsend. A few grains of opium not only wards off pain, but, what is more important, it will enable the poor man to pursue his daily avocations and earn his daily bread. To deprive these people . . . would be showing little consideration for . . . physical welfare. (GBOW [Bartholomeusz] 1894:IV:307)

Bartholomeusz did not believe opium cured any disease, most certainly not malaria. It was valuable because it relieved pain caused by many things. The drug was an all-purpose anodyne and he said natives thought the same way.

South India

Proponents of the "opium prevents 'malaria'" scenario also received no help from Surgeon-Major W. G. King during the seventieth day of the Commission hearings. King was a veteran of almost twenty years in South India's Madras Presidency, and its acting sanitary commissioner when he testified in Bombay. Sir William Roberts' question about natives using opium as a febrifuge, or for "purposes of relief or mitigation," elicited this response from King.

> No;[sic] the impression I gathered was that as a man got aged he regarded opium as a stimulant. I never had any direct evidence that it was taken to prevent malaria. A native will tell you that opium is taken as a prophylactic against all diseases by those who have passed the prime of life. . . . Resort to the use of the drug in malarious districts is probably more common than elsewhere on account of the relief afforded from neuralgic pains usual in malarial cachexia. (GBOW [King] 1894:IV:243)

For King, the principal reason prompting consumption among most natives in southern India, or at least Madras Presidency, was pain induced by "complications" or aftermath of the disease. Some elderly men might believe opium prevented the deterioration inevitable with advancing age, but they did not view it as a true febrifuge for 'malaria.' Younger people, and King himself, also did not believe the drug cured anything although he acknowledged it could make the suffering of a victim more tolerable.

The sixteen witnesses introduced thus far believed the only value opium possessed was its ability to relieve pain.[10] There was disagreement among the remaining ten witnesses who mentioned the sensation. These people claimed opium's status as an anodyne either proved or implied that the drug had additional importance, and that it performed other functions. They also provided sufficient information to illuminate the reasons for their contentions.[11]

Opium Was More Than an Anodyne

Middle India

Dr. M. C. Freeman Underwood received his medical degree in Brussels, Belgium, and was a licentiate of King's and Queen's College, Ireland, and the College of Physicians in Edinburgh, Scotland. He came to South Asia in 1875 whereupon Grant's Medical College of Bombay (the controversial Sir George Birdwood's institutional affiliation) certified him to practice in India. Freeman Underwood, testifying on the seventy-fourth day, said he had spent most of the ensuing years in a territory whose erstwhile rulers were Maratha. Marathas, whom he described as a "military caste," lived primarily in central India during the latter part of the nineteenth century. Drawing upon his experience among people of the region, Freeman Underwood offered this flowery tribute.

> Opium has for centuries been used as a household remedy for young men and old . . . [and is] much in vogue as a prophylactic against malarious fevers, neuralgia, dyspepsia, and diseases incidental to life in malarious districts. Opium again is habitually resorted to for alleviation of all pain . . . [and it is] considered by [the poor] . . . as 'as one of Heaven's choicest blessings'—a gift from the gods for the alleviation of suffering . . . (GBOW [Freeman Underwood] 1894:IV:328)

Other medical professionals working in South Asia, according to Freeman Underwood, dispensed opium for various diseases. They had excellent results, and "last, but not least, [for] the prophylactic treatment of fevers" (GBOW [Freeman Underwood] 1894:IV:328). The physician had no doubt, and according to him all people of central India concurred, that opium performed at least two invaluable functions: it qualified as an all-purpose anodyne and it prevented 'malarial fevers.' The drug might be a pain reliever and a prophylactic, but Freeman Underwood did not support this effusive endorsement with documentation that the drug could cure the disease once a person had it. In other words, he offered no evidence, circumstantial or otherwise, that opium also was a febrifuge.

West India

Surgeon Lieutenant-Colonel T. H. Hendley's positive opinion of opium was based upon experience in western and eastern India. He had previously worked in Bihar Province, adjacent to Bengal Presidency, and was currently stationed in Rajputana on the other side of the country (GBOW [Hendley] 1894:IV:8). In the city of Jeypore during the fifty-eighth day of the hearings, Sir William Roberts asked him about the status of the drug in this arid province. Hendley replied that almost everyone in the locales where he had worked thought it "protects against the prevailing disease" (GBOW [Hendley] 1894:IV:9). In Jeypore State, the heaviest use of opium as a prophylactic occurred near Fort Ranthambhor, and among malnourished inhabitants of the "very malarious districts" in the southeast corner of the state between the Bannas and Chambal rivers. Everywhere, he said, the

> poor suffer to an enormous extent from malarious fevers, as well as from their sequelae . . . [such as] chronic dyspepsia (due to malaria). . . . In all such cases, and especially when they are accompanied by aching and pain, opium is the sheet anchor . . . one can get it without difficulty, and, in the vast majority of instances, the sufferer obtains relief. (GBOW [Hendley] 1894:IV:10)

The people of Bihar, especially the destitute, also viewed the easily procured drug as a preventive of 'malaria.' And it provided relief from the painful consequences of 'fever' attacks. Hendley's description hints that plasmodia might have caused some of these attacks. He then claimed the Indians about whom he spoke believed opium's status as an anodyne qualified it as a febrifuge. This statement suggested that natives considered the alleviation of the sensation was tantamount to curing the affliction. Hendley accepted the notion.

Sir John Tyler, inspector-general of prisons for the Northwest Provinces, also had no doubt about the worth of opium when he testified on 11 January 1894. Natives told him it was a valuable febrifuge when he first came to India thirty years ago. They had never stopped saying it. Tyler, who had spent his entire career in the NWP, agreed.[12] For this witness, 'malarious conditions' pertained to a milieu of tangible and intangible variables. All of them were highly detrimental to health. In this vague assortment of negative entities, he said that differences in 'malarial conditions' produced different ailments. This in turn generated "certain cases of malarial fever" for which opium was "the only thing" that acted as a prophylactic. It was even superior to quinine. Tyler elevated the drug to almost panacea status for several maladies prevalent in some 'malarial conditions' because it had a "double action, namely, as a therapeutic agent, an anodyne, and hypnotic, and an action as a restorer and comforter" (GBOW [Tyler] 1894:III:110). For Tyler, *Papaver somniferum Linn* was a multifaceted weapon to alleviate misery and to prevent death.

Tyler's clear recognition that quinine cured some ailments whereas opium was a more effective medicine for other maladies is illuminating. Although the inspector-general recognized different types of afflictions responding positively to different drugs, he placed all these afflictions in the category of 'malarious' conditions. In this perspective, opium does cure 'fevers' emanating from 'malarious conditions.' The latter included variables responsible for malaria as we know it today and for which quinine is most efficacious. Tyler's notion of 'malarious conditions' also included diseases that quinine did not cure or prevent.

East India

Dr. Juggo Bundo Bose, retired after twenty-five years of government service in Calcutta and its environs, had an "independent practice" in the city. He testified on Tuesday, 28 November 1893, the fourteenth day of the hearings (GBOW [Bose, J. B.] 1894:II:90). His responses to Sir William Roberts' questions are a clue to what some educated and uneducated citizens in this part of India thought about the drug and its alleged powers. Bose said that his teachers in medical school and textbooks stressed the importance of opium. A long career subsequently confirmed it was indeed "a sovereign remedy for malarial diseases such as fever, malarial cachexia, and other malarial complaints which people suffer from" (GBOW [Bose, J. B.] 1894:II:90). Every physician Bose had met prescribed the drug for 'malarial fevers' because it enhanced the anti-periodic effects of quinine. However, he did acknowledge that opium could not replace the latter (GBOW [Bose, J. B.] 1894:II:91). For Bose, malaria was not a specific disease; it was an assortment of ills with somewhat similar symptoms. Opium influenced some phase of a few maladies, thereby gaining the attention of established physicians such as Bose and prompting them to accord significant therapeutic power to the drug.

Bose also commented about the drug in the everyday lives of poor people and among rural dwellers. Many of the former, he said, "take small doses of opium to keep off the effects of malarial diseases" (GBOW [Bose, J. B.] 1894:II:90). The wording is significant; although Bose believed the drug had much value, he realized that the destitute distinguished between a symptom and a disease. This suggested that the uneducated, the malnourished, the ill-clothed and poorly sheltered population of Calcutta and adjacent locales consumed the drug to suppress the overt signs of suffering from a serious illness. They knew the sickness would run its course, and that the malady could not be quickly eradicated. In other words, they cannot purge themselves of 'malaria,' but they might avoid unmitigated suffering from its consequences. Eating opium offered psychological well-being and physical comfort.

Surgeon-Lieutenant-Colonel Hugh Johnstone, senior civil surgeon and director of the General Hospital in Rangoon, Burma, voiced his opinion during the twenty-fifth session. Similar to Bose, Johnstone was a veteran of government service with twenty-three years spent in Burma and two years at the Medical College of Calcutta. Johnstone said Chinese, Burmese, and Indian inhabitants of Burma all viewed opium as a prophylactic for 'malarial fevers' and "bowel complaints." Natives also told him that Burmese and Indians in the 'malarious districts' smoked and ate opium as a "domestic remedy," which meant it was a common household item. Johnstone prescribed the drug for treating "malarious fevers" and was delighted to find it "often staving off an ague fit if given an hour before its usual period of seizure, and at least modifying its severity and adding greatly to the patient's comfort." For Johnstone, the drug was a "great boon" because it suppressed a symptom. This capability enabled natives to inhabit locales where they suffered from "malarial cachexia . . . malarial neuralgia [and] racking pains" (GBOW [Johnstone] 1894:II:207–08).

Johnstone attributed more power to opium compared to the aforementioned witnesses discussing Burma. No one disputed the drug being an anodyne for diverse ailments, but Johnstone said he and the Burmese population knew it also prevented an individual from getting the disease. This meant that opium was more than just a prophylactic. It also qualified as a febrifuge because it lessened the discomfort of 'malarial fevers.' Johnstone, and perhaps Burmese citizens, made no distinction between an anodyne versus a 'cure' for 'malarial fevers'; relief from the pain of a disease and curing a disease were the same thing.

Western Coast

Four witnesses from the Western Coast region of the country also said opium was more than an anodyne. The first, Mr. Rao Bahadur Dulerai Girdharlal, testified in Ahmedabad on the sixty-seventh day. Girdharlal had almost twenty years of government service to his credit. When appearing before the Royal Commission, he was the personal assistant to the British Political agent in Mahi Kantha Agency. Mahi Kantha was an administrative entity composed of separate native states. His previous assignments included being an administrator in the native state of Baroda and the superintendent of Palinpur for ten and eight years respectively (GBOW [Girdharlal] 1894:IV:199). Sir Arthur Pease asked if natives consumed opium to prevent or cure 'fever.' Girdharlal replied that "it rather acts as a preventive." Pease then asked whether natives who had not had 'fever' ingested the drug to avoid the malady. The witness said it was "taken under certain circumstances—generally to ward off fever which people think is due to moisture" (GBOW [Girdharlal] 1894:IV:200). Haridas Viharidas Desai pursued the topic later in the session. He inquired if people also used the drug to combat pain. Girdharlal said

> [s]ometimes they take it before the fever is on, and sometimes after the fever has left them. There are various modes in which opium is used. It is used as a medicine. (GBOW [Girdharlal] 1894:IV:200)

Girdharlal did not reveal his opinion about the relationship between opium and 'malaria,' but his comments suggest agreement with natives' convictions. Opium was a medicine that alleviated pain, and this capability qualified it as a prophylactic. There was little difference, for Girdharlal, between the nature of an anodyne and a prophylactic; relief from an unpleasant sensation and preventing the source of pain from establishing itself in a human being were synonymous.

Mr. B. H. Nanavati did reveal his preferences. Opium was a general anodyne because it relieved "neuralgic pains of all kinds" and prevented their recurrence. Nanavati had sufficient experience to support his statement. This Bombay University graduate held the rank of assistant surgeon in the Bombay Medical Service. He also had been a regional director of dispensaries in Gujerat for twelve years. When testifying on the seventy-first day of the Commission hearings, Nanavati was teaching surgery and midwifery at Byramji Medical School in Ahmedabad (GBOW [Nanavati] 1894:IV:273).

Nanavati was convinced opium qualified as a prophylactic against 'malarial fevers' because it usually gave "immunity" to consumers. This was especially applicable for poor people since they used it the most in "districts where [these fevers] are widely prevalent." An incident during 1886–1887 in a small village eighty miles from Ahmedabad illustrated his contention. Nanavati was "struck with the fact that whilst the residents of that little place—almost to a man—suffered from malarious fever and its effects, the only class of people who almost enjoyed immunity from them were men who manufactured the salt [sic], and a few others." Nanavati was curious. Further investigation revealed that "most of them were in the habit of eating opium habitually, and that they had a belief in its efficacy as a prophylactic." Their belief strengthened his conviction about the drug's "prophylactic virtues" (GBOW [Nanavati] 1894:IV:273). Nanavati provided no data from other villages or locales to support his idea. He also was oblivious to the possibility that distance within the community from 'malarial conditions' (the breeding places for malarial vectors), might have been a factor explaining the male salt makers' immunity from 'fevers.'

The Secretary of the Royal Commission on Opium described Surgeon-Major K. R. Kirtikar as an expert for all classes, primarily Muslims and Hindus, in Bombay, Sind, and the district of Thana. Kirtikar's current posting was Thana district's Civil Surgeon (GBOW [Kirtikar] 1894:IV:304). The statement about this physician having more expertise than other witnesses about specific groups in India is moot, but Kirtikar did say the drug was a prophylactic for many diseases. It was also very valuable for "all kinds of neuralgia, especially the headache caused by malarial poisoning" (GBOW [Kirtikar] 1894:IV:305).

Opium, Kirtikar continued, was well known to "eminent European writers on *materia medica* as an anti-periodic, and as such it is invaluable in a country like India where malaria is so much prevalent." Some Indian citizens felt the same way because local native doctors prescribed opium frequently. And, according to this witness, people became addicted only because they desired "the relief of pain in some of the maladies mentioned above" (GBOW [Kirtikar] 1894:IV:305). Kirtikar provided no details about what was included under 'malarial poisoning,' and he gave no information to determine if the category differed from his conception of 'malaria.' Nonetheless, opium was beneficial because it prevented recurring, remittent fever. The drug also relieved pain caused by diverse maladies, thereby qualifying the substance as an anodyne and a type of febrifuge. For Kirtikar, opium both 'cured' and relieved pain, but he did not address the question of its ability to end a disease and to ameliorate one of its common, overt symptoms.

Surgeon-Major D. N. Parakh, a surgeon at Gokaldas Tejpal Hospital in Bombay, testified on 12 February 1894, the sixty-ninth day of the hearings. Like Kirtikar, Parakh purportedly was an expert about Bombay's Muslims and Hindus who could speak with assurance about inhabitants in the city of Poona. Sir William Roberts asked what natives thought about opium. Parakh replied that they believed it was a general prophylactic, especially for "diarrhoea, ague, and cholera." He agreed with natives because of "instances in which it appeared to me that persons otherwise predisposed to malarious fevers escaped them because they were opium eaters." When asked about reasons for beginning the habit, Parakh said it was to "relieve aching of limbs, feelings of chilliness, and symptoms which are best expressed by the phrase 'general malaise.'" These symptoms, Parakh surmised, often preceded "an attack of some forms of malarious fevers." For indigenous inhabitants and this witness, the drug occupied the status of an all-purpose anodyne. Opium, however, did more: its ingestion prevented a person from getting 'malarial fever,' it cured 'malarial fever' if that person succumbed to the malady, and the drug relieved the pain experienced during a paroxysm (GBOW [Parakh] 1894:IV:215).

South India

In Bombay on the seventieth day of the hearings, the comments of the civil surgeon for Negapatam, a district in southern India, also implied that opium was more than an anodyne. Assistant surgeon Mohammed Osman Sahib Bahadur had worked for the Government of India in four districts in Madras Presidency after earning a medical degree from Madras Medical College (GBOW [Bahadur, M. O. S.] 1894:IV:244). Bahadur declared he was "aware of [opium's] true prophylactic action against any disease." He acknowledged it having "limited power" as a cure because he obtained excellent results when the drug was combined with other febrifuges. The latter were ineffectual when administered alone (GBOW [Bahadur, M. O. S.] 1894:IV:246). He also said that in

> unhealthy and malarious tracts . . . [opium] use is a necessity to the poor to abate suffering, to cheer their spirits, and to render them fit for work. It saves them money and lengthens their life. (GBOW [Bahadur, M. O. S.] 1894:IV:246)

For Bahadur, the drug was a febrifuge because it relieved pain. The status stemmed from his assertion that opium could 'cure' when combined with other substances. The mixture apparently liberated the capabilities of each ingredient to eliminate ailments. Nothing else can be said because Bahadur said no more. And he did not specifically mention malaria or any affliction that might have been classified as 'malaria.' Bahadur suggested opium was more than a pain reliever but submitted no data to support the claim other than mentioning the drug's morale-building capability.

Opium as an Anodyne—Summary

Two kinds of witnesses specifically mentioned opium and pain. Splitters realized the only thing that different diseases might have in common are what human beings feel when they have an elevated temperature. For these skeptics, the ability of opium to relieve pain was not proof that it prevented or cured any disease that lumpers subsumed under the category of 'malaria.' The drug was an anodyne and nothing more. The witnesses influenced by miasmatic and tellurian views of disease tended to disagree; opium's ability to relieve pain was proof that it 'prevented' and 'cured' the numerous and diverse afflictions that they, and other lumpers, referred to as 'malaria,' 'malarious fevers,' and related terms.[13]

IS OPIUM A FOOD?

The Royal Commission solicited comments from eighteen witnesses about the "opium as food" scenario that Sir William J. Moore and Sir George Birdwood had proposed the previous decade. There was no agreement about the nutritional benefits of India's *Papaver somniferum Linn.*

Opium Is a Food

Moore and Birdwood testified in London on Thursday, 14 September 1893, the fourth day of the hearings. Sir Arthur Pease asked Moore if he thought "there is anything nourishing in opium, or [does it offer] only a staying power for a while until [a person] could obtain solid food?" Moore replied that camel herders in the arid deserts of Rajasthan survived because they consumed opium and camel's milk. And consumption of the drug alone, he added, "prevents what we used to call . . . eremacausis, or waste of tissue" (GBOW [Moore] 1894:I:74). No one else on the Commission asked Moore about opium being a type of food because it prevented fatigue, a capability that, according to his publications, qualified the drug as a 'malaria' prophylactic.

Birdwood replied at length to queries by Brassey, Wilson, Mowbray, and especially Roberts, about the dangers of eating opium compared to smoking an extract of the substance. Birdwood reiterated his conviction about oral consumption being more detrimental. Commission members, however, did not ask for his opinion about the connection between opium eating and the prevention or cure of malaria (GBOW [Birdwood] 1894:I:77–80). Birdwood had enough sense not to mention his 1880 statements about gastrointestinal differences between Anglo-Europeans and South Asians. Brassey, Wilson, Mowbray, and Roberts avoided the topic.

The witnesses agreeing with Moore and Birdwood thought that opium provided nourishment to people who did not have enough to eat or subsisted on a vegetarian diet. Their logic was similar; consumption prevented a person from experiencing fatigue. And fatigue was a prime factor in the appearance of 'chill' that soon evolved into 'malaria' and 'fever.' Opium, therefore, was a prophylactic and a food because it inhibited development of a condition conducive to sickness. Other witnesses ridiculed the idea or accepted it using a definition so broad that the term was meaningless.

Dr. Ram Moy Roy was in the latter category. Roy, a medical officer at Sambhunath Pundit's dispensary in Bhawanipur, a town near Calcutta in East India, had no doubt when Sir William Roberts and Lord Thomas Brassey asked him about the drug's dietary value. Roy even declared the Commission's raison d'être was to establish opium as a kind of food. He agreed with both the idea and mission, and declared the controversy about the drug's effectiveness in malaria's prevention and cure was unimportant compared to its nutritional importance (GBOW [Roy, R. M.] 1894:II:114–17). Mr. A. F. Maconochie echoed Roy's statements. Maconochie, an eleven-year veteran of the Indian Civil Service with virtually all of it spent in the Western Coast Province of Gujerat as a magistrate and assistant collector, said that opium ingestion compensated for natives' "bad food." Maconochie did not specify what constituted detrimental cuisine but he claimed this also was the reason natives' gave for consuming the drug (GBOW [Maconochie]:IV:130–33).

Mr. Chintamanrao Vinayak Vaidya, a judge from the poppy-growing Malwa region of Gwalior state in Central India, also was favorable. To Brassey's inquiry Vaidya said yes; he and fellow Indian citizens did view opium as having dietary importance because it was indeed a form of food (GBOW [Vaidya] 1894:IV:110–11). No one asked for details. Mr. Manekji D. Cama, a medical doctor with impressive credentials, repeated Vaidya's comments for Middle India. Cama was in private practice in Bombay, on the western coast of the subcontinent. A licentiate of Medicine and the Joint Honorary Secretary of Grant Medical College Medical Society in Bombay, Cama said natives with whom he had contact definitely believed opium possessed nutritional value. When questioned by Roberts and Haridas Viharidas Desai about his own thoughts, Cama said the idea should not be dismissed out-of-hand (GBOW [Cama, M. D.] 1894:IV:268–70). Dr. Kailas Chunder Bose offered a similar comment for East India, specifically the city of Calcutta. This medical doctor in private practice and president of the influential Calcutta Medical Society thought there just might be some merit in viewing opium as a form of supplemental nutrition. However, he admitted medical men did not prescribe opium for dietetic purposes. Sir William Roberts failed to ask Bose what natives thought about the idea (GBOW [Bose, K. C.] 1894:II:87–90).

Several non-Indian citizens also endorsed the opium as food scenario. Some of them were in private medical practice. Other people were physicians employed in some capacity by the Government of India. The remaining witnesses held nonmedical administrative positions in the bureaucracy. The Honorable T. D. MacKenzie was in the last category. He was a high-ranking official in the Opium and Excise Department of the Government of India but had no medical credentials. In response to queries from Brassey and Lyall, he declared that yes, opium qualified as a kind of food. He then implied that natives also believed it had nutritional value (GBOW [MacKenzie] 1894:IV:279–287). The résumé of Mr. T. Gordon Walker, another bureaucrat, was equally impressive. Walker, Commissioner of the Opium and Excise Department of Punjab Province in Northwest India, also implied natives viewed opium as a food. No Royal Commission member asked if Walker agreed with the idea (GBOW [Walker] 1894:III:235–37).

One physician in private practice and two medical doctors working for the Government of India also thought the nutrition perspective was credible. Dr. G. R. Ferris, in practice for more than forty years (most of the period in Calcutta), was a member of the Royal College of Surgeons in London. He thought the drug did function to a "certain extent as food" when Arthur Pease asked him about the topic during the fifteenth session. Pease did not request specifics. No one asked Ferris what native Indians thought and he volunteered no information about their beliefs (GBOW [Ferris, G. R.] 1894:II:105–08).

The two medical professionals employed by the Indian Medical Service had much less field experience then the venerable G. R. Ferris. Two days before Ferris' appearance at the Royal Commission, Sir William Roberts and Henry Joseph Wilson had interrogated Surgeon-Lieutenant-Colonel E. G. Russell. Russell, who after seven years of labor in Assam and India, accepted the opium-as-food idea but neglected to tell the Commission members if natives accepted the notion (GBOW [Russell] 1894:II:84). And on 7 February 1894, shortly before the hearings ended, Surgeon-Major Gimlette said the same thing. He had spent five years with Indian regiments and nine years in native states located in Middle India. His assignments included agency surgeon in Baghelkhand and tutor to his Highness the Maharaja of Rewa. This fourteen-year experience convinced Gimlette that opium had some value in satisfying human nutritional needs. It added something positive to a native's diet. The wording of Gimlette's response to Roberts' question suggests the Indian nationals he knew favored the same interpretation (GBOW [Gimlette] 1894:IV:95–97).

An official with no South Asia experience who responded to William Roberts' questions must have delighted Sir Lyall. Mr. H. N. Lay, a pensioned administrator, had spent his entire career in China in British Government service. He held several positions in the Consular Service. They included assistant in the Canton Consulate, and an interpreter as well as a vice consul at Shanghai. He also was the British inspector of customs and had been promoted to inspector-general of Chinese Customs in 1858. Lay then worked for the Imperial Chinese government for nine years before retiring (GBOW [Lay] 1894:I:81). He reported that the Chinese natives' vegetable diet did not provide adequate nutrition. Opium consumption corrected this deficiency. Inhabitants in the 'malarial districts' of China's middle and southern provinces also used the substance because they thought it prevented 'malaria.' Lay agreed about poor nutrition making people susceptible to the disease. Opium circumvented fatigue, which in turn gave them strength to ward off sickness (GBOW [Lay] 1894:I:81–6).

The aforementioned thirteen witnesses supported, with varying degrees of enthusiasm, the Moore and Birdwood contention that opium had a dietetic function in parts of two heavily populated Asian societies.

The Indian penchant for eating the drug, and the Chinese preference for smoking an extract, precluded the mental and physical exhaustion that is conducive to the development of 'malaria' and 'fever.' Opium, therefore, was a 'preventive' regardless of the mode of ingestion or the consumer's motive for indulgence. Unfettered accessibility was justified because any form of consumption of the drug served a "medical purpose."

Opium Is Not a Food

As noted above, skeptics of the opium-as-food scenario either rejected the idea or declared it plausible only if the definition of nutrition was so general the word lost meaning. Still other witnesses said opium did positive things, but nourishing people was not one of them.

Opposition to the food supplement notion was voiced early, the third day to be exact, in the Royal Commission hearings. Brigade-Surgeon R. Pringle, the previously introduced thirty-year veteran of India service, said in response to questions from Brassey that he considered opium "invaluable medicinally, but useless as a dietetic" (GBOW [Pringle] 1894:I:52). It also was erroneous to classify the drug as a febrifuge for 'malaria,' 'fever,' and disease in general. Pringle was emphatic, declaring that "any one who habitually indulges in opium in small doses in fever districts, instead of giving him some protection from the disease, absolutely produces a tendency to fever" (GBOW [Pringle] 1894:I:53). The only positive function it performed, and Pringle did not denigrate this capability, was sedation. He believed calming the emotions of distressed people, however, was not the same as curing the underlying cause of disease. Any person or administrator in fever-plagued districts who advocated daily consumption of small doses of the drug for such purposes was doing great harm to the sick person. Pringle was convinced that ample supplies of quinine in the "malarial districts of India" would preclude any need for opium as a febrifuge or prophylactic (GBOW [Pringle] 1894:I:56, see also 174).

Surgeon-Major Edwin F. Dobson was more charitable. This veteran of thirteen years of government service, and civil surgeon for Shillong in Assam Province of East India, was reluctant to acknowledge opium as a type of food when asked by Roberts, Wilson and Arthur Upshawe Fanshawe. Dobson replied "not directly," and the idea had plausibility only with a very loose definition of food. Opium did do something positive, but postulating nutrition as a principal benefit of opium ingestion was an overstatement. Natives, he continued, also felt the same way (GBOW [Dobson] 1894:II:282–85).

Surgeon-Colonel H. Cook, a doctor with past Government of India experience in Gujerat and currently stationed in Nagpur district (Middle India), did not dispute the ability of opium to replenish depleted energy and to prevent a person from experiencing fatigue. Cook, however, refused to specify that this capability was a demonstration of "medical value" and that it did not make opium a "food" as the term was usually defined. He contended the drug had medical utility independent of, or separate from, the question of fatigue prevention. Preventing fatigue merely involved dulling the feeling of exhaustion (GBOW [Cook] 1894:IV:214–15).

Thus far, the skeptical Pringle thought opium's reputation was exaggerated. Dobson provided no clue to how he could accept the drug as a kind of food, and Cook said preventing fatigue did not qualify opium as being nutritious. Surgeon-Major A. Adams, their colleague and the officiating residency surgeon and chief medical officer in the Rajputana Province, was more obliging. He provided an illustration when responding to the Sir William Robert's question about opium being a prophylactic in 'malarial areas.' Adams said yes, natives did believe it was a preventive and Henry Wilson later asked him to elaborate.

Adams replied that opium functioned as a prophylactic only for dysentery and bowel diseases in both malaria-plagued locales and places free from the malady. Opium, therefore, had only a highly indirect food value even if the phrase was vaguely defined, and if the phrase was even appropriate to use in the first place. Ingestion of the drug helped to prevent dysentery and "bowel disease" brought on by "exposure to damp, sun and cold." Among people subjected to these climatic variables that deprived the body of needed nutrition, the drug helped a digestive tract absorb nutrients by slowing the passage of food. So, opium was a 'food' supplement only in the most general, and not very useful, sense (GBOW [Adams, A.] 1894:IV:38–40).

Other medical practitioners in government service thought opium was useful in alleviating dysentery. This capability, however, still did not warrant the drug being classified as a food or a nutritional supplement. This was true regardless how broad the latter term was interpreted. One of these witnesses was Surgeon-Major D. F. Barry, a veteran of fourteen years of service at several places in India. He was the civil surgeon in Sitapur and superintendent of the District Jail when he testified. Sitapur was located in the United Provinces (North India) (GBOW [Barry]:1894 III:115).

Barry declared opium had no nutritional value. Furthermore, there is nothing in Barry's testimony to suggest he would accept the idea even if a wider definition of food became commonplace. Doses of the drug, however, might have therapeutic value in lessening the severity of bowel disorders among non-Europeans caused by 'malarial poisoning.' Like Surgeon-Major A. Adams, Barry was alluding to dysentery. He said this capability qualified opium as having a "therapeutic value" that was distinct from its status as an anodyne and a "hypnotic" (GBOW [Barry] 1894:III:117).

Surgeon Major T. R. Mulroney also perceived therapeutic merit in using opium. The benefit did not involve the question of nutrition. Mulroney had served only in Punjab Province (West India). Arriving in 1880, three years later he had been posted to the Medical College in the city of Lahore. He was promoted to civil surgeon for Amritsar city in 1887 (GBOW [Mulroney] 1894:III:163–64). Mulroney declared opium was not a type of food. Nonetheless, it did help to prevent sickness, perhaps 'fever' and 'malaria' specifically, for another reason. He accepted the role of 'chill' as a precursor to the 'disease,' and said one consequence of opium consumption in 'malarial districts' was that it "enables a man to resist cold; it prevents chills, and in that sense it acts as a preventative against malarial fevers, and their sequelae" (GBOW [Mulroney] 1894:III:163). He declared that in Amritsar district, "which is essentially malarial, it is the prevailing, the universal opinion" that opium was useful. Mulroney refrained from identifying for what Amritsar's natives believed the drug had value. He also said inhabitants in the native state of Nabha believed the drug had value for unidentified maladies. This witness admitted ignorance about the idea being prevalent elsewhere in the country because his exposure to such places was minimal (GBOW [Mulroney] 1894:III:163).

Mulroney, therefore, indicated opium might be an indirect prophylactic for 'malaria' because consumption helped a person to avoid 'chill.' 'Chill' preceded an attack of the malady. The drug did nothing more than hinder the arrival of a predisposing agent, but not because it was a nourishing food. Mulroney thought some natives also believed opium was a prophylactic albeit not in the sense of being nutritious.

Assistant-Surgeon Tribhovandas Motichand Shah presented a succinct rebuttal of opium as a form of 'food.' Shah did not dispute the drug's ability to prevent fatigue, but he suggested many things did the same thing. He mentioned sufficient sleep, better transportation, less arduous work, proper clothing and shelter, adequate amounts of food items, and so forth. Shah, chief medical officer of Junagadh state for eight years immediately before the Royal Commission on Opium hearings, and employed by the British government before that, suggested that one must conclude that all things preventing fatigue qualified as food supplements. This meant that numerous substances and behavior were prophylactic for 'malarial disease' and 'fevers' (GBOW [Shah, T. M.] 1894:IV:188). He said Indian nationals did not view opium as a type of nutrition. The idea was, at best, an exaggeration (GBOW [Shah, T. M.] 1894:IV:188–92).

Concluding Remarks Concerning Witnesses' Testimony about Opium as a Food

Witnesses commenting about the dietary significance of opium indeed had varied opinions. Eleven people said yes, the drug was a kind of food because a person consuming the drug avoided fatigue, and fatigue was a precursor to 'malaria' and 'fever.' Seven individuals said no, but they differed regarding how valuable opium was for human beings and for what purposes—if any—the drug was most useful.

A few witnesses agreed with Moore's old idea (and to some extent with the least facetious parts of Birdwood's scenario published in *The Times* [London]) about the ability of opium to prevent dysentery, thereby enabling complete digestion of food to occur. Prolongation in the intestines, in turn, resulted in the body absorbing more nutrients.

No witness, however, entirely accepted this aspect in Moore's rendition of the theory, but many of those predisposed toward accepting opium being a form of nutrition did say that consumption prevented 'chill.' The Moore and Birdwood notion of opium being 'food' received little support from medical professionals and lay persons commenting about the topic. And those receptive to the idea accorded credibility to only a few aspects of Moore's entire theory of disease and fever classification.

THE STATUS OF QUININE

Thirty-five witnesses were asked to comment about quinine. They testified on behalf of British India's administration as well as the SSOT. The presence or absence of their perspectives in Sir William Roberts' report indicates which interpretation of 'malaria' he favored and what the man thought was the most appropriate way to eliminate the malady in South Asia.

Six people commenting about *Papaver somniferum Linn* as a pain killer or a type of food also evaluated the merits of opium and quinine as prophylactics and febrifuges for 'malaria.' All of them believed that quinine had preventive and curative value but they disagreed regarding how much benefit and for what kind of paroxysm. The differences that these people perceived between the two substances, similar to opinions about opium as an anodyne, were reflections of how the commentators defined 'malaria.' The enthusiasts who realized that quinine could prevent or cure some—but not all—people suffering from 'malarial fever' were also indicating that etiologically-distinct maladies sharing only a common symptom were erroneously classified under the inclusive term 'malaria.' Doubts about simplistic diagnosis prompted them to reserve the malaria category for sick people who manifested the pattern of fevers attributable to plasmodia. Witnesses expressing reservations about quinine did just the opposite; the substance was more effective than opium for some 'fevers' but less beneficial for others.

Twenty-nine of the thirty-five people asked for comments concerning quinine were not asked about opium's status as an anodyne or a 'food.' And if they had been asked for opinions about the drug, there would have been sharp disagreement: the group consisted of lumpers and splitters. There was, however, no dispute among these witnesses regarding quinine. All of them said the substance had value. Seven of the thirty-five people commenting about quinine admitted following one of two procedures. They either administered both opium and quinine to prevent a person from developing 'fever' in 'malarious conditions,' or they prescribed the two drugs in combination to individuals already suffering from episodes of elevated temperatures. These seven witnesses implied, or clearly stated, that the two drugs complemented each other. Dispensing opium with quinine at the same time prolonged the effects of the latter; opium became a "fortifier," thereby enhancing whatever it was that quinine accomplished. Another version was that the presence of quinine increased the therapeutic capability of opium.

Members of the Royal Commission realized the opinions of a few witnesses might not be an accurate assessment of how indigenous people felt about quinine. They therefore asked some witnesses about natives' beliefs. Witnesses' responses reveal how available quinine was to the Indian citizens who appreciated its therapeutic value. These comments also illuminate reasons for the public's acceptance or rejection of quinine as a preventive and a cure for 'malaria.' Witnesses' replies indicate the "natives" were no different from the people testifying; some of the indigenous folk were splitters, and others were lumpers.

QUININE "DOES" SOMETHING DISTINCT FROM OPIUM

Brigade-Surgeons R. Pringle and D. F. Barry, Reverend J. Wilkie, as well as Drs. R. Wallace, W. Huntly, and Ram Moy Roy, supplemented their comments about opium as an anodyne and a food with observations about the special characteristics of quinine. With the exception of Roy, who mentioned the nutritional aspects of the drug, all had relegated opium to a minor prophylactic and febrifuge status while extolling quinine. Roy stated that people in his region were susceptible to 'malarious fever,' and that "opium may not be a prophylactic against malaria in the sense that quinine is" (GBOW [Roy, M. N.] 1894:II:115).

The other witnesses were less reticent. Wallace declared opium was in no way "a special prophylactic like quinine" and that this also was the prevailing opinion in the medical profession (GBOW [Wallace] 1894:II:19). Huntly proclaimed the Government of India effort to promote the "adoption [of opium was] indefensible so long as we have in quinine a drug which is admitted by all to be the best prophylactic in malaria, and can be discontinued at pleasure without discomfort" (GBOW [Huntly] 1894:IV:60). The natives, according to Reverend Wilkie, apparently felt the same way because "even with opium in their hands they prefer quinine for fever when they can get it" (GBOW [Wilkie] 1894:IV:164). Pringle articulated all these sentiments when declaring that in the "malarious districts" he visited "the natives have perfect confidence in [quinine]; . . . [their] constant request was for quinine . . . but never once was [he] asked for opium" (GBOW [Pringle] 1894:I:52–3, 56). Pringle then claimed, as stated previously, that Indians in "malarial districts" would have no need for opium as a febrifuge and prophylactic if a sufficient amount of quinine was available (GBOW [Pringle] 1894:I:56, 174). In contrast to most other witnesses whose comments were the result of experience in one or two locales in India, it bears repeating that Pringle's generalizations were the product of twenty years in the NWP (West India), eight years in Orissa (East India), and two years in Central India (Middle India). Thirty years of service in three different regions gave his evaluation of quinine a semblance of pan-India credibility. Witnesses from other regions of India also professed unqualified preference for quinine, or they declared it to be more effective than opium.

North India

One medical missionary and two surgeon-majors working in different locations of North India were quinine enthusiasts. Brigade-Surgeon D. F. Barry said that despite the ability of *Papaver somniferum Linn* to provide relief from "muscular pains accompanying malarial fevers," he still could "not put much confidence in opium as a pure febrifuge." Quinine was different. Supplied with as much as needed, Barry found that in "the many complications of malarial fevers—and one or more complications frequently occur—it is a most valuable drug." Barry also criticized the current state of fever classification when he challenged the number of fatalities attributed to 'malaria.' He thought the term was misused because it lacked specificity. Many deaths blamed on the "generic term" malaria were from pneumonia caused by "constitutions broken down by malarial poison" (GBOW [Barry] 1894:III:116).

For Dr. J. Anderson, a resident of Bareilly for fifteen years serving as Civil Surgeon for the district and superintendent of the district's "lunatic asylum" and jail, opium was not "comparable to quinine as a prophylactic against malaria." *Papaver somniferum Linn*, however, did reduce a person's "liability to chills, and thus diminishes the risks of attacks of ague" (GBOW [Anderson] 1894:III:114). Anderson believed opium was only an "indirect prophylactic" because it "fights" an environment conducive to the evolution of the malady. Quinine, however, attacked and eliminated the disease. *Papaver somniferum Linn* therefore contributed to health maintenance, but it did not specifically prevent or eliminate the source of misery.

The last witness from North India was Reverend F. J. Newton, a medical missionary with experience in China and a resident of India since 1870. While in India, this missionary worked for twelve years at a dispensary hospital in Ferozepor that treated between 10,000 to 12,000 people annually. This experience convinced Newton that opium merely "warm[ed] the system in cold weather" (GBOW [Newton] 1894:III:199–200). The only proven prophylactics for 'fever,' he asserted, were quinine and arsenic. The absence of a similar sentiment for these items among India's natives was disquieting. He lamented that

> people in villages do not use them at all except when they can get them from dispensaries. They never use quinine and arsenic as household remedies. They know nothing about arsenic as a remedy for fever, but they have begun to know something about quinine. (GBOW [Newton] 1894:III:200)

West India

A high-ranking member of the Government of India believed his experience in several parts of India left no doubt about the relative merits of opium and quinine. He held posts in the Province of Oudh (North India) and his jurisdiction included parts of West India. On 22 January 1894, Mr. T. Stoker, commissioner of Excise and Stamps, and inspector general of the NWP and Oudh, responded to Brassey's query about the value of opium. Stoker declared he had "no reason to believe that it acts directly as an antiperiodic like quinine" (GBOW [Stoker] 1894:III:276). In other words, Stoker believed *Papaver somniferum Linn* had little or no effect in halting the recurring fevers generated by malarial plasmodia. Surgeon-Major D. Ffrench-Mullen expressed the same reservation about opium in Ajmere (in Rajputana) on Friday, 2 February 1894, the sixty-second day of the hearings. Ffrench-Mullen, a civil surgeon in the opium-producing district of Udaipur for most of his sixteen years in the country, was not enthusiastic about opium. He thought it was "quite unnecessary" if quinine was available in "malarial conditions . . . [when a] mitigator or . . . a prophylactic" was needed. Ffrench-Mullen, like Dr. J. Anderson, thought opium worked indirectly "by preventing chills which leads to fever." (GBOW [Ffrench-Mullen, D.] 1894:IV:47–8)

South India

The Government of India's effort to promote opium as a prophylactic and febrifuge for malaria was also criticized by Surgeon-Major A. J. Sturmer in Bombay on Tuesday, 13 February 1894, the seventieth day of the hearings. Sturmer, a nineteen-year veteran of the Indian Medical Service, was currently stationed in Kistna district. It was located midway between Madras and Nellore cities on India's southeast coast. Sturmer repeated a question posed to him by a Dr. Thin, a colleague in England who was conducting malarial vector research. Thin had asked him

> . . . why the medical men in India did not give opium in malarial fever because they had been cracking it up so much. My [Sturmer] reply to that is that we have got quinine and arsenic, which are better. (GBOW [Sturmer] 1894:IV:244)

Thin and Sturmer were saying that British India's officials contradicted themselves. They now were talking so much about opium's value in combating malaria, but past behavior indicated these people never advocated prescribing the drug for such a purpose.

East India

"Better" indicated that Sturmer accorded opium some efficacy in fighting the malady although he provided insufficient testimony to determine if he was a splitter or a lumper. Brigade-Surgeon J. H. Condon, however, left no doubt that opium, and anything it might contain, was worthless.

> [N]either opium nor any of its products which have been tried by Government, have had any prophylactic or other beneficial effect. We have tried narcotine and various other drugs which the Government have made in the Quinine factory at Darjeeling, and every medical man in the country has stopped using them. They are not a bit of use. (GBOW [Condon] 1894:III:181)

Condon was not a fanatic evangelist hostile to unorthodox forms of sedation or stimulation. Similar to Pringle, his opinion should have carried considerable weight with Royal Commission members. In private practice when he testified, Condon had retired after thirty-four and a half years of Government of India service spent principally in jails and as a civil surgeon in East India (GBOW [Condon] 1894:III:181).

Two other witnesses from East India were slightly less negative than Condon about opium. The drug, according to Ram Dhurlabh Mazumdar and Kali Sankur Sukul, was useful for a purpose other than 'malaria' and natives were aware of the alternative. Mazumdar, a member of the legal profession from Nowgong in central Assam, said people ingested quinine and cinchona for "malarious fever, but opium is never prescribed" (GBOW [Mazumdar, R. D.] 1894:II:60). Assamese natives used *Papaver somniferum Linn* for rheumatism and dysentery. Sukul, a professor in the City College and current rector of the City Collegiate School (Sova Bazaar Branch) was a former principal of Narial Victoria College in Jessore, Bengal. This academician told the Royal Commission that he had "never heard of [opium] being believed to be protective against fever—it is certainly never so used . . . [by his] countrymen" (GBOW [Sukul, K. S.] 1894:II:269). Sukul declared this certainly was the prevailing attitude even in one of the "most malarial tracts" where he had lived for three years. He simply had "never heard of it being useful . . . nor did I hear anybody say so, although I met with hundreds of people coming to the dispensaries . . . and the doctor for medicine" (GBOW [Sukul, K. S.] 1894:II:269). Bengali natives wanted only quinine for malaria and so did Sukul.

The favorable response to quinine was not limited to people commenting about South Asia. In London on the first day of the hearings, the Royal Commission questioned a Dr. Maxwell. Maxwell, secretary of the London-based Medical Missionary Association from 1863 to 1885 and stationed in malaria-plagued Formosa during 1874 through 1883, viewed quinine as a mechanism enabling other medicines to function properly as therapies. He said he could not successfully treat disease unless the patient was given quinine because it enabled other remedies to work. Quinine also cured Maxwell's numerous opium-smoking patients suffering from malaria whereas other treatments were useless (GBOW [Maxwell]:1894 I:19–20). Two sessions later Dr. William Gauld offered a brief comment about the status of opium and quinine among inhabitants in the city of Swatow, China. Gauld, a medical missionary for sixteen years, said the Chinese "use different kinds of drugs for their fevers, and what they do use is so inefficient that they are only too glad to get our quinine." They did not, however, ingest opium as a cure for 'malaria' and according to Gauld, it would be no help if they did (GBOW [Gauld] 1894:I:60).

The Inhabitants of India Also Prefer Quinine to Opium

Four other witnesses hailing from different regions of the country supported the statements of Reverend Wilkie and Brigade Surgeon Pringle concerning Indians' preference for quinine over opium. The four witnesses also concurred with Reverend Newton's observation concerning growing public awareness about quinine's benefits. The gist of their comments was that natives preferred quinine after their initial exposure to the substance. Its popularity among the people with whom these four witnesses worked would continue despite opium's lower cost and greater availability.

Western Coast

During the sixty-fifth session at Ahmedabad on 7 February 1894, Arthur Pease asked one witness if people in the "jungle districts" of Baroda and Kari districts consumed more quinine than opium to avoid 'fever.' Anant Gangadhar Khote, a collector and magistrate in Baroda State for eighteen years, replied that quinine was preferred in these areas even though there was "not much malarious poison" (GBOW [Khote] 1894:IV:120). Lord Brassey's interrogation of a witness from Gujerat elicited a different response. Mr. Mansukh Lal told Brassey that quinine was the drug consumed precisely in the areas most plagued by the malady. Lal was an editor of a periodical called *Banner of Asia* and a member of the Salvation Army for the past ten years (six of them in India). The man said that between twenty and thirty Indian members of the Salvation Army had at their disposal a "few simple remedies for fevers," including quinine, when they toured the countryside. People never asked Lal and his colleagues "for opium and it was never hinted that opium was used in cases of fever [despite] Gujerat [being] a very malarious country" where he suffered "greatly from fever" (GBOW [Lal] 1894:IV:300). Quinine was the overwhelming choice among the inhabitants of Gujerat with whom Munsukh Lal and his associates worked, just as it was in two other regions of India.

West India and North India

Henry Wilson told one witness about hearing that natives of Rajputana (West India) had a "strong prejudice . . . against European medicine . . . generally," and that they were especially antagonistic toward quinine because it caused "headaches and unpleasant symptoms" (GBOW [Valentine] 1894:III:293). Reverend Colin S. Valentine, principal of the Agra Medical Missionary Training Institute and responsible for sending many of its graduates to Rajputana, disagreed.

> I have moved about for months at a time amongst the villages (i.e., in Rajputana), and I could have distributed pounds of quinine for the ounces that I did distribute. I have known men come 30 or 40 miles to Ajmere for quinine. So far from being prejudiced against it, they have the greatest belief in it. (GBOW [Valentine] 1894:III:293)

Dr. R. Glyn Griffiths, chief medical officer of the East India Railway stationed at Allahabad in the United Provinces (North India) for twenty years, concurred. He told Sir William Roberts that Indians were reluctant to accept European medicines and that residents of Dinapur district flatly refused to even consider doing so. The dislike of quinine and other allopathic medicines in these "unhealthy locales" also was present "sixteen or eighteen years" ago. Now, he continued, people "know the value of quinine [and] they take it" (GBOW [Griffiths] 1894:III:275).

Quinine Has Limitations

Quinine had detractors. The medical missionary Reverend F. J. Newton mentioned above also indicated that people relying upon quinine and arsenic still had attacks of 'malarial fever.' Newton viewed 'malaria' broadly and he was correct in criticizing quinine as ineffective for all the maladies he subsumed under that name. Other witnesses felt the same way, and one of them was the already introduced Sir John Tyler. Three decades of government service in the NWP enabled him to tell Roberts that quinine was best for "certain cases" but the variety of "malarial conditions" made opium "superior" or the "only prophylactic" for other instances of this misery. The drug also had a "double action" that quinine lacked. It was "a therapeutic agent, an anodyne, and hypnotic . . . [and acted] as a restorer and comforter." It was, therefore, understandable that natives valued opium as a "remedy" (GBOW [Tyler] 1894:III:110).

Surgeon-Lieutenant-Colonel A. Crombie, a veteran of eighteen years of service in East India's Dacca and Calcutta city hospitals, and superintendent of the General Hospital of Bengal Presidency during his testimony, had reservations about both substances (GBOW [Crombie] 1894:II:75). He never prescribed opium as a prophylactic, and said many natives eschewed quinine because it did not help "many fevers." It even aggravated some of them (GBOW [Crombie] 1894:II:77). Lord Brassey questioned him about the effect of opium use upon the "fertility of families." Admitting he was unable to comment about this topic, Crombie then provided an explanation for natives' avoidance of quinine and his interpretation of their attitude.

> I ought to say something more about the use of opium in malaria. When one comes to India the first thing that strikes one is what seems to be the rooted and unreasonable objection that the natives have to being treated with quinine. Even now

one has sometimes to prescribe quinine under a synonym, because the patients have very often a strong objection to it, that if they know there is quinine in the medicine they will not take it. After a time one finds out that this objection is not unreasonable, and that there are a great many fevers—I might almost say the majority of some cases I have to treat in Bengal—which are not only not benefited by quinine, but which are aggravated by it. That we find out after some years, and we are able after a time clinically to distinguish those cases which are aggravated by quinine from those which are benefited by it. I treat a large number of cases of fever without any quinine excepting in convalescence. (GBOW [Crombie] 1894:II:77)

Crombie supported his argument with an anecdote. It was about one Englishman in India suffering from fever who was helped by ingesting laudanum but not quinine. Brassey, puzzled by these comments about opium and quinine, asked if he "distinguishes more than one type of fever which is prevalent," to which Crombie replied,

not only more than one type. I believe there is more than one infection. Though they are lumped under the name 'malarial' and appear in the records of the hospital as malarial fever, I am convinced that they are not an aggravation of the symptoms. I think that is the common opinion of all medical men of any experience in India. (GBOW [Crombie] 1894:II:77)

Brassey then declared that Crombie's "remarks point to the conclusion that the distribution of quinine would not replace opium in these districts." Crombie responded "no, not at all; quinine is of very limited application." He said that Brunton, "a great authority upon therapeutics," and Garrod had also made this observation. Both individuals

mention circumstances in the treatment of malaria fever in which opium is beneficial. The same opinion is held in the Fen country in England where the people use large quantities of opium for the same purpose, both in the treatment and prevention of fever. (GBOW [Crombie] 1894:II:77)

Crombie's belief in the existence of two kinds of infections subsumed under a generic term made him cautious. He would consume both opium and quinine if traveling in a 'malarious district' (GBOW [Crombie] 1894 II:80–1).

Surgeon-Lieutenant-Colonel Hugh Johnstone, the senior civil surgeon and director of the General Hospital in Rangoon, Burma, shared Crombie's reservations about quinine. He frequently had

employed [opium] . . . in treating malarious fevers with good results, often staving off an ague fit if given an hour before its usual period of seizure, and at the least modifying its severity and adding greatly to the patient's comfort. (GBOW [Johnstone] 1894:II:207)

Quinine taken alone did not yield these benefits. Johnstone believed a combination of opium and quinine "will often be successful when quinine alone fails"

(GBOW [Johnstone] 1894:II:207). There was, therefore, something in opium that enabled quinine to perform its function but the reverse was not true. Again, the multifaceted capability of *Papaver somniferum Linn* ensured its continued popularity among the common folk despite the availability of quinine.

The medical officer in charge of employees at the Government of India's opium factory at Patna in Bihar Province (North India) also declared that quinine would never replace opium in 'malarial districts.' In this case, the reason is that it was beneficial for diseases other than 'malaria.' Dr. Frederic Pinsent Maynard, whose prior assignment was civil surgeon at Burdwan and Nuddea in Lower Bengal (East India), knew that Indian opium contained much narcotine. He believed this alkaloid had antiperiodic effects similar, but not equal, to quinine. Opium, therefore, was appropriate for all cases of 'malaria,' including those difficult cases for which quinine was most efficacious. Quinine lacked this wide-ranging capability (GBOW [Maynard] 1894:II:69–70).

Quinine Is Not Superior; Opium Is Not Inferior; They Complement Each Other

The Calcutta physician Dr. Juggo Bundo Bose told Sir William Roberts during an early Commission session that opium increased "the antiperiodic effect of quinine" (GBOW [Bose, J. B.] 1894:II:91). Other witnesses portrayed quinine and opium as complementary therapeutic agents. Each substance possessed different degrees of effectiveness for 'malaria fevers.' Roberts also heard from another physician in private practice. It was Bombay's Dr. J. A. da Gama and he testified on 14 February 1894, the seventy-first day of the hearings. This medical doctor claimed many years of success in shortening "both the cold and hot stages of the fever" by prescribing "a grain of opium with 10 grains of quinine" (GBOW [da Gama] 1894:IV:266). This had not occurred when quinine was administered alone. Another Bombay physician on the same day described a similar situation. Dr. J. Gerson da Cunha told Henry Wilson that he occasionally prescribed opium with quinine to enable both recovering patients and healthy people to avoid 'malarious fever' (GBOW [da Cunha] 1894:IV:262). The next day Dr. T. Blaney, yet another Bombay private practitioner, told the Commission about physicians who added "a little opium to a preparatory dose of quinine when the cold attack was expected, and it had a very good effect" (GBOW [Blaney] 1894:IV:292).

Surgeon-Major Dantra of the Indian Medical Service confirmed the da Gama, da Cunha, and Blaney comments about Bombay and its environs. Dantra served twenty years in that locale before working in Burma for the past two and a half decades. In charge of large prisons in Burma for twelve of these years, Dantra had been Mandalay's civil surgeon for the last two (GBOW [Dantra] 1894:II:209). Roberts asked if he ever used "opium in malaria conditions." Dantra replied "yes, with quinine very often, and I have found it answer [sic] better than increasing the dose of quinine alone" (GBOW [Dantra] 1894:II:211). A similar response was elicited from a Dr. Elizabeth Bielby on 19 January 1894, the fiftieth day of the investigation. Bielby was director of Lady Aitchison's Hospital in Lahore (West India) and holder of a Doctor of Medicine degree from the University of Bern, Switzerland. She acknowledged using opium in treating "malarial fever, but only in combination with quinine." Roberts then asked if it was her "opinion that [opium] rather fortifies the action of quinine?" Bielby replied,

> [Y]es, if you choose your cases. If a woman is very much weakened from any other disease, say pneumonia, and she gets an attack of malarious fever, and you give her opium with quinine, I have found that the effect of quinine seems to be more sure and more prolonged. (GBOW [Bielby] 1894:III:216–17)

Another interpretation portraying opium as a complement to quinine, in this case a faster-acting prophylactic, was provided by Brigade-Surgeon T. Ffrench-Mullen on Friday, 2 February 1894, the sixty-second day. Ffrench-Mullen was stationed in the city of Jodhpore in the Province of Rajputana. He was the "officiating medical officer" for the native states of the province (West India). This witness said that if he did "not consider that I had time enough [i.e., three hours before the 'fever' eruption] to stop that attack by giving . . . quinine alone, and from experience in my own person, I would give him laudanum with the quinine in solution" (GBOW [Ffrench-Mullen, T.] 1894:IV:65).

Why Quinine Is Not Used: The "Natives" Perspective

Three witnesses from East India and one from Middle India responded to the question about natives not using quinine that Henry Wilson had posed to Reverend Colin S. Valentine, principal of the Medical Missionary Training Institute in Agra. The Honorable D. R. Lyall, a Government of India administrator for thirty-two years, currently a member of the Revenue Board of the "Lower Provinces" of Bengal Presidency, told Sir Arthur Pease during the twelfth day of the hearings on 24 December 1893, that natives in 'malarious districts' of Bengal did not like quinine because it gave them headaches (GBOW [Lyall] 1894:II:65). Five days later the Royal Commission heard from the aforementioned Calcutta physician Dr. G. R. Ferris. Ferris declared that natives called Kabirijas in East India and Calcutta complained that using quinine for disease in general had

> no effect at all, but a little aphim (opium) has acted beneficially. This is especially so in cases of famine. If it were not for opium during famines I believe the death rate would be tenfold. (GBOW [Ferris] 1894:II:106–07)

Surgeon-Major Edwin F. H. Dobson from Assam, and Surgeon Major-General Rice did not blame unpleasant side effects for the absence of quinine use among natives. They said the culprits were cost and availability. Dobson told Henry Wilson that the British Government of Bengal was the main problem. Natives did not object to using quinine; they simply could not get it because government vaccinators in Assam would not distribute the substance. It also was not sold in post offices, and any ruling to the contrary had "only recently come into force in Bengal consequent on Sir Charles Elliott's order" (GBOW [Dobson] 1894:II:285).

Surgeon Major-General Rice commented about Middle India. He agreed with Dobson about unavailability as a reason for no use of quinine. Natives in the Central Provinces, according to this director of the Indian Medical Department, did not think opium was a preventive or curative for anything. Rice also was convinced the drug was no "intermittent fever" febrifuge. He and Indian natives believed the value of opium was its ability to relieve pain. Furthermore, local people used the drug for malaria, intermittent fevers, and other diseases, only because it was cheap and plentiful. In contrast, quinine was too expensive at the local level whenever it was available. It rarely was obtainable (GBOW [Rice] 1894:II:11).

Quinine—A Concluding Comment

The common folk of the country, consequently, were destined to suffer if they could not obtain quinine because of high cost or insufficient supply. They also would continue to suffer if opium did not prevent or cure 'malaria.' Anti-opiumists were adamant that *Papaver somniferum Linn* most certainly did no such thing, and their opponents labored to put forth a convincing argument that it did. How each side defined the malady was fundamental, and each group had to convince members of the Royal Commission, especially Sir William Roberts, that its interpretation was correct. The proclamations of still other witnesses suggest these arguments were of secondary importance. These people believed there was a solution to misery in South Asia and it had nothing to do with quinine or any of the cinchona alkaloids. The answer also was not opium; it was something in the mother drug. The ingredient was not morphine, the alkaloid that Western researchers and the medical community had already designated as the most important physiologically active component in *Papaver somniferum Linn*. The key substance was narcotine. Other witnesses thought this claim was as fallacious as the argument for opium.

DOES NARCOTINE PREVENT OR CURE 'MALARIA'?

Ten people volunteered comments or responded to questions about narcotine as a prophylactic or febrifuge for 'malaria.' Five of them—Huntly, Condon, Nanavati, Anderson, and Maynard—were introduced earlier in the chapter.

The medical missionary Dr. William Huntly had declared opium prevented or cured nothing. The only benefit a consumer in Rajputana obtained was a slightly more tolerable existence during one phase of a paroxysm if the person actually suffered from the disease. Huntly was equally reticent about narcotine. Sir Roberts asked if he was "aware that even 50 years ago . . . opinion [about opium for disease treatment] was prevalent amongst the professional circles in India, and that narcotine, the most abundant constituent of Bengal opium, was provided for the dispensaries." Huntly said that he heard about the opium hypothesis only from "European medical men," but no native ever mentioned it to him at any time during his career in India (GBOW [Huntly] 1894:IV:61). And, if natives did not use opium for 'malaria' or the plasmodia-induced disease because it was worthless, the same indifference applied to the alkaloid. The everyday life of South Asian citizens, for Huntly, demonstrated the reputation of narcotine as therapy for 'malaria' or for malaria had credibility only in the minds of a few westerners.

Brigade-Surgeon J. H. Condon ridiculed the idea. His experience in the "rotting vegetation" and malaria-infested Tarai districts of the Province of Oudh in British India during 1863–1864 had convinced him that opium, narcotine, and other ingredients were worthless for preventing 'malaria' and useless for anything else. He correctly observed that Government of India administrators realized the same thing years ago when they stopped manufacturing the alkaloid and its distribution to dispensaries (GBOW [Condon] 1894:III:181).

Dr. J. Anderson's response to Sir William Roberts' query about this opium alkaloid was slightly more charitable, as were the answers of B. H. Nanavati and Dr. F. P. Maynard. Anderson said he knew that narcotine was "sometimes used in fever cases, but I have no experience as to its efficacy or otherwise" (GBOW [Anderson] 1894:III:113–15). Nanavati told Lord Brassey that he was "of the opinion that [opium] was a prophylactic against malarial fevers," but he specified narcotine as the responsible agent in the mother drug (GBOW [Nanavati] 1894:IV:274). Maynard said the inherently high narcotine content of Indian opium benefited victims of malaria because the alkaloid had "anti-periodic effects similar to quinine" but not equal to it (GBOW [Maynard] 1894:II:70). The remaining five witnesses also had varying opinions about narcotine.

In Bombay on Tuesday, 13 February 1894, the hearing's seventieth day, the Royal Commission interrogated Surgeon Lieutenant-Colonel Mayne, a twenty-year veteran of the Indian Medical Service. Currently stationed at Bangalore in South India, his previous duties included civil surgeon and superintendent of jails in four districts of the Central Provinces (Middle India). Mayne spent 1891–1892 in "Upper Burma" as the "medical charge" of the Regimental Detail Hospital in the city of Rangoon. Besides observations made in three regions of the country, Mayne had also studied opium-smokers for the past two decades.[14] He responded to Lord Brassey's questioning by declaring that narcotine "used to be issued before the [sic] quinine was in force; but I believe that any prophylactic qualities of opium are due to the narcotine in it" (GBOW [Mayne] 1894:IV:241). Mayne did not explicitly state that narcotine was a prophylactic like quinine, but he did not dismiss the possibility. It was a hypothesis he was willing to test.

Dr. Surji Coomar Surbadhicari shared Mayne's perspective. This retired private practitioner had distributed narcotine at Ghazipur city in Bihar Province (North India) during the "Indian Mutiny" of 1857–58.[15] He had no choice because "disease" had erupted and there was no more quinine (GBOW [Surbadhicari] 1894:II:92). In Surbadhicari's mind, narcotine was, and remained, an acceptable substitute for quinine because it apparently did something similar to the former. He did not, however, specify what function narcotine performed during the uprising that prompted him to associate it with quinine.

Surgeon-Major S. H. Browne, principal of Lahore Medical College (West India), was also positive about narcotine when he spoke on 2 January 1894, the fifty-second day of the investigation. Questioned by Sir William Roberts concerning natives' consumption of opium, Browne replied that he lacked "absolute knowledge" about inhabitants of districts in which he worked. He did not know if they believed opium had a beneficial effect upon 'malarial fever.' Browne also could not say with certainty if the drug was found in many households and if it was used as a 'domestic remedy' (GBOW [Browne] 1894:III:237).

Browne, however, did say something definite about narcotine. He believed that its use was "first described by Sir William O'Shaughnessy." In 1874, Browne observed the alkaloid's effects upon 'malarial fever' in Calcutta and was impressed. He began using it, and "presume[ed] from the good results obtained from the effect of narcotine that opium has in itself a certain anti-malarial effect" (GBOW [Browne] 1894:III:237).[16] His description suggested that the alkaloid diminished paroxysm severity. However, his comments included no characteristics about the kind of fever he was talking about.

Mr. Pares N. Chatterjee had earned a degree from Calcutta Medical College. He then practiced medicine for sixteen years; five of them in Bhagalpore and the past eleven in Patna. Both cities were in Bihar Province (GBOW [Chatterjee] 1894:III:37–8). A total of thirty-two years of service (including the medical practice) enabled him to discuss the region of North India with conviction. Chatterjee was dubious about the prophylactic and febrifuge capability of opium and only a bit less so regarding narcotine. Opium, he stated, did not really prevent 'malaria,' he had never heard of it doing such a thing, and he knew of no other physician who thought it did either (GBOW [Chatterjee] 1894:III:37–9). Any effect the drug might have had was indirect or secondary due to its ability to "blunt physical susceptibility to external influences . . . [therefore it] may [have a] . . . protective effect . . . to some extent against malaria" (GBOW [Chatterjee] 1894:III:37–9). Narcotine, he continued, had a different effect upon people. He knew the alkaloid was sometimes given as an antiperiodic, although he had never used it himself (GBOW [Chatterjee] 1894:III:39).

Mr. D. M. Gregory was deputy opium agent for the Government of India when he appeared before the Royal Commission on 1 January 1894, the forty-first day. A fellow of the Chemical Society in London, England, Gregory's twenty-year career in the opium department of British India included two years in the Bihar Opium Agency and three years in the Chota Nagpur Division of Bengal where, until 1877, he was "opening up [opium poppy] cultivation" (GBOW [Gregory] 1894:III:90). Assigned to the Opium Factory at Ghazipur city in Bihar Province during 1879, he eventually became its superintendent. Gregory said that he had also visited Mirzapur and areas in the NWP to inspect poppy cultivation.

Gregory provided the Royal Commission with statistics about past production of narcotine in British India, its distribution, and level of consumption in the country. He also gave them some information concerning the chemical composition of the *Papaver somniferum Linn* cultivated in South Asia. Narcotine, he said, "represents the largest alkaloid in Indian opium, and the average is 6 percent in Bengal opium, with 4 percent for morphia" (GBOW [Gregory] 1894:III:90).

Gregory's testimony confirms that practitioners of allopathic medicine in India circa 1893–1894 agreed with their Anglo-European colleagues back home: the status of narcotine was insignificant. Furthermore, Gregory also said that the alkaloid

> was produced largely about twenty-five or thirty years ago . . . [and] medical officers in charge of the factory had great faith in its powers as a febrifuge. Large quantities were supplied directly to the Medical Department. With the introduction of quinine and the falling price of quinine[,] narcotine has been gradually superseded [sic]. The Medical Department refused to issue it to their medical depots, and the factory has ceased making it. (GBOW [Gregory] 1894:III:90)

The British decision during the mid-to-late 1860s to treat malaria victims in India with an inexpensive febrifuge, a mixture of the alkaloids created from the bark of species of cinchona trees capable of surviving in South Asia, eventually forced the administration to halt narcotine production. Old ideas, however, die hard, especially when stocks of a once-useful alkaloid remained. Lord Brassey asked for "how long has narcotine been sent out expressly as a febrifuge." Gregory responded that "there were indents on the factory from the Medical Department . . . [and] about fifteen or twenty years ago they use to indent regularly on the factory."

Brassey then inquired about what type of medical professional still seriously believed that narcotine could cure malaria. Gregory replied that, "I have not got the report, but Dr. Palmer, who was in charge of the factory, distinctly says that narcotine (he calls it anarcotine) is valuable as a febrifuge." Palmer ceased being superintendent in 1859 and he left India the same year. Gregory then told the Royal Commission that the Medical Department had classified the substance as a febrifuge and shipped it regularly "from the Ghazipur factory fifteen to twenty years ago." Brassey ordered him to find these documents and submit them to the secretary of the Royal Commission (GBOW [Gregory] 1894:III:90). Sir William Roberts incorporated much of this twenty-five-year-old material in his final report about the medical aspects of opium use in India.

Lord Brassey concluded the interrogation by asking, "I suppose you would naturally infer that if narcotine had that power, although not equal to quinine, crude opium itself would possess the same power in a very much less degree?" Gregory replied,

> [Y]es, I have been told by doctors, although it is not supplied by the Medical Department, that in some descriptions of fever, they prefer narcotine. Narcotine has effects where quinine has no effects. I have been told that by doctors. (GBOW [Gregory] 1894:III:90)

Summary Statements about Witnesses' Views Concerning Narcotine

The oral evidence for narcotine's status as a 'malarial fever' prophylactic and febrifuge or an alternative to quinine was unconvincing. B. H. Nanavati said the alkaloid did have medicinal value. He believed narcotine was responsible for any capability that opium possessed for mitigating the effects of 'malarial conditions.' Surgeon-Major Browne, although articulating a vague rationale, concurred. Brigade-Surgeon J. H. Condon ridiculed the idea. Dr. William Huntly came close to saying the same thing whereas Dr. Frederic Pinsent Maynard considered the alkaloid inferior to quinine but not entirely useless. Surji Coomar Surbadhicari would administer narcotine only if quinine were unavailable. Surgeon-Lieutenant Colonel Mayne and Pares N. Chatterjee suggested there might be a use for narcotine. Lord Brassey elicited a similar response from D. M. Gregory. Dr. J. Anderson simply did not know enough to decide one way or the other, but he was aware that some people had used narcotine to treat maladies subsumed under the broad category of 'fever.'

Comments from these few witnesses asked specifically about the alkaloid, or volunteering information, indicate that narcotine had never been universally accepted in India as a 'malaria' febrifuge or prophylactic that was superior to quinine. The statement describes the situation in South Asia for at least three decades before the Royal Commission's creation. We do not know if these witnesses were aware of narcotine's modest reputation among researchers during the 1870s and thereafter. Nevertheless, there is a concurrence: narcotine was neither a prophylactic nor a febrifuge for the lumpers' and the splitters' version of the disease.

HOW DOES OPIUM HELP OR HINDER A VICTIM OF "MALARIA" OR "FEVER"? SOME IDEAS FROM WITNESSES

Sir William Roberts and fellow members of the Royal Commission also heard descriptions of exactly how opium aided a sufferer. Other scenarios portrayed how ingestion harmed the patient.

How Opium "Helped" a Sufferer

Four individuals provided support for the opium policy of the Government of India by viewing the clinical course of 'fever' and 'malarial fever' as a series of stages. Three of these witnesses asserted that *Papaver somniferum Linn* was beneficial for one stage. The fourth person suggested two stages. None of them identified the agent or agents responsible for the drug's effectiveness at the stage they specified. They also did not comment upon the status of narcotine. Like most other witnesses appearing before the Royal Commission, the four people were either ignorant about the composition of opium or they attached little or no significance to what Anglo-European physiologists, chemists, and pharmacologists already knew what the substance was capable of doing, and what it did not do.

Surgeon Captain W. E. H. Woodright, medical officer for the 10th Bengal Lancers, informed Lord Brassey on 18 January 1894 that members of the Sikh religion in the regiment took a daily dose of opium. The "Mahomedans and Dogra" sepoys were less indulgent. They occasionally used the drug, but only for relief from "dysentery and bowel complaints generally, and lung and malarial affections." All of them told this medical officer that opium was "an excellent drug" for "malarial fever" when "they get to the cold stage" (GBOW [Woodright] 1894:III:194).

Joseph Benjamin agreed, although he revealed little about how he arrived at the conclusion and did not mention the military. This veteran of ten years of government service as a physician only said that "in ague, it has been found very useful in the cold stage." Opium was, however, a medicine to be taken only in time of need. Healthy people should be encouraged not to use it (GBOW [Benjamin] 1894:IV:173).

Drs. J. C. Lisboa and Temulji Bhikaji Nariman, two private practitioners from Bombay, were more informative. Lisboa claimed he had expertise for Bombay and the city of Poona. For this graduate of Grant Medical College, opium was a valuable medicine because it had "saved many lives." It was especially helpful in enabling people with "chest, intestinal complaints, and malarial fever" to live "in comparative comfort." Unlike most witnesses, this physician was very specific. He said the drug "has an action in cutting short the cold stage of intermittent fevers, and lessening the intensity and duration of the second stage, if administered at the commencement of the first stage" (GBOW [Lisboa] 1894:IV:263).

Lisboa provided no more details about the two stages of intermittent fever and neither did his colleague, Temulji Bhikaji Nariman. Nariman, holder of a degree from the Bombay College of Medicine, had practiced in the city for twenty-one years. Sir William Roberts asked him if opium had value for treating 'malaria.' Nariman replied that

> it is used to cut short an attack of ague. Given in the cold stage, I have seen it cut short an attack of fever. It very often shortens or aborts an attack of coryza or cold and its subsequent effects. (GBOW [Nariman] 1894:IV:267–68)

Woodright, Benjamin, Lisboa, and Nariman realized the drug was not appropriate for all phases of the 'disease' but it did provide some help at certain times. And the people about whom they spoke apparently agreed.[17] This kind of testimony was congenial to the pro-opiumist position. The four physicians' statements could be used to argue that qualified medical personnel might not be available to administer the drug for all Indian citizens in the "cold" stage of a "malarial fever" induced by plasmodia or unrelated microorganisms. Continued unfettered availability of opium, therefore, was compatible with the SSOT insistence upon consumption being allowed only for legitimate medical purposes. Furthermore, people who ate the drug, and physicians who prescribed it, were certainly engaged in acceptable behavior; they were seeking to obtain, or to provide, relief from the discomfort that accompanied one or more periods in the duration of a malady.

A trained allopathic physiologist or physician during the 1890s might conclude that Woodright, Benjamin, Lisboa, and Nariman were describing opium's capability in suppressing symptoms. The four people were alluding to something in the mother drug's combination of alkaloid and nonalkaloid ingredients that prevented a sufferer from reacting to the sensation of being cold. Defenders of opium consumption in South Asia, however, viewed the absence of shivering as positive; it signified curing, the restoration of at least a semblance of health. For these people, opium did not mask the cause of sickness; the drug eliminated it.

How Opium Hindered a Sufferer

An equal number of witnesses described how smoking and eating opium were detrimental at all stages of any of the maladies they called 'malaria.' Like the four mentioned above, the respondents did not identify what was harmful in opium. They also dismissed, or were unaware of, the significance of physiological active and inert substances that comprised the mother drug.

The testimonies of the aforementioned Reverend Joseph Samuel Adams and the medical missionary Dr. William Gauld suggested that claims about the prophylactic value of opium, and the smoking extract specifically, were illusory. These witnesses were China veterans of fifteen and sixteen years respectively. Adams also had spent 1874–1879 in Bhamo. He called it "one of the most feverish districts" in "Upper Burma." The Reverend had a penchant for observing misery in unhealthy places; in China he found that "in the most feverish districts the opium smokers are the men who are first to suffer, whereas the healthier coolies who are not addicted to the habit can stand all day planting rice in the blazing sun with their feet in water and not suffer from ague" (GBOW [Adams, J. S.]:1894 I:24). Adams believed smoking the drug rendered a person more susceptible to 'fever.' Gauld thought the habit impeded recuperation because "the opium smoker when he takes the fever is less likely to get over it than a man who does not smoke opium" (GBOW [Gauld]:1894 I:60).

The remaining two witnesses used their experience in regions on opposite sides of India to educate members of the Royal Commission about the dangers of opium eating for people afflicted with 'malaria.' Dr. Edalji Nassarvanji was, like J. C. Lisboa, a graduate of Grant Medical College. Although Nassarvanji undoubtedly had much contact with drug users during thirty-five years of private practice in Bombay, he used the experience of only one opium-smoking patient suffering from dysentery and malaria to make his point. Nassarvanji had persuaded the man to reduce drug intake by seventy-five percent and to do so in only a few days. The patient showed no "ill effects" from this drastic change. Something quite different occurred. Nassarvanji claimed the man's "condition improved as regards his fever and his dysenteric symptoms," which led this physician to conclude that large quantities of *Papaver somniferum Linn* consumed in the past had "to a certain extent . . . interfered with his rapid recovery" (GBOW [Nassarvanji] 1894:IV:265).

Mr. Lalit Mohun Lahiri described himself as "pleader in the Judge's Court of Assam." Lahiri was born in a village located in Nuddea district of Bengal. The disease, he lamented, had killed millions of people in Bengal. Nonetheless, he had never heard of any native taking opium as a remedy or any physician prescribing it as a preventive. Ingestion, he continued, had the opposite effect because "habitual opium-eaters and smokers have largely and easily fallen victims to malarious fevers." Lahiri thought the fishermen of Gauhati were good examples of the drug's dangerous status. Their plight was so tragic that he had no hesitation in proclaiming "only the opium habit in certain men hastened their end" (GBOW [Lahiri]:1894 II:289).

Adams, Gauld, Nassarvanji, and Lahiri did not say that opium actually killed people. The consequences of consumption were more insidious. The drug inflicted indirect harm upon a victim of 'malarial fever' by retarding the speed of recuperation and decreasing 'immunity.' Both effects hastened the sufferer's demise. For these witnesses, a person ingesting opium, and especially a physician who prescribed the drug, was the antithesis of appropriate behavior for avoiding or alleviating misery.

CONCLUSIONS ABOUT WHY PEOPLE IN INDIA ATE OPIUM

Members of the Royal Commission sought no elaboration from more than two-thirds of the people asked about opium ingestion and 'malaria' therapy. A majority in this category thought the drug was beneficial in some way. (See Appendix B.) The remaining witnesses either ridiculed or voiced skepticism about the relationship. (See Appendix A.) The responses of many witnesses in both groups (especially Appendix B) consisted of little more than a yes or no to the questions they were asked.

The few people permitted to provide additional information about various topics related to the issue disagreed about the value of the drug in preventing or curing the splitters' or lumpers' interpretation of the disease. Although the majority of witnesses introduced in this chapter thought *Papaver somniferum Linn* was beneficial for something, Sir William Roberts and his colleagues heard contradictory comments about what the drug was good for. Witnesses did not concur about the wider significance of the capability of opium to alleviate pain. They also disputed its status as a 'food' or nutritional supplement. A few people identified narcotine as a preventive of 'malaria' or its cure while the majority said the claim was nonsense. There also was no agreement concerning the comparative merits of quinine and opium, and clinical descriptions of exactly how *Papaver somniferum Linn* consumption helped or harmed 'malaria' victims differed as well.

The conflict stems from these witnesses' definitions of 'malaria' and 'disease,' and what they viewed as 'curing' and 'prevention.' Some people thought pain was a disease unto itself. For them opium was both a cure and preventive because it dulled the sensation or precluded the feeling from even evolving. The same logic governed their interpretation of 'fever' and 'malaria'; *Papaver somniferum Linn* qualified as a prophylactic, or a febrifuge, or both because it lessened discomfort.

Splitters and people having less generous interpretations of sickness disagreed. Pain and 'fever' were symptoms, not diseases, and each was common to many different maladies. These skeptics declared that opium was a useful anodyne and nothing more. They also said the drug was most certainly not a 'food' or nutritional supplement. Those who claimed otherwise articulated variations of the Moore and Birdwood scenario about dietary deficiency leading to 'chill,' with 'chill' being a predisposition to 'malarious fevers.' According to skeptics, inadequate nutrition was only one of numerous variables that might produce sickness. The argument about narcotine being the agent responsible for the mother drug's prophylactic and febrifuge capabilities was attacked by critics. They demanded proof of the substance doing anything more than masking or suppressing symptoms. Unbelievers said the alkaloid either did little, or it did nothing, to eliminate disease. Splitters contested lumpers' disparagement of quinine being of limited value. Splitters asserted that the cinchona alkaloid was a specific for one of the distinct maladies that these misinformed people had subsumed under the category of 'malaria.' Quinine was the best, and the only answer, to malaria but it exacerbated the symptoms of other, unrelated ailments. The lumpers, they contended, were simply wrong about the cinchona alkaloid.

The SSOT and unaffiliated anti-opiumists had good reason to be hopeful despite Gladstone's change of heart. Thus far, witness testimony supporting the opium and malaria correlation was unconvincing and contradictory. The anecdotes were not fatal to the moralists' agenda to create a benevolent form of imperialism where a dangerous drug would be used to help, not enslave, people.

The Government of India needed data confirming that many—or better yet—all inhabitants of a 'malarious' locale ingested opium to prevent or cure the malady. It had a strong argument if a person's sex, age, religion, caste, ethnicity, and place of residence in an unhealthy locale did not determine consumption patterns throughout the country. The next chapter documents what members of the Royal Commission heard.

NOTES

1. Bhang is a "drug prepared from the leaves of the Indian hemp" (GBO [Glossary] 1895:VII:314). H. H. Wilson says that Bhang (also Bháng or Bhung), is an "intoxicating preparation of hemp (*cannabis sativa*), either an infusion of the leaves and capsules, or the leaves and stalks bruised and pounded, and chewed or smoked like tobacco." Furthermore, "the natives of Hindustan distinguish the Bhang from the Ganja plant; the former bearing female flowers only, the latter male." The composition of Bhang is different in Bengal (East India). Here the term "properly applies to the larger leaves and capsules, and Ganja [is the term given] to the dried plant with stalks. From the Bhang is prepared the infusion bearing the same name ([1855] 1968:404).

2. For examples, see the testimonies of Dr. Edalji Nassarvanji and F. B. Mulock. Nassarvanji, a private practitioner from Bombay, described one patient's abrupt abstinence from opium-smoking habit that resulted in his recovery from "fever" (GBOW [Nassarvanji] 1894:IV:264–65). Mulock, deputy commissioner for Lucknow in the United Provinces of North India, declared that small doses of opium produced a "marked im-

munity from malaria and . . . dysentery" and identified the head clerk in his office as a good example. He described this opium eater as having "the clearest head, and is the most energetic and indefatigable worker in [the office]" (GBOW [Mulock] 1894:III:97).

3. The Honorable A. S. Lethbridge only said that physicians in his "administrative region" consumed a lot of opium as therapy for diseases of "malarious origins" (GBOW [Lethbridge] 1894:II:135). Prince Wala Kadar Syed Husain Ali Mirja Bahadur from Calcutta and Raja Muhammed Salamat Khan from Bihar Province were equally uninformative. The Prince limited his comment to Bengali natives who were using the drug for "damp, malaria, cold, diarrhoea, and for their general health" (GBOW [Bahadur, Prince W. K. S. H. A. M.] 1894:II:247). Khan only said that opium helped people over the age of forty and that in "damp districts it is usually beneficial" (GBOW [Khan, Raja M. S.] 1894:III:72). This kind of testimony helped to confirm that people in some places in India did use the drug for "medical purposes." Members of the Royal Commission, however, asked for no more details and no documentation to support the witnesses' proclamations.

4. The Government of India mistakenly listed twenty-two occupational categories. There is no category 11 in the "Index to Witnesses Examined by the Commission: Part II Classed by Profession" (GBO [Occupation] 1895:VII:223–29).

5. Four Royal Commission on Opium volumes contain testimonies of the 149 witnesses volunteering information or asked to comment about opium and 'malaria.' Twelve witnesses are found in Volume I and fifty are in Volume II. Volume III and Volume IV have twenty-eight and fifty-eight testimonies, respectively. See "Witnesses Providing Oral Evidence" in the bibliography for an alphabetical list of witnesses in each volume.

In chapters 5 and 6, references to Indian witnesses having the same surnames are identified by including honorific title (if applicable), first-name initials, and initials of all other nonsurnames listed in the "Occupational Category" list compiled by the Government of India.

Sir William Roberts mentions one witness in his medical report who is not found in any of the Royal Commission on Opium volumes. The number of people commenting about the opium and 'malaria' connection, therefore, might be 150, not 149 as cited above. These volumes contain no explanation for the discrepancy.

6. One of these officials was D. M. Smeaton, an eleven-year veteran of various postings in Burma and Financial Commissioner of Burma when he testified. Smeaton did not think opium was a prophylactic for malaria and declared the idea also was doubted in "medical circles" (GBOW [Smeaton] 1894:II:238).

7. A tea planter from Assam by the name of C. Haviland exemplified this confusion while discussing an affliction he equated with malaria. Haviland read a prepared statement describing how opium eating among Assamese Hindus, Bengalis, and the Cachiris and Garos (two tribal groups) prevented them from "getting Kala-azar." The malady struck nonconsumers but not habitual drug users. He had cured several cases by encouraging sufferers to eat the substance.

A contradiction compounded the Haviland's diagnostic confusion. He admitted that the alcohol-using Cachiris people died from Kala-azar despite their consumption of *Papaver somniferum Linn*. The witness still defended the opium habit, however, because

> the Kala-azar is fearfully catching, and I do not think any cure for it has ever been found, but I think that if people round about had been opium-eaters, the disease would have passed over them, but it got among my Garos and then it spreads. It is infectious, or an epidemic, or something which spreads (GBOW [Haviland] 1894:II:291–92).

Haviland also admitted being unable to tell if opium eaters or smokers suffered more, or less, than nonusers when an "epidemic hit" (GBOW [Haviland] 1894:II:292). It is difficult to understand what this planter really believed; he implied alcohol might negate the resistance that opium provided to potential victims of kala-azar, a 'malarial' malady, but he was uncertain if the drug did anything for a severe outbreak.

The Royal Commission described kala-azar as "an epidemic disease peculiar to the Assam Valley (Anchylostomiasis)" (GBO [Glossary] 1894:VII:317). We now know it is found in Mediterranean countries and elsewhere in South Asia. The disease is caused by a protozoan parasite called *Leishmania Donovani*. The insect vector is a sand fly (genus *Phlebotomus*). Victims suffer from anemia and have irregular fevers and enlarged spleens and livers. Kala-Azar, therefore, had external and internal characteristics similar to plasmodial malaria.

8. See the next chapter for details about Wallace's medical colleagues in India and the wider significance of his comments. Another witness agreed about the absence in academia of opium depicted as a 'malaria' prophylactic. A Miss Carleton, an American medical missionary trained at the Women's Medical College in Philadelphia, Pennsylvania, told the Royal Commission on 16 January 1894 that nothing in her medical education had exposed her to the idea. Seven years in Umballa (Amballa), a city in Punjab Province, had provided no experience and no proof. There was therefore no "medical justification" for claiming that opium prevented 'fever' of any kind (GBOW [Carleton] 1894:III:169).

9. Huntly's comments are based upon personal experience as well as a survey he conducted in Rajputana. He queried 100 opium eaters. The report lists each person's age when starting the "habit," the amount of opium consumed (time frame is unspecified), the number of years the respondents have been eating the substance, and the affliction that prompted each individual to begin consumption. The day, month, and year that Huntly conducted the survey is not given. See GBO [Huntly–Appendix IX] 1894:IV:404).

10. Other witnesses rejecting the claim that Indian natives consumed opium to prevent and cure "malaria" are cited in Appendix A ("Opium Only Relieves Pain").

11. See Appendix B ("Opium Prevents and Cures Just About Everything, Including 'Malarial Fever,' 'Fevers,' and the Diverse Detrimental Consequences of 'Miasmatic Influences'") for witnesses' brief comments about the capability of opium to prevent and cure 'malaria.' These witnesses were lumpers; they defined 'malaria' broadly.

12. The Royal Commission occupational category appendix lists Tyler as a "Medical Practitioner (Government or Native State)" but his résumé denotes no medical education. He might have been a practitioner without formal training. However, it is doubtful he could have held the position of Inspector-General of Prisons for the Northwest Provinces if professional medical qualifications had been required (GBOW [Tyler] 1894:III:109).

13. Two witnesses are difficult to place in either category because they did not mention pain by name. It also is unclear if they believed that one of the drug's capabilities was providing relief from the feeling. The Royal Commission interrogated few people from South India compared to other regions in the country.

One South Indian they asked about the correlation between opium and "malarious diseases" was G. T. Vurgese, a minor official stationed in Malabar. Vurgese acknowledged that one of his duties as "executive officer [was] to collect the opium revenue" (GBOW [Vurgese] 1894:IV:255). He provided consumption statistics for "Native" Christians, Muslims, Jews, and people living in the "hill tracts" of Malabar, Travancore, and Cochin. Religious affiliation of the residents in "hill tracts" is unspecified, but he said that cultivators in such places use opium "with great effect as a protection against fever" as do some "boatmen" on the coast (GBOW [Vurgese] 1894:IV:253).

Roman Catholics, Syrian Christians, Church of England, "Not Stated," and "Other Sects" comprise the category of "Native Christians." The group had a total of 741,916 people. However, only 5 percent of "Native Christians," most of them Syrian Christians, used the drug for "diarrhoea, dysentery, diabetes, rheumatism [and] other diseases." Twenty percent of the 1,294 Jews ingested the drug, whereas only 3 percent of the area's 975,069 "Mahomedans" partook (GBOW [Vurgese] 1894:IV:253). All people consuming the drug did so only in moderation and the habit produced a "wholesome effect."

The Honorable Javerilal Umiashankar Yajnik, "Agent to His Highness the Rao of Cutch" and a member of "His Excellency the Governor's Legislative Council of Bombay," suggested Vurgese's "wholesome effect" was illusory. This longtime resident of Bombay declared that adults and old people who consumed opium "as a preventive and curative in malarial fevers" were misinformed. Yajnik, however, tempered his criticism with tolerance. "No sensible person," he continued, "contends that the habit of eating opium is good or to be commended or encouraged, but since people will have a stimulant such as opium, either as a prophylactic against disease in malarious districts, or as a stimulant, it is found to be less harmful when taken in moderation than many a drug" (GBOW [Yajnik] 1894:IV:225).

14. Mayne said he presented a paper entitled "Madak Smoking" at the nineteenth meeting of the British Medical Association (Burma Branch) in January 1893. He claimed to have published much correspondence in the *Indian Medical Gazette* during 1880–81 (GBOW [Mayne] 1894:IV:239).

15. Critics of British rule frequently do not call the event a mutiny. They refer to it as a nineteenth-century example of a desire for independence.

16. Dr. F. J. Mouat succeeded Sir William O'Shaughnessy as professor of Materia Medica and Chemistry in the early 1840s. O'Shaughnessy then stopped investigating the therapeutic qualities of opium that he had initiated at the Medical College Hospital in Calcutta. Mouat continued the work. He concluded that opium's "properties as an intoxicant and anti-periodic were chiefly due to the morphia content contained in it, but that it could not be substituted for quinine, which was at that time a very expensive curative agent" (Mouat 1892:959–61). He accorded narcotine no importance. O'Shaughnessy eventually completed his own study and published the results. Browne apparently was referring to the latter.

17. Mr. G. B. Prabhakar said that in Bombay and Kathiawar, opium sometimes acts as an "antiperiodic, and when taken in cold stages it cuts short the cold stage." It is unclear if this witness was referring only to the disease caused by plasmodia because he claimed that opium yielded "considerable beneficial results" for rheumatism, diabetes, neuralgia, dysentery, diarrhoea, dyspepsia, cold, and for what he called "malarial fever" (GBOW [Prabhakar] 1894:IV:272).

6

More Hope for the Moralists? Witnesses' Observations about Who Eats Opium in India

THE SIGNIFICANCE OF HIGH PER CAPITA OPIUM CONSUMPTION IN "VERY MALARIOUS" LOCALES

The Royal Commission asked few witnesses to comment about a link between high per capita consumption rates and 'malarious regions.' The opinions of other individuals are found in their responses to related questions. Witnesses who confirmed the existence of the correlation were important to the pro-trade activists. Their positive responses could be construed as proof that people were ingesting the drug for a legitimate medical reason. Statistics verifying the link in unhealthy regions were especially helpful. The pro-traders were disappointed. With one exception, no witness nominated by the Government of India provided statistical data associating the prevalence of 'malaria' with high per capita consumption.

There also was no agreement whatsoever about the amount of opium ingestion in 'malarial' locales, who consumed the drug, and where they lived. The lack of accord is found even among people who *did* believe the correlation was valid.

Other witnesses rejected the correlation as spurious, not as significant as proponents claimed, or they asserted that a link proved nothing. These skeptics believed variables unrelated to deleterious environmental characteristics were responsible for per capita consumption rates. They also contended that drug use was not commonplace even among natives inhabiting 'very malarious regions' saturated with 'bad air,' 'swampy, rotting vegetation,' and so forth. Furthermore, areas of heavy consumption in an 'unhealthy' location did not dissuade these doubting witnesses from labeling the 'opium is a prophylactic and febrifuge' idea as nothing more than a tenuous hypothesis. The only inference an informed individual could draw from these statistics was that some people living in a particular place indulged themselves. Presence of the 'habit,' however, did not prove the drug prevented or cured 'fever,' 'fever diseases,' 'malaria,' or any other malady with similar overt symptoms.

This chapter is brief because few witnesses provided commentary about the topics. Brevity, however, does not signify unimportance. People affiliated with the Government of India as well as witnesses sympathetic to the SSOT cast serious doubt upon the alleged opium and malaria link. And several intrepid souls were bold enough to condemn this pro-trade position as hypocritical, blatant nonsense.

Like the previous chapter, witnesses testified at different times during the hearings. Hence, their statements are scattered throughout the Royal Commission volumes' numerous pages. Reading these disparate, often fragmentary, comments is a tedious undertaking. A partial solution to the problem is to place witnesses' observations under several headings. These are: "There *Most Certainly* Is a Correlation between High Per Capita Consumption and 'Malarious Locales'"; "Blame the Climate, Blame the Air: Supplementary Comments about Miasmatic and Tellurian Causation of High Consumption Rates"; There *Is No Correlation* Between 'Malarious Places' and Patterns of Opium Consumption." Other headings for witnesses' responses are: "The Urban-Rural Contradiction"; "Male-Female Consumption Patterns"; "Was Opium Prescribed for 'Natives' But Not 'Europeans' in India?"; "Did 'Native' as Well as Anglo-European Doctors Prescribe the Drug?"; and "Summary Statement: For Whom Is Opium Appropriate?" The last section of the chapter is entitled "Was Opium Eating and the Prevention and Cure of 'Malarial Fever' a Contrived Theory?"

THERE *MOST CERTAINLY* IS A CORRELATION BETWEEN HIGH PER CAPITA CONSUMPTION AND 'MALARIOUS LOCALES'

Sixteen witnesses queried about this topic had no doubt that a correlation existed. One of them was a high-ranking provincial administrator. Mr. T. Gordon Walker, the commissioner of Excise for Punjab, said natives often used opium "to counteract the bad effects of the climate in marshy or malarious tracts." He also told the Commission that "extension of canal irrigation has led to the use of opium for the purpose of counteracting the various ailments which had followed the change from a dry to a damp climate." The presence of canals, according to Walker, increased the amount of humidity, hence the need for opium among many people. His statement about heavy users of the drug being "mostly Mohammedans" indicated religion was also a variable affecting consumption rates in this part of West India (GBOW [Walker] 1894 III:236). Walker provided no comment about differences in consumption rates between Muslims living in 'malarious locales' and coreligionists occupying less 'humid,' hence less 'dangerous' places.

Walker implied the countryside was the location of many 'malarious' places in Punjab. Dr. Surji Coomar Surbadhicari, however, was explicit about rural areas in the Bengal Province. Natives in these unhealthy locales of East India were indeed habitual users, but Surbadhicari did not identify their religious orientation (GBOW [Surbadhicari] 1894 II:92). F. W. Brownrigg, settlement officer for the Sultanpur district of Oudh Province in North India, was also explicit about locations of high opium consumption. On 11 January 1894, he told Sir James B. Lyall that Crawnpore city, the "Manchester of Northern India . . . shows the highest average consumption of all," and that opium use also was common in "malarial tracts . . . or where canal irrigation is extensive, and intermittent fever [is] unusually prevalent" (GBOW [Brownrigg] 1894 III:117). Similar to Walker, Brownrigg also associated heavy use with a specific group of people.

> In eastern districts, where fever is comparatively less and the climate drier and more healthy, the amount consumed is not so great [but] the Mahomedan [sic] population of the eastern tracts also is thinner than away west, and this too is a factor which affects the amount consumed. (GBOW [Brownrigg] 1894 III:117)

Mr. A. A. Wace, a veteran of twenty-six years as commissioner of fourteen Bengal districts and one assignment in Assam, testified on 3 January 1894, the thirty-sixth day of the hearings. Wace furnished the Royal Commission with statistical data for six rural districts of Bengal. Lord Brassey asked him to "connect the consumption in Bengal with the physical circumstances of the districts," to which Wace replied that the "surroundings and habits of the people" were the primary variables affecting drug use. He introduced data from an 1892 Sanitary Commissioner's Report to support the "oft-asserted connection between life in malarious tracts and the need of opium." Wace said the "death-rate from fever for the whole province [of Bengal was] 16.37" but it was much higher for several other districts within the province. Mortality rose to 30.9 in Dinajpur, 31.3 in Rangpur, 28.4 in Purnea, 30.7 in Maldah, 25.4 in Murshidabad, and 25.2 in Hooghly (GBOW [Wace] 1894 III:5).

The statistics Wace included with his testimony indicated high levels of opium consumption per thousand people in these six "notoriously feverish" administrative entities. The district with which he was most familiar, however, convinced Wace that climate was the prime cause of consumption throughout Bengal and elsewhere. The Ganges river cut Bhagalpur district in half. Bhagalpur's northern section was "damp and malarious." The district's "three most malarious" subdistricts had 27 percent of the district's population but 42 percent of the licensed opium shops. In contrast, he continued, the "three driest [subdistricts] of the south, containing a population of about four-fifths of the damper [subdistricts], have only two opium shops, while the three damp [subdistricts] have seventeen." From these data Wace concluded that opium was a valuable prophylactic in these "damp districts" (GBO [Wace] 1894:III:5).

After admitting that two of his associates were addicted, he said only moderate amounts of the drug were helpful. Large quantities were detrimental to health (GBOW [Wace] 1894:III:5). Henry Wilson then inquired if Wace could cite "where that is recorded either in official statements or in any other statements until within the last two or three years." Wace acknowledged that he had not read it until the Royal Commission began its hearings, but he knew that it was "a common idea among the people." Wilson pursued the topic, asking if the witness did "not know anywhere it can be found recorded either in medical or popular works?" Wace said he did not review medical literature and did not have the time to read many "popular works" (GBOW [Wace] 1894 III:7).

Wilson's questions suggest he suspected the opium as a 'malaria' prophylactic and febrifuge scenario was an invention of the Royal Commission in collusion with the Government of India. Nonetheless, the man's skepticism did not dissuade other witnesses from supporting the statements of Surbadhicari, Walker, and Wace with comments about West, East, and North India.

Mr. W. H. Ryland, current president of the Eurasian and Anglo-Indian Association in Calcutta, mentioned two of the districts Wace had identified. Ryland said people in Dinajpore and Rangpore districts often used opium for relief. This retired official's observations were based upon forty years of government service in India (GBOW [Ryland] 1894 II:157).[1] Assistant-Surgeon Soorjee Narain Singh was teaching at the Patna Medical School in Bihar Province of North India when he testified. Singh said opium was rarely consumed by people under the age of thirty except in "damp, malarious places." He confirmed the Ryland and Wace observations about heavy consumption in Dinajpur, Rungpur, Purnea, Murshidabad, and Hooghly districts, and added Dacca and Burdwan to the list (GBOW [Singh, S. N.] 1894 III:39). Mr. Sita Nath Roy, a banker, landowner, and secretary to the Bengal Chamber of Commerce, generalized about many districts. Consumption rates in Bengal Presidency, he suggested, varied "mostly due to the great prevalence of malarial fever in Central and Western Bengal" (GBOW [Roy, S. N.] 1894 II:43). And, Maharaja Bahadur Sir Narendra Krishna's experience as deputy magistrate in the lowland regions of Bengal for almost forty-five years, prompted this declaration. Bengali natives living in "malarial, low-lying swampy areas" ingested small amounts of the drug as a "tonic" to maintain their health (GBOW [Krishna] 1894 II:169).

A man by the name of S. C. Naik was confident about a correlation between unhealthy areas and consumption elsewhere in East India. This assistant superintendent of the Tributary States in Orissa said natives in at least one part of this province used the drug, and local doctors also prescribed it to inhabitants of "malarial regions" (GBOW [Naik] 1894 II:110–11). The testimony of Munshi Rahmat Ali, a planter from Assam, suggested that 'tribal' affiliation determined who consumed the drug. Ali, vice president of the Mohammedan Literary Society of Calcutta and introduced to the Commission as a member of the "Muslim ruling class," said that Bengalis, Assamese, and people called Mikirs and Kacharis worked in "damp and malarial districts" of Assam. For Ali, the link between opium use and labor productivity was obvious and positive. The Assamese and Bengalis consumed little. Consequently, they had less "endurance for hard labor [and] privations" than the opium-using Mirkirs and Kacharis (GBOW [Ali] 1894 II:302).

The Honorable Gangadhar Rao Chitnavis admitted his experience was limited to wealthy people who ate opium for various reasons. One rationale was to prevent 'malarial fever.' This administrator and honorary magistrate from

Nagpur in Middle India also knew that opium was ingested in "malarial climates when people go on long journeys, or have to undergo exhaustion" (GBOW [Chitnavis] 1894 IV:367). Chitnavis did not indicate if he believed that fatigue was a prelude to 'chills' and 'malarial' fever.

Two witnesses from different sections of North India offered additional comments about rationales for consumption in unhealthy locales. Brigade-Surgeon Lieutenant-Colonel W. R. Hooper told the Royal Commission on 10 January 1894, the forty-second day of the hearings, that "malarial diseases" plague inhabitants in Lucknow district of the United Provinces and Oudh. Furthermore, the number of Muslims and Hindus who use the drug increases during the rainy season. Hooper's conclusion was based upon twenty-nine years of duty for the Government of India. He had spent part of this time as civil surgeon for Lucknow and superintendent of the city's lunatic asylum. Hooper said nothing about a correlation between drug use and unhealthy locales found elsewhere in North India. And no commissioner member at the hearing that day asked what he had encountered during postings as director of jails for the cities of Allahabad, Benares, and Azamgarh (GBOW [Hooper] 1894 III:102).

Mr. T. Stoker alluded to the role of caste, racial identity, and custom in affecting rate of consumption. He also identified exactly who used the drug within a 'malarious region.' Stoker, the previously introduced commissioner of Excise and Stamps, and "inspector-general" of the NWP and Oudh, said indulgence was "more general among the Aryan races," but "aboriginal races" use it only as a medicine. Stoker was not suggesting Aryans were genetically predisposed to consume whereas 'aboriginal' people were not. The difference was a consequence of "locality and surroundings, caste or social position [and] is probably a matter of tradition" (GBOW [Stoker] 1894 III:276). The man was also suggesting that "Aryans" ingest the drug for medicinal *and* nonmedicinal (recreational) purposes.

Caste, economic status, 'racial' status as an 'Aryan' or 'aboriginal,' for Stokes, were unimportant for determining consumption patterns in locations plagued by sickness. He claimed opium was mostly used in "malarial tracts" as a therapy because it prevented and cured disease. Stores in Meerut district that sold only opium provided him with evidence that consumption and miserable locales were inseparable, and that 'malaria' could debilitate any person. All these drug establishments, he observed, were "grouped either along the low stands of the Jumna [River], which is a notoriously malarial tract, or along the line of the main Ganges canal, where the rise of water-level has been most marked, and malarial conditions are most prevalent" (GBOW [Stoker] 1894 III:276). In Stoker's mind 'malarial disease' could strike anybody and opium helped everybody. Consumption of the drug enabled people of any caste, religion, ethnic identity, and income level to survive if they lived in an environment hospitable to misery.

Two witnesses representing the Western Coast region provided only vague generalizations about the significance of high per capita consumption. Mr. E. S. Gubbay was manager of the Opium Department for Messrs. David Sassoon and Company in Bombay and China. The firm was a major exporter of opium from the native states of Central India and Rajputana during the latter part of the century.

On 13 February 1894, the seventieth day of the hearings, he said opium was "generally regarded in unhealthy and malarial tracts as a preventive against the insidious attacks of fever and rheumatism" (GBOW [Gubbay] 1894 IV:233). Gubbay agreed with the idea but did not specify if he was talking about Indian or Chinese natives, or both. The second witness, testifying on the same day, offered a short comment applicable only to South Asia. Mr. Mirza Husain Khan, secretary of the Bombay National Mahomedan [sic] Association, said the reason for opium consumption in India's 'malarial districts' was prophylactic (GBOW [Khan, M. H.] 1894 IV:238).

Another witness testifying on 13 February declared the correlation between drug consumption and 'malaria' also existed in South India. Colonel C. A. Porteus, inspector general of police for Madras and a resident of India for thirty-seven years, knew that people in Madras Presidency used opium obtained from poppy cultivated on the Malwa plateau in Central India. They considered the Malwa drug to be invaluable. This sentiment, he continued, was especially prevalent among inhabitants of 'malarious tracts' in Madras. Members of the Royal Commission only had to ask a few people in these regions, Porteus remarked, and any doubt they had about a need for the drug would quickly end (GBOW [Porteus] 1894 IV:255). Commission appointees did not have the opportunity to do so because few people from South India testified.

BLAME THE CLIMATE, BLAME THE AIR: SUPPLEMENTARY COMMENTS ABOUT MIASMATIC AND TELLURIAN CAUSATION OF HIGH CONSUMPTION RATES

The depositions mentioned above indicate that T. Gordon Walker linked construction of irrigation canals to increased humidity. This created an environment that spawned more cases of 'fever' diseases. The result was natives' increased reliance upon *Papaver somniferum Linn* to survive in these humid locations of Punjab Province (GBOW [Walker] 1894 III:236). Brigade-Surgeon Lieutenant-Colonel W. R. Hooper also alluded to the negative consequences of moisture and 'dampness;' opium use among Hindus and Muslims in Lucknow district of North India increased during the monsoon season (GBOW [Hooper] 1894 III:102). Hooper provided no more details.

The Honorable T. D. MacKenzie was more helpful. Cited in the previous chapter as being amenable to viewing opium as a food, MacKenzie also implicated moisture in determining patterns of opium consumption. This well-placed Opium and Excise Department official said that per capita use was high because "the climate is very feverish and during the hot weather and the monsoon [it is] trying and depressing" (GBOW [MacKenzie] 1894 IV:282).

Witnesses introduced other versions of miasmatic and tellurian causation to explain the geographic distribution of high consumption rates. MacKenzie, for example, implicated dirt as a factor when Sir Lyall asked him why opium consumption in Broach district was more than double compared to the cities of Bombay, Ahmedabad, and elsewhere in Gujerat. MacKenzie replied that

Broach was "a black soil district, that is, it is liable with very little rain to become water-logged [and] it is the most feverish district in the whole presidency" (GBOW [MacKenzie] 1894 IV:284). A Bengal Civil Service administrator echoed MacKenzie's accusation. Mr. E. V. Westmacott had spent most of his thirty years of service in Lower Bengal, including Orissa. He claimed that Orissa's soil was suitable for 'malaria' and natives consumed much opium to survive. This Opium and Excise official did not give details about what made the soil so hospitable to the 'disease' (GBOW [Westmacott] 1894 II:127–28).

Anant Gangadhar Khote attempted to educate Sir Lyall about opium's status in the native state of Baroda. Natives' use of the drug "in anointing the Hindu Gods" made it indispensable for ensuring emotional well-being (GBOW [Khote, A. G.] 1894 IV:119–20). It also enhanced the possibility of survival in adverse environmental conditions because

> some parts of the territory under forest is [sic] abounding in malarious fevers . . . [and] all these diseases make their ravages. . . . Here, the sovereign remedy, the family doctor, the home *Vaid*, is opium. People in general never frequent public dispensaries till they finish the stock of the homemade medicines. (GBOW [Khote, A. G.] 1894 IV:116)

Later in the session Khote said people inhabiting "jungle districts of the region" believed opium prevented 'fever.' Arthur Pease then responded "I suppose that people . . . [in nonjungle areas] take quinine more than opium for that purpose?" Khote mentioned hearing about people consuming quinine in districts such as Baroda and Kari. These places had much less "malarious poison" because they were not heavily forested (GBOW [Khote, A .G.] 1894 IV:120). The statement suggests that in Khote's mind opium was the drug of choice to alleviate the misery in places ravaged by the lumpers' version of 'malaria.' Quinine was adequate for regions of less severity. Although he thought *Papaver somniferum Linn* possessed more inherent therapeutic utility than the cinchona alkaloid, Khote offered no clue about the reason for opium's superiority in places where trees abound. We are left to surmise that for this witness, the drug contained something that destroyed harmful emanations from dense, tall standing vegetation. The man, therefore, recommended opium for miasmatic and tellurian interpretations of the disease whereas quinine was effective for plasmodial malaria.

THERE *IS NO CORRELATION* BETWEEN 'MALARIOUS PLACES' AND PATTERNS OF OPIUM CONSUMPTION

Several proponents of the prophylactic and febrifuge scenario also offered explanations for the absence of high per capita consumption rates in 'very malarious regions.'

In London on Tuesday, 28 November 1893, the fourteenth day of the hearings, Mr. Khurgeshur Bose declared that village folk rarely use opium. Henry Wilson later inquired about who suffered "most in Bengal from malaria, the ryots or the well-off people in the cities?" Bose, a medical officer for the Eastern Bengal Railway, said it was the former. Wilson was puzzled. He then asked why people who "suffer the most . . . take the least," to which Bose responded that "a very few people know that opium is a preventive of malaria" (GBOW [Bose, K.] 1894 II:100). Bose was implying that consumption data collected in rural Bengal might be an inaccurate assessment of the drug's value. Country people also might increase per capita consumption if they were better educated. For this witness, opium was beneficial but segments of the population who needed it the most were uninformed.

Two days later, E. V. Westmacott told Wilson that residents in "malarial regions" of the "lower provinces of Bengal" did not ingest great amounts of opium because it was too expensive. He was convinced consumption would increase if it cost less (GBOW [Westmacott] 1894 II:129). Assistant-Surgeon Soorjee Narain Singh was surprised when Wilson told him on 5 January 1893 that the price of opium in India's "most malarious districts" was three times greater than it was in Patna city, Singh's place of work. Wilson again recognized a contradiction: if opium really did prevent and cure 'malaria,' then why did the Government of India allow the drug to be priced so high that many poor people living in 'very malarious regions' were unable to afford it? Singh could not answer the question.

Other witnesses rejected these explanations. Some of these people were introduced earlier; the rest were not. Nonetheless, all of them said that cost, education, and ignorance were irrelevant; there was no correlation between per capita consumption in unhealthy locales because opium neither prevented nor cured malaria. The drug had the same status for any sickness referred to as 'malarial fever.'

Dr. William Huntly said the correlation did not exist for parts of Rajputana in West India. He claimed the inhabitants "during the last two seasons of excessive rain . . . [and] opium-eaters suffered equally with the non-eaters" (GBOW [Huntly] 1894 IV:60). Dr. H. Martyn Clark expressed a similar thought for Punjab Province. He lamented the absence of immunity for both consumers and nonconsumers in the malaria-plagued city of Amritsar and its environs (GBOW [Clark] 1894 III:191–92). Mr. Mansukh Lal said opium did nothing to alleviate the disease in the "very malarious country" of Gujerat (GBOW [Lal] 1894 IV:300). Dr. Maxwell, secretary of the Medical Missionary Association in London, said the same thing about the disease-ravaged island of Formosa (GBOW [Maxwell] 1894 I:19–20). And, Brigade-Surgeon J. H. Condon said nobody in the Terai districts of Oudh Province (North India) ever prescribed or ingested opium to avoid misery. This avoidance characterized people constantly exposed to the "rotting vegetation" and the "very heavy dews" that caused "very bad malarious fever." Condon also said he had never even heard about any native mentioning opium consumed for this purpose (GBOW [Condon] 1894 III:181).

A similar response came from the physician Nil Ratan Sircar, a fellow of Calcutta University in the Faculties of Arts and Medicine and lecturer of Forensic Medicine in the Calcutta Medical School (GBOW [Sircar] 1894 II:162). Sircar had been practicing medicine for the past six years and provided the Royal Commission with details about visits to the eastern and central part of Bengal Presidency. He found no difference in the number of 'malaria' cases among opium eaters and abstainers. He also claimed to never having met any cultivator, fisherman, or member of the "lower classes" who lived in "marshy parts" and "malarious districts" consuming opium on a habitual basis for anything. Furthermore, none of these people ever told him about the existence of such behavior. Sircar told Henry Wilson that the Indian public, meaning residents of 'malarious' and healthy locales, including Calcutta, did not "have the idea that opium is a protection against fever" and that there is "no evidence to prove [its] supposed prophylactic action" (GBOW [Sircar] 1894 II:163).

Wilson then asked whether or not medical professionals other then Sircar thought that opium was especially useful in "malarious districts." The witness said no, it was not "a useful medicine in malarious districts, either as a prophylactic against fever, or as an antiperiodic during the course of a fever." He acknowledged Dr. William O'Shaughnessy having used the drug in the past, albeit for only a short time, as an "antiperiodic" for "the intermission [sic] stage [of] malarious fever." O'Shaughnessy stopped dispensing it upon discovering that only large, "unsafe doses" had any antiperiodic effect (GBOW [Sircar] 1894 II:163).

The message from Condon, Maxwell, Lal, Clark, Huntly, and Sircar was clear: no correlation existed between high consumption and unhealthy locales. The ingestion of opium did not guarantee freedom from 'malarial fevers' for anyone, anywhere, and at any time. The drug's alleged status as a prophylactic and febrifuge was erroneous.

Mr. Maung Hpo Hmyin, a member of the business community in Moulmein, Burma, also claimed the correlation was nonexistent. He told Lyall and members of the Royal Commission on 13 December 1893 that nobody thought the drug prevented 'fever' or that it was of any use in malarious districts. Hmyin had also visited "timber forests" where malaria was "most prevalent," but had never known, and had never heard about, any foresters using the drug to prevent the sickness (GBOW [Hmyin] 1894 II:204).

Dr. Donald Morison, a medical missionary, had been stationed for most of his sixteen years in the town of Rampore Bauleah (population 20,000) in Rajshahye district of Lower Bengal. Morison emphatically rejected the opium as a prophylactic and febrifuge scenario, and dismissed the "malarious regions" and high per capita consumption correlation as ridiculous. He also provided statistics to support the denial. On 29 November 1893, Morison told Lord Brassey that visits to the rural parts of the district "twice a year in the rainy season, and during the cold weather, and [occasionally] the districts of Maldah and Pubna," enabled him to have close contact with all kinds of people. He also had treated "six to 10,000 patients annually."

Morison described the dismal situation in Rajshahye district to prove his point. The entire district was "malarious, in some parts intensively so," and its 1.5 million inhabitants suffered badly throughout the year. The situation was at its worst during September, October, and November when "sixty to eighty percent of [his] patients suffer[ed] from malarious fever or their complications." Despite this misery, sick people in Rajshahye and inhabitants of the "districts of Maldah, Pubna and indeed I may say to Lower Bengal" did not ingest opium either as a "prophylactic or for the cure of fever." This included "Mahomedans" (GBOW [Morison] 1894 II:100, 104).

Morison then began reading from page sixty-eight of Sir William Roberts' book, *Dietetics and Dyspepsia*, to defend his contention about the addictive nature of opium eating. Roberts immediately interrupted to say he did not "see what relevance that has to the question before the Commission" (GBOW [Morison] 1894 II:101). Morison wanted to elaborate but Lord Brassey did not permit it.

Morison then told the Royal Commission that even Government of India personnel admitted that opium did not deserve its alleged status. "[F]our educated Hindus" working for the Administration had recently told him that the city of "Cuttack, and generally over most parts of Orissa . . . [was] peculiarly free from malaria with spleen and fevers as compared with Calcutta, Burdwan, Nadya, and other parts of Lower Bengal." They also told Morison about friends who migrated to Orissa because it was known to be malaria-free. Furthermore, they were convinced "the taking of opium in Orissa is not due to malaria, as the people themselves do not attribute the habit to that cause" (GBOW [Morison] 1894 II:102).

Another Hindu and a "European government official" Morison related, admitted the same thing. And then, a few days later, Morison had spoken to a deputy collector who had written a report about the drug. The official said that he never heard of opium used to "cure or ward off malaria, for here in Cuttack we have little or none." This gentleman, whose letter Morison had in front of him, said he knew of families who traveled from Calcutta "from Bengal with their members suffering from spleen and fever, and after residing here for some time without taking medicine, they have been cured of their malarial ailments" (GBOW [Morison] 1894 II:102). Morison continued reading statements from other native acquaintances. They all attested to the relatively healthy environment and opium's inconsequentiality as a preventive or cure among Orissa's inhabitants.

In response to Arthur Fanshawe's question about opium being a "necessity of life," Morison tried to teach the man about "the weak points of [the] theory of malaria accounting for the excessive consumption of opium in certain districts of India." First, it was erroneous that excessive consumption in Assam and Orissa "is due to the fact that these parts are more malarious than other parts of India, and that [opium] is taken as a prophylactic by the poor ryots." The inaccuracy is further demonstrated by realizing that opium consumption was virtually nonexistent in some "very malarious" districts of Bengal. Morison then contended that drug consumption was exceptionally high in malaria-free districts of India and China. He concluded that "malaria" alone was not the cause of excessive opium consumption in Assam and Orissa (GBOW [Morison] 1894 II:103). Morison ended the long response to Fanshawe by declaring that Orissa

> generally, instead of being a hotbed of malaria, is a kind of sanitarium for Bengal, where those who can afford to do so go to get rid of Bengal malaria and are not disappointed. That opium is not taken in Orissa as a prophylactic, for the people do not know the antiperiodic properties of the drug nor do they need it for malaria.

That opium is never taken by the people themselves to cure fever. That the opium-eaters, who are saturated with the 'prophylactic,' are at least as liable to fevers as others. That the use of opium is looked upon as a curse by all intelligent natives of Orissa who have the welfare of their people at heart. (GBOW [Morison] 1894 II:103)

Henry Wilson, following Fanshawe, inquired if Morison was adamantly opposed to associating opium consumption with "malaria." The witness said yes. Wilson then asked when the "doctrine" linking the drug and the 'disease' first appeared. Morison did not know who first advanced the notion, but replied "it was only within recent years that it has come before the public . . . [and that] "it was coincident with the agitation against opium" (GBOW [Morison] 1894 II:104). For Morison, the proclaimed correlation between the consumption of *Papaver somniferum Linn* and "very malarious regions" was a disingenuous tactic using nonexistent data and invalid geographic comparisons to defend a dubious official opium policy.

Deputy Surgeon-General W. P. Partridge cited personal experience in "malarious regions" as well as Morison's data to say no to Lord Brassey's question about opium being a 'fever' prophylactic. This thirty-year veteran of government service in India, whose career began in 1855 and ended in 1885, had completed a fourteen-year stint as superintendent of two Bombay jails. He then was twice appointed civil surgeon, a position that took him to different parts of Gujerat, Bombay and Upper Sind. Partridge identified Dr. Donald Morison as a preeminent authority about the drug. He told the Commission about Morison having treated between 6,000 and 15,000 patients "annually for fifteen years, and though 80 percent suffered from malaria he [Morison] never heard one native hint that opium prevented fever." Partridge's experience during the thirty-year career was identical. He had been in "malarious places" such as Gujerat and Sindh. Yet "never once [had he] been asked by any native for opium as an antidote for fever; they never hinted at such a thing, and [he did] not believe that any of the natives use it as a prophylactic for fever (GBOW [Partridge] 1894 I:127).

Reverend A. W. Prautch's statistics were much more impressive than Morison's numbers for Bengal and Partridge's commentary about the opposite side of the country (GBOW [Prautch] 1894 IV:294).[2] Prautch had been a Bible seller for nine and a half years in Bombay and its environs. He also had worked for a shorter period of time in Gujerat and Lucknow, the city in North India. He described one administrative entity on Bombay's border to invalidate the correlation between high consumption and 'unhealthy locales.' On 15 February 1894, the seventy-second day of the hearings, Prautch said Tanna district was

> considered very malarious because the chief crop is rice. I have made diligent inquiries from the villagers ever since I heard the surprising statement that opium was considered as a preventative and cure for fever. I have never met one Native who ever hinted that it might be good for fever, and when questioned as to whether they ever used opium for fever, the answer was invariably 'No.' I have made inquiries of the Free Church dispensary at Tanna. During 1893, 12,615 patients (aggregating

36,436 visits) were treated; of these over half were suffering from fever. The doctor uses opium as a drug, but using opium for fever, he said he never had. (GBOW [Prautch] 1894 VII:324)

THE URBAN-RURAL CONTRADICTION

It is difficult to imagine pro-trade activists being delighted by the statements of Soorjee Narain Singh, Surji Coomar Surbadicari, and Khurgeshur Bose. These witnesses told the Royal Commission that people living in malaria-plagued rural areas consumed less opium than inhabitants of urban areas where malaria was not a major problem. F. W. Brownrigg and Walker were also no help. Brownrigg's comment about the industrial city of Crawnpur, and then the Walker and Brownrigg identification of Muslims as heavy users, also indicated that high per capita consumption was not invariably associated with 'malarial' regions. People living in relatively healthy places consumed great amounts of the drug; inhabitants of 'malarious' regions did not. And some of rural people saw no need to begin the opium habit to avoid or cure the sickness.

Raja Udai Pratap Singh from the city of Lucknow in North India, and Calcutta physician Dr. Juggo Bundo Bose also noted the urban-rural contrast. Raja Singh owned a large estate in Bhinga of Bahraich district of Oudh Province. He appears to have been a very influential person. A member of the Viceroy's Legislative Council, Singh also was the chairperson of Lucknow's Municipal Board. His other public service activities included being a fellow of Allahabad University. Singh said the inhabitants of Lucknow habitually consumed opium whereas village people living in 'malarious' areas ingested it only as a "general tonic" for "malaria." Henry Wilson attempted to account for the surprisingly meager use of a substance that officials in British India proclaimed to be a preventive and febrifuge in areas "saturated" with malaria. He asked Singh several questions. One query was why did consumption remained modest in all but eight to ten of "malarious villages" located in the district Singh knew best (GBOW [Singh, Raja U. P.] 1894 III:102). Singh was unable to explain why.

Dr. Bose, a firm believer in opium's capability to prevent and cure 'malarial fevers,' unwittingly exposed contradictions in the Government of India's drug policy. Like other witnesses, he acknowledged less opium use in the countryside where the 'disease' was rampant in contrast to high consumption in urban areas where 'malaria' was less prevalent. Bose then said rural-dwelling females ingested the drug less often and in smaller amounts compared to men. The reason for the difference between the sexes is that women did not like the drug even though they were as susceptible to 'malaria' as males.

Bose's speculation raised issues that Sir William Roberts and other members of the Royal Commission would have to address. The first was just how far natives' ignorance and high prices could explain the inverse ratio between level of consumption and prevalence or severity of the disease. The second issue involved other factors that might account for higher per capita consumption in urban areas where 'malaria' was less prevalent compared to villages.

One explanation for the contradiction is that opium might be useful for many ailments unrelated to 'malaria,' with which people living in cities and towns had to contend. Far more people lived in an urban milieu than in a village. People in a city, therefore, needed a greater quantity of the drug than residents of rural areas, and the rural-urban difference in total amount of opium consumed was to be expected. Another interpretation is that opium for urban residents was a remedy for many complaints; it was an all-purpose tonic. The countryside was different; many villagers did not use the drug because they realized it was ineffective for 'malarial fevers' and for the disease caused by plasmodia.

MALE–FEMALE CONSUMPTION PATTERNS

The difference between male and female drug consumption also needed an explanation if one assumed (as did Bose and some of his medical colleagues) that opium was a potent prophylactic and febrifuge for 'malarial fevers.' It was logical to conclude that females would consume the drug as much, and as often, as males, regardless of how distasteful they found the drug to be. Both sexes in India lived in unhealthy locales and a person's sexual identity did not determine susceptibility to mosquito bites and infection. The one possible exception was lactating or pregnant women. All females in rural areas, however, were not continuously pregnant, and some did not bear children because they were too young or menopausal. No evidence existed during the 1890s demonstrating that lactating or pregnant females were less susceptible to the lumpers' version of 'malaria' or the splitters' definition of the disease.[3] The ignorance and poverty of natives might explain some incidents of low opium consumption in locales plagued by 'malaria.' However, the two factors were inadequate for explaining all examples of urban-rural disparities, and most certainly not the male-female contrast identified by Bose. The only way to explicate the latter peculiarity is to assume that Indian females *chose* not to consume a substance that cured a serious disease or prevented their demise. In other words, they preferred to be miserable or die rather than swallowing pieces of opium. This was an unlikely occurrence.

Another verification of the idea that opium prevents and cures 'malaria' was to compare consumption patterns among natives, Anglo-Europeans, and other foreigners in India. It was also logical to assume that *everybody* living in South Asia would want to consume the drug if it did the things the defenders of the status quo proclaimed.[4]

WAS OPIUM PRESCRIBED FOR 'NATIVES' BUT NOT 'EUROPEANS' IN INDIA?

There are two ways to verify the malaria-opium hypothesis using witness testimonies. The first is to ascertain how many Western medical doctors working in India prescribed opium for fellow occidentals suffering from the 'malarial' maladies. The second is to determine how many native-born physicians trained in

Western medical schools dispensed the drug to English, American, and European residents of India experiencing 'fever.' Defenders of the status quo welcomed oral testimony indicating physicians recommended opium to *both* foreign-born and Indian nationals. It meant their contention about the benefits of eating the drug had credibility among medical professionals who were products of the same cultural traditions as members of the Royal Commission. Anglo-European or Western-trained doctors telling occidentals in India to use the drug might convince Sir William Roberts and his colleagues that more restriction of public accessibility was unnecessary and unwise. The substance prevented 'fever' and cured its victims, and if some of the fortunate individuals were Anglo-Europeans, others were probably Indian natives. The ability of suffering people to obtain opium when needed was the important issue, and the present distribution system in India was sufficient. The SSOT and other misguided Christian moralists should leave well enough alone.

Why Was Opium Prescribed for Natives But Not Europeans?

There are three answers to the question. The first is lack of money. The second is availability. The last is natives' preference for eventual self-medication.

Surgeon-Major D. F. Barry recommended opium to poor Indian natives only because nothing else was available. Wealthy Indians and Anglo-Europeans were able to afford treatment more appropriate for their afflictions. Barry's conviction was the result of fourteen years of experience in various regions of India. This included his present assignment in the Sitapur district (GBOW [Barry] 1894 III:117). Dr. Hari Bhikaji, chief medical officer for Gondal State in Kathiawar on the Western Coast, also mentioned the drug being a therapy of last resort for the unfortunate. He told Sir Lyall that opium really was useless as a febrifuge and that its primary therapeutic value was symptom relief. Bhikaji knew of no Western-trained physician telling a person to consume the drug for 'malarial fevers.' However, he continued, "in India there are millions of people beyond the reach of skilled medical aid [and] . . . [i]n such cases they use opium" (GBOW [Bhikaji] 1894 IV:188). Mr. Kunwar Jaswant Singh, a regent of Sailana State near Bombay, testified on 8 February 1894, the sixty-fifth day of the hearings. He declared that people throughout the country used opium as a medicine. It enabled citizens to save money by medicating themselves. This enabled them to avoid having to rely upon what he called "medical men" (GBOW [Singh, K. J.] 1894 IV:157). The previously mentioned Anant Gangadhar Khote generalized about the common folk in Baroda State. He said they considered crude opium to be "the sovereign remedy, the family doctor, the home *Vaid*," and they "never frequent public dispensaries till they finish the stock of the homemade medicines" (GBOW [Khote] 1894 IV:116).

Barry, Bhikaji, Singh, and Khote provided no evidence about opium's prophylactic and febrifugal superiority for any disease or for people of a particular nationality. Socioeconomic status, not drug efficacy, determined to whom a physician dispensed the substance. Foreigners and wealthy Indians were better served by different resources and more effective therapies.

DID 'NATIVE' AS WELL AS ANGLO-EUROPEAN DOCTORS PRESCRIBE THE DRUG?

The Government of India's opium argument was strengthened if everyone involved in health maintenance recommended the drug for 'malarial fever.' Everyone included the "home *vaids*" mentioned by Anant Gangadhar Khote. Many of these people were undoubtedly trained in Unani (of Islamic origin; also called Tibb) or Ayurvedic medicine. Some were quacks. Nonetheless, Indians frequently consulted them. Evidence that these 'native' doctors *and* Anglo-European trained physicians dispensed the same thing for the same disease was proof that opium was indeed beneficial, and that people following different medical traditions in India knew it.

Mr. Sudan Chunder Naik, assistant superintendent of Tributary States in Orissa, claimed that European doctors never recommended opium for any case of elevated temperature. People living in 'malarial' and healthier locales in at least one part of Orissa, however, initiated opium ingestion themselves. Individuals whom Naik called "local, native doctors" in the region also prescribed the drug to prevent 'fever.' After prodding from Henry Wilson, Naik admitted being unsure if these local physicians administered it to a person already suffering from 'malarious fever' (GBOW [Naik, S. C.] 1894 II:111). Naik's comments suggest that in this part of East India, rural doctors untutored in Western allopathic medicine apparently accepted opium as a prophylactic but not as a febrifuge for 'malaria.'

Wilson obtained a similar response from Reverend Dinnonath Mazumdar, minister of Bankipur's Brahmo Samaj New Dispensation Church. Mazumdar believed local doctors did not need to prescribe opium because both consumers and abstainers had few paroxysm episodes. This equivalence prompted him to declare the drug did not protect a person from 'fever' (GBOW [Mazumdar, D.] 1894 III:33). No one questioned his logic.

Dr. Kailas Chunder Bose, the previously cited physician in private practice and president of the Calcutta Medical Society, told Roberts that opium eaters in North India were known for being healthy people. He specified the inhabitants of the "malarious" Terai region (Himalayan foothills) and Darjeeling (also in the highlands). Natives in the region who ignored opium eaters' advice to consume the drug succumbed to "malarious fever" and developed abnormal (enlarged) spleens. These tragedies convinced Bose that the drug "and its preparations are powerful antidotes against malarious fever" (GBOW [Bose, K. C.] 1894:II:87). Roberts continued to interrogate. He eventually elicited criticism from Bose about the "medical men" who did not prescribe the drug for "daily dietetic use" among Anglo-Europeans. Bose said they were mistaken. He would recommend to a foreigner who was living, or traveling, in a "marshy region" to eat a small, daily amount of the drug. This also was the advice he gave to Indian nonconsumers who inhabited "malarial regions" and were ignorant about the drug's value (GBOW [Bose, K. C.] 1894 II:88–9). Bose, however, never prescribed crude opium alone as a "malaria cure." He believed it prevented people from getting 'malaria' but could not cure them if they already had the 'disease.' The drug needed other substances to function as a febrifuge (GBOW [Bose, K. C.] 1894 II:89).

Bombay physician J. Gerson da Cunha told Roberts that he had no opinion about opium being able to do anything. He also had "no idea" if any of his patients used the drug "as a prophylactic [against 'fever']" (GBOW [da Cunha] 1894 IV:262). The witness changed his mind when responding to a question from Henry Wilson. He admitted to occasionally prescribing opium with quinine for "malarious fevers in order to prevent [native and foreign-born] patients from getting the fever as well as to prevent it from returning" (GBOW [da Cunha] 1894 IV:262).

Mr. Babu Madhav Chandra Bardalai, whom the Royal Commission described as an "extra-assistant commissioner at Barpeta" in Assam, had no doubts about opium (GBOW [Bardalai] 1894 II:302–03). On Friday, 29 December 1893, the thirty-fifth day of the hearings, Henry Wilson asked if he thought "that opium is one of the choicest gifts of God" (GBOW [Bardalai] 1894 II:303). Bardalai said yes albeit not for 'malarial fever.' Although not a physician, Bardalai would refrain from advising a young man going to "malarial country" to take opium on a regular basis. He doubted the drug prevented 'malaria' because no doctor ever recommended consuming the substance when he had been working in "fever" regions. Allopathic medical practitioners did not ingest opium themselves because they knew it was useless. This sentiment is shared, according to Bardalai, by Indians aware of "the advantages of medicine" (GBOW [Bardalai] 1894 II:304). This Government of India administrator, however, was sympathetic to his uninformed opium-consuming "countrymen because they do not care for any other medicine, and who regard other medicine, allopathic or homeopathic, as poison" (GBOW [Bardalai] 1894 II:304).

Mr. S. Peal, a planter from Assam, and Mr. Appaji Govindrao Kale, a "medical officer" in Palitana State (Western Coast) confirmed Bardalai's observations about allopathic medical practitioners. Peal, whose thirty-year working career in India included poppy cultivation, told Haridas Viharidas and Arthur Fanshawe that he knew of no European physician or Indian national practicing Western medicine ever recommending "habitual use of opium as a prophylactic against malaria." And if they did give this advice, according to Peal, the Assamese would refuse to follow instructions because they "will not take medicine from a practitioner as a rule" (GBOW [Peal] 1894 II:154). All Assamese natives,' however, really did believe *Papaver somniferum Linn* was a 'malaria' prophylactic and that it cured 'fever.' Peal admitted to never having seen boys consume opium for malaria or for anything else. Nevertheless, he accepted the natives' beliefs. For ten to twelve years, he had regularly distributed the drug to employees upon request (GBOW [Peal] 1894 II:153).

On 9 February 1894, Sir James Lyall asked Appaji Govindrao Kale if Indians ingested opium "as a prophylactic, or because of the pains which follow malarious fever." Kale replied yes to both queries because they believe it is "a prophylactic-preventive." He first observed the practice at the Chamadari dispensary in Kathiawar district. The area was "rather malarious, and most of the people take opium as a prophylactic . . . with good result." Kale himself, however, had never prescribed opium to prevent 'malarious fever' during his twenty-six year career in Kathiawar as director of dispensaries in 'malarious districts.' He said his behavior had not changed since arriving in Patilana State (GBOW [Kale, A. G.] 1894 IV:192–93).

In Lower Bengal and Orissa, the aforementioned Dr. Donald Morison insisted opium "was never prescribed by any European or native doctor to ward off or cure malaria" because they realized opium eaters suffered from the disease as often as abstainers (GBOW [Morison] 1894 II:100).[5] His associates also said malaria was not the reason that consumers in Orissa proffered for their habit. Natives of Lower Bengal, however, used the drug as a domestic remedy for rheumatism and syphilitic rheumatism, but not for fever or "withstanding chills" or to ameliorate the accompanying pain (GBOW [Morison] 1894 II:102, 105).

Surgeon-Lieutenant-Colonel A. Crombie was not one of Morison's opium-disdaining occidental physicians. He told Sir William Roberts about good results obtained during almost eighteen years in Dacca and Calcutta hospitals (GBOW [Crombie] 1894 II:77). Crombie did not tell the Commission how many of his patients were English, American, or European. Furthermore, his testimony indicates the 'malarial fevers' responding to opium were the etiologically-different maladies he recognized as causing diagnostic confusion. Crombie admitted never having prescribed opium as a prophylactic for one type of 'malarial fever.' His comments indicate it was caused by plasmodia. So for this witness, *Papaver somniferum Linn* was beneficial for the lumpers' 'malaria' but not for the splitters' version of the disease. Crombie also was cautious; he would ingest quinine and opium if required to travel in a 'malarial' region (GBOW [Crombie] 1894 II:80–1). He said nothing about prescribing the same regimen to fellow occidentals.

Brigade-Surgeon Lieutenant-Colonel James Arnot, a physician with the Bombay Medical Services and St. George's Hospital for a total of twenty-seven years, told Sir Roberts that excessive amounts of opium were indeed injurious to human beings. This *might not* be true if people (regardless of nationality) consumed moderate quantities. Arnot had been

> in the habit of prescribing it, variously combined, in fevers and inflammations, and with marked benefit. I am quite certain that it is a valuable remedy in malarial fevers, and though I have not used it as a prophylactic, preferring other remedies, I believe it would be a useful prophylactic. (GBOW [Arnot] 1894 IV:211)

SUMMARY STATEMENT: FOR WHOM IS OPIUM APPROPRIATE?

Witnesses evince no unanimity about 'local' doctors and allopathic-trained Indian or Anglo-European physicians recommending opium to indigenous people. They furnish meager evidence documenting physicians dispensing opium by itself to Anglo-Europeans in India who suffered from "fever" or to other foreign nationals wanting to avoid attacks. These individuals also reveal that allopathic-trained personnel, or people preferring this medical orientation, often prescribed opium combined with different medicines to English, Canadian,

American, and other non-Indians. For indigenous people, however, *Papaver somniferum Linn* mixed with something else was the best way to alleviate the episodes of elevated temperature that accompanied different maladies.

Several Anglo-European doctors and physicians trained in allopathic medicine had no hesitation in prescribing opium to natives. These witnesses did not believe opium was admirably suited to eliminate whatever was making the person sick. They also did not think the drug was uniquely appropriate for purported idiosyncratic physiological and psychological characteristics of patients. And they did not believe the biological endowment of Anglo-Europeans cautioned against dispensing opium to treat their ailments. These Western-trained physicians prescribed the drug for natives because there frequently was nothing else to give. More efficacious medicines such as quinine were frequently unavailable or too expensive. So, many natives ingested opium because they had no alternative. The drug also was usually available in the local market and it was cheap. These two factors enabled people to avoid patronizing nonnative doctors, thereby saving money and time in obtaining some relief from the symptoms of disease.

WAS OPIUM EATING AND THE PREVENTION AND CURE OF 'MALARIAL FEVER' A CONTRIVED THEORY?

Some witnesses admonished the Government of India for its recent advocacy of opium eating.[6] They claimed the argument was not prompted by a concern about the welfare of India's population but rather by political and economic expediency. British India's administrators were responding to the SSOT's attack upon all aspects of the opium trade. The drug and disease argument was merely a cynical tactic to continue a policy that made the drug available to the public.

Few witnesses were asked to comment at length about the allegation. Others volunteered an opinion. Only two people refused to condemn the British administration's initiative. The first was Mr. A. A. Wace, the previously mentioned commissioner of Patna. The second was Mr. Ram Moy Roy.

Wace's many years in Bengal and Assam made him very aware that natives consumed the drug for 'malarious fevers.' He had always dismissed the custom as worthless until people associated with the Royal Commission on Opium told him that moderate consumption of the drug was *indeed* a valuable prophylactic. This prompted Wace to chastise anti-opiumists such as Joseph Alexander for insisting upon regulating who can obtain the drug in India (GBOW [Wace] 1894 III:7).

Ram Moy Roy had no problem with the advocacy. It meant that an indigenous custom had scientific merit. As mentioned in the previous chapter, Roy believed the Royal Commission's real purpose was to validate Indians' contention about opium having nutritional value. According to this witness, continued production and distribution of the drug in the country guaranteed that people who lived in unhealthy conditions would have a food supplement. Its ingestion enabled them to avoid chill, the precursor to 'malarious fever,' and possible death. Opium's classification as a type of food qualified the substance as an indirect prophylactic "by giving greater power of endurance and a power to resist the effects of cold and dampness" (GBOW [Roy, R. M.] 1894 II:115).

The other witnesses rejected Roy's assessment. Reverend M. B. Kirkpatrick, the medical missionary from the Shan States of Burma, told the Royal Commission on Friday, 15 December 1893, that the drug was merely a pain reliever and its current acclaimed status as a prophylactic was surprising. "It is only within the last few months that I have heard of it. I never heard it advanced by a native" (GBOW [Kirkpatrick] 1894 II:219).

According to this witness, only several confirmed opium smokers he had treated in an urban hospital claimed the drug was a prophylactic. And he was unaware of any European physician stating the drug prevented and cured 'malarious fever' (GBOW [Kirkpatrick] 1894 II:219). Henry Wilson elicited a similar response from another missionary. Reverend T. J. Scott, principal of the Bareilly Theological Seminary of the American Methodist Episcopal Church, had lived in North India for the past thirty-one years. During this period, he had never heard of opium being given or taken in "malarious districts" for "fevers." The idea began circulating only several months before the Royal Commission's arrival in India (GBOW [Scott] 1894 III:107). For Reverends Scott and Kirkpatrick, the notion was an excuse presented as a medical fact to maintain the status quo. And Dr. Donald Morison, the contentious medical missionary from Bareilly, had no doubt about it; he told Lord Brassey and Brassey's associates that the opium and malaria "doctrine" was linked to the rise of anti-opium agitation (GBOW [Morison] 1894 II:104).

Members of the Royal Commission who were antagonistic to the SSOT could dismiss Scott's statements as an example of religious zeal replacing objectivity. Although this Christian missionary had more than a typical layperson's knowledge of medications, he still lacked formal education in an Anglo-European medical institution. His contention, therefore, was suspect. The criticism was less appropriate for Kirkpatrick and Morison. These medical missionaries were qualified medical doctors, although doubters claimed religious beliefs made them irrational in judging the therapeutic utility of opium.

Using religious ideology to denigrate witnesses' testimony was far less effective when evaluating the comments of medical practitioners who were not missionaries. These were the people employed by the Indian Medical Service or other departments within the Government of India, or by a native state. All of them were licensed physicians, all were trained in allopathic medical schools, and all had experience treating disease in India. Their reputations and careers were linked to officialdom. Only with justification would they give testimony detrimental to the interests of the Government of India. Some of these medical professionals did just that, or came close to it when asked about opium's prophylactic and febrifuge status.

On 15 January 1894 Surgeon Captain S. E. Jennings told the Royal Commission that nothing in his medical schooling warranted prescribing opium for the maladies mentioned during the hearings. Describing himself as the "medical charge of the 32nd Pioneers," Jennings in the past was either oblivious or gave no credence to native doctors and civilians in India who advocated using the drug for malaria and fevers. He told Sir William Roberts that only "since the Commission started" had he "tried opium medicinally for fevers with beneficial results, and if it is useful in fevers, it must be a prophylactic also" (GBOW [Jennings] 1894 III:159). Jennings said evidence for this was a significant reduction in the number of opium eaters from "damp" locales being admitted to hospitals for ague. The protection, however, was only temporary because he realized opium consumers constantly developed "malaria fever" (GBOW [Jennings] 1894 III:158–59).

Jennings remarkable reeducation about the drug also illuminated a paradox that Commission members ignored or did not comprehend; how could opium be a prophylactic if consumers were constantly suffering from the malady? And if the drug did help to prevent sickness, the transient relief it provided meant it was not a potent, long-lasting preventive.

On 13 February 1894, Surgeon-Major A. J. Sturmer, the district surgeon from South India, stated that people in the highlands of Jeypore in Madras consume great amounts of opium because

> it is a highly feverish district, but the inhabitants are a very healthy race, strong, and very keen sportsmen. They told me that they took opium as a preventative against fever, and the people who live at the foot of the ghats gave me the same reason. (GBOW [Sturmer] 1894 IV:243–44)

Sturmer had no problem with this folk practice and its consequences. He then told Sir William Roberts that he "always thought it was one of the peculiar ideas which natives get about various drugs; for instance, they say that buttermilk is very cooling but I do not know that there is any fact to prove it" (GBOW [Sturmer] 1894 IV:244). And Sturmer was unimpressed by the evidence presented to the Royal Commission thus far. No witness or official from any Government of India had proved opium was a prophylactic and febrifuge for 'malaria.' For this witness, the idea was based upon conjecture, not science, regardless of recent announcements from people closely affiliated with the Royal Commission on Opium. The native peoples' folk belief might be accurate but the Anglo-European evidence had not yet convinced the man.

Surgeon-Major T. R. Mulroney's dialogue with Arthur Upshawe Fanshawe revealed how the Government of India's endorsement of a folk belief could generate so much disagreement among educated people. Mulroney had been stationed in Punjab Province since 1880. But it had taken time for him to realize that all natives thought opium prevented 'fever' or 'malaria' (GBOW [Mulroney] 1894:III:163–64). Fanshawe then said "we have been told by some witnesses that the belief in opium as a prophylactic is a new doctrine, but you do not agree with that in 1887 and in subsequent years you found it a prevalent belief among the people themselves?" Mulroney said this was correct. He then told the Commission why people could reject the Government of India's position. Defenders of the custom were part of the problem. They had failed to inform skeptics to make a distinction between an "attack" and "a predisposition to an attack." For Mulroney, the difference was crucial. All apologists and consumers believed opium "does indirectly protect them inasmuch as it prevents a man running the risk, when going out on a cold night, of catching chill; chill is an exciting cause of fever; anything which lowers the system predisposes to an attack of malarial fever; that is how opium acts as a prophylactic" (GBO [Mulroney] 1894 III:164).

Mulroney was declaring that opium might ameliorate conditions necessary for a possible appearance of the affliction. The drug, however, did not end malaria once an attack began, and it did not guarantee prevention of an attack if predisposing factors were present (GBOW [Mulroney] 1894 III:164). The man also implied that the Government of India, or the Royal Commission on Opium, was condoning sloppy science if they decided that opium eating prevented and cured 'malaria,' 'fever,' and so forth. For this witness, *Papaver somniferum Linn* had limited therapeutic value for the affliction or afflictions classified as 'malaria.' Advocates for the notion also embraced an increasingly contested theory of disease causation.

Mulroney's testimony provided the SSOT with an argument negating reliance on opium. Anti-opiumists could construe his comments as suggesting that anything preventing a human being from developing "chill" was an "indirect prophylactic." Examples were a sweater to retain heat in the chest, shoes to protect feet from becoming cold, mittens to keep hands and fingers warm, a scarf and hat to prevent heat loss from the neck and head, and four walls and a roof to enhance the protective capability of each of these items. All the above qualified as malaria preventives, all prevented "chill" from disabling the body's extremities, and all enabled the heart and brain—two vital organs—to conserve energy and continue functioning. Arguing about a correlation between opium ingestion and malaria's prevention and cure now becomes far less important, perhaps irrelevant; people could avoid the disease using something other than a controversial drug. Anti-opiumists would welcome the Government of India providing citizens with warm clothing and adequate shelter to help end the problem of 'malaria' in India. This was unlikely to occur.

The SSOT still had reason for optimism if defenders of the status quo insisted upon classifying the drug as a direct or indirect prophylactic, and as the best solution to 'malaria.' Anti-opiumists then could argue that motives other than alleviating misery were the foundation of government policy regarding the Indian public's ability to obtain *Papaver somniferum Linn*.

Two Calcutta-based physicians in private practice also disagreed with the Government of India's agenda. Support for the "new doctrine" in local newspapers disturbed Mr. Atool K. Datta.

> I was astonished to find the Bangabasi, a largely circulated vernacular newspaper in Bengal, extolling its prophylactic powers, against fever, etc., and likewise its habitual use, because when all fever remedies in the case of one of the compositors of the Bangabasi staff failed, two grains doses of opium succeeded in speedily curing him. No argument can be more frivolous than this. (GBOW [Datta, A. K.] 1894 II:311)

He knew of no medical authority who encouraged habitual use, or who claimed that the drug protected "against malarious fever." Datta, an honorary member of the Homeopathic Medical Society in Philadelphia, Pennsylvania, did not dismiss the drug entirely because his colleagues "know that opium is of use in intermittent fevers where the paroxysms come every three days and manifest symptoms similar to those produced by opium eating in a normal state of health, but its action then is homeopathic" (GBOW [Datta, A. K.] 1894 II:311).[7] The second Calcutta physician identified the source of Datta's concerns.

Dr. James R. Wallace's testimony undermined the Government of India's argument. He agreed with Sir William Roberts' remark about eating a good breakfast being a better preventive than eating opium. Wallace told Lord Brassey that "orthodox" eminent physicians practicing in India never prescribed opium as a prophylactic "or as a remedy in malarial fever." He was referring to Drs. Norman Chevers and David B. Smith, Surgeon-Colonel R. Harvey, Surgeon-Lieutenant Colonels F. P. McConnell, Coates, McLeod, and Ray. They were all, Wallace said, "men whose lectures and practice I have attended and seen," but they had never uttered a "word of commendation" for the practice (GBOW [Wallace] 1894 II:117–18).[8] Lord Brassey asked if he had anything else to add about the views of allopathic doctors in India. Wallace mentioned the "frequent condemnations" and "recorded opinions against the use of opium" from Chevers, his former teacher and the author of *Medical Jurisprudence in India* and *Diseases of India*, two influential books published during the 1880s (GBOW [Wallace] 1894 II:118–19).

Henry Wilson then inquired if Wallace was acquainted with the report of a discussion that occurred about one and a half years ago during a meeting of Calcutta Medical Society. Wilson also asked if Wallace was a member of the organization.[9] The witness said yes to the first question and no to the second. Roberts asked why he did not belong. Wallace responded that he had been secretary of the Society "some years ago" but that "it came to be of a very official nature, and I resigned." Henry Wilson then inquired if he was correct in assuming that Wallace did "not agree with the majority of the gentlemen who spoke" during the Calcutta Medical Society discussion. Wallace replied that he disagreed with the speakers. The tone of his response suggests strong disagreement (GBOW [Wallace] 1894 II:119). The conversation continued with Wilson asking most of the questions.

(Wilson)   "Am I right in supposing that the gentlemen of that Society represent substantially the opinion of the orthodox medical practitioners in Calcutta?"

(Wallace)   "I believe they do not."

(Roberts)   "Can you quote any names in support of that?"

(Wallace)   "Very recently Dr. Lall Madhab Mukerjee, a past president of the Calcutta Medical School, called on me and gave me his deliberate opinion that he himself and the staff of the institution with which he is connected were wholly against the opinions that were being expressed before this Commission."

(Roberts)   "Are they orthodox practitioners according to the European method?"

(Wallace)	"Yes, they are graduates of the Calcutta University."
(Wilson)	"When you say that the Society partook of an official character, what do you mean by official?"
(Wallace)	"I do not like to go into details, but I may say that the Society practically expresses its views through the official medical journal, the *Indian Medical Gazette*, in which its reports appear. At the time in question it was very largely membered by officials, and less so by general practitioners. That is why in a limited sense I say that it has been largely an official society, the official element predominating."
(Wilson)	"Does it represent the profession in Calcutta necessarily?"
(Wallace)	"Not necessarily nor in fact."
(Wilson)	"Can you clear up that point as to the number of orthodox practitioners in Calcutta? Do you know anything about the numbers outside?"
(Wallace)	"Yes, I do."
(Wilson)	"Can you tell us how far the society represents medical opinion in Calcutta? I am sorry that the question was not asked of those who belong to this Society."
(Wallace)	"If I must mention it, I may say that the Society numbers according to its last report, December 1892, 117 members, twenty-five of whom did not reside at Calcutta, but in other parts of India. The Medical Register and Directory of the Indian Empire shows there are 780 or more medical practitioners in Calcutta."
(Roberts)	"Qualified?"
(Wallace)	"Qualified."
(Brassey)	"European?"
(Wallace)	"European and Native. This Society is supposed to represent the medical profession, whether European or Native."
(Wilson)	"You mean according to the European system?"
(Wallace)	"Yes; they are graduates of the Calcutta University."

(GBOW [Wallace] 1894 II:119–20)

The dialogue continued after William Roberts asked how much it cost to be a member of the Society.

(Wilson)	"Did I understand you to say that there are between 700 and 800 practitioners at Calcutta according to the European method?"
(Wallace)	"Yes"
(Wilson)	"The Society numbers about 117, of whom twenty-five are nonresident; so there are something less than 100 members in Calcutta?"
(Wallace)	"Yes."
(Brassey)	"Yes. Out of 780 in Calcutta how many have graduated in the United Kingdom?"
(Wallace)	"I could not tell, unless I went through the registered list of practitioners which is given in the *Indian Register and Directory* for 1892."
(Wilson)	"Do I rightly gather from this statement of yours that you think this doctrine about the use of opium in malaria is a comparatively modern doctrine?"
(Wallace)	"Yes, a comparatively modern doctrine."

(Wilson)	"May I ask you to define 'comparatively modern'?"
(Wallace)	"I first heard of it in connection with the discussion at the Calcutta Medical Society when I read the report; since then I gave the theory a trial."
(Mowbray)	"With regard to the *Indian Medical Gazette*, do I understand that it is an official publication?"
(Wallace)	"Official in this sense, that it is supported by Government."

(GBOW [Wallace] 1894 II:119–20)

Wilson's questions and Wallace's insinuations intrigued Robert Mowbray, the other Parliamentarian appointed to the Royal Commission. He inquired about the status of another periodical, the *Indian Medical Record*. Wallace said that he started it five years ago, and that it was "supported entirely by the medical profession in India." The periodical, therefore, did not depend for survival upon funding from either the Government of India or administrators in the Bengal Presidency (GBOW [Wallace] 1894:120). It was not a vehicle for advancing official opium policy in the guise of allopathic medicine as was the *Indian Medical Gazette*, a function that Wallace said now characterized the Calcutta Medical Society and the report about which Wilson inquired. The aforementioned Sir William Moore had published many articles about 'fever,' 'malaria,' and the nutritional value of opium in the *Indian Medical Gazette*. Mayne had done the same for opium smoking. Wallace was, in effect, labeling their views about *Papaver somniferum Linn* and disease as Government of India propaganda.

Wallace told Lord Brassey earlier in the session that he had given "the [opium and malaria] theory a fair and honest trial during the past ten or twelve months" after reading the Society's report. Other than relief of some pain from "malarial fever," Wallace found that opium "in no way prevents or shortens its paroxysms," and "its administration in many . . . cases would be undoubtedly harmful" (GBOW [Wallace] 1894 II:117). He assumed that Indians felt the same way about using the drug. It was to be expected, therefore, that he had never heard of even uneducated urban dwellers, or natives living in remote rural areas, taking "opium to protect themselves against malaria" (GBOW [Wallace] 1894 II:120). The "new doctrine" being discussed "among men practicing on the European system" and hailed in some literature was, for Wallace, bad medical science and clever politics (GBOW [Wallace] 1894 II:120). He wanted no part of it.

Wallace testified during the sixteenth day of the hearings. Five sessions earlier, on Monday, 23 November 1893, Lord Brassey had asked Reverend T. Evans what he thought about opium preventing 'malaria.' The man's response was as damaging to the Government of India as Wallace's rejection of its "new doctrine." Evans, a missionary for thirty-eight years who remained in India after retirement to "do temperance work," admitted he did not have the qualifications "to give a reliable opinion." Nevertheless, if opium was indeed a prophylactic, he continued, then

> it seems strange our benevolent government, which supplies cholera pills free of charge to people living in places where that sickness prevails, should not be

equally liberal in supplying opium pills to its poor subjects residing in malarious districts. And further, if opium is such a powerful prophylactic, how is it that, while the Chinese in Burma may enjoy the boon, it is strictly forbidden by law to allow the Burmans either to sell or to purchase it?

Another strange mystery about this question is this, that, while it is supposed that opium is good to those who live in British territory, strange to say, the subjects of native states are forbidden to enjoy this boon by the cultivation of it in their own native country. The Government of India has made a treaty with the State of Mysore in Southern India by which the cultivation of opium in that country is strictly prohibited, and if I am not misinformed, the same restriction is enforced upon other native princes in India. (GBOW [Evans] II:47)

Evans' tactful allegation that the British India administration was illogical and hypocritical has merit. There is a discrepancy between official policy in the past and what pro-trade supporters proclaimed during the hearings. Assume that Dr. William Huntly had grossly underestimated the drug's capability. This occurred when he had told Lord Brassey that "the grain of truth underlying all this talk of the beneficial use of opium in malaria is its power of lessening the discomfort felt in the cold stage of the attack" (GBOW [Huntly] 1894 IV:60). Further assume that everything the SSOT's opponents said about the drug was accurate. This includes arguments uttered *before* the Commission's first hearing on 2 February 1894. It also includes declarations from all witnesses in London and India who endorsed the opium and 'malaria' correlation.

The following assertions then comprise the pro-trade position. The first is that eating opium really did prevent and cure 'malaria,' and that the nosological confusion some witnesses identified was irrelevant to the discussion. Thus, the drug was both a prophylactic and febrifuge for etiologically distinct maladies that shared a common symptom. Opium also was a type of food, a nutritional supplement that precluded the development of 'chill,' and 'chill' was the precursor to 'malaria.'

Other proclamations uttered during the decades-old controversy were also correct. The poppy cultivated in India yielded opium that was indeed more effective for 'fever' disease than quinine. This cinchona alkaloid might be useful for one manifestation of 'malaria.' At best, quinine was a 'specific' only for a type of 'fever' that misinformed anti-opiumists and some witnesses nominated by the Government of India were blaming on miniscule bugs. Data from South Asia did not confirm the existence of microbes or plasmodia. The proclamation, therefore, was incautious speculation or simply ridiculous.

Another 'fact' in the pro-trade stance is that narcotine was the substance responsible for opium's therapeutic power in 'malaria.' The correlation between high per capita consumption and 'malarious' environments also is valid. Inhabitants of such places ingested nonaddictive opium only for legitimate medicinal reasons. The 'opium habit' enabled them to avoid misery and probable death. Furthermore, a modest rate of consumption was the norm for all other regions of British India and the native states.

Still another fact in this scenario is that people throughout the country ate opium, drank pieces of it dissolved in liquid, or absorbed the drug through anal insertion. And people consumed the substance regardless of sexual identity, age, religion, economic status, ethnic identity, caste affiliation, or nationality. In other words, opium was good for everybody, in all places, and for lots of things. The drug was not a panacea but it came close to being one.

Now, if opium was all these "things," and if it performed all these functions, then how did the Government of India answer Reverend Evan's question? Its administrators had controlled poppy cultivation and opium processing for decades in territories under their direct control. Furthermore, British regulation of commerce in many native states commenced in the early 1800s. Treaties had prevented these entities from cultivating poppy and manufacturing opium for sale within British India and within their own territories. Reverend Evans wanted to know why there was a contradiction between past and present official policy if opium *really* was a cure-all? What explains this administrative inconsistency when 'malaria,' 'malarious environments,' 'miasmatic conditions' and 'rotting vegetation' are responsible for so much misery in India? And why had the Government of India not used *all* these facts to eliminate restraints on production and intra-India distribution that were already in place during the years prior to the Royal Commission's creation in 1893? In brief, why was the 'medical' argument *not* a centerpiece in the pro-trade offensive against the misinformed moralists from the earliest days of opposition?

Reverend Evans testified early in the Royal Commission hearings. No other witness in the ensuing months stated the paradox so succinctly. With the possible exception of Henry Wilson, no Commission member in attendance that day, or at any other session, addressed Evan's critique. That would be the responsibility of Sir William Roberts after conclusion of the hearings. The task involved evaluating oral evidence and documents submitted by the antagonists, reviewing statistics, and examining the scant experimental data provided by the Government of India. The guideline Roberts followed to accomplish this task was "knowledge" accumulated during his long, eminent career in aspects of Anglo-European research and practice.

NOTES

1. These are the districts of Dinajpur and Rangpur in Wace's testimony. There are numerous instances of location names ending in "pur" also spelled as "pore" elsewhere in the volumes. The author adopts the spelling used in each Royal Commission on Opium testimony.

2. Prautch also accused Mr. Rustomji Pestonji Jehangir, the "chief opium inspector of Bombay," with at least four instances of sending his own police staff to protect "illegal smoking shops" from interference by Bombay city authorities. Prautch wanted the Royal Commission to disregard Pestonji Jehangir's publications about opium smoking in Bombay, and to investigate the man's recent efforts in London to discredit SSOT activities.

Prautch was not through complaining. Pestonji Jehangir's intimidating visits to the Bombay "medical men" who had signed an anti-opium memorial presented to Parliament especially upset him. The Royal Commission on Opium later refused to consider this document as evidence because "the visits were followed by the alleged repudiation of a number of the signatures" (GBOW [Prautch] 1894 IV:295). The signatories claimed they did not know what they were endorsing.

3. An early investigation of the topic was conducted less than a decade after conclusion of the Royal Commission hearings. F. H. Edmonds studied the effects of "simple intermittent," "bilious remittent," and "cachexia malaria fever" (i.e., "complications") on Indian females during pregnancy. He concluded "malaria fever" was the cause of many stillbirths, and that a "high fever" led to "aborted fetuses and miscarriages" (1900:259–60).

See A. Baer for malaria's effect upon female fertility (A. Baer 1988:909–15), and Nina L. Etkin and associates for the relationship between indigenous "native" diets and male-female susceptibility to malarial infection (N. Etkin 1979:401–29; N. L. Etkin & Paul J. Ross 1983:231–59).

4. How does a person explain Surgeon-Lieutenant Colonel R. Caldecott's statement of 6 February 1894 when he said malaria and dysentery caused men in western Malwa to consume opium for protection and relief? All natives, he declared, "have a very firm belief in [its] efficacy" but in the same conversation he admitted it was "comparatively rare for young men to consume it" (GBOW [Caldecott] 1894 IV:94). An impartial observer would conclude that youthful males in this part of India had an enhanced, inherent genetic immunity to malaria plasmodia, to 'miamastic influences,' 'fevers,' and to any of the terms identifying the etiologically distinct afflictions called 'malaria.' Caldecott furnished no evidence for this genetic immunity, and neither did anyone else. This leads one to speculate that perhaps young males in western Malwa were either stupid, careless, or that they knew this "very firm belief" had dubious credibility.

5. Three other East India witnesses said the same thing. See Satyanath Borah for comments about a village in Assam (GBOW [Borah] 1894 II:286). Lalit Mohun Lahiri claimed that doctors in Bengal never prescribed the drug as a preventive or remedy despite malaria having "carried off millions of people" in the province (GBOW [Lahiri] 1894 II:289). Kali Sankur Sukul told the Royal Commission that he had never heard of medical professionals of any kind ever dispensing or recommending the drug during the three years of residency in Jessore. He described Jessore as "one of the most malarious tracts" in Bengal (GBOW [Sukul] 1894 (II:269).

6. Kali Sankur Sukul was more surprised than dubious. He did not think opium prevented 'fever.' He also said that not even the Government of India recommended it for such a purpose (GBOW [Sukul] 1894 II:269).

7. See Volume II, page 311, for Atool K. Datta's homeopathic description of opium's effect upon human organs, tissues, and 'fever.'

8. See the previous chapter for Wallace's comments about medical colleagues in India. The commentary is found in his discussion of opium's status as an anodyne. Miss Carleton, the American medical missionary, mentions the absence of the opium and malaria "doctrine" from her medical school training in the United States (GBOW [Carleton] 1894 III:169).

9. Wilson was referring to the 11 May 1892 event chaired by Dr. Kailas Chunder Bose, another witness. The report is entitled "Discussion on the Effects of the Habitual Use of

Opium on the Human Constitution." It was published as a supplement to the August 1892 issue of *The Indian Medical Gazette*. As mentioned in the chapter entitled "The Gathering Storm," the opinions of Surgeon-Lieutenant Colonel A. Crombie comprise almost 50 percent of the document. The rest of the report contains Indian physicians' comments about the body's reactions to the drug. See GBO [Calcutta Medical Society] 1894:II:407–25. Crombie's testimony at the Royal Commission also indicates he believed opium had value for the lumpers' view of 'malaria.'

7

Sir William Roberts' Evaluation of the Opium and 'Malaria' Evidence

THE REAFFIRMED PREMISE

William Roberts' review of witness testimony and additional documents submitted by the Government of India delighted supporters of the status quo. He concluded eating opium was beneficial in general, that the habit was widespread, and that one ingredient in the mother drug was able to cure 'malaria.' The man's brief experience in India had reinforced a belief that "consumption of articles of a stimulating and restorative character" was almost ubiquitous in human societies because they satisfied some "profound instinct of human nature." What was ingested to experience the sensation varied from place to place. Inhabitants of South Asia used some items. Natives elsewhere resorted to different substances. The oral ingestion of opium, therefore, was no different from consuming Indian betel nut and hemp, or cocoa, alcohol, tobacco, tea, and coffee. Roberts also recognized that these items were useful, albeit not indispensable, to "man's animal life" because people in still other parts of the world might abstain from all of them. And within a particular society "individuals, even whole classes of people," were able to "forgo their use, either wholly or in part" (GBO [Roberts] 1895:VI:99).

Being able to choose to indulge or to abstain at any time meant these substances were nonaddictive "when legitimately used" (GBO [Roberts] 1895:VI:99). Roberts did not clarify what he meant by "legitimate use," but the implications were obvious. Which article was selected and how much of it was ingested to feel good or rejuvenated varied according to societal customs, to availability of the item, and to idiosyncrasies of the person. Overindulgence was a voluntary act, a consequence of personal choice, a matter of moral character.

Roberts was predisposed not to ignore the few Moore and Birdwood-inspired witnesses who claimed opium was a type of food. Before the South Asia trip he had stated that tobacco, alcohol, tea, and coffee were not "true articles of food" because they did not "possess, in their essence, nutritive properties" (GBO [Roberts] 1895:VI:99). These witnesses' comments about Indian opium modified his position. Roberts now claimed such substances might have a "collateral use," one being "dietetic." Implicit in this acknowledgment was an acceptance of a very loose definition of food and nutrition, a view that critics testifying before the Royal Commission had condemned as meaningless, if not ridiculous. Roberts did not think so and cited two witnesses' brief comments as proof. The first, not mentioned in previous chapters because he said nothing specific about the relationship between opium and malaria, was a Dr. Cobb.[1] According to Roberts, Cobb observed that natives in the "damp climates" of Eastern Bengal, whose diet was primarily rice, suffered from loose bowels. The condition was especially prevalent as they grew old. Cobb had told Roberts that opium prevented "diarrhoea, dysentery, and other allied affections." The drug, therefore, maintained health and prolonged life. The benefits of oral consumption were found elsewhere in the country. The only example Roberts' cited was Dr. Elizabeth Bielby's statement about women in Lahore eating a little opium before meals because it functioned as a "digestive" (GBO [Roberts] 1895:VI:105).

The written evidence was little help to Roberts. Only one Government of India document sent to the Royal Commission provided scant support for the "opium as food" scenario. One hundred and thirty-six occidental people living in China were asked what made "Asiatics more liable to contract the [opium] habit?" A mere seven respondents from different parts of country perceived a correlation between drug intake, nutrition, and food (GBO [Her Majesty's Minister in China] 1894:V:212–343).[2]

Roberts also had no doubt about the "essential purpose" of opium consumption; these substances were taken to "modify, in a favourable sense, the action of the nervous system." Roberts meant "'favourable' as judged by the sensations of the user." This "natural group of (nonnutrient) physiological substances" generated "an enhanced sense of well-being" although the actual effect of each "euphoric agent" differed in degree and kind (GBO [Roberts] 1895:VI:99). For Roberts, opium apparently made Indians feel good because it actually was doing something positive. It slowed passage of food through the body, thereby enabling more thorough digestion, and it was a form of nourishment needed to maintain nervous system equilibrium. Disequilibrium rendered some inhabitants of this predominantly vegetarian society susceptible to 'chill,' the precursor to 'malaria.' He said nothing more about the dietary status of opium.

SIR WILLIAM ROBERTS' DISMISSAL OF ANTI-OPIUMISTS' ACCUSATIONS

Roberts then rejected SSOT accusations about the Government of India encouraging addiction to a substance responsible for various social ills. The India natives' "higher tolerance for opium than Europeans," he concluded, was "congenital" (GBO [Roberts] 1895:VI:101). The statement implies that a high consumption rate is benign. Opium eating also was primarily a male habit in South Asia, and "commonly begun between thirty-five and forty-five" when men realize they are getting old (GBO [Roberts] 1895:VI:102–03). Roberts, however, acknowledged a "tendency to a progressive increase of the dose" among people starting the habit. This also was no cause for alarm. The amount remained stable once an individual's tolerance level had been reached. Meager doses (two to eight grains daily) then became the norm. Ending the habit most often had only modest, temporary consequences because after a "few days, or a week or two, [negative physiological and psychological] symptoms subside and health is restored" (GBO [Roberts] 1895:VI:104). And moderate consumption most certainly did not shorten the life span of South Asian natives.

The testimony of witnesses also enabled Roberts to declare that opium saved many more people then it killed. Giving small amounts of the drug to children, an "ancient" custom prevalent in some castes, also was harmless. The practice usually started when a child reached the ages of three to five, and cases of accidental poisoning were rare. He concluded there was no justification for discouraging the habit. The reasons cited were Indian mothers' "vigilant maternal instinct" not to harm their infants, the adverse conditions under which all natives live, and their "unquestioning faith in the wholesomeness" of the custom (GBO [Roberts] 1895:VI:112–15).

The drug also was not "responsible for any disease peculiar to itself," it damaged no tissues or organs, and opium eaters recovered from surgery as well as nonconsumers (GBO [Roberts] 1895:VI:105). And under no circumstances did opium cause insanity. Roberts cited testimony suggesting that consumption was even beneficial for precluding development of this mental condition (GBO [Roberts] 1895:VI:105). Furthermore, "official statistics" from different provinces in India indicated no correlation between the habit and suicide (GBO [Roberts] 1895:VI:106–07). Moralists' condemnation about opium indulgence leading to increased lewd and immoral sexual behavior also had no credibility. Testimony and numerical data indicated that the Indian product possessed no "special power" as an aphrodisiac. Just the opposite prevailed; the sexual drive decreased (GBO [Roberts] 1895:VI:107–08).

Roberts admitted that opium, like any other substance, could be misused. However, the problem was so minimal in the subcontinent that official drug policy was blameless. Defective human beings, not irresponsible leadership or inherent detrimental qualities of chemicals, were responsible for the alleged social problems. So Roberts concluded that opium consumption was an innocuous habit for most Indians.

Declaring a behavior or a drug harmless, however, was not synonymous with proving it did anything sufficiently beneficial to warrant continued Government of India support and encouragement. And saying a substance was innocuous was a weak defense for drug policy when confronted with a decades-old vigorous opposition armed with medical data. Roberts, in response, "proved" the value of opium by revealing its central and unappreciated role in combating 'malaria.' He first argued for continued consumption of the mother drug itself, and then the production of one of its components.

CONFRONTATIONS WITH A HORRIBLE DISEASE: THE PURPORTED UBIQUITY AND CONTESTED BENEFITS OF EATING OPIUM IN SOUTH ASIA

Roberts declared that the usefulness of opium "in the complaints of damp and malarious regions is very widespread." He mentioned the immense popularity of laudanum in the Fens region of rural England as one example. Two other examples were along the "swampy shores of the Caspian Sea" where inhabitants consumed the drug as a "protective against malaria," and in ancient Persia among people "exposed to the miasmata of marshy regions." Members of the Royal Commission, Roberts claimed, had been exposed to evidence proving the same was true for India. Local consumption of the drug "bore a close relation to the greater or less prevalence of malaria" in some districts in South Asia. Roberts cited Mr. Wace's testimony regarding vastly different rates of consumption in the dry and "damp" parts of Bhagalpur district of British India's Patna district. For Roberts, the man's comments were "a striking illustration" of the correlation between 'malarious' locales and opium consumption (GBO [Roberts] 1895:VI:109).[3]

Roberts mentioned no witnesses discussing other parts of British India or the native states. Immediately after publication of the Royal Commission volumes, he was chastised for the omission and condemned as biased. An 1895 commentary in the *Indian Medical Record* declared Wace's argument was erroneous and Roberts erred in relying upon it. People in the southern subdivision of Bhagalpur use of lot of opium but they have cultivated it themselves for the past twenty years. So, the reason for few opium shops is that people produce their own drug. These establishments simply are unnecessary. The crucial factor responsible for the opium habit was availability of the drug, not the locale's healthiness or lack thereof. Roberts' assertion about a "close relationship" between opium consumption and the "greater or less prevalence of malaria" had no credibility (*IMR* 1895:18).

Roberts also was accused of ignoring the significance of contradictory oral as well as written evidence concerning the correlation between opium use and "malarial" environments. The previous chapter clearly demonstrates there was no consensus about the issue. And the 1895 *Indian Medical Record* editorial board is incredulous that Roberts had "allowed himself to be so completely under the influence of Government officials." There was no "definite relation" between consumption and distribution, and the existence, "far less the intensity, of malarial fevers in different parts of India" (*IMR* 1895:18). Some healthy locales had high consumption rates and several unhealthy regions indicated the opposite. The inhabitants of almost malaria-free Darjeeling, for example, consumed "15.7 grains per head per annum" while "Jalpairuri, including the deadly feverish Dooars, [used] only 6 grains" (*IMR* 1895:18). And Balasore, "considered one of the healthiest districts in Bengal, shews [sic] a consumption of 86 grains per head" whereas statistics from Dacca and Mymensingh, those "terrible swamps of Eastern Bengal" described by Dr. Crombie, indicated only 5.4 grains per individual. The natives of Simla were another example. One would expect inhabitants of this hill station in the western Himalayas to consume little opium because they lived "far above the malarious zone" and cultivated only a little poppy. This was not the case; the natives of Simla ingested a formidable "136 grains per head" but in "Rajshahi and Jessore, the two most malarious districts in Bengal," the average consumption per head per annum was only 10.3 grains (*IMR* 1895:18–9). The periodical's editors were adamant; "[t]hese figures shew[sic] clearly that malaria has absolutely nothing to do with the prevalence and distribution of the opium habit" (*IMR* 1895:19).

The *Indian Medical Record* was actually attacking Roberts' extensive citation of Dr. Vincent Edward's 1877 study of 613 opium eaters (414 males and 169 females) in Balasore, Orissa (East India). The journal's argument is caustic and credible because Edwards was not a neutral investigator. He had conducted the study to expose the "absurd extravagance" of anti-opiumists and to discredit their "fiery declamation" about opium eating. Edwards also wanted to "test the accuracy of Dr. William James Moore's conclusions" about "no appreciable ill effect" caused by moderate consumption of the drug. He also wanted to verify Moore's contention that, in some instances, the habit had beneficial consequences (GBO [Edwards] 1894:II:436).

The *Indian Medical Record* critics also identified 'fever' as only one of many reasons that Edward's informants gave for beginning the habit. Other rationales of equal importance were "elephantiasis, dysentery, colic, rheumatism," and enabling a person to "undergo fatigue, and to make long journeys" (GBO [Edwards] 1894:II:437). Daily consumption ranged from two to forty-five grains, the average being seven grains for men and five grains for women. The average age at which a man first consumed the drug was thirty-five years or older. Many women did not begin eating opium until they were over fifty "and not a few sixty" (GBO [Edwards] 1894:II:436). Males before the age of thirty-five, and women before their early fifties in Balasore, were no more immune to 'malaria' and 'fever' than anywhere else in the country. The *Indian Medical Record* contended that if Edwards' subjects typified the wider population, avoiding 'malaria' and 'fever' were not salient reasons for drug use in this part of East India. Roberts, however, had concluded otherwise (GBO [Roberts] 1895:VI:100).

Other documents from India submitted to the Royal Commission also provided minimal support for Roberts' drug use and 'malaria' correlation. He ignored their contents. Surgeon Lieutenant-Colonel Hendley's two investigations of opium consumption in Jeypore State of Rajputana are illustrative (GBO [Hendley–Appendix I] 1894:IV:376–81). The first study involved fifty-five Indian and European medical and nonmedical respondents (twenty-eight medical and twenty-six "nonprofessional" people). Some respondents were splitters and others were lumpers. In either case, informants furnished meager evidence for natives ingesting opium to prevent or cure 'malaria.'

Two questions elicited the pertinent information. The first (question #12) was "[w]hat induces a person to begin the habit?" The second (question #17) asked if the reader thought that use of the drug "protects against any disease" or "the effects of cold and "[i]f so, what diseases?" No respondent said 'fever' prevention was a reason for beginning the habit. The second question elicited the following responses from these fifty-five individuals. Only two English ministers believed the drug prevented 'fever.' One of them declared it also was a cholera prophylactic. Forty-nine people thought the substance "offers protection from cold" but they did not elaborate. Only five Indian nationals were slightly more informative; they said opium was useful for warding off the effects of "cold" but several of them acknowledged that very large doses were needed to accomplish the task. Hendley also mentioned the "Vaids [native doctors who] say it protects against . . . disease of the phlegmonous humour," which were the "cold diseases, and against corpulency." Another question addressed the practice of giving opium to children. Some "nonprofessional" respondents defended the custom. They claimed it helped to prevent diseases. One was 'fever' (GBO [Hendley–Appendix I] 1894:IV:380–81).

Hendley's second document is an 1894 investigation of why 4,409 opium eaters in Jeypore began the habit. The Government of India considered Jeypore and Rajputana to be a 'malarious region.' Nonetheless, Hendley found that only 480 individuals, or 9.18 percent, cited 'malarial fevers' as the reason for beginning the habit (GBO [Hendley–Appendix II] 1894:IV:381–82).

Discussions with indigenous opium smokers also indicated no correlation between 'malaria' and drug use. Mr. Rustomji Jehangir's inquiry about the health of sixty-six madak smokers and 162 chandu smokers in Bombay found only two people associating the habit with avoidance or cure of 'fever' (GBO [Jehangir] 1894:IV:485–95). One informant was a beggar by the name of Ebrahim Balaram. He admitted having smoked an anna's worth of madak for 'fever' during the past two years (GBO [Jehangir] 1894:IV:487). The other respondent was Kisimgu Barogir, whom Rustomji Jehangir described as "strong, bright, and healthy." Barogir admitted that

> [t]wenty years ago I suffered from enlargement of the spleen and piles and was advised by a friend to take opium. I took it and have been much better ever since, but [if] I leave off taking it my old complaint returns. I smoke two or three pice worth [of] madak every day. (GBO [Jehangir] 1894:IV:487)

Data from the middle part of the country also cast doubt upon Roberts' contention, and a document from South India is only slightly more supportive. Lieutenant-Colonel D. Robertson solicited replies to sixty-two questions from thirty-two "native" leaders, military men, cultivators, medical practitioners, and other people. They all lived in the native states of the Central India Agency (GBO [Robertson–Appendix X] 1894:IV:405–06). Only two respondents cited opium being useful in preventing 'malarial fever.' Four other witnesses merely implied the substance was useful for unspecified illnesses (GBO [Robertson–Appendix XIII] 1894:IV:417–24). No informant indicated awareness of any difference between kinds of fevers, 'malaria,' and 'malarious diseases.'

Representatives of the Government of Madras [South India] interviewed twelve people. The respondents were two police inspectors, two people with unspecified occupations, one British collector (district commissioner), three surgeons, one superintendent of a "lunatic asylum," one chemical examiner, one professor of pathology, one hospital assistant, and one tahsildar (a native who collected land revenue.) Few people in this region of South India associated consumption with 'malaria.' One police inspector said the drug "helps to check the effects of malarious climate," that it was "a safeguard against the evil effects of malaria . . . [and was] used . . . by all classes of people" (GBO [Government of Madras] 1894:IV:448, 450). The second inspector said the drug was consumed in solid form as a prophylactic but did not indicate what it prevented (GBO [Government of Madras] 1894:IV:450). The English surgeon declared opium was used "very largely in native medicines; it is the sheet anchor of the native practitioner in all diseases of the bowels . . . and malarious fevers which are only too common" (GBO [Government of Madras] 1894:IV:451). The Indian hospital assistant, a veteran of twenty years of experience in Madras, believed opium was "extremely useful for medical purposes . . . [i]t has a beneficial effect . . . in malarious fevers" (GBO [Government of Madras] 1894:IV:451). He said nothing more about the disease or the drug, and neither did anyone else questioned by the Madras authorities. For one of the remaining witnesses, any association between opium consumption and 'malaria' prevention was unheard of. This chemical examiner declared that his district (Ganjam) was

> notably a feverish district, and some of the worst forms of malarial fever are to be met with there, but I have never heard that, or came across any instance in which opium was taken as a prophylactic or cure for malaria. Either its reputed action against malaria is unknown here, or I am badly informed. (GBO [Government of Madras] 1894:IV:452)

The Royal Commission did not consider Robertson's studies and the Madras Government document when formulating its recommendations for the final report to Parliament. No reason was offered for the omission. It is unknown if Roberts examined the two documents.

Thus far, a more accurate evaluation of witness testimony and documents indicates there was minimal support for Roberts' contention about opium's status as a prophylactic and febrifuge. Data from other Asian locations provides additional confirmation that the man's argument was tenuous.

Two documents concerning drug consumption in Southeast and East Asia were available to Roberts. Each one contains data germane to opium and malaria (GBO [Singapore, Penang, and Hong Kong] 1894:V:145–212; GBO [Her Majesty's Minister in China] 1894:V:212–343). Roberts mentions neither source in the 1895 report.

Early in the hearings (and previously mentioned), Lord Brassey ordered a questionnaire be sent to British officials in the colonies and dependencies of Singapore, Penang, and Hong Kong. Singapore, Penang, and the "native states of the Malay Peninsula" comprised the "Straits Settlements" (GBO [Singapore,

Penang, and Hong Kong] 1894:V:145). He had the same questionnaire sent to Her Majesty's Minister in China. Copies were then forwarded to each of the twenty-one British Consulates in the country. Each consulate sent the document to individuals deemed qualified to respond.

Several questions in both documents elicited natives' and European residents' opinions about opium, and the prevention and cure of 'malaria.' People in China, Hong Kong, Singapore, Penang, and the native states of the Malay Peninsula were asked if

> opium, within your knowledge, [is] a prophylactic against fever, or rheumatism, or malaria? Or is it so regarded by any Asiatic race with whom you are conversant? (GBO [Singapore, Penang, and Hong Kong] 1894:V:145; GBO [Her Majesty's Minister in China] 1894:V:212).

The questionnaire was sent to forty-three individuals living in Singapore, Penang, and the native states. Thirty-five people returned a completed, or partially completed, form. Twenty-nine respondents were British or European. The remaining eight were Chinese or Malay (GBO [Singapore, Penang, and Hong Kong] 1894:V:145–84).

Examination of the responses reveals weak support for opium's alleged therapeutic status in this part of Asia. Eighteen people answered the questions. Sixteen (thirteen British and European, three Malays, and Chinese) said that only Chinese inhabitants of the "Straits Settlements," Singapore, and Penang believed opium was a prophylactic against 'fever' or 'malaria.' Two other Chinese respondents disagreed. One said his countrymen did not take opium to protect or relieve the misery of 'fever' or 'malaria,' and neither did anyone else. The second informant thought the idea was fallacious.

Only one of the British or European "medical" (i.e., physician) respondents believed the drug provided protection from 'malaria.' Five other Western physicians were among the twenty-nine respondents. One doctor said the idea was unfounded. The other four were reluctant to confirm it. No respondent answering the questions claimed that *Papaver somniferum Linn* 'cured' people who were already suffering from 'fever' or 'malaria' (GBO [Singapore, Penang, and Hong Kong] 1894:V:153).

Sixty-one residents of Hong Kong received the questionnaire.[4] Thirty-six people returned completed forms. Twenty-three respondents answered the question concerning how "Asiatics" in the colony viewed opium and 'malaria.' Twelve people said yes; Asian people (meaning Chinese) believed the drug prevented 'malaria' or 'fever.' Eight individuals said natives did not ingest the drug to prevent either malady. Two other witnesses said they were ignorant about what "Asiatics" thought. Another person said that natives in India consumed the drug for these afflictions, but he did not know about Hong Kong. An affirmative answer from only twelve people out of a total of thirty-six respondents is not overwhelming support for the validity of Roberts' contention in Asian locations beyond India's border.

The respondents willing to reveal their personal beliefs about the ability of opium to prevent 'malaria' and 'fever' were even less supportive. Seven people said opium eating or smoking had a prophylactic function (GBO [Singapore, Penang, and Hong Kong] 1894:V:145–209). Only one of these respondents had medical training. The person had earned a diploma in public health from an unidentified institution in London (GBO [Singapore, Penang, and Hong Kong] 1894:V:198, 205). Eleven respondents rejected opium's alleged prophylactic status (GBO [Singapore, Penang, and Hong Kong] 1894:V:145–209). One person in this group of unbelievers also had medical training. He was a physician and a member of Hong Kong's legislative council (GBO [Singapore, Penang, and Hong Kong] 1894:V:199–200, 205).

In China, British officials, and bureaucrats in Imperial Government service, were asked to respond. The invitation was also extended to "[m]edical men, merchants, and other residents in [the country] or natives . . . who are especially conversant with any part of China in which opium is grown or consumed" (GBO [Her Majesty's Minister in China] 1894:V:212). One hundred and thirty-six people did so. There was even less support for the opium as a prophylactic and febrifuge for 'fever' and 'malaria' notion than among the Straits Settlements respondents. Twelve people had no doubt that opium ingestion prevented both maladies, although the endorsement of one individual from Ningpo was highly qualified. Six respondents, all from Formosa (Taiwan), said natives believed the idea. However, with the exception of one European, these respondents thought that the natives were mistaken. Most respondents from mainland China shared the skepticism. Only twenty-two out of 136 other respondents said that Chinese natives accepted the idea. And one of these people acknowledged indigenous folk believing the drug was useful for only some kinds of 'fever.' Not other details were provided.

Lord Brassey must have been disappointed if he thought these responses were going to lend support to the alleged link between consumption and disease prevention and cure in India. The data simply were not there. Sir William Roberts would have to find confirmation some other way. He did, and the argument was based upon a selective use of evidence.

Sir William Roberts' Conceptualization of 'Malaria'

Sir William Roberts concluded that India was "more or less malarious from end to end, and suffers severely from the disease incidental to such climates" (GBO [Roberts] 1895:VI:109). The man construed 'malarious' as a synonym for a locale detrimental to human health. It was a vague, ambiguous category of environmental components that included heat, humidity, standing water, vegetation or lack thereof, the presence or absence of human sanitary practices, perhaps elevation above sea level, and who knows what else. The prevalence of certain maladies in 'malarious' regions jeopardized life almost anywhere in India. Roberts claimed to have numbers to prove it.

Official statistics cited 'fevers' as the principal cause of death in British India.[5] Roberts said authorities were actually referring to 'malarial fevers' but he listed no defining symptoms or characteristics for his interpretation. These documents indicate a staggering mortality rate. It was approximately 70 percent in the provinces of Bengal (East India), Bombay (Western Coast) plus Punjab and the

NWP (both in West India), 60 percent in the Central Provinces (Middle India), 50 percent for Assam (also in East India) and 45 percent in Berar (Western Coast). Madras Presidency fared little better; "fever" accounted for 38 percent of the "total deaths" in this region of Southern India where opium consumption, according to the Royal Commission, had always been minimal. Roberts realized these numbers for India might be excessive. Medical officers with whom he conferred admitted that "pneumonia and other acute diseases are sometimes erroneously included under the heading 'fever'" (GBO [Roberts] 1895:VI:109). Here, Roberts expresses cognizance about the problem of faulty nosology: flawed classification of maladies that generate elevated temperatures in victims.

The situation in India was grim regardless of diagnostic confusion and possibly exaggerated numbers. The "main fact," Roberts insisted, was "that malarial fevers dominate the death-rate in every province of British India."[6] The "next most prolific" killers were dysentery, "endemic diarrhoea," and cholera. These "account for only 12 percent of the total deaths." It should be no surprise, therefore, that Indians view opium as a "general panacea for their health troubles." They have "learnt from long experience" that opium "alleviates their sufferings, and, more or less . . . prevent[s] a recurrence of their feverish attacks" (GBO [Roberts] 1895:VI:109). Consumption of the drug prolonged existence and helped to make bearable whatever time they had left on earth. For Roberts, the "opium habit" was a demonstration of common sense, not a manifestation of moral decadence as the anti-opiumists pontificated.

Roberts then generalized from the opium and 'malaria' evidence given during the Royal Commission sessions. He said there was a "consensus of opinion" about the drug being "an invaluable mitigator of, and prophylactic against, the prevailing complaints" besieging Indians. There also was "no doubt" about "its general therapeutic value" and that no "other known remedy" could replace opium (GBO [Roberts] 1895:VI:109–10). Both assertions are at best overstatements, if not inaccurate. With few exceptions, witnesses testifying before the Royal Commission in England and India did acknowledge the therapeutic value of the substance. But, there was no concurrence for exactly what the drug was beneficial and to what extent it prevented or cured anything other than alleviating pain and discomfort.

Roberts dismissed the opinions of splitters who insisted that opium was no more than a useful anodyne for their definition of malaria, and for other 'fever maladies' subsumed under the same category. Roberts' stance was paradoxical; he used some information about *Papaver somniferum Linn* accumulated by Anglo-European medical researchers throughout the nineteenth century to support his argument. He was either oblivious to, or intentionally ignored, other insights that challenged his position.

SIR WILLIAM ROBERTS' UNDERSTANDING OF *PAPAVER SOMNIFERUM LINN*

Roberts was only partially aware of what Western scientists knew about opium in 1894–1895. He correctly recognized *Papaver somniferum Linn* as "a very complex substance" consisting of "not less that sixteen or eighteen different active principles." Morphia was indeed one of its "two most important and abundant alkaloids" and the drug's remaining alkaloids were found in "very minuscule [sic] amounts." Morphia relieved pain, it was responsible for the "hypnotic properties" attributed to the mother drug, and it was highly toxic in small amounts (GBO [Roberts] 1895:VI:110).

Roberts also knew the "opium used in England for medical purposes [was] called Smyrna opium" but he glossed over the significance of this point. It is difficult, however, to imagine him not knowing that genetic endowment was one reason why both English and European chemists and the pharmaceutical industry preferred the Symrna product for most of the nineteenth century. He did say that opium from British India and the Malwa plateau in central India was morphia-poor (3.98 percent and 4.61 percent) compared to an average of 8.27 percent for the "very rich" Symrna product (GBO [Roberts] 1895:VI:110).[7] Since the principal value of opium in western markets was morphia content, the Indian product (as mentioned earlier) was considered to be inferior to imports from the Middle East.

A liability in one place can be an advantage in another. This was true of India's morphia-poor drug, at least up to a point. Roberts was confident that opium prevented 'fever' and that oral consumption was an efficacious way to do it. The problem in India was that "only large consumers [were] absolutely protected against the malarial poison." An amount ranging from sixteen to forty-five grains consumed at one sitting or over a three-day period to effect a cure could be lethal to the average person, especially if he or she were not already habituated. Morphia was so toxic that even the meager amount in the Indian drug "puts an absolute bar" to the amount of opium required to guarantee immunity from 'malarial fever' (GBO [Roberts] 1895:VI:111). And consumers of moderate quantities of the drug had only partial protection. This, according to Roberts, explained why some witnesses were able to claim opium eaters suffered as much from 'fever' as abstainers. The unfortunate victims simply were not ingesting enough of the drug and they would kill themselves if they did so.

IF OPIUM DOES NOT HELP YOU, NARCOTINE WILL

Narcotine was the other "most important and abundant" alkaloid.[8] Roberts was correct about abundance; the British India product averaged 6.36 percent, the Malwa drug was slightly less at 5.14 percent, whereas Symrna opium had a meager 1.94 percent (GBO [Roberts] 1895:VI:110).

Roberts now turned water into wine. Again, the man's awareness of Anglo-European research was selective. He correctly observed that narcotine was a "crystalline alkaloid resembling quinine" and that both substances had a crystalline structure and very bitter taste (GBO [Roberts] 1895:VI:110). Everything else he said was incorrect. He claimed that narcotine-rich Indian opium made it uniquely suited to prevent and cure 'genuine malarial fever.' Furthermore, just like quinine, narcotine had "tonic and anti-periodic properties" (GBO [Roberts]

1895:VI:110). Western chemists and physiologists had already concluded that the alkaloid prevented and cured no disease.

Narcotine might qualify as a "tonic" as the term was commonly defined during the 1890s. This is not saying much because numerous substances made people feel better. Any equivalency between the two substances ends here. Roberts also ignored the voluminous literature about cinchona and its alkaloids. The message circa 1893–1895 was unequivocal: quinine occupied a position of prime importance in malarial therapy.

There was nothing similar in the history of narcotine. No Anglo-European medical publications prior to 1894–1895 attempt to prove that narcotine prevented or cured the kind of malaria envisaged by splitters. Almost all published literature addresses merits of opium, not its alkaloids, in treating cases of the lumpers' interpretation of 'malaria.'[9]

Three items from British India, however, convinced Roberts that narcotine was equal to, or better than, quinine as a solution to the 'malarial fevers' plaguing the subcontinent. And narcotine, extracted from the mother drug and administered in small doses, circumvented the danger of morphia toxicity. Roberts was claiming to have rediscovered the value of a substance that western physicians and chemists mistakenly forgot or overlooked. To support the contention, Roberts uses a document that dates back fifty-seven years. The publication describes the work of Dr. William B. O'Shaughnessy and several associates. Roberts selected some information from O'Shaughnessy, ignores the rest, and says nothing about other people's observations in the document. A brief description of the article's contents, and then what Roberts chose to say about the material, suggests that the man wanted to make as strong an argument as possible for the importance of narcotine.

THE LEGACY OF DR. WILLIAM B. O'SHAUGHNESSY

The excitement generated by the discovery of alkaloids in opium during the 1820s and early 1830s spread to South Asia. Attendees at the Pharmacopoeia committee's panel during the 4 August 1838 meeting of the Calcutta Medical Society first listened to speakers relating how narcotine 'cured' twenty-six out of twenty-seven cases of 'remittent' and 'intermittent' fevers. Then Dr. William B. O'Shaughnessy of the Indian Medical Service described the thirty-two cases in which narcotine failed to 'cure' only one individual. The cumulative success rate, fifty-seven out of a total of fifty-nine cases, was remarkable (AJMS 1838:194).[10]

O'Shaughnessy was not finished. After listening to other speakers' comments, he provided the audience with two anecdotes. One was about narcotine curing two of his servants. The second item involved fifteen cases he "extracted from the journals of the Medical College Hospital." Although unspecified, O'Shaughnessy implies the fifteen patients had been treated with narcotine. Five of them were given the alkaloid after failing to respond to quinine and arsenic.[11] Eleven of the fifteen also had enlarged spleens or livers, and one person suffered from "inflammation of the knee joint." The hospital records indicated only two fatalities. The first was a patient admitted into the hospital on the seventh day of "violent fever . . . [who] died the next day." The second mortality was a child whose "spleen, liver, pancreas, and mesenteric gland, were immensely enlarged, and the case hopeless from the beginning." O'Shaughnessy concluded this Calcutta Medical Society gathering by reminding attendees that "more than 100 ague cases had been treated by his pupils and acquaintance with perfect success by this remedy" (*AJMS* 1838:195). The fifty-nine (not sixty) cases mentioned at the beginning of the panel made the achievement even more impressive. He said nothing more about the two servants and Medical College Hospital anecdotes, although a success rate of thirteen out of fifteen for the latter is impressive.

Dr. William B. O'Shaughnessy's fellow participants also praised the alkaloid's effectiveness for patients in the eastern region of India. Four speakers merely expressed delight. A Dr. Smith had a memorable experience with three sick people in a place called Hidglee. He exclaimed "[a]s far as these cases go, I cannot speak too favorably of narcotine and am very desirous of trying it more extensively" (Smith, quoted in *AJMS* 1838:194–95). He did not describe paroxysm characteristics and was silent about the course of treatment prompting his enthusiasm. The same limitation applies to Mr. O'Brien, "apothecary of the native hospital" whose location was not stated, plus a Mr. Evans and the "Pundit Modoosoodona Gupta." O'Brien successfully treated three patients. The other two individuals each administered to one. Gupta's subject was suffering from dysentery at the time narcotine was administered, and Pundit Gupta implied this alkaloid also ended the bowel disorder. They offered no corroborating data (*AJMS* 1838:195).

The remaining participants illustrate the level of diagnostic sophistication prevalent in South Asia at the time. A Captain Marshall of Calcutta administered narcotine to three servants with 'severe ague' whereupon "all were rapidly cured." Marshall was impressed albeit cautious about the 'cure.' He admitted that it "would be presumptuous in me to offer any opinion as to the virtues of narcotine; all I can say is, that if ever I am ill of fever I shall unhesitatingly and confidently prefer it to sulphate [sic] of quinine or any other medicine I know of" (*AJMS* 1838:195). He did not describe characteristics of the 'ague' involved and if quinine had been given before narcotine.

Dr. J. Chapman, Mr. R. O'Shaughnessy, and Mr. Gooeve *did* clarify the status of quinine in their work. Chapman, Assistant-Surgeon of the Calcutta General Hospital, talked about a "European" who "contracted violent remittent fever at Kedgeree on the 16th of July." This patient entered the hospital on 19 July. The year was not identified. Quinine "was used in the usual manner on the first remission on the 20th, and again on the 21st, but the symptoms were rather aggravated than improved." Narcotine was then administered. Except for a slight headache and for restlessness . . . on the 23rd . . . [a] complete remission" occurred and the "fever never returned." On 28 July, the patient received no more medicine and was discharged as "convalescent" (*AJMS* 1838:195).

Mr. R. O'Shaughnessy operated on a patient for "stone . . . [who] was attacked by virulent ague on the day of the operation" (R. O'Shaughnessy, quoted in

AJMS 1838:195). The 'ague' returned the next day at the same hour. O'Shaughnessy deemed it unwise to administer quinine but no rationale for this reluctance was cited in the *American Journal of Medical Science* article. He decided to give the person four doses of narcotine, and observed that the "fever did not return, [and] the wound was not in the slightest degree affected" (R. O'Shaughnessy, quoted in *AJMS* 1838:195). The patient also had no headache and displayed no "excitement." O'Shaughnessy implied the alkaloid also acted as a sedative. The patient had not slept soundly for two nights before receiving the first dose. That night he did so, and was discharged "cured of the effects of the operation" fourteen days after the operation (R. O'Shaughnessy, quoted in *AJMS* 1838:195).[12]

The *American Journal of Medical Science* article includes comments from a Mr. Gooeve concerning two cases. The first instance was the late deputy-collector of Chittagong, who most likely was an Englishman. The patient suffered from an enlarged spleen and a "[q]uotidian of several months standing." Gooeve had no success with quinine despite administering it in "every possible form" for the daily recurring fever. Arsenic was substituted. It "checked the fever [but] did much mischief to the patient's good health" (Gooeve, quoted in *AJMS* 1838:194).

Quinine, therefore, was of no use whatsoever for a persistent fever. Arsenic halted the paroxysm but almost killed the patient. Narcotine was given "with such success" that Dr. Gooeve had no hesitation "in saying that this patient owes his life to the remedy in question" (Gooeve, quoted in *AJMS* 1838:194). The second patient was suffering at the same time from "inflammation of the bowel." Giving quinine was "inadmissible" although Gooeve provided no reason for his decision. Narcotine was administered, and the patient apparently was cured.

At the end of the 1838 article, the *American Journal of Medical Science* editor(s) included a note written by a Mr. Green, the civil surgeon in Howrah, India. Green's statements about narcotine were as positive as the comments of William B. O'Shaughnessy and others at the 1838 conference.

> I have now employed the [sic] narcotine in sixteen cases of remittent fever, and such is my opinion of the efficacy of the remedy, that in instances of fever, intermittents and remittents, in ordinary healthy subjects, and in whom there is no complication of severe organic disease, I give it with the full expectation of arresting the next periodic return of the fever. I have seen the result follow in ten of the cases of the fever alluded to [and] I consider narcotine a more powerful antiperiodic than quinine. The remedy does not act silently. I have observed a degree of general heat follow its use in the first instance, and subsequently, perspiration, so that it appears to excite in the system a salutary and powerful counteraction as to stop the morbid concentration that issues in fever. I have not observed narcotine to lead to local organic disturbance in the case in which I have used it. In short, even from my scanty experience, I consider the remedy an invaluable one. (Green, quoted in *AJMS* 1838:195)

Some facts that people mentioned in the *American Journal of Medicine* lent credibility to narcotine's purported antiperiodic capability for plasmodia-induced paroxysms. These were the "enlarged spleen" of Gooeve's deputy-collector, Dr. Chapman's comments about 'violent remittent fever,' and Green's successful treatment of ten of the sixteen patients suffering from 'intermittent and remittent fevers.' Gooeve's second case was irrelevant because quinine had not been administered. The alkaloid's capability, therefore, was not evaluated. Marshall and R. O'Shaughnessy's proclamations about narcotine stopping "severe ague" and "virulent ague" respectively only suggested that, in some way, the alkaloid affected an unknown number of fever-inducing maladies subsumed under the inclusive term 'ague.'

Sir William Roberts, however, viewed Dr. William B. O'Shaughnessy's 1838 observations about 159 patients in India as the earliest proof of narcotine's "curative power in malarial fevers" (GBO [Roberts] 1895:VI:110). Roberts' 1895 report contains only five sentences about the man. There is no mention of O'Shaughnessy's fellow participants' doubts about the alkaloid being equal or superior to quinine as an "anti-periodic." The omission is understandable. Roberts was advancing a case for narcotine; negative comments and qualifying statements were not helpful. William O'Shaughnessy also cited more cases as proof, and his interest in exploring the substance's therapeutic potential did not end with the 1838 observations. One year later O'Shaughnessy criticized the "only process yet published by which pure narcotine can be obtained" as "tedious, troublesome, and apt to fail, unless in very expert hands" (AJMS 1838:248). The doctor was referring to one of three techniques available during the 1830s: Derosnè's method of extracting narcotine from the mother drug, the Merck process, and the Thiboumery and Mohr process (Barbier 1947:121–24). O'Shaughnessy believed he had perfected a totally new "process which is at the same time simple, economical, and productive, which ensures the separation of the febrifuge narcotine from the powerful sedative morphia, and which can be performed in every locality where opium can be found" (AJMS 1839:248). He did not indicate how it differed from the other methods.

O'Shaughnessy's continued interest in alkaloid extraction and his 1838 narcotine data prompted Sir William Roberts to declare that "[t]hese results, and others of a like character caused the Indian authorities to institute further experiments, and these, proving favourable, they caused anarcotine to be prepared in quantity at the laboratories of Ghazipur and Patna and distributed to the medical depots throughout India" (GBO [Roberts] 1895:VI:111).[13]

THE GHAZIPUR EXPERIMENTS

Roberts was far more impressed by two obscure experiments conducted in Ghazipur City (North India) during the late 1850s. W. J. Palmer was responsible for the first undertaking and Dr. A. Garden supervised the second experiment. The Palmer data, and other narcotine correspondence, is the material that Lord Brassey had ordered D. M. Gregory (the aforementioned deputy agent in the Opium Department) to forward to the Royal Commission. Garden's work was published elsewhere. Roberts proclaimed the

246   Chapter 7

Palmer and Garden research deserved "resuscitation" because the large number of people tested left no doubt that "anarcotine [narcotine] is scarcely inferior—and, in some cases, is superior—to quinine as an antiperiodic" (GBO [Roberts] 1895:VI:110). All other comments in Roberts' discussion about the two experimenters were positive. The content of the Palmer and Garden documents, however, do not justify Roberts' enthusiasm for the alkaloid.

W. J. PALMER'S 1857-1859 INVESTIGATION

Sir William Roberts' Comments about the Palmer Experiment

Roberts credited W. J. Palmer with renaming narcotine as anarcotine because Palmer found it had no "narcotic qualities" (GBO [Roberts] 1895:VI:110 [footnote]).[14] Nonetheless, it was still a remarkable substance. Palmer recorded amazing results after giving one to three grains to each of 546 people suffering from what he called "malarial fever" during 1857–1859. Five-hundred forty-one patients were 'cured.' Only five died. Roberts claimed these "officially reported cases" did not tell the whole story because Palmer also treated many other cases of 'malarial fever' with similar consequences. The total number of anarcotine recipients was slightly less than one thousand. Palmer included no more data about this larger sample. Roberts said the omission was irrelevant because the man's encounter with the first group was typical of his "general experience" (GBO [Roberts] 1895:VI:110).

Palmer's general experience was indeed gratifying. Patients with an "intolerance to quinine, and where quinine has been given without any effect for a long time," responded favorably to anarcotine (GBO [Roberts] 1895:VI:110–11). Ninety percent were eventually "cured" albeit at different rates. In

> 70 percent the fever was permanently arrested at the second paroxysm after the medicine was arrested; in 20 percent the arrest was equally sure, but was not quite so quick; and in 10 percent the medicine did not appear to have any curative result. (GBO [Roberts] 1895:VI:110)

Roberts felt that nothing more had to be said about Palmer's research. The latter had proven that the alkaloid was a potent weapon in the battle against 'fever' and 'malarious diseases.' The assertion is moot because Palmer's statements were taken out of context.

What W. J. Palmer Said about His 1857-1859 Ghazipur Experiments

W. J. Palmer was not convinced that O'Shaughnessy's work during the 1830s had confirmed narcotine to be a "remedy against the common fevers" of India and a "substitute for quinine." Although O'Shaughnessy's proclamations generated much excitement in England, the "actual value of the remedy could not well be tested because cases of the same classes of disease were not very common" (GBO [Gregory–Enclosure 79] 1895:V:77). In other words, the 'fever' diseases in both countries were dissimilar. Palmer claimed that O'Shaughnessy's failure to document enough cases, combined with no verification forthcoming from Great Britain, resulted in anarcotine falling into disuse after his departure from India.[15] Twenty years later Palmer viewed O'Shaughnessy's work as an unconfirmed, flawed, albeit intriguing hypothesis that deserved more investigation. Another limitation is that the pioneering O'Shaughnessy might not have succeeded in separating anarcotine from the mother drug's other alkaloid and nonalkaloidal components. This meant that O'Shaughnessy's conclusions about the capabilities of the substance were suspect. He actually might have been observing the consequences of several ingredients comprising the mother drug.

Palmer's Positive Results from Early Tests of Anarcotine in British India

The source of morphia produced in India at midcentury was opium confiscated from smugglers. Extraction of the alkaloid left a waste product called "dregs" which opium officials destroyed. They considered it useless. Palmer disagreed. Convinced these "dregs contained a considerable portion of anarcotine," he successfully petitioned his superiors to use the meager quantity of opium confiscated during the 1856–1857 season to extract the residual alkaloid.

Palmer sent some of the salvaged anarcotine to a Dr. Gibbon, the director of a local military hospital. Gibbon used the substance to treat "all fevers of [sic] his hospital and reported most favorably upon it." Results from the Ghazipur Charitable Dispensary and the Ghazipur Jail Hospital and Civil Station were also positive. Administrators at the latter two locations even reported using 50 percent less quinine during the twelve months despite having to treat "a much larger number of fever cases . . . than in previous years." And surgeons who traveled waterways near Ghazipur periodically were given samples to treat sick people but "in consequence of the unsettled state of the country no record of these has been obtained." Palmer did not doubt the results were positive (GBO [Gregory–Enclosure 79] 1894:V:77).

Palmer then obtained permission from Mr. H. C. Hamilton, his immediate superior and the Benares opium agent in Ghazipur, to "extract the whole of anarcotine, as well as the morphia, from the opium confiscated during the current season." There was no guarantee of success. Palmer suspected that O'Shaughnessy's technique as well as current methods of extraction were not the "most economical mode of separating anarcotine on a large scale." This limitation, however, did not prevent him from estimating how much of the substance was procurable and what should be done with it. All of it should be "distributed so as to obtain the most carefully observed results as to its medicinal properties" (GBO [Gregory–Enclosure 79] 1894:V:77). This would confirm, or refute, O'Shaughnessy's 1838 conclusions about anarcotine's purported curative power.

Palmer's experiments intrigued Dr. J. Forsyth, the director-general of the Medical Department. And in a 12 March 1859 note to the secretary to the Government of Bengal, Forsyth "pointed out the necessity of estimating the cost of manufacturing both morphia and anarcotine" (GBO [Gregory–Enclosure 169] 1894:V:77). Ordered to conduct "careful experiments" at the Benares and Bihar Opium Agencies, Palmer sent the results to Hamilton on 15 November 1859. He also informed Forsyth and Dr. Grant, apothecary-general for the Government of India, that the amount of anarcotine obtained from confiscated opium during the past year fell short of his December 1858 estimate because a

> large proportion of the anarcotine is lost in our present method of preparing morphia, or rather in the present state of our knowledge it would be very expensive to extract it; this is one cause of the diminution, secondly, a number of experiments were made to extract anarcotine without the aid of spirit; and in trying which form of the alkaloid could be produced most economically this was another cause of the diminution. (GBO [Gregory–Enclosure 169] 1894:V:78)

Quality was as serious a problem as quantity. The two batches of hydrochlorate of anarcotine sent to Forsyth and Grant for examination represented the highest degree of purity obtainable after a year of experimentation. Palmer was dissatisfied, admitting that at "first much difficulty was found in making the anarcotine pure and up to the present time there is a difficulty in extracting the whole of it" (GBO [Gregory–Enclosure 169] 1894:V:78). In other words, it was probably contaminated by the presence of other opium alkaloids.

Palmer's reservation about the amount and purity of anarcotine after almost twelve months of concentrated effort to find a solution is even more applicable to O'Shaughnessy. The 1838 method of extracting anarcotine was obviously not cost effective, and O'Shaughnessy had not separated the alkaloid from other opium ingredients. The pioneer's proclamations about anarcotine's 'fever' efficacy, and the favorable comments of his copresenters at the Calcutta Medical Society conference, did indeed lack credibility. In 1859 Palmer recognized the limitations of O'Shaughnessy's endeavors and Government of India officials concurred. Thirty-six years later Sir William Roberts did not mention the problem.

Palmer knew that fluctuating, and always small, amounts of opium confiscated per season might yield insufficient anarcotine to fill all future requests from dispensaries in India. A new source of the mother drug had to be found. And if this was not possible, then a more effective process for extracting maximum amounts of anarcotine from a given quantity of morphia had to be perfected. In either case, the Government of India would have to bear the expense of guaranteeing an uncontaminated, adequate, and uninterrupted supply of the alkaloid. Palmer needed extensive and careful documentation of patients 'cured' by anarcotine to persuade his superiors. He recommended the substance be given only "on special indent" to medical officers "required to keep records of its therapeutic effects" (GBO [Gregory–Enclosure 169] 1894:V:78).[16]

Palmer still viewed anarcotine as a rational medical and economic investment despite the technical difficulties involved in procuring it. The alkaloid had "been used very extensively here as a remedy in fevers, especially during the late severe visitation, from which so large a proportion of the population has suffered; it appears to me hardly inferior to quinine in its power of arresting the attack of fever; indeed, in many cases it appears superior, and as the dose required is rather smaller than that of quinine, I estimate its commercial value as at least equal to that of that drug" (GBO [Gregory–Enclosure 169] 1895:V:78). And in a 14 February 1860 report to Dr. Forsyth, Palmer supported the optimistic evaluation with some statistics collected during a two-year study of the therapeutic effects of anarcotine for 'malarious fever' patients.

Palmer, as Roberts noted, administered anarcotine to 546 people at several locations in Ghazipur. Between 6 November 1857 to the end of September 1859, 188 cases of "malarious fever" were admitted into the Gaol [Jail] hospital.[17] The alkaloid therapy 'cured' 184 patients. Four people expired. Three hundred fifty-eight people were admitted to the Ghazipur Military Hospital between July 1858 and the end of September 1859. Only one mortality was recorded and 357 were discharged free from the malady (GBO [Gregory–Enclosure 192] 1894:V:78). A success rate of 541 out of a total of 546 victims was indeed amazing.

Palmer provided additional evidence for anarcotine's efficacy. It came from "a large number of fever patients . . . under my medical charge" at the Ghazipur Charitable Dispensary while in charge of the 2nd Sikh Infantry Hospital between July and October 1858. Then there was data collected from the end of September to the end of November 1858. He obtained it during his duty as hospital supervisor for soldiers of the "4th Madras Light Cavalry and the regiment of irregular cavalry, called the Benares Horse." Palmer claimed that in "all cases the results were exactly similar to those reported above, and the total number treated falls little short of 1,000 cases" (GBO [Gregory–Enclosure 192], 1894:V:78).

What Sir William Roberts Did Not Include from Palmer's Experiment

Three components of Palmer's research challenge the credibility and feasibility of Roberts' anarcotine argument. Roberts does not mention them in the 1895 report. The first is Palmer's partial recognition of the biased nature of the documented cases, the second is his awareness of the potential toxicity of anarcotine, and the third is the variable rate of 'curing' Palmer observed among patients.

Palmer's Acknowledgment of Patients' Atypical Status

The people responsible for Palmer's remarkable success with anarcotine were not representative of the population of India. No females or children participated in the experiment. Second, Palmer admitted that the Military Police hospital patients were well fed and adequately housed males "in the prime of life." They comprised almost two-thirds of the cases for which he provided some data. A mortality rate of one out of 357, while still impressive, loses a little luster. Four deaths among the 188 jail hospital male patients translate into a mortality rate four times higher than the Military Police tally. These prisoners, frequently old and diseased, were slightly more representative of the general population. Palmer also said that two of these inmates had been admitted in "dying state, and a third was an enfeebled old man" (GBO [Gregory–Enclosure 192] 1894:V:78). Palmer provided no demographic details about the remaining individuals in the 1,000 sample.

Toxicity and Therapy Schedule

Palmer viewed anarcotine as a "very powerful remedy [that] must be used with great care." He recommended a "uniformly simple" initial step. All people complaining of "any one of the forms of malarious fever" were first given a "purgative" to determine if constipation was the cause of fever.[18] Dispensing the alkaloid followed a strict protocol. Mr. G. Osborne, subdeputy opium agent at Gorakhpur in Bihar, was told that hydrochlorate of anarcotine should then be ingested in doses of "one grain every six, four or two hours according to virulence of the fever [and] [i]t may be taken in a little water." At what point anarcotine became toxic varied among participants. Dosage level, therefore, had to be adjusted for each patient because too much caused "giddiness" and vomiting, in which case the physician must immediately reduce the amount (GBO [Gregory–Enclosure 103] 1894:V:77).

The schedule was slightly different for a person claiming to have "fever" but showing no signs of sickness during consultation with a physician. The patient "was allowed to remain without more medicine until the attack came on, and was examined." Upon verifying that the person was suffering from "malarious fever," the examiner should then administer "one, two, or three grain doses, either alone or dissolved in a little dilute [sic] sulphuric acid and water, three or more times a day in proportion to the severity of the attack" (GBO [Gregory–Enclosure 192] 1894:V:78).

Establishing a patient's tolerance for anarcotine was a paramount concern for Palmer. An amount suitable for one person might cause death or debilitation in another. And as described below, some people showed no change regardless of total dosage received during a course of therapy.

Variable "Curing" Rates and Dosage Levels among Survivors

Virtual Ineffectiveness of the First Dose of Anarcotine Patients were introduced to anarcotine at the beginning of the first "fever" episode following the purgative. The amount of alkaloid received depended upon the severity of an individual's attack. This initial dose rarely "cured" anybody, although the physician and perhaps the victim thought the experience was less violent. In Palmer's own words, the "first expected return of the paroxysm after the medicine was commenced, usually came on, sometimes as if no medicine had been taken, generally with less severity than before" (GBO [Gregory–Enclosure 192] 1894:V:78). His statement that 'fever' attacks usually erupted after the initial dose of anarcotine implied that some did not reappear. Palmer provided no details to explain these exceptions. He apparently concluded their rarity made them insignificant.

The Benefits and Inconsequential Effects of More Than One Exposure to Anarcotine with Adjusted Dosage Each day all patients continued to receive from one to three grains administered alone or in solution. The number of grains in each exposure, as cited above, was adjusted for severity of 'fever' and physiological idiosyncrasies of the person. Palmer placed each patient in one of three categories. The categories referred to time required to effect a 'cure,' ranging from complete and quick to never being 'cured.' How many days passed before a recurrence of fever determined the rapidity of 'cure.' He briefly described a few cases "typical" of each category and indicated the percentage of patients comprising the group.

Category 1: The Nonappearance of Another Paroxysm

Palmer was ecstatic about six cases that he said "fairly represent" 70 percent of the patients treated. He found that the "second expected return seldom came, the paroxysm had been arrested [and] [s]o constantly was this the case that I would scarcely refrain from assuring the patient that the second return of the paroxysm would never come" (GBO [Gregory–Enclosure 192] 1894:V:78–81). While a substantial majority of 'malarious fever' victims enjoyed a complete and quick cure, others were not so fortunate.

Category 2: Hampering the Onset of a Subsequent Paroxysm

Anarcotine was far less effective in four cases. Its effects upon these individuals were first seen [in] postponing the attack. While no medicines are being given it is not uncommon to see each succeeding paroxysm commence a little earlier, continue a little longer, and with more severity than the former ones. When these three signs are reversed under the influence of the medicine, a rapid cure may be predicted (GBO [Gregory–Enclosure 192] 1894:V:78). Twenty percent of Palmer's patients were in this category.

Category 3: Anarcotine Exacerbated 'Malarious Fevers'

The remaining 10 percent perplexed Palmer because anarcotine had "no curative effect" whatsoever despite careful dosage adjustment. In fact, the recipient's condition worsened. Each "succeeding paroxysm of fever commenced earlier and lasted longer, or [came] with more violence." Palmer was forced to choose other antiperiodics. He was convinced there "must be some difference in the character of the fever" and searched unsuccessfully for "any pathognomonic symptom by which they may be distinguished before the treatment is commenced" (GBO [Gregory–Enclosure 192] 1894:V:78).

Palmer's success with anarcotine, consequently, was not as remarkable as Roberts asserted.[19] The alkaloid rarely prevented the onset of a second bout of elevated temperature, and continued dosage only moderated symptoms in many instances of recurring paroxysms. Treatment was ineffective, even harmful, in at least 10 percent of Palmer's subjects.

Roberts ignored another limitation: Palmer's results were obtained under highly controlled circumstances. Patients were closely monitored and received amounts of anarcotine tailored to their level of tolerance and severity of 'fever.' It was unrealistic to assume adherence to a similar protocol would be feasible if anarcotine were dispensed to India's population as a substitute for the mother drug. Facilities and personnel for such care were nonexistent in the country. And it was equally unrealistic to expect the positive results from this atypical test group would be the norm for a wider audience of recipients.

THE 1859-1860 ANARCOTINE RESEARCH OF DR. A. GARDEN

Sir William Roberts needed more evidence to strengthen the anarcotine argument. He thought a physician, whose name was A. Garden, had provided it.

W. J. Palmer's effort to persuade the Government of India to finance alkaloid extraction improvement did not end with his 1 October 1859 departure from Ghazipur. He instructed his successor, Dr. A. Garden, to continue the anarcotine endeavor (Garden 1860:400). Garden did not have to wait long for a good opportunity to do so. Ten days later he confronted "a severe outbreak of intermittent fever, of quotidian and tertian type" and then administered the alkaloid to 684 cases. Garden discusses the experiment in "Report on Anarcotine." The article appears in an 1860 issue of the *Indian Annals of Medical Science*.

Sir William Roberts' Comments about Garden's Research

Garden's publication contains much more data than the Palmer document but Roberts used only a fraction of it. He also said that Garden's results were as remarkable as those documented by Palmer.

Doses ranging from one and one-half to three grains "rapidly cured" 187 out of the total of 194 patients for whom Garden maintained records. Only seven people, or 3.6 percent, failed to respond. Furthermore, the substance cured some individuals who were unresponsive to quinine. Garden concluded, and Roberts reported, that anarcotine might not be as valuable as quinine, but it had a strong claim to occupy "the next place in the ranks of antiperiodics is, I think, an undoubted fact" (Garden, quoted in GBO [Roberts] 1895:VI:111).

Roberts cited nothing more from Garden's carefully documented experiment. He ended the commentary by declaring that the significance of the Palmer and Garden work regarding the "prophylactic powers of opium against malarial fevers" was in providing proof that "anarcotine in doses of 1 to 3 grains rapidly (in about three days) cut short the paroxysm of intermittent fever and completely arrested the disease" (GBO [Roberts] 1895:VI:111).

Roberts was wrong. Garden's minimal number was one and one-half grains, not one grain. The importance of a half-grain difference is discussed later in the chapter. And the Garden data that Roberts did cite exaggerated anarcotine's power.

There Was Nothing Special about Anarcotine

Dr. Garden's first caveat is that anarcotine was not the only antiperiodic administered to "fever" patients unresponsive to quinine. He found none of the substances better, or worse, in lessening duration of an attack or ending the malady (Garden 1860:403). There was, therefore, nothing unique about the alkaloid providing relief or a cure for sufferers of 'malarious diseases.' It was merely one of several possible therapies. Anarcotine might be only slightly inferior to quinine, but so were other substances. Garden did not name the other antiperiodics.

A related point is the number of Garden's subjects who had actually been unresponsive to prior quinine therapy? His statistics identify only two individuals, and both were suffering from daily recurring fevers (quotidian fever). The first received a total of nine grains of anarcotine over a period of nine days after quinine proved to be "ineffectual" (Garden 1860:413 [Table A]).[20] The patient apparently recovered. The second was a "Goorka Sepoy, of the Military Police Battalion" (Garden 1860:412). The reaction to anarcotine given in six-grain doses was not much better. The patient became constipated and remained sick. Garden then administered a purgative which "seemed to act like a charm" and "[f]rom that day, he had no return of fever" (1860:412). The policeman had been relieved literally and figuratively. How many other test subjects, if any at all, were in this "quinine-resistant" category is unknown. Roberts implied all of them but Garden offered no confirmation whatsoever.

The Nonrepresentative Nature of Garden's Subjects

There was nothing special about the alkaloid but there was something atypical about the people to whom anarcotine was administered. Garden recruited patients from a Military Police Hospital and from a Jail Hospital.[21] Like Palmer's research, members of the Military Police comprised almost two-thirds of Garden's test subjects. Garden, aware of the consequences of this nonrepresentative status, admitted that the Military Police sepoys were in much better shape, being "young men, well fed, and well clothed." In contrast, a higher rate of anarcotine ineffectiveness culminating in a higher mortality rate among patients from the Jail Hospital should be expected because of "the general condition of the prisoners as to age, previous habits and method of life, and the general state of depression, mental and physical, which occurs during imprisonment" (Garden 1860:401).

The significance of this recognition is that generalizing about anarcotine predicated primarily upon responses from an elite group such as military police personnel was dubious science because not everybody in India was a young male. Even fewer people in the country were well fed and adequately clothed. And the kinds of individuals populating the Jail Hospital were, at best, only slightly more typical of the general Indian population. Garden realized that the atypical demographic characteristics of test subjects qualified his success with anarcotine. Roberts, just as he did with Palmer, ignored the problem and remained silent about inherent bias.

What Dr. Garden Actually Said about the Anarcotine Experiment

Sir Roberts was right about one thing. Upon arrival in Ghazipur, Garden was indeed confronted with an emergency. A "most severe and fatal epidemic of fever" began on 10 October 1859 and "raged throughout this and the surrounding districts for four months" (Garden 1860:400). Garden labeled this period—from October 10 through January 1860—the "virulent" phase. A less lethal phase lasted until 30 June 1860. He claimed to have administered anarcotine to nearly 700 patients admitted to the two hospitals during these nine months (Garden 1860:400, 402). The exact number was 684. A total of 238 patients in the Jail Hospital received the alkaloid. Eight individuals died. The Military Police Battalion Hospital provided Garden with 446 test cases. Anarcotine ostensibly 'cured' all but one of these policemen. Sir Roberts in 1895 proclaimed this nine-month experiment involving 684 people with only nine fatalities to be an unequivocal demonstration of the alkaloid's therapeutic power. A review of the two phases of the nine-month epidemic, each one considered separately, as well as the kinds of 'fever' Garden treated, indicate that Roberts was wrong. Even Dr. Garden had recognized the significance of these factors.

Two Phases of the Nine-Month Experiment

Garden attached greatest importance to results obtained from 525 men during the first or "virulent" period dating from 10 October 1859 to the end of January 1860. The "fever was raging" with "rapid fatality" among the wider population during these months. The Military Police Battalion Hospital provided 352 soldiers for this phase of the experiment whereas only 173 male inmates in the Jail Hospital participated. Most people in the entire study, therefore, were treated during the "virulent" period. It was in these months that all of them "were more than ordinarily difficult to cure, and especially prone to relapse" (Garden 1860:401). Table 2 ("Patients Receiving Anarcotine During the Two Periods of Dr. Garden's Nine-Month Study") lists the number of anarcotine recipients in each category during the two phases of Garden's experiment.

One hundred and fifty-nine men participated in the less significant or "nonvirulent" phase of the study that began during February 1860. Garden reluctantly ended the entire project on 30 June of the same year. No anarcotine remained for the ninety-four Military Police Hospital and sixty-five Jail Hospital patients because "the whole quantity manufactured had to be sent to the different medical Depots" (Garden 1860:400–01).

Garden's Mortality and "Cure" Rates

The ability of anarcotine to 'cure' 675 out of a total 684 patients, a 98.4 percent success rate or 1.6 percent rate of ineffectiveness, appears remarkable. But as Garden acknowledged, the military policemen were younger, healthier, better fed, better clothed, and more adequately housed than Jail Hospital patients. These traits, combined with the medical care available to members of such organizations, enabled the policemen to respond more rapidly and with greater success to therapy than their less fortunate brethren (Garden 1860:401). The policemen, 352 during the "virulent" period, and ninety-four during the "nonvirulent" phase, represented two-thirds of the total number of test cases over the nine months. The presence of this elite group of 446 males in the study inflates the alkaloid's therapeutic potential for the nonprivileged in India. What happened to the Jail Hospital participants might be a more accurate depiction of what Indians of both sexes and all ages could expect from anarcotine consumed under nonlaboratory conditions. The match, however, is not at all perfect because inmates did receive food, clothing, shelter, and at least some medical care from the state. Nonincarcerated citizens had no such guarantees.

The mortality rate among anarcotine recipients in each hospital differed drastically; only one of the 446 policemen expired compared to eight among the 238 jail patients. This means the inmate population, which provided almost 50 percent fewer test subjects, experienced a death rate eight times higher than the military police subjects. Adjusting the number of inmates to approximate the number of military police almost doubles the probable mortality rate among jail patients, a group more representative of the "common folk" in the country.

This depressing assessment is moderated by the Jail Hospital mortality to 'cure' ratio. Eight deaths signify a 3.3 percent rate of ineffectiveness. The other way of saying this is that 96.7 percent of the 238 inmates were restored to 'health.' The figure is only slightly less than the 98.4 percent 'cure' rate proclaimed for the entire 684 participants during the nine months. These statistics are still striking; they seem to be a dramatic demonstration of the therapeutic value of anarcotine until more details of Garden's study are examined.

The Kinds of 'Fever' Garden Was Treating

Palmer and Garden investigated the therapeutic capability of anarcotine to persuade the Government of India to improve alkaloid extraction technology. It stands to reason that Garden would have enhanced his contribution by citing more examples of successful or 'cured' patients. Providing statistics for all 684 patients is a logical inclusion if their rate of 'cure' approximated that of the 194 people for whom records were kept. But details for the remaining 470 anarcotine recipients are absent because Garden did not bother to collect them. And the far fewer 194 documented cases raise questions about the kinds of 'fevers' Garden actually treated.

Garden limited his study to ascertaining the effect of anarcotine upon two types of "Intermittent Fever." He labeled them "*Febris Intermittens Quotidiana*" and "*Febris Intermittens Tertiana*" (1860:402). Henceforth, they are called quotidian and tertian. Quotidian fevers recur daily. Tertian fevers occur every other day, or every third day if occurrence and recurrence are counted. Garden prohibited people with "Quartant Fever" from participating in the study. These were people whose paroxysms appeared every fourth day, or every third day after the day the fever first appeared. Garden also excluded individuals suffering from "Remittent Fevers" and other kinds of "Intermittent Fevers." He cited no reason for these exclusions, he did not specify what other "Intermittent Fevers" meant, and he neglected to describe the characteristics of "Remittent

Fever." Garden did say that anarcotine's effect upon "Remittent Fevers" was very unimpressive. His conclusions, therefore, pertain to only two types of fever. And during the nineteenth century, both were often subsumed under the broad, ambiguous category of 'malarious diseases' and 'malarial fevers.'

Garden maintained records for 154 patients with quotidian or daily occurring fever. But he did this for only forty people who experience tertian paroxysms. Thirty-five years later, the splitters who testified before the Royal Commission insisted that the term 'malarial fever' was misleading and too inclusive. Etiologically-distinct ailments, they argued, caused episodes of elevated temperature that are only superficially similar. Some ailments also might generate a continuous or uninterrupted low-grade, barely detectable fever with a flare-up every day. The same criticism applied to quotidian fever; some etiologically-distinct maladies might have daily paroxysms or a twenty-four hour cycle of waxing and waning of elevated body temperature. This increased the number of maladies that opium or anarcotine might effect in some way. Splitters' criticism implied that Garden was an example of the fallacy. Garden's error, can be excused because of limitations imposed by the diagnostic standards of 1859–1860. Roberts had less excuse after hearing testimony from the aforementioned critics three and a half decades later in an environment of increasing sophistication. One of the plasmodia responsible for malaria as it is now understood does produce a daily paroxysm. The reactions of Garden's quotidian fever patients to quinine would have shown a difference between plasmodia-induced malaria and the amorphous 'malaria' category that skeptics testifying before the Royal Commission had rejected. But Garden was documenting reactions to anarcotine, not quinine, so the question cannot be answered.

Far fewer maladies generate tertian fever. One type of malaria plasmodium does just this. There is, therefore, a possibility that a greater percentage of Garden's tertian fever patients did have plasmodial malaria compared to the number registered for quotidian sufferers. These tertian victims would have responded favorably to quinine if it had been given. And treatment with anarcotine should produce a higher "rate of ineffectiveness" among these people compared to quotidian fever sufferers. In other words, responses of tertian fever patients to anarcotine should reveal a longer period of treatment required before any "cure" occurred, a greater number of "incurable" people, and more incidents of serious negative reactions during a course of therapy.

The preponderance of quotidian fever patients (154) compared to only forty for tertian indicates Garden's study was biased toward a positive evaluation of anarcotine. Test results confirm it. The alkaloid failed to "cure" four out of 154 quotidian fever sufferers. Garden presented this as one in 38.5 cases not restored to health, a 2.59 percent failure rate (1860:7:402 [Table 1]). This becomes a 98.41 percent "cure" rate for people suffering from daily occurring paroxysms.

Quotidian fever subjects outnumbered tertian patients almost four to one but the latter had only one less instance of anarcotine failure (three "no cures" out of forty cases). In other words, one out of 12.33 patients remained sick. This is a 7.5 percent failure rate, or a 92.5 percent rate of effectiveness (Garden 1860:402 [Table 1]). The data appear impressive. But a more accurate interpretation is that a physician had a 250–300 percent greater chance of either not relieving or exacerbating misery for a hypothetical 154 tertian patients than for an equal number of quotidian fever sufferers. And for "one case out of every 27.71" in both fever categories, Garden had to cease administering the alkaloid because it either produced an "increase in severity of symptoms" or the fever ceased to abate "after a fair trial" (1860:402–03). Four quotidian and three tertian fever subjects were in this group. Garden henceforth excluded these seven cases from his discussion. This lowers the number of quotidian and tertian patients reacting to the drug in some way other than violent or severely negative to 150 and thirty-seven respectively.

Rapidity of Cure: The "True" Test of Anarcotine's Therapeutic Capability

Garden considered "rapidity of cure" to be the "true test" for the therapeutic capability of anarcotine. A patient received no alkaloid until constipation was eliminated as the cause of the paroxysm. Garden, however, was more cautious than Palmer. He did not begin therapy for quotidian fever cases until after the fourth paroxysm. Some tertian fever victims received their initial dose of the alkaloid after the third episode. Other patients received nothing until the fourth paroxysm had subsided (Garden 1860:403 [Table 2]). This protocol guaranteed that the test subject was firmly in the grip of whatever was responsible for the fever. Depending upon how soon a purgative was given after being admitted into the hospital, quotidian participants were forced to wait four days or more before receiving any of the alkaloid. The corresponding period for tertian patients ranged between three and twelve days.

Quotidian subjects experienced an average of 2.48 paroxysms after the first dose of anarcotine and tertian patients slightly more at 2.54. The numbers pleased Garden. He was even more pleased upon discovering that in "nearly one-fourth of all cases, and in more than one-fourth of the quotidian fevers, the first doses checked the fever so that it never returned" (1860:405). The alkaloid thus far seemed to be a panacea for 'fever'; it very quickly 'cured' one-quarter of all cases and greater than 25 percent of 'quotidian fever' subjects. Garden then emphasized the speed with which anarcotine worked its magic with some complicated summary statements about "the average return of fever in the whole number of cases cured" for quotidian and tertian victims. The way in which the data are presented accentuates the power of anarcotine while deflecting attention away from its limitations.

Garden's Summary Statements: Accentuating the Positive

As stated above, quotidian fever subjects had an average of 2.4 paroxysms after their first dose of anarcotine. The number for tertian patients was 2.54 episodes. But 64 percent of the 154 quotidian individuals did not even reach the average of 2.4 and 67.57 percent of the forty tertian people also fell below the average for their category. Garden combined the two sets of data to conclude that "in 64.7 percent of the whole cases; that is, in nearly two-thirds of the cases treated, the fever was cured after the return of the second paroxysm" (1860:406).

Ten percent of quotidian victims experienced yet another paroxysm after the initial dose. The alkaloid was again slightly less effective for tertian patients; 10.81 percent suffered a third outbreak of elevated temperature before Garden declared them "cured." The number of people in both categories having the third bout was 10.16 percent of the entire sample. He was delighted with the results; 74.86 percent of the patients whose responses were documented experienced three or fewer episodes of "fever." Garden's summary statement now ends. Other than listing statistics, he says nothing about the remaining 25.98 percent less fortunate patients. The reactions of these people—more than one-fourth of his test subjects—did not dissuade him from proclaiming that anarcotine "as an anti-periodic" still "deserves well at the hands of the profession" (Garden 1860:406). The patients in this more "resistant" group of patients did have to ingest greater amounts of anarcotine over a longer time compared to their "cured" colleagues. They also suffered additional fever episodes. A majority was eventually 'cured'; the remainder would have remained sick even if Garden had not been forced to conclude the experiment at the end of June 1860. However, the data Garden introduced before these summary statements yield a less glowing evaluation of the alkaloid.

The Limitations of Garden's Analysis

The criterion W. J. Palmer used to evaluate anarcotine was its effect upon the intensity plus the duration of each paroxysm appearing after the initial dose. Dr. Garden provided no comparable information about intensity and duration. The closest approximation to this kind of information is found in table 4 of the 1860 article. It is entitled "Shewing [sic] the Number of Paroxysms After the First Administration of Anarcotine with Percentage." This book's table 3 ["Condensation of Statistics in Dr. Garden's Table 4: 'Shewing [sic] the Number of Paroxysms After the First Administration of Anarcotine with Percentage.'"] condenses statistics in Garden's table. It is referred to in the following discussion as table 3 [Condensation]. Several paragraphs require citation of data from Garden's more detailed table 4. These occasions are identified by Garden (Garden 1860:405 [Table 4]).

Dr. Garden excluded the aforementioned seven failures from his tabulations. They are not mentioned in his table 4, and are therefore absent from table 3 [Condensation]. This omission suggests that severity was a more serious problem for the entire group than his statistics indicate. There is no question that the number of paroxysms all patients experienced before their 'cure' was of paramount importance for judging the value of anarcotine. But just as significant was documenting the length of time a patient had to endure a recurrence of misery as well as an estimation of its intensity, or how much discomfort the victim was experiencing during each paroxysm. Garden's argument for the alkaloid would have been stronger if he had addressed these issues. His experiment had other limitations.

Garden's exclusion of the four quotidian and three tertian patients who either experienced increased severity of symptoms, or were completely unresponsive to "further treatment," is not insignificant. These cases might be examples of what witnesses testifying before the Royal Commission suggested thirty-five years later; that people reacting negatively or not at all to opium (hence to anarcotine) were suffering from a disease etiologically distinct from the malady affecting individuals having positive responses. Four of Garden's seven negative cases were tertian patients compared to only three for the far more numerous quotidian sufferers. It is possible that some of these thirty-seven tertian victims did have the kind of malaria envisaged by splitters testifying before the Royal Commission during 1893–1894. Anarcotine does something to people with daily fevers of diverse origins. But a high probability exists for it being far less instrumental in restoring health to victims suffering from plasmodia-induced malaria.

There is no question, however, that the omission of these seven subjects exaggerated the ability of anarcotine to combat 'fever.' The percentages in each of the "response" categories become more modest with the inclusion of these people. Table 3 [Condensation] lists a total of thirty-nine quotidian fever patients suffering four to twelve paroxysms after initial exposure to the alkaloid. The number for tertian fever patients is eight. The total for both kinds of fever, therefore, was forty-seven people. Adding Garden's seven excluded cases increases the number of individuals demonstrating "varying degrees of recalcitrance" (including "complete imperviousness") to a grand total of fifty-four individuals. This means that 27.83 percent of the 194 people participating in the entire study responded neither as favorably nor as rapidly to the alkaloid as Roberts proclaimed in his 1895 Royal Commission report.

Garden's failure to indicate what phase of the nine-month study these seven individuals were involved in also complicates the issue. Their participation in the experiment, and failure to be restored to "health" during the "virulent" phase, further weakens any claim that anarcotine was a potent remedy for an outbreak of severe proportions. The alkaloid was even less impressive for periods of moderate intensity if the seven individuals' involvement in the study was restricted to early February through 30 June 1860. The responses of a group representing almost 28 percent of the participants in the experiment should have qualified Garden's optimism and tempered Sir William Roberts' enthusiasm about anarcotine. It did not.

Garden's lack of specificity raises other questions. He tells us how many military police Battalion Hospital participants and Jail Hospital patients (684) were treated during the entire nine months. He does not do this for the 194 individuals for whom he kept records. Yet, these were the patients who enabled him to make conclusions. We do not know how many of these 194 documented cases were members of the elite, atypical category of subjects, or how many were prison inmates who more closely approximated the physical and psychological condition of the general population.

There is another problem with the 194 subjects. Garden indicated the nine-month experiment involved 154 quotidian and forty tertian fever patients but he did not cite the number of each fever type appearing in each of the study's two phases. How many quotidian and tertian policemen were treated during either the "virulent" months or the less severe months after January 1860 is not indicated. We therefore cannot conclude if anarcotine was more potent for quotidian sufferers during the "virulent" period as compared to the more moderate months. We also are unable to say anything definite about tertian patients' experiences in each of the two phases.

The gaps in Garden's analysis, therefore, are significant. The absence of data specifying how many jail patients and policemen had quotidian and tertian fever, respectively, detracts from the study's applicability to a wider audience. The problem is compounded by not knowing how many of the 194 subjects for whom records were maintained were military policemen or in jail. Inclusion of these statistics, especially for prison patients, would have provided a more accurate estimation about the average Indian citizen's responses to the alkaloid for either kind of fever. The absence of such material renders Garden's work much less useful for predicting the impact of anarcotine upon people inhabiting a nonlaboratory, nonhospital environment.

Sir William Roberts' Selective, Misleading Use of Garden's Statistics

Sir William Roberts used fragments of Garden's data about averages to portray anarcotine in a very favorable way. He said Garden "rapidly cured" 187 of the 194 patients with doses ranging from only one and one-half to three grains (GBO [Roberts] 1895:VI:111).[22] A quick reading gives an impression that miniscule amounts restored almost everybody to health. The key word is "doses." Roberts was referring to an individual dose, each one varying from one and one-half to three grains. He said nothing about the number of doses each patient required before being declared "well." Roberts also ignored Garden's important distinction between "cure" and "convalescence," and he said nothing about the amount of anarcotine administered in each of these categories.

The Number of Doses Required for Restoration of "Health"

Garden's numbers do not support Roberts' claim about one and one-half to three grains. Garden said the initial dose of anarcotine "checked the fever so that it never returned" in "nearly one-fourth of all cases, and in more than one-fourth of the quotidian fevers" (1860:405). Table 3 [Condensation] specifies that thirty-nine of the 150 quotidian and three of the thirty-seven tertian fever patients were "rapidly cured"; forty-two cases from a total of 187. This indicates 26 percent of quotidian and only 8.1 percent of tertian sufferers, a combined average of 22.46 percent of participants in the nine-month study, were ostensibly free from subsequent attacks after their first dose of the alkaloid. Being able to quickly cure slightly more than one out of five people looks good, but Garden needed much anarcotine to do it.

Table 3 [Condensation] indicates thirty-nine quotidian and three tertian patients were 'cured' after one dose of anarcotine. In other words, they had no recurrence of 'fever.' Garden classified the people as "rapidly cured." Table 4 (a reproduction of table 5 in Garden's 1860 article) lists the amount of anarcotine required for the "rapidly cured" thirty-nine quotidian and three tertian patients. Quotidian fever sufferers needed 6.19 grains for their 'cure.' Tertian victims required five grains. Each group needed much more than Roberts' one and one-half to three grains. His statement is an exaggeration of the alkaloid's therapeutic status.

Garden's category of "rapidly cured" patients included more than the thirty-nine quotidian and three tertian fever victims. An unnumbered table in his article reveals that people having one to as many as three paroxysms after initial exposure to anarcotine are also in the category (Garden 1860:405).

According to table 3 [Condensation], ninety-eight out of a total of 187 patients (for whom Roberts had data) experienced one to three episodes of elevated temperature after ingesting the alkaloid for the first time. Table 3 [Condensation] also indicates that the number of quotidian fever sufferers in the one-to-three paroxysm category was seventy-two (out of a total of 150 people in the quotidian category). The tally for tertian fever victims experiencing one to three episodes before their 'cure' was twenty-six (out of a total of thirty-seven tertian patients).

Table 3 [Condensation], however, does not specify how many "rapidly cured" people in each category (quotidian and tertian) suffered one, two, or three bouts of 'fever.' Table 4 in Garden's 1860 article does have these details. These statistics further challenge the veracity of Roberts' statement about the power of anarcotine to "rapidly cure." Thirty-three (22 percent) of the 150 quotidian patients and twelve (32.43 percent) of the thirty-seven tertian sufferers experienced one attack after their initial dose of anarcotine before becoming "healthy" (Garden 1860:405 [Table 4]). These people should have ingested an average of three to six grains (two doses of anarcotine) according to Roberts' scenario. Garden's anarcotine data (table 5 in the 1860 publication) indicate otherwise.

As mentioned above, Garden's alkaloid tabulations are reproduced in this book's table 4. The title of table 4 is "Statistics in Dr. Garden's Table 5: 'Shewing [sic] Average Amount of Anarcotine Taken Before and After Cessation of Fever According to the Numbers of Paroxysms.'" Henceforth, citations from this source are identified by an abbreviated title: table 4 [Statistics].

Table 4 [Statistics] denotes that thirty-three quotidian sufferers required an average of 10.17 grains. The average tertian patient needed 17.54 grains; an amount more than 300 percent higher than their more fortunate tertian colleagues who were 'cured' after only one five-grain dose, and much higher than Roberts' calculation of no more than six grains.

Twenty-four quotidian and ten tertian patients suffered two attacks after initial exposure to anarcotine (Garden 1860:405 [Table 4]). Their experience also challenges Roberts' proclamation about small, incremental dosage. These people—16 percent and 27.02 percent of their fever types, respectively—should have consumed an average of only four and one-half to nine grains before enjoying a 'cure' if Roberts was correct. They did not; the quotidian group averaged 15.70

grains and the tertian subjects needed 26.40 grains (table 4 [Statistics]). The quotidian total is almost 400 percent, and the tertian figure is 300 percent, higher than Roberts' assessment.

The last category Garden considered as "rapidly cured" were people having three paroxysms after the first dose of anarcotine. Table 4 in Garden's 1860 article (page 405) shows that he placed fifteen quotidian and four tertian patients in this category. The fifteen quotidian patients consumed an average of 19.26 grains (table 4 [Statistics]). They represent 10 percent of the total number (150) of Garden's documented quotidian participants. The four tertian victims, or 10.81 percent of the thirty-seven individuals, had to ingest much more—32.37 grains—before they were "healthy" (table 4 [Statistics]). Roberts' scenario, however, posited a minimum average of six and a maximum average of twelve grains for victims of both types of 'fever.'

Roberts' Misplaced Enthusiasm about "Rapidly Cured" Patients

Table 3 [Condensation] indicates 74 percent of the quotidian and 78.36 percent of the tertian patients were "rapidly cured." The number of 'fever' attacks these people experienced following the initial dose of anarcotine ranged from zero to three. Thirty-nine quotidian sufferers (26 percent) of the total of 150 patients in this category were free from 'fever' after the first exposure to the alkaloid. Seventy-two quotidian patients (48 percent of the total) experienced one to three paroxysms before their 'cure.' The 74 percent "rapidly cured" quotidian statistic is impressive. So are the numbers for tertian fever victims. Table 3 [Condensation] reveals that out of a total of thirty-seven patients in this category, three victims (8.10 percent) suffered no recurrence of 'fever' after first ingesting anarcotine. Twenty-six people (70.26 percent) suffering from tertian fever endured from one to three paroxysms after their initial dose of the alkaloid.

Garden combined these quotidian and tertian cases. Then, as stated above, he declared that 74.86 percent of the 187 participants in the nine-month study had been quickly restored to "health." Furthermore, far fewer victims in either 'fever' category endured more than three episodes of misery before they were 'cured.' Thirty-nine quotidian and nine tertian victims experienced from four to twelve recurrences. This small number of alkaloid-resistant cases (48 people) and the 74.86 percent "rapidly cured" figure is persuasive. It undoubtedly prompted Roberts' celebration of the potency of one and one-half to three grains of anarcotine. However, entries in table 4 [Statistics] for quantities required to 'cure' in each category of "number of returning fevers" do not support Roberts' declaration. The discrepancy between the scenario that Roberts wanted the Royal Commission to accept as valid and what occurred during 1859 and 1860 is huge.

The data Garden obtained from people experiencing more than three subsequent fevers contradict Roberts' assertion about requisite minimal and maximum amounts of anarcotine to 'cure.' And the fate of two admittedly exceptional tertian patients in this four-to-twelve paroxysm category truly challenges Roberts' argument. One man had five recurring fevers. The other person endured six episodes. The first subject should have needed an average of seven and one-half to fifteen grains of anarcotine if Roberts was right; the second between nine and eighteen grains. The actual amounts Garden cited for the first and second victims are 151 and 150 grains respectively. Roberts ignored the startling discrepancy and he said nothing about another issue that Garden had identified. The reason for his silence is that it also challenged the anarcotine argument's credibility.

Garden's Distinction between "Cure" and "Convalescence"

None of Garden's 187 patients enjoyed permanent relief from fever. Each man suffered a relapse. These episodes were especially common during the "virulent" phase from 10 October through January 1860. The unexpected reappearance of paroxysms in people seemingly restored to health made it necessary to give more doses of anarcotine. The amounts were equal to the quantities ingested for the initial 'cure,' and some cases required from three to eleven times as much.[23] Garden referred to this "relapse" period as "convalescence." The aforementioned unfortunate tertian patient with six recurring fevers who needed 150 grains for a 'cure' required the same amount for his "convalescence," a grand total of 300 grains. The other tertian sufferer ingesting 151 grains needed thirty-nine more, or 189 grains, before being diagnosed as "healthy." They were not the only tertian individuals exceeding 100 grains for both periods. One person with eight recurring fevers consumed 157 grains; 118 in the first period and thirty-nine grains during "convalescence." Still another person required eighty-two grains, and an additional twenty-seven for a combined total of 109 grains. He had survived eleven paroxysms after the first exposure to anarcotine (Garden 1860:417–18 [Table B, Patients #9 and #20]). Both men far exceeded the amount needed for a 'cure' if Roberts' one and one-half to three grain scenario is accepted. The discrepancy is exacerbated when consumption totals for the two men during their "convalescence," as well as amounts for the two "exceptional" tertian cases, are added to the tally.

These statistics show that Roberts was not uttering an untruth; he simply was not saying anything profound about the power of anarcotine to 'cure' tertian 'fever' victims. The "relapse" statistics for Garden's documented quotidian patients further illuminate the mundane status of Roberts' conclusion.

One quotidian patient 'cured' with a single dose of three grains required thirty-eight more during "convalescence" (Garden 1860:414 [Table A, Patient #60]. Forty-one grains seem modest, but it was much greater than the amount predicted by Roberts' definition of 'cure.' Consumption statistics for other quotidian patients during "cure" and "convalescence" periods also dispute the "rapid" therapeutic capability of anarcotine. Garden cited total amounts of 133, 115, 108, 99, 93, 90, 88, 85, 82, 79, 77 grains plus two people requiring 76 grains. Another person needed 75 grains and one required 70.5. Two more people ingested 70 grains (Garden 1860:413–17).[24] Many patients fell within the 50 to high-60 grain range for the two periods, but Garden's use of averages minimized their significance.

Garden calculated the average amount of anarcotine required for a 'cure' among quotidian patients at 19.37 grains plus another 15.8 during "convalescence." The combined average was 35.17 grains (Garden 1860:407). A tertian sufferer needed 39.5 grains just for a 'cure,' almost double the amount for a quotidian patient, and still greater than a quotidian individual's "cure" plus "convalescence" periods. Tertian patients were clearly more resistant to whatever anarcotine was thought capable of doing. These people consumed an additional 18.3 grains during an average "convalescence," culminating in a total figure of 57.8 grains for both periods. Garden glossed over the contrast by merging the quotidian and tertian statistics. This resulted in an average requirement of 22.7 grains for one person's "cure" and 16.3 grains for a "convalescence," a total of only "39 grains per case" (Garden 1860:407–08). Roberts did not mention Garden's discrete or averaged high consumption requirements.

Cognizance of pre-1895 plasmodia research also did not alter Roberts' conception of 'malaria' and the status of *Papaver somniferum Linn* in eradicating it. He looked favorably upon the discoveries of Laveran, Marchiafava, Bignami, and Mannaberg in Germany. But their work, he contended, would likely increase, not decrease, the importance of Indian opium, specifically anarcotine, "in the treatment of Indian fevers in the future." These researchers had identified a microorganism with several types as "the infective material of malarial fevers" and each type, according to Roberts, caused a distinct kind of fever. Furthermore, he concluded that the testimony of witnesses, and the Palmer and Garden experiments, proved that anarcotine was superior to quinine as an antidote for most of these 'malarial poisons.' This capability would eventually elevate the substance to a position of importance equal to the cinchona alkaloid (GBO [Roberts] 1895:VI:112). Roberts said nothing about vector research. This omission included the pre-1895 pioneering investigations of Patrick Manson in China, Manson's work in England before 1895, and the man's collaboration with Ronald Ross in India. The Royal Commission did not summon these two qualified men to testify, and the opium volumes contain no references to their research.

SIR WILLIAM ROBERTS: A MOST SUITABLE PERSON AT THE MOST APPROPRIATE TIME?

Lord Brassey and fellow members of the Royal Commission attached "great weight" to the testimony of the "medical witnesses." And lest anyone question the accuracy of what Indian Medical Service personnel said, the final report describes their rigorous training and extols their impeccable competency (GBO [Final Report] 1895:VI:15–16). Sir William Roberts' reliance upon these people, therefore, could not be faulted. His positive evaluation of the opium habit and its efficacy in combating the misery engendered by 'malarial diseases' was incorporated into the Commission's final report. The Commission, however, was silent about the credentials of the many nonmedical witnesses selected by the Government of India to testify.

Henry J. Wilson, the Commission's one Member of Parliament, was the exception. So obvious during the hearings, his dismay and skepticism culminated in a written objection to the Commission. He complained that

> the whole of the facts were [not] presented to us with the impartiality and completeness due to such an inquiry. The Report adopted by my colleagues appears to me to partake more of the character of an elaborate defence of the opium trade of the East India Company, and of the present Government of India, than of a judicial pronouncement on the immediate questions submitted to us. On this ground also, as well as for the reasons already given, I am unable to join in it. (GBO [Wilson–Minute of Dissent] 1895:VI:151)

Wilson also condemned the Government of India for intimidating witnesses, and for doing nothing to ensure that witnesses with different viewpoints could, or would, appear before the Commission. He also chastised British officials for deliberately withholding documents germane to making an accurate assessment of the opium situation in India (GBO [Wilson–Appendix C] 1895:VI:161–62). He claimed that Lord Brassey, upon being informed of these sentiments, prohibited him from participating in writing the Commission's Final Report. Lord Brassey responded by saying this had been a suggestion, not an order. In any case, Wilson refused to sign the document (GBO [Wilson–Minute of Dissent] 1895:VI:151).

Wilson's objections to Roberts' analysis were just as pointed. He lamented the man's reliance upon dubious witnesses and rejected all conclusions based upon their pronouncements. The evidence regarding opium eating in British India was, at best, contradictory. Most Indians themselves did not agree about how widespread the habit was in the country and how useful it was for maladies. Furthermore, Wilson asserted, "from the evidence on which they are founded . . . the popular ideas which seem to prevail among Europeans in India are entirely irreconcilable with the actual facts" (GBO [Wilson–Minute of Dissent] 1895:VI:143).[25] He acknowledged that some people in India consumed the drug on a daily basis, but most of them did so

> with the object of relieving pain, although it may have no permanent effect on the cause of the pain. The theory was advanced [that opium eating] . . . originated . . . [for the] purpose of repressing some positive ailment, or to avoid disease which climatic or other conditions render probable. In accordance with this theory evidence was given . . . [o]n the other hand, this view was strongly controverted by other witnesses . . . who disputed the value of opium as a prophylactic against fever, or as a remedy in the disease, and as regards many parts of India there was no such belief amongst the natives. (GBO [Wilson–Minute of Dissent] 1895:VI:143)

Wilson's knowledge of allopathic medicine strengthened the negative evaluation of Roberts' medical report. He said claims about moderate consumption of opium being beneficial, especially as a preventive against 'malarial fever,' had no credibility. Another excerpt from Wilson's dissent clearly conveys his feelings about the hearings. He declared that "[c]opious references to important medical evidence will be found in the Notes, showing that this prophylactic theory is an entirely new one; not taught in the medical schools; never heard of by many practitioners; that opium is not used or recommended by many of those who have heard of the theory; that many practitioners who profess to believe in it prefer other remedies; that other practitioners, both pro-opiumists and anti-opiumists, deny altogether that opium does possess any such prophylactic properties; and that vast numbers of the people have no knowledge of or belief in opium as a preventive of fever" (GBO [Wilson–Minute of Dissent] 1895:VI:145).

Wilson then implied that policy makers for the Government of India were either ignorant or hypocritical. This accusation included Roberts.

> It is incredible that if the highest medical and other authorities in India seriously believed in this prophylactic use of opium that they should have allowed so many members of the medical service to remain in ignorance of it. The opinion of the Government of Madras was indicated when a complaint was made that they were teaching the people of certain tracts to rely on opium as a febrifuge, for they replied that so far from that 'we are doing all we can to gradually wean them from their hereditary habit of using it on all occasions.' (GBO [Wilson–Minute of Dissent] 1895:VI:145)

Wilson was decidedly unimpressed with the witnesses who claimed that opium eating was a prophylactic or febrifuge for 'malaria' or 'fever.' Supported by insights from Anglo-European medicine, he concluded the drug provided only a temporary relief from pain (GBO [Wilson–Minute of Dissent] 1895:VI:150). Wilson's condemnation of Roberts and the dubious 'evidence' became part of the post-1895 anti-opiumist effort to discredit the Royal Commission's recommendations (Johnson 1975:315).

The Enduring Condemnation of Sir William Roberts and the Royal Commission's Medical 'Evidence' in the Post-1894–1895 Era

According to the *British Medical Journal*, Sir William Roberts "always looked back on his experience in India on this Commission as one of the most interesting events of his life" (1899:1065). It most likely was also the most controversial public engagement because Roberts defended himself soon after returning from India. He reiterated the anarcotine argument in London. The occasion was his address at the opening of the Pharmacology and Therapeutics section of the annual meeting of the British Medical Association. The presentation was brief and contained nothing new (Roberts 1895:405–06). It also did not dispel the hostility of his detractors.

The earliest critiques discrediting the Royal Commission hearings about all topics pertaining to the trade also implicated Roberts.[26] Medical professionals and civilians in India and in other countries immediately condemned his logic, naiveté, and lack of objectivity. The aforementioned *Indian Medical Record* publication, for example, included a very negative commentary of Roberts' analysis. The periodical's editors asked why he had been selected as the Royal Commission's medical authority. Roberts also was criticized for creating a bogus theory to resolve obvious contradictions in the oral evidence he deigned to consider. And his argument for anarcotine was chastised as outdated and basically nonsense.

Much of the evidence to which Roberts was exposed, according to these skeptics, was "unreliable, erroneous, and misleading." He also was too ignorant about India to realize he was being duped. Even knowing what was occurring might not have made a difference; the man was committed to one side of the controversy before arriving in India. He held a position in medical circles analogous to that of Sir W. B. Richardson in Great Britain. If Richardson, who was famous for "having very pronounced views regarding the effects of alcohol upon the human organism, were to be selected as an expert to weigh evidence and finally to write an authoritative report which would settle the scientific, social and physiological aspects of the alcohol question, an outcry would immediately be raised that the whole question had been put at the mercy of a bigoted temperance advocate" (*IMR* 1895:2).

Roberts was no different. His mind was not a *tabula rasa* and, according to his critics, he ignored facts that challenged his scientific outlook. He had already declared that dietary customs were a reflection of profound instincts, and that they satisfied fundamental wants in human beings. People consumed things because they had to do so, and what they ingested rarely was harmful to most of them. To think otherwise—even more so to act upon contrary beliefs—was to engage in "ignorant meddling" (Roberts, quoted in *IMR* 1895:3). The Royal Commission evidence that Roberts valued justified opium being added to the list of acceptable entities to ingest.

Roberts also was condemned for being "absurd" as well as hardheaded. In the 1880s dietetic lectures, he claimed that Europeans' consumption of tea, coffee, and cocoa was harmless. Eating meat also was beneficial. Proof for these assertions, according to Roberts, was the "continued progress of these nations, and their increasing ascendancy among the nations of the world" (Roberts, quoted in *IMR* 1895:3). Roberts' statements were now used to ridicule his opium argument.

> If we substitute 'opium' for 'tea and coffee' and Asia for [European] 'Nations' . . . it might read thus: That the effects of opium have not been favorable to the material progress and advancement of Asia (especially India) is demonstrated by her backwardness, poverty, degeneration, and continued dependence among the nations of the world. (*IMR* 1895:3)

Roberts' critics asserted that the India Office in London had indeed made a wise decision to select him for the Royal Commission appointment. The man had "pronounced and fixed views entirely in favor of [the aforementioned] food accessories" and it was improbable that anything would make him "undo his lectures" or "reject opinions which had gained . . . him a certain reputation." The scientific community, furthermore, was not told about his possible appointment, and it would have rejected the man as "eminently disqualified to sit on any such Commission." Witnesses nominated by the Government of India were aware of Roberts' intellectual proclivities and they tailored their comments accordingly. This "medical expert" had been "misled, hoodwinked, and betrayed into the most glaring errors" (*IMR* 1895:4).

The *Indian Medical Record* was being diplomatic when it blamed others for Roberts' behavior. He could have avoided these deficiencies by allowing contradictory evidence to modify his convictions. He instead invented theory to resolve the difficulty. Roberts' critics said an illustration of this trait was his discussion about "irregularities and anomalies" involving heavy opium consumption in areas of minimal "malaria" and meager use of the drug in very unhealthy locales. The "dual character of the opium habit with its medicinal side and its euphoric side" partially explained the contradiction (Roberts, quoted *IMR* 1895:3–4). Roberts used "euphoric" to signify a person "feeling perfectly well and able to bear pain and anxiety easily" (*IMR* 1895:5). People wanting only to feel good explained why large amounts of the drug were consumed in the 'malaria-free' areas of the Punjab and Rajputana. This idea, according to the *Indian Medical Record*, was a new—and questionable—way of classifying the drug. Western scientists had "been accustomed to look upon opium as possessing various distinct properties—anodyne, hypnotic and sedative . . . here it is divided into 'euphoric' and medicinal or antiperiodic [and] only its antiperiodic properties . . . would cause a demand for its use in low-lying, damp and malarious districts" (*IMR* 1895:5).

Roberts also concluded that enclaves of South Asian citizens had evolved different reactions to the drug. This had occurred during many centuries of opium use. These variations were now a consequence of genetic endowment, and they were drastically different from the responses of people belonging to "European nations." Critics chastised Roberts for engaging in such speculation. How could it be, the *Indian Medical Record* asked, that "whole provinces and races have developed this peculiar instinct for appreciating only one side of the drug, and that it is not anodyne, hypnotic or sedative qualities, but a new quality called 'euphoric,' or 'making to feel well'?" (1895:6). Roberts provided no proof, but the notion enabled him to explain why communities of Sikhs and Muslims in healthy locales indulged themselves whereas Hindus, Buddhists, Christians, animists, and atheists living in the same place might abstain from the habit. Roberts' antagonists said his idea was nothing more than a convenient way to rationalize demographic inconsistencies.

Roberts' opponents continued to express outrage into the twentieth century. The Crafts and Leitch 1911 condemnation about the Commission and the "stinking sepulcher of 'infernal revenue'" was harsh, but these missionaries did have a point. The Royal Commission's mission was indeed linked to revenue and so was Roberts' anarcotine argument.

NOTES

1. Surgeon-Major R. Cobb testified on 25 November 1893, the thirteenth day of the hearings. See GBOW [Cobb] 1894:II:84–85.

2. See question twelve and the responses of Mr. Hare (page 226), Dr. B. C. Atterbury (page 232), Mr. Thomas W. Duff (page 259), Reverend H. J. Brown (page 284), Consul R. W. Hurst (page 322), Consul R. W. Mansfield (page 335), and Dr. J. H. Lowry (page 336). See GBO [Her Majesty's Minister in China] 1894:V:212–343.

3. Roberts quotes Wace in a footnote in the section "Opium as a Remedy and Prophylactic Against Malaria" (GBO [Roberts] 1895:VI:109).

4. Sixty-one residents of Hong Kong received the questionnaire (GBO [Singapore, Penang, and Hong Kong] 1894:V:205). British authorities classified them as "Orientals," "Officials," "Medical (nonofficials)," and "Merchants and others." The "Orientals" (a total of twenty-eight) consisted of eight Indians, five Parsees, five Persians, and ten Chinese. There were twelve "Officials"—all were British. The six "Medical (nonofficial)" respondents included one Chinese doctor. The other five were British or European medical practitioners. The category of "Merchants and others" included British nationals, Europeans, and people from each group of "Orientals." Fifteen individuals were in this category (GBO [Singapore, Penang, and Hong Kong] 1894:V:184–212).

A "government analyst" for the British consulate also answered the questionnaire. The person is not listed as having been sent the document and the source of his comments is unstated. Nonetheless, he says that Hong Kong natives do not believe opium prevents 'malaria' or 'fever.' Furthermore, no European or British resident of the colony (with or without medical training) believes opium consumption (eating or smoking) functions as a prophylactic for these afflictions (GBO [Singapore, Penang, and Hong Kong] 1894:V:208–09).

5. The data do not include mortality rates for the native states.

6. Roberts was also mistaken. In a discussion about diagnostic sophistication in South Asia as of 1908, the *Indian Medical Gazette* reveals why. The editors "must emphasise [sic] the fact that as in modern days up till a dozen years ago many other specific fevers were included in the comfortable and comprehensive term 'malaria.'" Furthermore, although in "recent years the tendency has been to exclude many fevers from the category of malaria . . . we have not completely done this even yet." An example of the mistake still being made is a malady they identify as "Leishman-Donovan Infection." "Up 'til a few years ago," they tell us, "thousands of cases of this infection were called 'malaria,' and in every case where the vital statistics of an Indian village or district have been checked, the result has been to show that malaria as a factor in mortality has been grossly exaggerated." (*IMG* 1908:24). The implication of these 1908 comments is clear. Many cases of the sickness that Roberts believed to be malaria actually were the product of a discrete, fever-producing malady. This sickness was unrelated to many other afflictions that were classified under the term 'malaria.'

7. Malwa opium is the name of the drug produced by quasi-independent native states located in two administrative agencies. A small portion of Malwa opium came from two districts under direct British jurisdiction.

8. Roberts used the word anarcotine instead of narcotine. The reason for the change is explained at the beginning of the section of this chapter describing W. J. Palmer's research. The term "anarcotine" is then used in the rest of this chapter.

9. See especially the previously mentioned J. MacCulloch 1830; G. M. Sternberg 1884:113–14, 179–80; W. J. Moore 1886b and *JAMA* 1887:265–66 for paroxysms of etiologically distinct maladies subsumed under the category called 'malaria.' Also consult T. W. Jetson 1832–33:41, and E. H. Janes 1862:149. W. Tully (1832:1–12, 37–44, 56–63) describes the effects of the alkaloid upon healthy individuals, including himself. The remaining pre-1895 articles discuss the alkaloid's chemical composition. As mentioned in the opening chapter, these include G. H. Beckett & C. R. Wright 1875:537–85; J. Blyth 1843–45:33–39; A. Matthiessen & G. C. Foster 1863–64:153:345, 1867, 1868:157:687, 1869, and 1870:159:66. Other sources are W. Tully 1832:1–12, 37–44, 56–63; T. G. Wormley 1859–60:277–85, and 1860:158, 170.

10. Dr. William O'Shaughnessy's name is spelled differently in the 1838 authored by him and in the 1839 *AJMS* comment. Both publications were consulted. The *AJMS* material indicates "O'Shaughnessey," and the 1838 article spells it "O'Shaughnessy." The latter version is used because the 1838 publication is the principal source of data for the topic.

O'Shaughnessy's comment was published as "On Narcotine as a Substitute for Quinine in Intermittent Fevers" in the *AJMS* 1838:194–95). The periodical's editors say the total number of cases was sixty. Adding twenty-seven and thirty-two results in fifty-nine individuals, not sixty.

Sir William Roberts might have read the original Calcutta Medical Society transactions. They were unavailable to this author. See 1838 "Quotidian of Nine Months' Duration Cured by Narcotine" *IJMPS* 3:New Series:710–11) for details of O'Shaughnessy's narcotine research. Abstracts are found in *BFMR* 1839 1839:8:no. 263:839, and in *LAN* 1839:2:606.

11. Arsenic during the era was a remedy for 'malarial fever' and other ailments.

12. The *AJMS* article does not indicate if R. O'Shaughnessy and Dr. William B. O'Shaughnessy were related to each other.

13. Roberts overstated the case. In a letter dated 7 October 1875, T. W. Sheppard, principal assistant of the Benares Opium Agency, says "there was but a very small demand for this alkaloid" before 1858–59 (GBO [Gregory–Enclosure 74] 1894:V:81–82).

14. W. J. Palmer held several positions in Ghazipur. He was "civil assistant surgeon" from 6 November 1857 until the "end of September 1859" and more than likely held the position after the latter date. As of 15 November, he also was the "1st assistant and opium examiner" (GBO [Gregory–Enclosures 169 & 192] 1894:V:78–9).

15. Roberts did not mention this disenchantment in his discussion about O'Shaughnessy. See GBO [Gregory–Enclosure 74] 1894:V:81–82). Roberts also is silent about the relevance of the administration's early 1860 decision to establish cinchona plantations for quinine extraction. See Appendix C for details of cinchona cultivation in South Asia.

16. The indents between 4 April 1860 and 23 January 1894 are found in "Statement Showing the Quantity of Narcotine issued to the Medical Department before 1878," and "Statement of Narcotine supplied from 1876 to January 1894" (GBO [Gregory–Statement] 1894:V:82).

17. The Palmer and Garden spelling and capitalization of experiment locations and sources of patients is followed in the chapter narrative. The slight difference in style between the two is also honored.

18. Dr. A. Garden did the same thing. His rationale was that the "only other possible negative consequence in giving anarcotine to fever patients" is the need to pay "careful attention to the state of the bowels." The alkaloid has a "great tendency to produce constipation, whereby its favorable action is impeded." Garden describes a patient "suffering from Quotidian fever who was not responding to anarcotine, as much as doses of 6 grains per administration. The patient was constipated, but [t]he purgative . . . seemed to act like a charm [and] [f]rom that day, he had no return of fever" (1860:412).

19. Palmer did not try to determine if anarcotine was a prophylactic: that ingesting the substance prevented a healthy person from becoming sick with 'fever,' 'malarial disease,' and so forth. He concentrated upon establishing the alkaloid as a febrifuge or cure for people already sick. He wanted to know if the substance precluded, with varying degrees of success, the recurrent bouts of elevated temperature. Palmer obtained his results by following a careful, controlled protocol with a nonrepresentative group of patients.

20. This is quotidian fever patient #1 in table A. Table A is located between pages 413 and 417 of Garden's 1860 article.

21. Garden frequently capitalized Jail Hospital when identifying the source of patients. The trait is retained in the chapter narrative.

22. Roberts used one to three grains of anarcotine when discussing the combined effort of Palmer and Garden. But in a separate review of Garden's work, Roberts acknowledges that the man's success resulted from employing one and one-half to three grains. As mentioned before, the difference of one-half grain seems insignificance but it has a significant cumulative consequence. This point is addressed later in the book.

23. The title of table 3 is "Condensation of Statistics in Garden's Table 4: 'Shewing Average Amount of Anarcotine Taken Before and After Cessation of Fever According to the Numbers of Paroxysms.'" The table lists no relapses for tertian patients having seven, nine, ten, or twelve paroxysms after their first dose of anarcotine. At first glance this suggests that tertian sufferers fared better than their quotidian colleagues did. This is not the case. Garden documented no tertian subjects experiencing these numbers of recurring fevers. Everybody treated by Garden, therefore, had a relapse after their 'cure.'

24. See table A in Dr. A. Garden 1860:413–17. These are patient numbers: 104, 73, 118, 123, 115, 14, 63, 103, 128, 120, 27, 76 and 80, 11, and 14.

25. Henry Wilson lists the names and page locations of witnesses whose testimony he claimed Roberts intentionally ignored. He says these witnesses' comments illustrate opium's alleged status as a 'malarial' prophylactic and febrifuge was contrived and imaginary (GBO [Wilson–Note A. to par.2] 1895:VI:159).

26. See Joshua Rowntree (1895). Also see his 1905 publication and its 1908 edition. Arnold Foster said much "evidence" found in the "seven volumes, weighing together over fourteen pounds, and containing 2,550 pages, of which nearly 2,000 are closely printed in double columns and small type," was biased in favor of the Government of India, inaccurate or fabricated (1896:2). Two other articles appearing in the same periodical (*China Medical [Missionary] Journal*) support and refute Roberts' observations. P. B. Cousland said the man's observations about the effects of opium smoking were inapplicable to China (1896:10:1:21). In a 1908 issue of the same publication, Dr. J. A. Otte presented comments from a few individuals agreeing with Roberts' notion about the usefulness of anarcotine and opium for "malaria." Otte quoted sentences out of context. Many of the comments also date from the 1890s. The difference between Otte and Roberts is that Otte accepted the malarial parasite idea (1896:22:4 [July]:225–29). The contents of the *China Medical* [Missionary] *Journal* during the 1890s indicate that Roberts' broad conceptualization of 'malaria' was not the dominant perspective among contributors.

8

The Anti-Opiumists' Nightmare

INTRODUCTION

Sir William Roberts was a godsend to the Government of India. His evaluation justified the existence of all opium produced and distributed for consumption within India. It portrayed all activities associated with each phase of the industry and responsible for such quantities as having prevented the premature demise of some people in the subcontinent. More inhabitants would live if individuals' consumption of the mother drug increased and a person susceptible to morphia toxicity could obtain a sufficient amount of anarcotine.

The second part of this chapter describes what Roberts succeeded in defending by addressing two issues: the quantity of opium manufactured in India and how much its citizens consumed. Stating an accurate figure for each topic is difficult. The obstacle is clandestine production and smuggled opium. The data in several documents provide an estimate for these "activities" during the late nineteenth century. And for Roberts, any statistic cited for total amount of the licit and illicit drug represented a situation that had to change. His program for minimizing mortality entailed more per capita consumption of the mother drug and additional *Papaver somniferum Linn* for extraction of the alkaloid. Calculations about approximate anarcotine quantities needed for India's 'malaria' sufferers and potential victims are found at the end of the chapter. The first part documents the status of anarcotine in India by comparing victims' requirements with supplies actually manufactured in British India and distributed between 4 April 1860 and 23 January 1894.

SMALL DOSES OF ANARCOTINE
REQUIRE LARGE AMOUNTS OF OPIUM

Roberts' 1895 report contains minimal information about crude opium requirements for his anarcotine argument. He only said that sixteen grains of crude opium were needed "to equivalize the minimum dose of one grain of anarcotine, which was found effective in arresting the paroxysms of intermittent fever, and forty-eight grains to equivalize the maximum dose" of three grains (GBO [Roberts] 1895:VI:111). In other words, sixteen pounds of crude opium were needed to procure one pound of the alkaloid, or each three-grain dose of anarcotine used in 'fever' therapy was extracted from forty-eight grains of the mother drug. Roberts' use of the 16:1 ratio to evaluate the significance of the Palmer and Garden experiments is misleading.

First, Roberts used only the average anarcotine content of the product from the major poppy-cultivating region in British India to arrive at the 16:1 ratio. The amount was 6.36 percent, roughly one-sixteenth. Average anarcotine content of *Papaver somniferum Linn* from the second major location, the Malwa plateau region of the Central India and Rajputana Agencies, was 5.14 percent (GBO [Roberts] 1895:VI:110). More crude opium was required to obtain Roberts' minimal and maximum single doses when, or if, confiscated opium manufactured in Malwa supplemented supplies available in British India. Second, only Palmer advanced the one grain to three grains "effective" amount; Garden's minimum number of one and one-half grains was 50 percent higher. A one-half grain increase for each person per exposure seems insignificant. It is not when prospective consumers number in the hundreds of thousands or millions. Palmer and Garden also stipulated that restoration of health required more than one exposure to the alkaloid. Multiple doses of the drug for numerous users entail much anarcotine and a huge amount of crude opium from which it is obtained.

Another limitation is that alkaloid extraction was not as easy as Roberts implies. Neither Palmer nor Garden was able to obtain one unit of anarcotine from sixteen units of opium. As Palmer indicated, morphia first had to be extracted and then treated to obtain anarcotine. The sequence was unavoidable in the early years due to the absence of technical sophistication and a reliance upon opium deemed unsuitable for other use (GBO [Gregory–Enclosure 169] 1895:V:78). The criteria used throughout most of the nineteenth century to judge the suitability of cultivators' opium sent to British factory officials was aroma, color, texture, taste, volume, weight, and consistence (i.e., the percentage of solid material remaining after being dried at 200 degrees Fahrenheit). Chemical analysis to ascertain actual percentage of any alkaloid in the sample was too expensive and rarely conducted.[1] Again, a large quantity of the mother drug produced a little bit of morphia that yielded even less anarcotine. Grossly adulterated crude opium resulted in poor quality or smaller amounts of salvageable morphia. This precluded extraction of any anarcotine, or reduced the amount procured. Administrators eventually adopted, and slightly modified, the Gregory–Robertson system to manufacture morphia at the Ghazipur factory. In the early years of the 1890s, anarcotine was extracted directly from the mother drug.[2] The quantity obtained still depended upon the quality of crude opium (i.e., aroma, consistence, and so forth). Throughout the period of anarcotine production in India after the Palmer and Garden experiments, the alkaloid came from opium classified as unsuitable for the export and domestic market (GBS [Watt] 1891:65; GBO [Rivett-Carnac] 1894:II:322). Garden's anarcotine consumption statistics and some data in the Palmer correspondence are much more helpful in calculating the amount of *Papaver somniferum Linn* required for Roberts' alkaloid advocacy.

THE CRUDE OPIUM TO MORPHIA TO ANARCOTINE SEQUENCE

The amount of opium confiscated during the 1859/60 season was 818 pounds. This yielded between twelve and thirteen pounds of "pure muriate of morphia" and seven pounds of "pure anarcotine" (Garden 1860:409).[3] The crude opium to anarcotine ratio was 116.85714 to 1, or 116.9:1 when rounded off to the nearest tenth. Palmer and Garden, therefore, had to process approximately 116.9 grains of the mother drug confiscated during 1858–1860 to obtain one grain of anarcotine. Garden expressed hope that future efforts would produce "one ounce and a half [of anarcotine] as the average amount obtained from every seer [two pounds] of opium" (1860:410). His anticipated opium to anarcotine ratio is 32:1.5; only thirty-two ounces of the mother drug would be required for one and a half ounce of anarcotine. Another way of saying the same thing is that Garden expected twenty-four ounces of crude opium to produce one ounce of the alkaloid. Hereafter, Garden's adjusted figure of 24:1 is used instead of the 32.5 figure. Keeping the amount of anarcotine constant rather than alternating between the 1 and 1.5 ratio simplifies calculations and comparisons.

A restatement is in order: the two researchers were able to extract only one grain of anarcotine from 116.9 grains of opium. Garden thought the ratio might improve to 24:1. The first calculation was reality as of 1860 and the second was a possibility sometime in the future.

ANARCOTINE CONSUMPTION AND CRUDE OPIUM REQUIREMENTS FOR DR. A. GARDEN'S DOCUMENTED PATIENTS

The 116.9:1 Ratio

Garden's 154 quotidian and forty tertian patients consumed 5,456 and 2,158.5 grains of anarcotine, respectively, during their "cure" and "convalescence" periods (1860:413–17 [Table A], 417–18 [Table B]). The grand total was 7,614.5 grains, or 1.0877 pounds (slightly less than 1.09).[4] This means the 194 patients for whom Garden maintained records during the nine-month study required 890,064 grains, or 127.152 pounds, of crude opium to satisfy their anarcotine needs.

Garden provided no reason to think the percentage of quotidian compared to tertian cases among the 490 undocumented participants was different from the documented 194 individuals. The undocumented group would have used approximately two and one-half times (2.5257731 or 2.526) more anarcotine. The exact total of alkaloid is 2.74753 pounds; a figure slightly less than 2.75 pounds, or 2 pounds, 12 ounces, during their "cure" and "convalescence" compared to their 194 colleagues. The 116.9:1 ratio for the 490 men produces a crude opium requirement of 321.1859 pounds.[5]

The consequences of the 116.9 ratio are startling; the 684 men participating in Garden's nine-month experiment needed 448.34 pounds of opium to provide them with the 3.84 pounds of anarcotine consumed during their "cure" and "convalescence." His patients, representing a tiny percentage of the numerous people suffering from 'fever' in British India, would have "used" more than 50 percent (54.809 percent to be exact) of the drug confiscated over a two-year period.

Garden's "Wished-for" 24:1 Ratio

Garden's second figure is based upon the assumption that the mother drug was free from gross contamination. This rarely was the case. There are two ways to state the 24:1 ratio calculation. More anarcotine is extracted from a given quantity of crude opium with the 24:1 ratio. Or, less opium is required to obtain a specified amount of anarcotine compared to the amount for the 116.9 ratio. The 684 patients' need for approximately 3.84 pounds of anarcotine (1.0877 or 1.09 for 194 participants and 2.7475302 for 490 people) remained the same. Their opium requirement is now 92.16 pounds. The amount is 11.266 percent of the drug confiscated during the 1858–1860 seasons.

Garden's study offers a perspective absent from Roberts' report. The medical needs of only 684 males who were arguably atypical Indian citizens exhausted slightly less than 55 percent of the opium accumulated over two years and stored at the Ghazipur factory. A very optimistic assessment reduces this to a fraction more than 11 percent. In either case, a miniscule number of quotidian and tertian "fever" victims in the subcontinent required a minimum of 92.16 pounds if the 24:1 ratio had been applicable, or a more realistic 448.34 pounds of opium to experience some relief.

HOW MUCH ANARCOTINE AND OPIUM FOR HOW MANY SUFFERERS?

The anarcotine and opium needs of Garden's 684 subjects provide a rough estimate of alkaloid and mother drug requirements for a much larger number of 'quotidian' and 'tertian' sufferers in India. These ratio calculations, admittedly only suggestive, are useful for two reasons. First, victims' projected needs can be compared to amounts of anarcotine actually used in India in the years after the Palmer and Garden experiments. Comparing projected need with recorded demand becomes a statement about the status of the alkaloid among medical practitioners and Government of India policy makers from 1860 to 1894–1895. In other words, the two figures measure the credibility that British personnel bestowed upon the experimenters' conclusions about the alkaloid before the arrival of Sir William Roberts. Second, estimates based upon statistics from Garden's experiment illuminate the implications of Roberts' anarcotine argument for Indian opium production, distribution, and consumption in 1895 and subsequent decades.

Garden's 684 victims require 3.84 pounds of anarcotine, and the extraction ratio determines how much opium is needed to obtain this amount of the alkaloid. Garden's 116.9:1 ratio produces a figure of 448.34 pounds of crude opium and the 24:1 ratio yields a requirement of 92.16 pounds. Sir William Roberts' 16:1 declaration, however, produces a figure of 61.44 pounds of opium needed to obtain the 3.84 pounds of anarcotine for 684 "malarial fever" sufferers. Multiplying the number of Garden's patients yields the mother drug and anarcotine requirements for a greater number of sufferers. These data are found in table 5, "Estimate of Anarcotine and Opium Requirements for Quotidian and Tertian Fever Patients Based upon Dr. A. Garden's 1859/60 Ghazipur Experiment." For example, one table 5 entry shows that the 684,000 victims need 3,840 pounds of anarcotine. The 116.9:1 ratio indicates that the Government of India had to use 448,896 pounds of the mother drug to obtain the amount of anarcotine. The figure is 92,160 pounds if the 24:1 ratio was operative. Sir William Roberts' 16:1 calculation translates into a need for 61,440 pounds of opium for these 684,000 sufferers. An increase in the number of 'malarial fever' victims in British India also increases the total required amount of anarcotine and opium. According to official documents, there were millions of sick people in the subcontinent during the latter part of the nineteenth century. These data are introduced elsewhere in the chapter.

THE STATUS OF ANARCOTINE
FROM 4 APRIL 1860 TO 23 JANUARY 1894:
MINIMAL DEMAND AND GOVERNMENT INDIFFERENCE

The Palmer and Garden experiments did not persuade the Government of India to dramatically increase the availability of anarcotine. The opposite occurred. The Ghazipur factory temporarily stopped manufacturing it, as well as morphia, in 1865. The opium in stock, amounting to 160 pounds confiscated during three years, was destroyed (GBO [Gregory–Enclosure 2] 1894:V:81). When production resumed, the popularity of anarcotine peaked between 1871/72 and 1874/75.[6] More than one hundred pounds of the alkaloid were issued to each of three Presidencies in British India as a "febrifuge for malarious fevers" during these three years (GBO [Gregory–Enclosure 74] 1894:V:81–2). Demand then plummeted. In a letter dated 27 March 1877, T. W. Sheppard claimed there was a steady call for the alkaloid but his statistics show no one was clamoring for it. Only 142 pounds were issued to locations throughout India during the 1875/76 season. One year later, in the 1876/77 season, the amount had decreased to 137 pounds, leaving twenty-two pounds, seven ounces in storage. The 1875/76 and 1876/77 distribution quantities were a "slight increase over the issues of 1873–1874 and 1874–1875" (GBO [Gregory–Enclosure 175] 1894:V:82).

Available documents do not specify exact amounts issued to the three Presidencies between 1871/72 and 1874/75. A generous estimate would be substantially more than 300 pounds, perhaps even as high as 384. Garden's statistics for 384 pounds of anarcotine (see column 3 in table 5) indicate the three-year supply of the alkaloid is sufficient for only 68,400 people (column 2 of table 5). This is an average of 22,800 citizens per year in the three Presidencies combined, or only 7,600 sufferers per year in each location during the thirty-six month period. The 142 pounds in 1875/76 and the 137 pounds for 1876/77 distributed throughout India would have helped about 25,000 and 23,500 people respectively. If Roberts' depressing observations in 1895 about mortality rates (as high as 70 percent in several British provinces) are applicable to the 1870s, medical personnel were dispensing anarcotine to very few of the numerous 'malarial fever' victims in India.

The Ghazipur factory extracted 188 pounds of the alkaloid in 1879/80 but demand was negligible. Beginning with the 1881/82 season, anarcotine for domestic consumption was no longer manufactured in India (GBS [Watt] 1891:65). As of 1883, the Ghazipur authorities had on hand 433 pounds, ten ounces and four drams of a product that nobody in the country wanted. It remained in storage until sometime in late 1892 or early 1893 when all but thirty pounds, one ounce was sold in London, England (GBO [Rivett-Carnac] 1894:II:322, 330).

Statistics submitted to the Royal Commission by G. M. Gregory on 14 February 1894 clearly show the lack of enthusiasm among Government of India policy makers. Gregory documented what the Medical Department of India did with anarcotine supplied by the Ghazipur plant.[7] The Medical Department was responsible for supplying the alkaloid to personnel and institutions affiliated with the Indian Medical Service and from medical practitioners not in government service. The first entry for an order is 4 April 1860, and the last is 23 January 1894. The locations are widely dispersed in the northern half of the country. Nothing was sent to southern India.

A total of 1,290 pounds had been allocated as of 12 August 1880, the final season of anarcotine production at Ghazipur. The medical department then received no requests for more than three years. Sometime during October 1883, it sent one hundred pounds of the unused alkaloid to the secretary of state in London. Between 21 May 1886 and 23 January 1894, a mere three pounds, ten ounces were issued to four locations in India. A Mr. Francis of Durbhanga received almost all of it (three pounds) (GBO [Gregory] 1894:V:82–3).

The medical department data provide no support for Roberts' argument about the benefits of anarcotine. The 1,290 pounds were distributed over a period of twenty-four years, from 1860 to 1883. This is an average of only 53.75 pounds of anarcotine for each year, enough to "cure" perhaps 8,000 'malarious' individuals. Roberts' aforementioned 'fever' percentages suggest the number of sufferers each year was many times this number. The significance of such a modest demand for such a long time is obvious: allopathic medical practitioners in India held anarcotine in low regard for the "cure" and "convalescence" of 'fever' victims when the substance was available. And the miniscule amount of three pounds, ten ounces (less than Garden's 684 patients' requirements for only twelve months) issued from the remaining stock between 26 May 1886 and 23 January 1894 indicates their opinion had not changed for almost another nine years.

British administrators in India were neither stupid nor void of compassion. They would not have ignored a valuable and abundant product found in an indigenous plant to alleviate the misery of India's multitudes for thirty-three years without good reason.[8] The alkaloid also promised monetary rewards. Palmer calculated the value of morphia and anarcotine obtained from opium confiscated during the 1858/59 and 1859/60 seasons at 18,933 rupees. The cost of preparing the two alkaloids was only 1,737 rupees, leaving a handsome profit of 17,196 rupees (GBO [Gregory–Enclosure 2] 1894:V:81). Government of India financial support for improved extraction facilities would further reduce expenses incurred for anarcotine, thereby increasing the return on its investment. The administration did nothing after 1860 because the venture lacked credibility. In 1894–1895, Sir William Roberts disagreed.

Roberts' assessment of the alkaloid and mother drug had profound implications. As alluded to in the introductory comments above, all activity leading to the consumption of opium among Indian citizens served a "medical purpose." This meant that the cultivation of poppy, collection of raw latex, processing of raw opium, and distribution of the drug to vendors and government departments in the country were beyond reproach. So were consumers of the drug. Each person ingesting opium, be it small pieces of a cake or in any other form, was "taking medicine." Regardless of reasons for indulgence that the SSOT found so offensive, all habituates had some protection against misery and possible death. Roberts, in effect, had legitimized the status quo of all opium production, all manufacture, all distribution, and all consumption everywhere in South Asia. 'All' includes licit and illicit *Papaver somniferum Linn*. The Government of India furnished the Royal Commission on Opium with varying, sometimes contradictory, statistics about legal use but very little about the clandestine commodity. Data about both types indicate the people of India were consuming much more opium than the Government of India was willing to acknowledge or able to confirm. And from the perspective of Sir William Roberts, all consumers were benefiting from the mother drug's inherent anarcotine. The problem confronting Indian citizens, he argued, was that they still were ingesting insufficient amounts of opium and virtually no anarcotine whatsoever to mitigate the prevalence and severity of 'malarial fever' in the subcontinent.

Roberts' awareness about morphine toxicity preventing many 'malarial fever' victims, or prospective victims, from ingesting sufficient amounts of opium had equally profound ramifications. Additional *Papaver somniferum Linn* had to be procured for the extraction of anarcotine. Satisfying this need by tapping into current production reduced the amount of opium available to the public for oral consumption. This step, according to Roberts' logic, would result in even higher mortality rates from 'malarial fever.' A situation leading to more deaths was unacceptable to both pro-traders and their antagonists.

The remainder of this chapter offers commentary and statistical data that show what Sir William Roberts was defending. It discusses how much opium British India produced, and the quantities manufactured in regions over which the central government had nominal control. It also documents the amount of licit *Papaver somniferum Linn* that Indian citizens everywhere in the country really did consume, and the complications created by the ubiquity of smuggled opium. The production and consumption data are then linked to mortality rates in the subcontinent. This illuminates the economic and political consequences of advocating anarcotine as a prophylactic and febrifuge for 'malarial fever.' In brief, Sir William Roberts provided the Government of India with a medical justification to protect, even to increase, opium production, consumption, and revenue.

THE PRODUCTION AND CONSUMPTION OF OPIUM IN INDIA

"Medical Opium"

Satisfying the SSOT demand for restricting opium consumption in India to "medicinal purposes" presented a problem to the Government of India. Only a minute fraction of yearly production in the country placated critics. This was "cake" and "powdered" opium made at the Patna factory.[9] The two products, collectively called "medical opium," were prepared from "opium especially selected from the season's supply on account of its excellence in colour, aroma, and texture" (GBO [Rivett-Carnac] 1894:II:322). Some of this drug was the result of the administration's desire to comply with western pharmaceutical standards for manufacturing "cake" and "powdered" opium. Starting in the early 1880s, opium department administrators selected small plots of land that they thought had advantageous soil type, wind, and moisture conditions. This land was reserved for careful cultivation of poppy to ensure the highest quality latex. High quality was synonymous with a morphine content exceeding the average found in the Indian drug. And morphine, as mentioned previously, was the prime criterion for calculating the worth of most opium sold in the western market during the 1800s.

Opium factory officials carefully monitored each phase in processing the selected raw material. While the "cakes" and the dry, pulverized form of the raw drug complied with Great Britain's pharmaceutical requirements of the time regarding purity, high manufacturing costs combined with the inherently low morphine content of Indian opium during the 1800s did not make the project commercially viable on a larger scale. Production throughout the second half of the nineteenth century remained modest and distribution was limited to locations within India (Eatwell 1851–52:310–11; PuIB 1966:239).[10] Both kinds of "medical opium" were supplied only to the Indian Medical Department and to "charitable medical institutions" in the country to be administered under supervision by trained personnel. One source says the average quantity of "cake opium" and "powdered opium" manufactured annually at Patna from 1890/91 through 1894/95 was 410 pounds and 677 pounds respectively (GBS [Godley] 1897:5)

A document prepared for the Royal Commission on Opium contains "medical opium" data for a longer time. The average amount of "cake opium" manufactured per year from 1883/84 through 1892/93 was slightly more than 742.421 pounds. The annual average distributed to Government of India and "nongovernment" medical depots for the same period came to a bit more than 758.053 pounds. A "medical opium" reserve initiated prior to 1883/84 accounts for the difference between the amount manufactured and the number of pounds distributed. The reserve consisted of opium held over from the previous year. A part of it was dispensed if the special poppy crop failed to yield enough of the drug to satisfy demand during that season. The administration's Indian Medical Service depots received slightly more than 713.002 pounds of "cakes" during each season in the ten-year period. Medical depots unaffiliated with the Government of India received no "cakes" before 1886/87 and they got very little thereafter, approximately 60.889 pounds per year from 1887/88 through 1892/93 (GBO [Rivett-Carnac] 1894:II:329).

The Government of India manufactured much less "powdered opium" during the ten years; an average of slightly more than 322.874 pounds per season. And only 272.979 pounds per year was supplied to the medical establishments cited above. Again, Indian Medical Service depots received the most, a yearly average of more than 255.699 pounds. Institutions unaffiliated with the government were supplied with "powdered opium" beginning only in 1886/87, and shipments per season averaged slightly more than 16.25 pounds (GBO [Rivett-Carnac] 1894:II:329).[11] These figures are miniscule compared to the amount of "nonmedicinal" *Papaver somniferum Linn* processed for export and for sale to the public within India.

Two areas in India produced virtually all opium for both export and the "nonmedicinal product" consumption within the country. The Benares and Bihar Agencies in British India comprised the first locale. The second was the Malwa plateau region of the Central India and Rajputana administrative agencies. All other opium consumed in India during the nineteenth century came from several other locations on the subcontinent. The most prominent of these secondary locales was the British-controlled Punjab Province.

SECONDARY LOCALES OF OPIUM ACTIVITY

Production, Consumption, and Smuggling in Punjab Province

Punjab was the only locale under direct British control permitted to grow the plant in significant amounts other than tracts in the Benares and Bihar Opium Agencies. Its inhabitants cultivated poppy in almost every administrative unit. Shahpur was the principal drug-producing district and the "chief Sikh centres of Lahore and Amritsar" received most of what the district manufactured (Watt [1908] 1966b:854). Male members of this religious group consumed much opium.

George Watt's claim about the area under cultivation in Punjab being "regularly declared" suggests that provincial officials knew how much poppy had been planted. He calculated annual production in the province at "about 1,400 maunds" and said that all of it was consumed locally. The 115,199.98 pounds per year, however, was insufficient to meet demand (GBS [Watt] 1891:36, 38).[12] Inexplicably, only a small amount of Bengal Excise opium was imported to help meet consumer demand during the twenty-year period from 1873/74 through 1892/93. The grand total of 1,207 maunds is equivalent to an annual average of only 60.35 maunds (4,965.941995 pounds) (GBO [Rivett-Carnac] 1894:II:327).[13] Equally peculiar was the Government of India's policy of prohibiting Punjab administrators from importing more than 935 maunds (76,937.1295 pounds) per season of the Malwa product from Central India and Rajputana (GBO [Finlay–Appendix X] 1894b:II:355).[14] These supplementary legal supplies (i.e., an annual maximum of 935 maunds) had failed to satiate consumer desire because drug smuggling from Nepal and the Malwa region into Punjab had been commonplace for decades. A total of 192,137.1095 pounds (equivalent to 2,335 maunds or slightly more than 1,556.7 Bengal Excise or Malwa chests) was consumed legally each twelve-month period in Punjab. The exact amount of illicit opium entering the province to placate demand was unknown despite diligent "efforts to suppress this contraband trade" (GBC [Consumption] 1892:62). Then there were Punjab administrators in 1889 who complained about the "disproportionately small amount of opium" obtained from many acres under cultivation in nine districts (GBC [Consumption] 1892:62–3). Too much land in several poppy-growing locations apparently was producing far too little opium. Watt's claim about the area being "regularly declared" is too optimistic. Something was remiss; farmers were keeping part of what they incised from ripe poppies and either ingesting it themselves or selling the raw latex clandestinely. In either case the Government of India was losing revenue and the citizens of the province were consuming more opium than official statistics indicated.[15] The situation in South India was very different.

Production and Consumption of Opium in South India

The Opium Agent at Indore, a city in the Central India Agency, supplied the Malwa drug to destinations in South India. The locations included British-controlled Madras, Mysore, and the large native state of Hyderabad. Apart from a small annual acreage of poppy with insignificant yields in Madras Presidency and several places for Mysore Province, all licit opium consumed in this part of the country during the latter part of the nineteenth century originated in the Malwa plateau of Central India (GBS [Watt] 1891:38; GBO [Finlay–Appendix X] 1894b:II:355–57; IDRA 1900:II:102–04; Hastings 1895:10).[16]

Other Opium Consumed in India

The principal producers of India's opium were the Benares and Bihar Opium Agencies in British territory, the Malwa plateau of Central India and Rajputana, and Punjab Province. Poppy, however, was grown "[t]hroughout the length of the Himálaya" (GBS [Watt] 1891:36). In Nepal, for example, opium production during the early 1890s was viewed as "a modern branch of agricultural enterprise." Acreage devoted to the plant was "very extensive" and "smuggling into British territory" had become a frequent and serious problem (GBS [Watt] 1891:38). And in Himalayan regions under direct British control, the Government of India imposed no restrictions upon acreage, and local people consumed virtually all the latex that was collected. Administrators thought the rest of it was smuggled into adjacent British provinces. The amount was insignificant and the British lost very little revenue (GBS [Watt] 1891:36).

The Government of India, in fact, adopted a "habit of noninterference" and permitted limited poppy cultivation anyplace where "semi-independent native States and wild mountainous country occur" (GBS [Watt] 1891:36). The northeast frontier was illustrative. Some of the opium consumed in South Asia came from "tracts outside the limits of British possessions" in Assam and Burma. While cultivation was "severely punished in 'Assam proper,'" nothing was done to stop it within the "aboriginal tribes" that inhabited the "mountainous country" (GBS [Watt] 1891:38). An unknown amount of this opium, as well as the drug produced by "aboriginals" in Burma, was available to people in the British dominated-districts of Assam and Burma.[17]

Poppy acreage and opium production elsewhere in India was minimal. Besides the aforementioned enclaves in Madras and Mysore in South India, there also was a "small annual acreage" reserved for poppy in the Central Provinces. However, no reliable data concerning amount of opium obtained existed in the early 1890s (GBS [Watt] 1891:38). The city of Bombay periodically obtained some of what it needed from the "territories of His Highness the Gáekwár" of Baroda (GBS [Watt] 1891:74). What percentage of Baroda's annual production Bombay absorbed (and how much poppy the native state of Baroda cultivated) was unknown (GBS [Watt] 1891:38). Opium from Central India and Rajputana also contributed to satisfying demand from the citizens of Bombay. Available records, however, do not identify specific place of drug origin. Bombay bought a total of 1,575 chests from these locations during 1887/89 and the next year it was 1,571.5 chests. Imports increased to 1,741.5 chests in the 1889/90 season (GBS [Watt] 1891:74). Baroda, therefore, apparently manufactured enough for its own consumers and had a surplus to export. The situation changed two years later; this native state imported 338 maunds of opium from Malwa during 1891/92 (GBO [Finlay–Appendix X] 1894b:II:355).

The only other opium legally consumed in India came "from beyond the Frontier." The exact place of origin is unspecified and only three seasons are indicated, these being 1888/89, 1889/90, and 1890/91. The amounts were 19,330 seers (39,761.810 pounds), 5,509 seers (11,332.013 pounds), and 1,094 seers (2,250.358 pounds) respectively (GBC [Consumption] 1892:20).

THE PRINCIPAL LOCALES: THE BENARES AGENCY, THE BIHAR AGENCY, AND 'BENGAL OPIUM'

'Bengal Opium' Administrative Framework

The collective name for the Benares and Bihar Agencies' product was 'Bengal Opium.' The Benares Agency was responsible for twenty-nine poppy-cultivating districts in the Northwestern Provinces and Oudh. Its headquarters and opium factory were located in the city of Ghazipur. The Bihar Agency obtained opium from eleven districts in the Patna, Bhagalpore, and Chota Nagpur administrative divisions. They all were located in the western part of the 'Lower Provinces' of the Bengal Presidency.[18] The Bihar Agency headquarters and its opium factory were in Patna city. Both factories processed the crude opium collected each season in British India. Their product was exported or sold within India for domestic consumption.

The drug manufactured at both factories and scheduled for shipment overseas was called 'Bengal Provision.' This was often shortened to 'Provision.' Provision chests were exported from Calcutta, and each chest contained 140.43 pounds of the drug. The technical name for the product prepared for sale and consumption within India was 'Bengal Excise' or 'Abkari' (GBO [Finlay–Appendix IX] 1894a:II:345). A chest of Bengal Excise held 123.4257 pounds of opium.[19] Most Excise chests were sent to warehouses in Calcutta. They were then distributed to Assam, Burma, and all district and subdivision treasuries in Bengal. Districts in Bihar were supplied directly from the Patna factory. Ghazipur distributed the Excise drug to the Northwestern Provinces and Oudh, Punjab, and the Central Provinces (GBO [Rivett-Carnac] 1894:II:321). The administration of the Central Provinces in turn supplied opium to native states within its jurisdiction. No Bengal Excise opium was issued to the Madras Presidency or any other location in South India (GBS [Watt] 1891:38).

Malwa Opium—Historical Context and Administrative Setting

The Malwa plateau was the other major source of opium in India. Most often referred to as Malwa opium, the exported and domestically consumed commodity was produced by native states in the Rajputana and Central India Agencies.[20] A small portion came from the native state of Baroda. Baroda and Bombay had a common border. With the exception of two small districts called Ajmere-Merwara, no Malwa opium was produced in British territory.[21] Merwara (a narrow strip of land) and Ajmere were entirely surrounded by semi-independent, poppy-cultivating native states. The Government of India had no success in preventing clandestine shipment of Ajmere-Merwara opium into a neighboring native state and vice versa (GBO [Finlay–Appendix IX] 1894a:II:345; IFCD [Meyer] 1900:24–5). The effort's utter futility also dissuaded the administration from even attempting to regulate consumption and production in rural areas within the two districts despite inhabitants being "much addicted to the use of opium" for a long time (IFCD [Meyer] 1900:24). In fact, the local population consumed most of its own product. The Government of India collected some money from Ajmere-Merwara opium by taxing chests shipped to a weighing station in the city of Ajmir (sometimes spelled Ajmere or Ajmeer). These chests were then sent to Bombay for export overseas. The Ajmir city weighing station also supplied the opium factory at Ghazipur with a portion of the crude opium required for manufacturing Bengal opium. This occurred for twelve years during the period from 1881/82 through 1894/95.[22]

The native states situated on the Malwa plateau accounted for the remaining yearly overseas shipments of the Indian drug. They also produced a substantial part of the opium legally consumed throughout the country in any year. All opium that the native states prepared for consumption outside the country and for legal sale in British territory was sent to one of three Government of India weighing stations situated on the plateau or next to it. As mentioned above, one station was in Ajmir city (Rajputana Agency). Another weighing station was located at Indore (Central India Agency), and the third was in the city of Ahmedabad (Bombay Presidency).[23] The transit tax ("pass-duty") imposed at Ajmir also was levied on each chest (one chest held 140.25 pounds of opium) arriving in Indore and Ahmedabad before a container was allowed to enter British territory en route to Bombay for shipment overseas. A small percentage of Malwa chests reaching Bombay were periodically diverted prior to export for local consumption in the Bombay Presidency.

The "pass-duty" for Malwa opium destined for sale anywhere within British India was higher. Each of these Malwa chests also contained 140.25 pounds of the drug (GBO [Finlay–Appendix IX] 1894a:II:346–47).[24] Some of the Malwa product paying taxes in any year might be kept in "reserve" (i.e., held back). It remained in a government warehouse for distribution to the Indian public during another season.[25] The British kept detailed records of all these transactions. Opium export data from the Ajmere-Merwara districts and the "pass-duty" statistics were the only consistently accurate information available about opium production in the Malwa region throughout the 1800s.[26]

Treaties negotiated earlier in the century prevented the Government of India from regulating the production and consumption of Malwa opium within these native states (IFCD [Meyer] 1900:2; GBO [Clarke] 1894:II:446).[27] Noninterference posed problems for British administrators. They had no reliable statistics for total amount of poppy cultivated, opium manufactured, and drug consumption within each native state. The policy also meant not knowing the quantity of opium available for smuggling into British territory. The situation in 1891 prompted George Watt to declare that

> [t]he accuracy of the returns of area furnished by the chief native states that produce the Malwa opium, is doubtless, open to suspicion. Further, the amounts registered at the weighment stations cannot be used as a factor to check these returns, since it is well known that, in spite of all precautions, considerable quantities do actually percolate illicitly into British districts. At the same time the local consumption within native states is not known, so that the returns, such as they are have to be accepted. (GBS [Watt] 1891:36)[28]

EXPORTS OF BENGAL PROVISION AND MALWA OPIUM

In his 1891 report to Parliament, George Watt calculated that the average annual production of Bengal Provision opium from 1860/61 through 1890/91 exceeded 93,500 maunds. The "1 maund is 82.2857 pounds" equivalency was used during the second half of the nineteenth century. The Patna and Ghazipur factories, therefore, manufactured an average of more than 7,693,712.95

pounds of the drug every year for foreign consumption beyond India during the thirty-year period. (GBS [Watt] 1891:37). Both figures convert to an average of 54,899.017 Bengal Provision chests manufactured each year for overseas export beginning in 1860/61 through 1890/91.[29]

A Parliamentary paper prepared by Mr. Arthur Godley of the India Office in 1897 includes data for the period during which the Royal Commission on Opium conducted its work. Godley's document also has amounts of the Malwa drug exported from Bombay as well as the number of Bengal Provision Opium chests leaving Calcutta from 1885/86 through 1894/95. And a report written especially for the Royal Commission on Opium by J. F. Finlay (secretary to the Government of India in the Department of Finance and Commerce) provides Bombay-Malwa export figures for the two seasons preceding 1885/86 and then through 1892/93. Data from both documents are reproduced in table 6 ("Bengal and Malwa Exports.")[30]

The SSOT had good reason to be appalled by the amount of opium exported from India. George Watt's calculation of 93,500 maunds of Bengal Provision is equivalent to more than 7,693,712.95 pounds sent overseas during each of the thirty years between 1860/61 and 1890/91. Godley's data are just as sobering. With each Bengal Provision chest holding 140.143 pounds of the drug, the average annual export of 51,928.8 chests from Calcutta between 1885/86 and 1894/95 represents 7,277,457.818 pounds.

The numbers are staggering when Malwa export data are included. An average of 32,574.25 chests left Bombay each twelve months of the twelve-year period from 1883/84 through 1894/95. Since a chest of Malwa opium contained 140.25 pounds of *Papaver somniferum Linn*, a conversion yields 4,568,538.5625 pounds per season. A summary statement about the years addressed by both administrators (1885/86–1894/95) is possible if Finlay's entries for 1883/84 and 1884/85 are omitted. A grand total of 313,959.5 chests left India during the ten years and the annual average for the period amounts to 31,395.95 chests or 4,403,281.9875 pounds per season.

The combined average amount of Indian opium (Malwa export and Bengal Provision) reaching foreign shores each year from 1885/86 through 1894/95 now increases to 11,680,739.805 pounds.[31] An amount exceeding eleven and three-quarter million pounds every year is a lot of opium. The SSOT condemned all of it (and the pre-1885/86 exports as well). Except for "cake" and "powdered" opium, anti-opiumists also considered the smaller quantities of *Papaver somniferum Linn* processed for consumption within India equally objectionable. The question now is how much of the domestic product was manufactured, and how much of it did Indian citizens ingest?

THE MANUFACTURE OF BENGAL EXCISE (ABKARI) OPIUM FOR CONSUMPTION IN INDIA

Table 7 lists the amount of Bengal Excise opium manufactured at each Agency factory, the combined total, and the quantity distributed within British India each season from 1873/74 through 1892/93. The territories were Bengal, the Northwestern Provinces and Oudh, the Central Provinces, Assam, Burma, and Punjab. The original document expresses amounts in maunds. These are cited in table 7: "Statement Showing Quantities of Excise Opium Manufactured at the Bihar and Benares Agencies and the Quantities Supplied to the Several Local Governments During the Last Twenty Years." The following comments also specify maunds but include approximate equivalents in Bengal Excise chests and pounds.[32]

The Patna and Ghazipur factories manufactured an amount of opium equivalent to slightly more than 89,080.7 chests during the twenty-year period. The average amount of Bengal Excise product available every twelve months for legal distribution in the country was, therefore, a fraction more than 4,454.5 chests.[33]

THE DISTRIBUTION OF BENGAL EXCISE ("ABKARI") OPIUM FOR CONSUMPTION IN INDIA

The quantity of opium that British India's two factories issued to provincial governments varied from year to year. The volume depended upon consumer demand, the need to maintain a reserve to offset possible failure of a poppy crop, restrictions about amounts permitted for the provinces, and other factors.[34] Entries for columns 3 and 4 in table 7, therefore, differ. For example, 1877/78, 1878/79, 1882/83, 1882/83, as well as from 1886/87 through 1889/90 and again during 1892/93, indicate that demand was met by including Excise opium held over from past seasons.

The total amount of Bengal Excise supplied to British India during the twenty-year period was 126,118.5 maunds (column 4). This is equivalent to a fraction more than 10,377,749 pounds or a bit less than 84,081 chests. The yearly average for the period was about sixteen ounces shy of 6,306 maunds, which is equivalent to almost 518,887.5 pounds or slightly more than 4,204 chests.

The greatest amount of Excise distributed during any season for the period, a total of 9,621.5 maunds, was 1889/90. This is almost 791,712 pounds or slightly less than 6,415 chests. The smallest amount issued to provincial governments occurred during 1874/75. It was equivalent to only 2,880 maunds (about 236,982 pounds, twelve ounces or a fraction more than 1,920 chests) (GBO [Rivett-Carnac] 1894:II:327).[35]

The Rivett-Carnac document consulted in creating table 7 has no data about amounts of opium that the provincial governments of Bengal, Punjab, and the Northwestern Provinces and Oudh redistributed to a native state situated within their respective borders. A Parliamentary paper submitted on 6 February 1893 to the British Parliament by Arthur Godley, undersecretary of state for India, does have this information for the period 1881/82 through 1890/91. For reasons adumbrated in the Malwa discussion below, these data exclude the poppy-cultivating, opium-producing native states associated with the Malwa plateau region of the

Central India Agency and the Rajputana Agency. However, Godley's entries incorporate statistics from the two small Malwa districts of Ajmere-Marwara directly administered by the Government of India.

This 1881/92–1890/91 data is useful although possibly qualified. The material reveals the percentage of Bengal Excise consumed by residents in British territories compared to citizens of native states. The limitation is that Godley's statistics about yearly amounts of Bengal Excise sent to provincial administrations differ from the Rivett-Carnac entries cited in column 4 of table 7. Rivett-Carnac identified amounts supplied to British India. He did not indicate if the entries include opium to be redistributed to native states located in these provinces. Godley, however, did separate the opium that a provincial administration provided to its native states. After deducting the amount reserved for native states, Godley's entries still differ from Rivett-Carnac's statistics for at least three seasons. The small differences suggest that Rivett-Carnac's province-to-native state redistribution numbers, had he included any, would be slightly less than Godley's statistics.[36] Despite the discrepancy, Godley's 1881/82–1890/91 data show that a very small amount of the Benares and Bihar Agency product was distributed to the non-Malwa native states in three provinces of British India. These were the Central Provinces, Bengal, and the Northwestern Provinces and Oudh. The amount averaged slightly more than 89.5 chests per season compared to an average that was a fraction more than 4,204 chests issued to administrations in British territory during each season for the ten-year period (GBS [Godley] 1893:6).[37] Residents of the native states undoubtedly consumed more than an average of 89.5 maunds of opium each year from 1881/82 through 1890/91. All documents indicate smuggled opium was commonplace.

THE PRODUCTION AND DISTRIBUTION OF MALWA OPIUM FOR LICIT AND ILLICIT DOMESTIC CONSUMPTION IN INDIA

The Government of India did not know exactly how much opium the poppy-cultivating native states on the Malwa plateau produced in any year during the nineteenth century. It had no way to obtain reliable data. Besides the aforementioned treaties precluding interference with drug consumption, the administration collected no money from the internal opium trade of any of these Central India and Rajputana entities. It also was prohibited from disrupting drug commerce between native states that shared a common border. Commentators could only speculate about per capita consumption and they could only estimate total production for any or all years (Hastings 1895:10, 16–7). The only thing the British could do with confidence was fret about that portion of the drug not consumed within the area and not paying pass-duty.

The enduring problem confronting the Government of India was the ubiquity and quantity of Malwa opium smuggled into British India and the native states located beyond the region. Estimates and reports portray the amount as huge. The pro-traders' claim about moderate consumption of opium in the subcontinent was therefore qualified. The Government of India was able to calculate per capita consumption of Benares and Bihar Agencies' Bengal Excise product as well as Malwa opium paying pass-duty with some degree of accuracy. The reason for the capability was access to detailed records and occasional reliable reports from licensed vendors in the provinces to whom the drug was sold for eventual public consumption. This did not characterize the relationship between British officials and rulers of the poppy-cultivating native states of the Central India and Rajputana administrative agencies. Accurate information was scarce and access to whatever data existed was infrequent. Some skilled Government of India officials stationed in a few locales might be able to gather information about some aspects of local production. Most were not so lucky.[38] The Government of India and its defenders had nothing to gain by suggesting, especially in the vicinity of its critics, that Indian citizens might be consuming far more opium than acknowledged. Administrators and pro-opiumists uttered vague generalities when referring to the probability of underestimated all-India consumption rates. This did not prevent them from citing the prevalence of smuggling to discredit SSOT insistence that curtailing the illegal trade required little effort.

Legal Distribution of Malwa Opium in British Territory

Records of pass-duty transactions from the weighing stations at Indore, Ahmedabad, and Ajmir can reveal the amount of Malwa opium *exported* from Bombay and quantities distributed throughout British India from these three Malwa locations. But, compilations of data about the Malwa drug's distribution *within* India are rare. Table 8 is a partial replication of material from a report prepared for the Royal Commission on Opium. The title of table 8 is "Chests of Malwa Opium Weighed/Taxed at All Stations and Number of Chests Manufactured for Sale in British Territory and native states."

The difference between column 6 ("Diverted or Weighed for Local Consumption in British Territory and native states") and column 5 ("Total Chests") for each year is the number of Malwa chests exported from Bombay to overseas destinations between 1883/84 and 1892/93. Table 8 entries are identical to amounts listed in column 3 of table 6 ("Bengal and Malwa Opium Exports") for these years. Both tables indicate a total of 334,589 chests leaving the port between 1883/84 and 1892/93. This is an annual average export of 33,458.9 chests of Malwa opium during each season of the ten-year period.[39]

Column 6 in table 8 represents the amount of Malwa opium available for legal consumption in British provinces and non-Malwa native states from 1883/84 through 1892/93. Compared to the number of chests departing Bombay, the figures are modest. Levies were imposed upon a grand total of 30,929.7 chests for the ten-year period at the Indore, Ajmir, and Ahmedabad weighing stations. This means the average annual amount of *licit* Malwa opium available to provincial governments for eventual distribution to consumers in their territories from 1883/84 through 1892/93 was 3,092.7 chests (GBO [Finlay–Appendix IX] 1894a:II:347).[40]

A summary clarifies the serious problem confronting Government of India administrators: they did not know what percentage of the total amount of Malwa opium produced in any year, or for any period, was available for illegal sale within British India. The Malwa plateau was a geographical area conducive to the cultivation of poppy. Native states in the Central India and Rajputana Agencies comprised most of the region, and they accounted for virtually all the drug manufactured every season. The erection of custom barriers on roads and paths linking the native states to British India and constant patrolling of the border, which was "between 2,000 and 3,000 [total] miles in length," was the only way to curtail smuggling. Pro-traders, many witnesses testifying before the Royal Commission, and the Government of India, contended these measures were not viable because the prohibitive cost and ensuing "discontent . . . would constitute a serious political danger" (GBO [Batten] 1894:I:143).

The native state of Baroda, which was not under the jurisdiction of either the Central India or Rajputana Agency, contributed only a small portion of the non-Bengal opium product. *Papaver somniferum Linn* originating in Baroda went to the Ahmedabad weighing station in Bombay Presidency, as did the small quantity produced by the small state of Dungapore. Dungapore was in the Rajputana Agency (GBO [Finlay–Appendix IX] 1894a:II:347). Column 4 ("Total Malwa Opium at Ahmedabad [Bombay]") of table 8 indicates a ten-year total of 2,558.5 chests, and an annual average of only 174.3883 chests. The original document does not have separate shipment entries for Baroda and Dungapore. Residents of Bombay city and its environs purchased all Baroda and Dungapore opium that had been taxed for domestic consumption at the Ahmedabad weighing station. The only other administrative entities producing Malwa opium were the two small British districts of Ajmere-Merwara. To reiterate, the residents of Ajmere-Merwara consumed most of the drug they produced. Cultivators sent some of their yearly production to Ajmir city. The remainder was smuggled into neighboring native states.[41] All other opium processed at the Ajmir weighing station came from native states under the jurisdiction of the Rajputana Agency. Those in the Central India Agency sent their product to Indore city. A rough approximation of the percentage of Malwa opium manufactured exclusively by the native states in each Agency (including Dungapore) can now be made. The reason for the delineation follows.

The Government of India had records documenting the arrival and taxation of a grand total of 365,518.7 Malwa chests for the ten-year period. This is an average of 36,551.87 containers per year available for sending overseas, or for sale to British provinces and to native states distant from the Malwa plateau. The Central India Agency native states contributed 321,602.19 chests during the ten years to this total; an annual average of 32,160.219 (see column 2 "Total Malwa Opium at Indore [Central India Agency]"). All entries for column 3 ("Total Malwa Opium at Ajmir [Rajputana Agency]") are counted as originating in the native states of Rajputana despite some of each year's product coming from the British districts of Ajmere-Merwara. The exact amount originating in these two districts is unspecified, as is the amount that the Rajputana Agency native state of Dungapore sent to Ahmedabad. For the sake of convenience, assume the respective quantities are approximately the same. The "Total Chests for 10 years" and "Average Chests Per Season" statistics for column 3 (1,743.883 and 174.3883 chests respectively) now approximate the amount of opium that the native states in the Rajputana Agency forwarded to Ajmir city for eventual overseas exports or sale within British India.

Combining the Indore and Ajmir weighing station entries yields a total of 323,346.073 chests from 1883/84 through 1892/93. This is an average of 32,334.6073 chests per season; it is equivalent to 4,534,928.6738 pounds or 55,111.989979 maunds (one Malwa chest held 140.25 pounds of the drug and one maund was equal to 82.2857 pounds). The average annual number of chests, maunds, and pounds is useful for calculating how much of the Central India and Rajputana Agencies' native states' annual opium production served a purpose that was detrimental to British monetary interests. Stated again, the Government of India documented an average of almost 55,112 maunds (55,111.989979) per season produced in the Central India and Rajputana Agencies. The amount of Malwa opium for which it could not account was formidable.

The Problem with Malwa Opium and the Poppy-Cultivating Native States of the Central India and Rajputana Agencies

George Watt's review of Indian opium statistics for 1860/61–1889/90 (gleaned from unspecified sources he alludes to elsewhere in the report) enabled him to conclude the native states of Central India manufactured an annual average of 65,000 maunds (5,348,570.5 pounds) of the Malwa drug per year. The Rajputana states produced 40,000 maunds annually, a figure equivalent to 3,291,428 pounds (GBS [Watt] 1891:38).[42] The combined total is an annual average of 105,000 maunds or 8,639,998.5 pounds.[43] Using the Government of India's Malwa weighing stations' standard (140.25 pounds per container), the native states of Central India produced an average of 38,135.975045 chests per year. The figure for the Rajputana Agency native states is 23,468.292335. The combined total is 61,604.268395. Slightly more than 61,604.25 chests (105,000 maunds or 8,639,998.5 pounds) accessible every twelve months for consumption within India and elsewhere in the world is an enormous quantity of opium.

Bombay exported an average of 33,458.9 chests of Malwa opium each year during the 1883/84–1892/93 period. The addition of 3,092.97 more containers available for distribution in British territory (mentioned above) raises the amount of the drug whose destination the Government of India was able to confirm to an annual average of 36,551.87 chests. This leaves a total of 25,052.398395, or almost 25,052.4 chests.

At first glance, 25,052.4 chests appear to be a huge average amount of opium produced in the native states every season. Watt's calculations, however, are correct, and they can be verified. Assume that his figure of 105,000 maunds of Malwa opium is the total amount for the thirty-year period, not the average per year he claimed and cited above. The 105,000 maunds (8,639,998.5 pounds) divided by thirty years yields an average annual production of 287,999.95 pounds. This translates into an average yearly manufacture of *only* 2,053.4755793 chests of Malwa opium (using 140.25 pounds per chest) available for *both* overseas export *and* licit or illicit consumption anywhere in India. This number—slightly less than 2,053.5 chests—cannot be correct. The next two paragraphs explain why not.

All documents indicate that the total amount of Malwa opium produced per season for use within British India or overseas (sent to Bombay from the Ajmir, Indore, and Ahmedabad weighing stations) was identical or similar to the data found in one column of two tables. These are column 3 entries ("Exports from Bombay [Malwa]") for 1883/84–1892/93 in table 6, and the statistics in column 5 ("Diverted or Weighed for Sale in British Territory and Native States") of table 8. According to Finlay (table 8), the smallest number of Malwa chests paying a pass-duty for export from Bombay or for sale within British territory was 2,856.75 during the 1885/86 season. This entry represents the quantity that was available for sale within India for only one year. It is more than the average total amount (2,053.5 chests) of Malwa produced for both overseas export and consumption with India during that year if Watt's thirty-year total was 105,000 maunds rather than the average for a single season. Furthermore, exports from Bombay accounted for 90 percent to 95 percent of the Malwa opium weighed annually at Indore, Ajmir, and Ahmedabad.

There is another reason for accepting Watt's average annual production statistic of 105,000 maunds. The "maximum revenue from minimal production" policy, a victory for the SSOT in the previous decade, continued unchanged.[44] The Benares and Bihar Agency officials during the early 1890s still regulated the number of acres allocated to poppy cultivation. The same thing applied to the amount of opium distributed annually to the provinces and ultimately to the public. Charging customers in India as high a price as possible further regulated consumption. However, poppy cultivators under contract to the Benares and Bihar Agencies were capable of producing a yearly average amount of the drug equal to or exceeding Watt's 105,000-maund calculation.[45] The opium-producing native states were free to plant as much poppy and to manufacture as much opium as the market would bear. They did so, especially the larger ones such as Gwalior, Indore, and Bhopal (GBO [Griffin] 1894:I:105; Hastings 1895:14). The Government of India had only one mechanism for controlling the distribution of any native state's Malwa opium within British territory. It was the aforementioned quota governing the quantity issued from the weighing stations and warehouses in each province. So, the 105,000 maunds per year is a lot of opium and the Government of India, apart from the mandated allotments and complaints about smuggling, had little control over what the native states did with a substantial percentage of it.[46]

Smuggling and Consumption in the Poppy-Cultivating Native States of the Central India and Rajputana Agencies

An estimate of the annual amount of Malwa opium available for smuggling into British territory is possible. George Batten, for example, told his 1891 Society for the Arts audience that "a vast amount of opium is smuggled out" of the Central India and Rajputana Agency native states every year (GBO [Batten] 1894:I:133). He was unable to give a specific number for the illicit drug. Nonetheless, it can be inferred from the man's comments about total annual profits from poppy cultivation. The annual value of the "Malwa crop, licitly consumed in British India and exported by sea," he claimed, was worth £4,000,000. Batten then assigned a value of £2,000,000 for the Malwa drug "consumed in Central India, Rajputana, and Baroda, and smuggled thence." The number of chests consumed, not merely distributed by the Government of India to British Provinces, was "about 2,000 chests . . . chiefly in the Bombay Presidency . . . [T]he Madras Presidency, Hyderabad, and Mysore are also supplied from this source, and some . . . [go] to the Punjab" (GBO [Batten] 1894:I:135–36). And as previously cited, the province of Punjab was permitted to legally import no more than 935 maunds (76,937.1295 pounds) of the Central India and Rajputana Malwa product per season (GBO [Finlay–Appendix X] 1894b:II:355). This is equivalent to 548.57 chests of the Malwa drug manufactured for consumption within the country.[47] This indicates that Bombay and locations in South India received less than 1,500 chests of *legal* Malwa opium annually.

The native states' average annual production of 25,052.4 chests provides a clue to the amount of smuggled opium in British India. Subtracting Batten's calculation of approximately 2,000 chests of licit consumption in all British territories (including Punjab) leaves 23,052.4 chests possibly smuggled from the native states every year. Batten could say nothing more precise about the clandestine product. Neither could the British: they were as unsuccessful in confiscating substantial amounts of the illicit drug as they had been during the 1859/60 Palmer and Garden anarcotine experiments.[48] Although Batten did not suggest it, a percentage of the 23,052.4 chests probably remained in the region. Native states were known to retain some of their annual production. They used it to supplement a drug shortage created by a poor harvest the next year, or a future season. This is a 'reserve' similar to the British system for Bengal Excise and Provision opium, and for the licit Malwa drug. A native state also might have withheld some of the substance to sell sometime later when local market conditions ensured a higher price, hence greater profit (GBS [Watt] 1891:68). Which states did this, for what years, and how much manufactured opium was retained in any season before 1894/95, is not accurately known. In 1894 for example, Lieutenant-Colonel D. Robertson could only offer an estimate. He said merchants of the major towns of Malwa (especially in the native states of Gwalior and Indore) had been storing approximately 55,000 chests in warehouses. The amount was also growing each season (GBO [Robertson] 1894:IV:88).[49]

REGIONAL, PROVINCIAL, AND PER CAPITA CONSUMPTION OF LICIT OPIUM IN BRITISH INDIA AND THE NATIVE STATES, 1860/61–1892/93

Consumption of Malwa Opium in the Poppy-Cultivating Native States of the Central India and Rajputana Agencies

Residents of the drug-producing native states of Central India and Rajputana obviously ingested a portion of their own product.[50] People who lived in a non-poppy-cultivating native state sharing a border with the former also consumed some of it. The exact amount for either situation is, however, unknown (GBS [Watt] 1891:36; Hastings 1895:10). George Batten was more assertive; the region's 21,750,000 people—10 percent of India's population—ingested much opium (GBO [Batten] 1894:I:136). Other than Batten's statements, the closest thing to estimates are statements applicable to all native states in the country. One example is that the opium "habit" was more entrenched in native states than in British territory. This generalization, however, did not apply to the British provinces of Burma and Assam. Another example is that the population of native states increased 20 percent compared to only 11 percent elsewhere in the country (i.e., British India) between 1881 and 1891 (GBO [Clarke] 1894:II:447). The implication is that the number of heavy drug users might have risen in all locales over which the Government of India had minimal jurisdiction or presence.

Steady Rate of Opium Consumption in British India

George Watt produced two reports containing much data about consumption of *Papaver somniferum Linn* in India. The first, cited in preceding paragraphs, was written to educate members of Parliament about many aspects of drug production and distribution. He also argued against interfering in opium commerce within the country and stressed Indian citizens' modest use of the substance. His comments concerning consumption are different in the second publication. This is a multivolume dictionary about economic products in India. It was not written exclusively for influential politicians. Both documents offer a perspective about amount of consumption and provide data for calculating per capita ingestion of opium in the country. Watt's observations about all-India rates, and commentary from other sources, are cited first. Calculations for per capita consumption of opium follow this section.

In the informative and decidedly nonneutral or pro-trade 1891 Parliamentary Paper, Watt said the consumption of Bengal opium remained "practically stationary" from 1860/61 through 1889/90. Each year Indian nationals throughout the country used "less than 2,500 maunds" (GBS [Watt] 1891:37–8). This is approximately 222,500 pounds, or 1,802.7 chests, every twelve months during the thirty-year period. Watt was talking about consumption of the Benares and Bihar Opium Agencies' product in both British India and the native states. Inhabitants of the Malwa native states had access to sufficient opium without buying the Bengal product. His statements are therefore applicable only to the quasi-independent political entities not located on the Malwa plateau. Watt's second perspective is found in a chapter of one book that is in a ten-volume series entitled *The Dictionary of the Economic Products of India*. The series was published between 1885 and 1894.[51] This time Watt said considerable fluctuation characterized opium consumption in British India for the past thirty (or more) years. According to this British official, the "minimum has been 2,243 chests, and the maximum 5,554 chests . . . [and this range] represents the total Indian consumption, less the supplies produced within the native states" (Watt [1908]

1966b:852). There is no way to determine if Watt (in the [1908] 1966b publication) was referring to the Malwa drug taxed at the weighing stations or to the illicit product flowing from the poppy-cultivating native states of the Central India and Rajputana Agencies.

Watt's observations allow a generalization applicable to British India for a period beginning in 1860/61 and continuing for at least thirty years: the all-India rate of consumption of the Benares and Bihar product had not risen in proportion to population growth. Consumption varied, perhaps from year to year or for brief periods, but there had been no overall dramatic increase as SSOT members proclaimed. The Government of India could even argue that per capita ingestion or regional consumption of Bengal opium had declined during the second half of the nineteenth century because the population of "British Territory" increased 11 percent between 1881 and 1891 and 20 percent in "native territory" for the same period (GBO [Clarke] 1894:II:447). In other words, a substantial growth in population had not been accompanied by an equivalent increase in opium consumption.

Another document supports Watt's assessment, at least for British India from 1880/81 through 1889/90. On 17 December 1891, the Secretary of State for India reported to the Governor-General of the country that there had been no great rise in the quantity of licit opium consumed in British India, although the amount had fluctuated during the ten-year period. And in some provinces, especially Bombay and Madras, the expansion was "largely due to the substitution of licit for illicit opium" (GBC [Consumption] 1892:108).

Per Capita Consumption of Licit Opium in British Provinces and in Native States Beyond the Malwa Plateau

George Watt's 1891 comments permit a rough estimate of per capita opium consumption in British India during the first half of the century's last decade. The per capita calculation includes residents of those native states not situated on the Malwa plateau. The 1891 census lists 221,172,952 people living in British territory and 66,050,479 residents of "native territory" (i.e., native states) (GBO [Clarke] 1894:II:447). Subtracting George Batten's estimated 21,750,000 inhabitants of the Malwa plateau's poppy cultivating and nonproducer native states of the Central India and Rajputana Agencies leaves a total of 44,300,479 people in "native territory." Adding the latter statistic to the population of "British Territory" produces a grand total of 265,473,431 people. According to Watt, these 265,473,431 people ingested less than 2,500 maunds of opium (less than 222,500 pounds or 1,802.7 chests) during 1890/91. There are 7,000 grains (avoirdupois) in one pound. Since one maund contains 82.2857 pounds, one maund of opium is equivalent to 575,999.9 grains of the drug. The 265,473,431 Indian citizens ingested 2,500 maunds, or 1,439,999,750 grains of the mother drug. Dividing the last statistic by 265,473,431 consumers yields an average per capita consumption of slightly more than 5.4 grains.[52] This is not a daily dose; it is the amount of opium one person consumed in one year. The quantity is miniscule and the anarcotine ingested during the twelve months is virtually nonexistent. The amount of each substance is actually smaller because Watt is unclear regarding exactly how much less than 2,500 pounds was consumed per year.[53] Watt's 1891 exceptionally modest figures, obtained from more than one source, do not reflect reality in the subcontinent during the decade; data in other documents suggest his numbers are too low.

Other Calculations of Per Capita Consumption of Licit Opium in British India

Statistics about total consumption of nonsmuggled opium in British India circa 1892 enabled one official to illustrate the drug's minimal role in the lives of India's citizens. If distributed in equal amounts to every individual, the quantity would suffice to "furnish a moderate daily dole of . . . one-tenth of an ounce . . . to about 400,000 people, that is, to two persons in every thousand of the population." (GBC [Consumption] 1892:108). This statement can be interpreted as meaning that if only one person out of every five hundred in British India consumed opium, the intake per day for each of these consumers was one-tenth of an ounce. Since there are 437.5 grains in one ounce, at least one individual in every five hundred Indian citizens was ingesting 43.75 grains of opium. The person also was absorbing whatever anarcotine was inherent in this amount of the mother drug.[54] The remaining 499 people were unprotected because they were nonconsumers. The per capita quantity of drug ingested was negligible even if everyone received an equal share of the one-tenth of an ounce instead of only two in every thousand (or one out of 500 people).[55]

Yet another perspective about licit consumption in the country is available. It is provided by commentary and data from a Government of India document submitted to the Royal Commission on Opium. The material was available to Sir William Roberts when he wrote his medical report. The document is Memorandum VII: "Tables Showing the Distribution, by Districts, of the Opium Habit in India" (GBO [Memorandum VIII] 1895:VI:178–84). The licit consumption referred to involves two kinds of opium. The first is the Malwa drug that was sent to the weighing stations of Ajmir, Indore, and Ahmedabad. The second type is the Bengal Excise product manufactured at the Ghazipur and Patna factories.[56] The memorandum has consumption statistics for the districts comprising the British provinces of Assam, Bengal, Berar, Bombay, Sindh, Central Provinces, Madras, Northwest Provinces and Oudh, and Punjab. This document, however, does not indicate if figures for a province included shipments of Bengal Excise opium that were redistributed to any native state within the jurisdiction of that province.

Comments preceding the statistical data in Table I of Memorandum VIII indicate the amount of opium consumed in Coorg (a small province in South India) was so meager that its statistics were omitted from the tables. Data for the "British territory of Balochistan" in the Northwest Frontier (frequently spelled "Baluchistan" and occasionally "Baloochistan" in the literature) also are not cited. The reason given is that "the population over which the consumption is distributable is not on record" (GBO [Memorandum VIII] 1895:VI:178). Consumption figures for Ajmer[e]-Merwara also are absent from the table because the Government of India did not collect them. The last qualification mentioned in the memorandum is that opium consumption in Punjab was underestimated. Approximately "6,000 Baloch wanderers, encamped at the time of [the] census in the Dera Ghazi Khan district" were excluded from the compilation because they were not part of the "settled population" in the province (GBO [Memorandum VIII] 1895:VI:178). The exact number of "Baloch wanderers" was 5,934 (GBO [Memorandum VIII] 1895:VI:180).

"Hill tracts" located in several districts of Assam and Bengal were a problem for data collectors. The issue is not explained but the districts were North Lushai, Chittagong, Angul, and Cuttack. Average yearly consumption of licit opium in these locales, therefore, is slightly incorrect. The wide range of per capita consumption and regional distribution of the "opium habit" is obvious from table 9, "Total Population Grouped by Provinces, with Average Yearly Consumption of Licit Opium Per Head."

DOCUMENTED CONCENTRATION OF THE 'OPIUM HABIT' WITHIN INDIA: THE NORTH-SOUTH AND URBAN-RURAL DICHOTOMIES

Geographic Distribution of the Opium Habit in British India, 1892/93

Peninsular (Southern) India

Table 9 confirms what many witnesses appearing before the Royal Commission acknowledged: the 'opium habit' was much more prevalent in the northern part of the country than in the South. While per capita consumption for Madras (South India) was a modest fourteen grains per year, parts of the province registered much higher rates. Supplementary data cited elsewhere in the memorandum from which table 9 is taken (but not included in the table) indicates that Godavari district (Madras Province) was an abnormality for South India; its residents consumed an average of 130.6 grains during 1892/93. The entry closest to Godavari was the district of Vizagaptam (40.7 grains). Inhabitants of the Nilgiri Hills districts were far behind with only 27.1 grains and even Madras city registered a modest 26.5. Yearly consumption in the other districts ranged from meager to almost nonexistent; the smallest amount was 0.6 and .08 grains consumed per year in the districts of Tinnevelly and South Arcot respectively (GBO [Memorandum VIII] 1895:VI:179). Consumption in other regions of South India was inconsequential.

Non-Peninsular (Northern) India

The 'opium habit' also was not evenly distributed within the northern half of the country. And one province, this being Assam [East India], was truly exceptional.

Its Lakhimpur district (population of 254,053) had the highest annual average amount of the drug consumed per person registered for the entire country by far (747.4 grains). Three other districts in the province also indicate high per capita consumption: Darrang district (374.9 grains; population of 307,761), Nowgong (353.7 grains; population of 344,141), and Sibsagar (442.2 grains; population of 457,274.) Amounts were much lower for the eight remaining Assamese districts. The smallest tally recorded was 5.6 grains for the 121,570 residents of the Garo Hills district (GBO [Memorandum VIII] 1895:VI:178). Calcutta city and its environs in Bengal Province [East India], the district with the highest consumption anywhere in the country if Assam Province is excluded, was far behind Nowgong district's tally of 353.7 grains.

The province-by-province data found in table 9 tend to support George Watt's 1908 claim that the "mean consumption expressed to head of population in British India (including the high rate prevalent in Assam) comes to 38 grains per head per annum and if Assam be excluded it is under 30 grains" (Watt [1908] 1966b:857).[57]

The Urban-Rural Distribution of the Opium Habit in British India

Entries in Memorandum VIII for individual districts in British provinces also indicate that high per capita yearly consumption was an urban phenomenon. In Bengal, for example, the greatest amount cited for the forty-six districts was 276.1 grains in "Calcutta and suburbs." No other location came close. The nearest were Balasore district with 86.3 grains and the 41.4 grains ingested by the inhabitants of Hughli (GBO [Memorandum VIII] 1895:VI:178–79).

The situation was almost identical for Bombay Province. Residents of Ahmedabad city ingested 114.7 grains, the people occupying "Bombay Island" consumed on average 155.2, and the population of Broach used 179.6 grains per year. People in Ratnagiri district were almost complete abstainers; they admitted to ingesting only 1.7 grains every twelve-month period. Urban dwellers in Punjab and the Northwest Provinces and Oudh also were the heaviest users: the urbanized district of Lucknow was far out front with 106.8 grains. The densely populated district of Benares was in second place with 87.7 grains. With the exception of Crawnpore district (urban) and the Himalayan foothill district of Dehra Dun, consumption in the Northwest Provinces and Oudh ranged from low to slightly more than average (i.e., the low thirties). In Punjab, the residents of Ludhiana city registered the highest consumption levels for that province (176.8 grains). The next was Ferozpur city with 144.5 grains. Simla district (British India's summer capital in the foothills of the Himalayan Mountains) registered 136.8 grains, the third highest consumption locale in this part of India. Opium consumption in the Punjab cities of Amritsar, Lahore, and Ambala (also referred to as Umballa in the Commission hearings) was far behind other places in the Province. The numbers were 81.2, 75.5, and 74.8 grains respectively (GBO [Memorandum VIII] 1895:VI:179).

Berar Province was the one exception to high consumption rates being an urban phenomenon; its six districts all indicated considerable amounts per season. The lowest was 34.7 (Basim district) and the highest 154.4 grains per year in Elichpur (GBO [Memorandum VIII] 1895:VI:179).

OPIUM IN INDIA: THE PROBLEM AND ITS SOLUTION ACCORDING TO SIR WILLIAM ROBERTS

Abstinence and Underconsumption of Opium: The Problem and Its Solution

The presence of illicit opium from Burma, Assam, Punjab, Nepal, and other Himalayan locales precludes an accurate assessment of actual per capita consumption in any district, province, or native state in British India. The problem is compounded by not knowing exactly how much opium the poppy cultivating native states on the Malwa plateau manufactured and what percentage of this drug was smuggled into British territory. One consequence of clandestine distribution is that the pro-opiumists' proclamation about modest consumption being the norm throughout the country was moot. The generalization might be appropriate if it pertains only to the Bengal Excise product for which tax records existed. The pro-opiumists' contention is questionable when all sources of opium in India are included in their assessment. The Government of India's reluctance to publicize statistical estimates about the smuggling problem also deprived the SSOT from citing quantitative data to refute opponents.

Sir William Roberts' evaluation of opium relegated the debate about quantity to irrelevance. Consumption of all *Papaver somniferum Linn* was medically justified regardless of where the substance came from, where it was processed, the legal status of its dispersal, the rationale for its ingestion, and how much was consumed. In all cases, people were defending themselves against a horrendous malady whereas abstainers had no protection whatsoever. The problem confronting the country was far too few people consuming far too little opium, licit or illicit, to do any good. This was, in Roberts' mind, a rationale for promoting greater per capita and regional consumption of the drug. The SSOT had a different interpretation; the statistical data indicating a lack of widespread use invalidated claims about opium's efficacy to prevent and cure any disease. The SSOT's logic was simple: if the drug was so good, then why were not more people in all provinces and districts of India ingesting more of it?

Roberts was not the only participant in Royal Commission on Opium activities to cite 'malarial fever' data illustrating the tragic consequences of abstinence and underconsumption in British India. Mr. S. E. J. Clarke, secretary of the Bengal Chamber of Commerce, submitted equally sobering and more informative data to the Royal Commission on 3 December 1893. Table 10 contains Clarke's compilation of 'fever' mortality rates found in the correspondence. The title of table 10 is "Population and 'Fever' Mortality Statistics in Five British Provinces Compiled by Mr. S. E. J. Clarke, Secretary to the Bengal Chamber of Commerce, 4 December 1893 and Submitted to the Royal Commission on Opium."

The Significance of S. E. J. Clarke's Data

Clarke complained about too many people in India dying needlessly. He claimed that at least 4,393,353 out of a population of 149,795,398 residents in five British provinces expired during 1891. This was a mortality rate of 2.93 percent. Among the deceased, Clarke's "fever," which Sir William Roberts said was really "malarial fever," killed 3,062,031 people. This represented almost 70 percent (exactly 69.69 percent) of the fatalities. Roberts calculated that 'malarial' deaths accounted for 50 percent of the mortality in Assam Province whereas Clarke's figure was a bit more at 50.59 percent. Clarke's totals for Bengal, the Northwest Provinces and Oudh, and Punjab were 70.31 percent, 70.72 percent, and 73.85 percent respectively. Roberts slightly underestimated all of them by declaring the affliction was responsible for "about 70 percent" in each province. Both men almost concurred about deaths in the Central Provinces; Roberts said 'malaria fever' was responsible for about 60 percent. Clarke's tally was 61.71 percent. Roberts also concluded that 'malaria' dominated the death rate in every province of British India (GBO [Roberts] 1895:109). Clarke provided no statistics for the remaining British provinces to support Roberts' assertion but agreement was implicit in Clarke's comments.

The Roberts and Clarke assessment for five provinces, however, covered only 52.15 percent of India's population.[58] The total number of people living in both 'British Territory' and 'native territory' was 287,223,431 (GBO [Clarke] 1894:II:447). Since 47.85 percent of India's population was excluded, the actual number of individuals dying from the malady was much higher than indicated in Clarke's comments about 3,062,031 people perishing in only five provinces.[59]

Clarke and Roberts also contended that low per capita consumption of opium guaranteed a high number of deaths from 'fever' or 'malarial fever' throughout the country. Statistics for five provinces (see table 9: "Total Population Grouped by Provinces, with Average Yearly Consumption of Licit Opium Per Head") are illustrative. The average per capita ingestion of 141.4 grains per year in Assam had resulted in 'malarial fever' blamed for only 50 percent of all deaths in that province. The percentage, although still high, was far more preferable than the dismal situation associated with lower per capita consumption rates elsewhere in the country. The malady was still responsible for 73.85 percent of all deaths in Punjab despite an annual average per capita opium consumption of forty-two grains. Bengal fared no better; 70.31 percent of all deaths due to 'malarial fever' was accompanied by an average ingestion of fifteen grains per person over twelve months. The same assessment applied to the Northwest Provinces and Oudh, where a modest annual average of eighteen grains for each individual generated a 70.72 percent fever mortality rate.

The conclusion was obvious to Roberts, Clarke, and pro-opiumists. Residents of the Northwest Provinces and Oudh, Assam, Bengal, Punjab, and the central provinces were consuming insufficient amounts of the mother drug. Exacerbating a dismal situation was the absence of anarcotine to either prevent an attack, or to ensure what Dr. Garden referred to as a victim's complete "cure" and "convalescence" after the first paroxysm. Life was the same elsewhere in India.

Statistics from another table (Table III) in Memorandum VIII can be interpreted to conclude that all ten British India provinces suffered from the consequences of insufficient consumption of licit *Papaver somniferum Linn* and anarcotine in 1892/93 (GBO [Memorandum VIII] 1895:VI:184). And this, more than likely, is how Roberts viewed the data. A total of 39.2 percent of the combined populations of Assam, Bengal, Berar, Bombay, Sindh, Central Provinces, Madras, Northwestern Provinces and Oudh, and Punjab consumed less than seven grains of opium per person during 1892/93. At the opposite extreme were the mere 2.1 percent citizens in British India ingesting more than 145 grains during the year. These "heavy consumers" were concentrated in those locales where registered mortality from 'fever' or 'malarial fever' was relatively low; 25.4 percent of Assam's population ingested more than 145 grains per season. The quantity was responsible for keeping the mortality rate to only 50 percent. People consuming small amounts of the drug were to blame for the 50 percent figure. Almost 42 percent of the population of Assam (precisely 41.9 percent) ingested less than seven grains per year, an amount that rendered them more susceptible to the disease. Berar was similar to Assam; only 10.9 percent of its population consumed more than 145 grains during 1892/93. Everyone else ingested no less than thirty grains (GBO [Memorandum VIII] 1895:VI:184). Sir William Roberts reported 45 percent of Berar's annual mortality rate was the result of 'malarial fever.'

Another illustration ostensibly supports the Roberts, Clarke, and Government of India contention about an obvious and undeniable correlation between substantial opium intake and fewer deaths.[60] In 1892/93 the percentage of people in the Central Provinces consuming between ninety-seven and 144 grains, or more than 145 grains, was zero. A mere 19.1 percent of the population ingested from forty-nine to ninety-six grains. The majority absorbed only twenty-five to forty-eight grains, a situation that pro-opiumists could claim was responsible for the depressing figure of 70 percent of all deaths due to 'malarial fever.' Statistics for each province can be presented in different ways yet still lead to the same conclusion: 'malarial fever' deaths in a population decreased as per capita consumption of opium increased. Anomalies did not invalidate the conclusion.

Roberts calculated the 'malarial fever' mortality rate for Madras Presidency was 38 percent. Statistics in the Royal Commission on Opium document indicate that 74.3 percent of Madras residents each ingested less than seven grains of the drug during the entire season of 1892/93 (GBO [Memorandum VIII] 1895:VI:184).[61] Since so many people consumed so little over a period of twelve months, the SSOT or any skeptic argued that Madras invalidated the correlation between opium eating and 'malarial fever.' Pro-opiumists responded by asserting that 'malarial fever' did not plague the region so there was no need to consume the drug in great amounts. Furthermore, a 38 percent mortality rate was still significant, albeit moderate compared to the rest of the country. The reason for the relatively low percentage was that 5.8 percent of the citizens of Madras Presidency (Province) consumed between ninety-seven and 144 grains of the drug during 1892/93. A total of 9.4 percent of the population ingested between twenty-five and forty-four, and 5.2 percent of the population absorbed thirteen to twenty-four grains during the twelve-month period. Another 5.3 percent consumed between seven and thirteen grains. The people (25.7 percent of the total population) who ingested six grains or more during 1892/93 were responsible for keeping the death rate at only 38 percent. There would have been fewer deaths if 74.3 percent of the people in the Presidency had indulged more often or consumed greater quantities when they did so (GBO [Memorandum VIII] 1895:VI:184).[62] They did not, and the result was too many people suffering needlessly.

ALLEVIATING MISERY AND REDUCING 'MALARIAL FEVER' MORTALITY

Roberts' assessment provided the Government of India with a tactical flexibility to neutralize SSOT opposition that it lacked prior to creation of the Royal Commission on Opium. The administration could adopt one of several options concerning the future of the mother drug and the alkaloid. All options were "medically justified" because they involved two substances that helped to prevent and cure a horrendous malady. Every program involved no diminution in poppy cultivation, and no decrease in the manufacture, distribution, and consumption of *Papaver somniferum Linn* within India. Each option also protected or had the potential for raising the percentage contribution of money earned from the domestically consumed drug to the general opium revenue (i.e., income from *both* the Provision and Excise commodity).

The Benefits of Changing Nothing

From Roberts' point of view, avoiding a reduction in the production and distribution of opium was essential to preventing an escalation of 'malarial fever' deaths in British India. A continuation of present policy helped to keep provincial mortality rates at current levels if serious epidemics over wide areas in the country did not occur with greater frequency. One option for the Government of India, therefore, was to preserve the status quo; the prospect of needless deaths did not disappear but at least the situation would get no worse if luck prevailed.[63] The administration was beyond reproach if its post-1895 opium policy promulgated no drastic decline in poppy acreage or diminution in the aforementioned production, distribution, and consumption statistics for Bengal Excise opium.

Sir William Roberts' conclusions about opium consumption also assailed the credibility of an SSOT issue. This was the insistence upon ending smuggling from the unregulated poppy-cultivating native states of the Malwa plateau into British-controlled territory. Eliminating the amount of clandestine opium consumed in British India would increase the 'malarial fever' mortality rate because the deaths which Roberts and Clarke lamented occurred in a population ingesting *both* licit and illicit opium. Less opium consumed, regardless of its origin or its legal status, guaranteed diminished protection and a multiplication of tragic consequences. The SSOT's opponents could now argue with even greater conviction that a policy of noninterference concerning the illicit drug was most appropriate. The presence of smuggled opium was an unappreciated variable preventing the documented mortality rates from rising still higher. The clandestine drug's availability provided the Government of India with another benefit; it reduced pressure upon the British administration to augment efforts to reduce or minimize 'malarial fever' fatalities.

Before 1893, representatives of the Government of India, and then numerous witnesses testifying before the Royal Commission on Opium, claimed that ending the annual amount of illicit Malwa circulating in India was not economically and politically viable. Although inaction ensured lost revenue for the Government of India, critics said that the cost of implementing a successful antismuggling program exceeded the amount of money acquired from taxation. Roberts' logic provided these people with a medical justification for inertia. And Mr. S. E. J. Clarke echoed many skeptics when he asserted the Government of India "would look to be reimbursed for the enormous Police and Preventive establishments she would have to keep up in all the provinces" (GBO [Clarke] 1894:II:450). Citizens in Great Britain or the inhabitants of British India's provinces had to finance this impossible undertaking. Roberts' declarations circumvented the problem of politicians and administrators confronting inevitable protests from the tax-paying populations of both locations.

Different strategies were necessary if the Government of India wanted to reduce the 'malarial fever' mortality rate rather than merely prevent it from increasing. This required the resolution of two problems: the amount of opium to be consumed, and identifying where in India use of the drug had to be encouraged.

Ending Maldistribution of the 'Opium Habit'

The 'opium habit' in India circa 1893–1895 was maldistributed in two ways. As cited above, official documents concerning licit consumption indicated that 'eating opium' and other forms of ingestion were concentrated in urban locales, not in the countryside where 'malarial fever' was rampant. It was imperative, therefore, for the Government of India to make consumption as commonplace in rural areas as it was in the cities.

The regional distribution of consumption also needed correction. The 'opium habit' was a "North India" phenomenon. It had to evolve into a more 'all-India' custom with citizens in the southern half of the country also benefiting from the drug's prophylactic and febrifuge capability. There was no reason to assume that people in South India would continue to escape serious episodes of the 'disease' in the years to come. One way to minimize misery and premature death throughout the subcontinent was to encourage opium consumption before an outbreak of the malady. This would not happen unless the Government of India, in cooperation with all provincial bureaucracies and the rulers of native states within the jurisdictions of the latter, took steps to make it a reality. The cooperation of different departments within the central government also was required to solve the problem of underconsumption among two kinds of people: the individuals who did indulge, and the many inhabitants who needed to but refrained from doing so.

Reducing 'Malarial Fever' Mortality

Past and present high death rates were ample evidence that Indian citizens' ingestion of licit, as well as illicit, opium had protected and cured few of them. Many consumers needed to use much more of the drug per day, per week, per month, and per year to avoid suffering and demise. People with no 'opium habit' had to acquire one if they wanted to help themselves. It was neither immoral nor irresponsible, therefore, for the Government of India to relax, or to abolish, restraints affecting any phase of providing licit opium to Indian citizens. The opium factories, for example, should manufacture as much drug as the market will absorb, and the cultivators sanctioned to plant as much poppy as they deemed feasible. There also should be no limitation upon the amount of nonsmuggled Bengal Excise and Malwa drug that each provincial administration was permitted to allocate to native states within its borders or to licensed vendors for eventual sale to citizens of the province.

Quotas for the maximum amount of opium each person was allowed to purchase at one time also had to end in all provinces where these regulations existed. The benefits of consumers' unrestricted access to opium exceeded the liabilities of such a change. Overindulgence by some individuals was to be expected, but many more citizens now had the opportunity to provide themselves with an inexpensive 'malarial fever' prophylactic and febrifuge. The far higher number of people prolonging their lives in the subcontinent, therefore, eliminated the onus of a minimal increase in deaths due to excessive use.

The steps mentioned thus far helped to increase per capita consumption of the mother drug and absorption of its inherent anarcotine. The problem of underconsumption, however, was not solved. It is one thing to propose greater use of opium; it is quite another to find a way to obtain the substance. And then there is the problem of morphia toxicity forcing most people to ingest inconsequential, hence ineffective, amounts of the mother drug.

The Need for More *Papaver somniferum Linn*

The Government of India needed more opium if it decided to reduce mortality in India by raising per capita consumption or by persuading nonusers to begin the 'habit.' Additional opium also was necessary to correct the north–south and urban–rural maldistribution. One solution to meeting future higher demand was to expand poppy cultivation and drug production above current levels.[64] An alternative was to use the opium reserves maintained at the two opium factories and by the provincial governments. At best only a temporary solution, diminishing these stocks was a precarious undertaking. The reserves guaranteed availability of the drug in case of crop failure in the Government of India's Opium Agencies. Depletion or these stocks, followed by one or two successive poor seasons, would result in insufficient *Papaver somniferum Linn* to meet demand throughout the country; a repetition of the situation partially responsible for creation of the reserve system. It was absolutely necessary, therefore, for the Ghazipur and Patna factories and the provincial governments to increase their respective reserve holdings. And the amount had to be large enough to supply the substance to a greater number of people, these being former underconsumers and abstainers, potential future victims in South India, and rural inhabitants throughout the country.

The SSOT would object to the Government of India's expansion of poppy acreage regardless of the medical and humanitarian rationale proffered. The organization viewed its opponents as hypocritical and duplicitous. Opium use was beneficial, but only under strict supervision. The Government of India, according to the SSOT, had demonstrated insufficient awareness about the drug's limitations and contempt for anyone who tried to warn them about this shortcoming.

One way for the administration to temper, but not to end, opposition was to use the chests that were scheduled for export to provide the population with its additional *Papaver somniferum Linn* requirement. This program entailed a change in destination for what was already produced. It did not require an increase in cultivation for manufacturing more opium. There was another benefit from using Provision opium. Money earned from increased sales of the drug in India would compensate for the decline in exports to China and other parts of the world. The unpleasant reality of a shrinking overseas market in 1894–1895 might evolve into something less disquieting.

Another reality confronting the administration was the possibility of needing more than one option to obtain the enormous amount of *Papaver somniferum Linn* required to reduce 'malarial fever' mortality throughout the country among people already consuming the substance and those who had to begin. The exact quantity necessary for the populations of British India and the native states is impossible to calculate. Roberts and Clarke had documented 'malaria' deaths in five provinces where people consumed licit and illicit opium. The Government of India had statistics regarding amounts of the legal substance supplied to this public but no comparable data for smuggled opium. This means an unacceptable number of deaths occurred in an area having 52.15 percent of the country's total population despite consumption of legal and possibly large quantities of the illegal drug. The remaining 47.85 percent of India's people also consumed licit and illicit opium. And Sir William Roberts' 'malarial fever' most likely accounted for a substantial percentage of total mortality in this second group whose number also represented almost one half of the country's total population. British officials, therefore, had to manufacture an amount of opium that exceeded the quantity available legally and illegally in all locales if they were serious about preventing unnecessary deaths in the subcontinent. The amount needed would be known only when the percentage of deaths attributable to 'malarial fever' began to decline in a milieu of easy access to the drug.

BENGAL EXCISE OPIUM AND THE ANARCOTINE EXTRACTION RATIOS

Procuring Anarcotine for 'Malarial Fever' Victims in India

The anti-opiumists' nightmare was not over. Regardless of the option (or options) selected regarding future production and distribution of the mother drug, the Government of India had to procure an additional supply of opium for extracting the anarcotine that morphia-intolerant individuals required. The amount of *Papaver somniferum Linn* needed for Roberts' recommended alkaloid dosage is calculated by increasing the 'number of sufferers' (column 2 entries) cited in table 5 ("Estimate of Anarcotine and Crude Opium Requirements for Quotidian and Tertian Fever Patients Based upon Dr. A. Garden's 1859–60 Ghazipur Experiment"). The quantities required for extracting sufficient anarcotine for 1,500,000 to 4,000,000 victims are listed in table 11: "Anarcotine and Bengal Excise Opium Requirements Using the Three Ratios for More than One Million Sufferers." Quantities of the mother drug (columns 3–5 of table 11) are cited in Bengal Excise chests because Roberts specified using the Benares and Bihar agencies' product.[65]

Roberts and Clarke presented similar mortality figures. Assume, however, that Clarke was one of the individuals whom Roberts said had incorrectly classified some fatal cases of pneumonia as 'fever' deaths. The actual number of fatalities attributable to 'malarial fever' in the five British provinces is now less than Clarke's 3,062,031 total for column 5 ("Number of Deaths in Province") in Table 10.[66] Further assume that Clarke, or whomever Roberts had in mind, made either many or a moderate number of mistakes. A substantial diagnostic error might be 62,031 people succumbing to maladies different from those Roberts included in his 'malarial fever' category. Subtracting 62,031 from Clarke's original number leaves a total of 3,000,000 'authentic' cases of 'malarial fever' in Assam, Punjab, Bengal, the Central Provinces, and the Northwest Provinces and Oudh. Table 11 indicates 3,000,000 morphia-intolerant sufferers required 16,842.21 pounds of anarcotine for their complete "cure" and "convalescence." A modest number of mistakes for Clarke—12,031 for example—increases the real 'malarial fever' fatality statistic in the five provinces from 3,000,000 to 3,050,000 victims and a need for 17,122.91 pounds of the alkaloid.[67]

The number of 'malarial deaths' in the five British provinces increases to 3,062,031 upon dropping the assumption about miscalculations, and accepting Roberts' suggestion that Clarke erred only in using an incorrect name. The amount of anarcotine these 3,062,031 morphia-intolerant patients afflicted by "malarial fever" required for a complete "cure" and "convalescence" is 17,190.45 pounds.[68]

A summary of these statistics illuminates the steps the Government of India had to take to prevent the death of large numbers of morphia-intolerant 'malarial fever' sufferers. Three million people required 16,842.21 pounds of anarcotine for a complete "cure and "convalescence." The amount increased to 17,122.91 pounds for 3,050,000 individuals. The 3,062,031 victims that Clarke and Roberts documented had to ingest 17,190.45 pounds to avoid death. Three and one-half million people needed 19,649.24 pounds of the alkaloid whereas 4,000,000 patients had to use 22,456.28 pounds (see column 2 of table 11). The last two statistics (3,500,000 and 4,000,000) are not unrealistic. Clarke and Roberts cited *reported* deaths in the five provinces, not the higher number of undocumented people who were sick and likely to die in the not-too-distant future. It also must not be forgotten that the Roberts and Clarke 3,062,031 mortality statistic applied to only 52.15 percent of India's population. As mentioned before, Roberts and Clarke would have classified many deaths occurring beyond the borders of these five British provinces as additional cases of 'malarial fever.' Inclusion of a mortality figure for the remaining 47.85 percent of the nation's population, if the statistic had been collected, would raise Roberts' 'malarial fever' victims to a number substantially higher than 4,000,000. The Government of India then had a problem. It would have to procure anarcotine to treat more than 4,000,000 Indian people who suffered from the disease that Roberts called 'malaria.' The number of victims might be as high as 5,000,000. Furthermore, the British administration's data for per capita consumption indicated that very few people in the country ingested the mother drug anywhere near a level sufficient to either prevent or cure the malady. Roberts said the same thing in his report. The implication is that throughout India most people at some time needed to use the alkaloid, not opium itself, to prolong their existence. Qualifying statements aside, more anarcotine required more *Papaver somniferum Linn*, and the alkaloid extraction ratio determined how much more.

Bengal "Abkari" Chests and the Three Opium/Anarcotine Ratios

The 116.9:1 Extraction Ratio

Table 11 indicates a fraction less than 15,951.75 chests of Bengal Excise opium provides sufficient alkaloid for the "cure" and "convalescence" of 3,000,000 sufferers in the five provinces if the 116.9:1 opium-to-anarcotine yield ratio governed the extraction process during the 1890s.[69] Clarke's documented 3,062,031 sick people used 16,281.58 Abkari opium chests. The number increases to 18,610.36 Bengal chests for 3,500,000 victims who experienced only one outbreak possessing the virulence of Dr. Garden's 1859/60 encounter. Four million people need 21,456.28 containers.[70]

The 116.9:1 ratio calculations justify anti-opiumists' despair. Entries in table 12 list the quantity of Bengal opium the Government of India had to manufacture to supply 'malarial fever' sufferers and potential victims with Roberts' recommended small doses of anarcotine. The requirement for these four groups of alkaloid recipients is sobering. It ranges from slightly more than 358 percent to almost 482 percent of the average number of licit Bengal chests prepared per season (4,454.5) for domestic consumption during the two decades before the Royal Commission's existence.[71]

The other ratios (table 13 [24:1 figures] and table 14 [16:1 figures]) also promised little comfort to SSOT activists and their supporters. The titles for table 13 and table 14 are identical to table 12: "Quantity of Bengal Abkari (Excise) Opium Chests Required to Extract Sufficient Anarcotine for 'Cure' and 'Convalescence' of Four Groups of 'Malarial Fever' Sufferers. Entries Are Expressed as Percentage of Bengal Chests Prepared for Domestic Consumption During the Twenty-Year Period from 1873/74–1892/93."

The 24:1 Extraction Ratio

A more efficient extraction ratio did not change the amount of anarcotine required for several million sufferers. It did, however, reduce the quantity of opium necessary to obtain the substance. Three million victims needed 3,274.95 Bengal Excise containers to satisfy their alkaloid requirement if the 24:1 ratio was operative. The number of opium chests increased to 3,820.77 for three and one-half million victims, and Clarke's 3,062,031 sufferers needed approximately 3,342.67 chests.[72] Four million victims mandated the procurement of a grand total of 4,366.60 Abkari chests for their complete "cure" and "convalescence." Table 13 indicates the quantities for these groups of people were equivalent to more than 73.5 percent, and slightly higher than 98 percent, of the average annual number of Abkari chests manufactured at the Benares and Patna Agencies' factories from 1873/74 through 1892/93. The implications are obvious. Distributing sufficient anarcotine to sick Indians under 24:1 extraction ratio conditions required an approximate 75 percent to almost 100 percent increase in availability of Bengal Excise opium chests provided the number of people subjected to this therapy did not exceed 4,000,000.[73]

The 16:1 Extraction Ratio

Sir William Roberts' 16:1 proposal and table 14 yield the following numbers. Three million people required 269,475.36 pounds of opium for their alkaloid therapy. This was equivalent to the contents of 2,183.30 Bengal Excise chests. The total for three and one-half million sufferers was 314,387.92 pounds or slightly more than 2,547.18 chests. Four million individuals needed 359,300.48 pounds or 2,911.07 containers.[74] Clarke's 3,062,031 victims required 2,228.44 chests of the Bengal Excise mother drug for possible restoration of health if Sir William Roberts' opium-to-anarcotine ratio was valid for the mid-1890s.[75] According to table 14, the average annual production of Bengal Abkari chests had to expand from almost 50 percent to more than 65 percent. This increase would provide sufficient alkaloid for the three to four million 'malarial fever' sufferers unable to ingest adequate amounts of the mother drug to prevent or to cure their illness.[76]

These statistics and estimates demonstrate that Sir William Roberts' proposal was indeed good news for Government of India economists and provincial administrators.[77] The proposition's effect upon the post-1895 administration's drug policy and the SSOT, and its significance for the study of imperialism, is the subject of the next chapter.

NOTES

1. For a discussion of criteria observed during the nineteenth century, consult Impey (1848), Winther (1990), and GBS [Watt] 1891:57.

2. The steps in extracting narcotine, comments about alkaloid purity, and a description of the modified Gregory–Robertson system for morphia manufacture are found in GBS [Watt] 1891:65–66. A useful, albeit brief, review of nineteenth-century morphia extraction techniques and their limitations, is M. André Barbier (1947:5:2:121–40). Some comparable information about other methods of extracting alkaloids during the nineteenth and early twentieth centuries is found in Robert J. Bryant (1988:146–53).

3. The amount of confiscated opium was ten maunds and nine seers. This produced between six and six and one-half seers of morphia and three and one-half seers of anarcotine. Garden's maund is equivalent to eighty pounds. His seer is two pounds (1860:409).

A "maund" or "seer" does not guarantee a constant amount. Weights and measurements with the same name in India differed from region to region and might fluctuate over time in the same location. Garden provides numbers for deciphering occidental equivalents for his "maund" and "seer." For other conversion preferences, see R. N. Chaudhuri (ed.) 1971:iv; Binod Bhushan Chadhuri 1970:7:2:June:235; and H. H. Wilson [1855] 1968:474.

R. N. Chaudhuri says officials in British India used the following conversion figures between 1814 and 1858. One "factory maund" was equivalent to 74 pounds, 10 ounces and 10 drams (rounded off to 74 pounds and 11 ounces). A "factory maund" contained forty seers or 640 chattaks (Palmer's spelling is "chittak") (1971:iv). Garden was not referring to "factory maund." Wilson's volume is valuable for illustrating the various meanings of numerous terms used throughout the country.

Garden rounded off fractions to the nearest whole number when converting a maund or seer to pounds and ounces. Commentators during the 1890s were more precise. They converted one maund to 82.2857 pounds and one seer to 2.057 pounds (GBO [Watt] 1891:61; GBO [Clarke] 1894:II:447; GBC [Statistical Abstract–No. 42] 1896a:95. Garden therefore slightly underestimated the amount of crude opium needed to obtain the required anarcotine. The maund and seer conversion figures cited in the 1860 article, however, are used in this section when discussing his calculations.

4. One pound contains 7,000 grains (avoirdupois). Garden's 194 documented patients, therefore, needed 1.0877 pounds of anarcotine. The 116.9:1 crude opium to anarcotine ratio results in a total of 127.152 pounds of crude opium needed to produce the required amount of alkaloid.

5. The anarcotine and opium need of Garden's 490 undocumented participants using the 116.9:1 ratio is calculated as follows. One-hundred and ninety-four (the number of patients for whom Garden maintained records) multiplied by 2.525773 is 490 (the number of Garden's undocumented participants). This total (490) is 2.525773 (or 2.526) times greater than 194.

The 194 patients consumed 1.0877 pounds of anarcotine, or slightly less than 1.09. The 490 undocumented participants' anarcotine consumption is obtained by multiplying 1.0877 pounds by 2.526. The result is a total of 2.7475302 pounds. The number is a fraction less than 2.75 pounds, or two pounds, twelve ounces of the alkaloid. This amount of anarcotine requires 321.1859 pounds of opium. This figure is obtained by multiplying the 194 documented participants' opium requirement of 127.152 pounds by 2.526.

The 116.9:1 ratio, therefore, indicates that Garden's 684 patients consumed approximately 3.84 pounds of anarcotine. This in turn required 448.34 pounds of opium.

6. T. W. Sheppard's 1894 enclosure in the Gregory document cites no reason for the cessation of morphia and anarcotine extraction at the Ghazipur factory. If policy makers decided to halt anarcotine production because of the availability of cinchona alkaloids in 1865, Sir William Roberts' 1895 contention about anarcotine has even less credibility. The administration's decision three decades earlier is a tacit recognition of the superiority of quinine, and possibly other cinchona alkaloids, as a prophylactic and febrifuge for at least one kind of 'malaria.' This suggests that British officials' view of the malady in 1865 is similar to the version articulated by the splitters who testified before the Royal Commission during 1893/94. Both parties acknowledge that anarcotine does not prevent or cure the fever-producing afflictions subsumed under the inclusive term 'malarial fever.' Anarcotine production was resumed prior to 1870/71. Yet, only meager amounts were extracted despite numerous people suffering from 'malaria.' The Government of India stopped extracting the alkaloid from the mother drug after a few years.

7. Gregory first lists the amount of anarcotine issued to medical department locations and other institutions throughout the country. The period covered is seventeen years, from 4 April 1860 to 24 April 1876. The data are found on page 82 in "Statement showing the Quantity of Narcotine issued to the Medical Department before 1878." The next page continues the itemization to 23 January 1894 This table is entitled "Statement of Narcotine supplied from 1876 to January 1894."

Shipments of anarcotine over a period of seventeen years (from April 1860 through April 1876) went to medical officials in Gorakhpur, Benares Circle, Mean Meer, Calcutta, Allahabad, Umballa (Ambala), Sialkot, Saugor, and to several institutions. One of the earliest deliveries was four ounces to the "Medical-in-Charge" at the Ghazipur factory. This probably was Dr. Garden.

Destinations are also listed in the second table (from 15 December 1876 to January 1894). The table also mentions Mean Mccr, Calcutta, Allahabad, the civil surgeon at Ludhiana, the surgeon-general at Agra, the factory superintendent at Behar, and one "private individual." This last person is identified as Mr. Francis of Durbhanga. The October 1883 shipment of 100 pounds to the secretary of state in London, England is cited at the end of the table. Both tables are in GBO [Gregory] 1894:V:82–83.

8. There was minimal demand for anarcotine in India from 1860 through 1894/95 even though the cinchona industry had collapsed and quinine was virtually unavailable to the public until after 1880. The quinine came from Java, and it remained too expensive for most Indian natives to afford. For details, see *Appendix C: Cinchona Cultivation and Quinine Production in South Asia During the Nineteenth Century.*

9. "Cake opium" was distributed "in cases of 2 lbs. each" (GBO [Rivett-Carnac] 1894:II:322).

10. During the 1830s, the aforementioned Dr. O'Shaughnessy tried unsuccessfully to increase the inherent low morphine content of Indian opium. He relied upon selection of poppy varieties, and careful methods of cultivation and latex extraction. Additional comments about later efforts are found in Eatwell 1851–52:11:269–71, 306–11, 359–64; Eatwell 1852:118–33; and PuID 1966:VII:239.

11. Data are condensed from two tables in the Rivett-Carnac document. His quantities are stated in maunds, seers, and chittaks (page 329). The first table is Statement G–Table I: "Quantity of Medical Cakes Manufactured and Issued During the Financial Years–from 1883–84 to 1892–93 and Value of the Same." Rivett-Carnac's second table is

Statement G–Table II: "Quantity of Powdered Opium Manufactured and Issued During the Financial Years–from 1883–84 to 1892–93 and Value of the Same." Both tables are in GBO [Rivett-Carnac] 1894:II:319–35.

12. Another document covering consumption from 1879–1880 through 1889/90 yields a similar figure: an average of 1,460 maunds (120,137.122 pounds) per year. This is slightly more than Watt's calculation. Entries in this second document for 1879/80 and 1880/81, a total of 1,898 and 2,375 maunds respectively, denote a probable inclusion of "a large weight of poppy heads." And the 1886/87 citation specifies that 730 maunds were poppy heads.

A popular form of ingestion in Punjab was amul-pani. This was an infusion of opium poppy heads in water. Subtracting poppy head entries from the grand total of ten years yields a figure close to Watt's estimate. See GBC [Consumption] 1892:60.

13. The province of Punjab imported very little Bengal Excise opium from 1873/74 through 1892/93 compared to the Bengal Presidency, Assam, Burma, and the Northwest Provinces and Oudh. The Bengal product was sent to Punjab only in 1879/80, 1880/81, 1886/87, 1887/88, and in the four seasons from 1889/90 through 1892/93. The amount for each year was negligible: 10, 410, 200, 200, 80, 110, 147, and 50 maunds respectively (GBO [Rivett-Carnac] 1894:II:327). Total amount of the Benares and Bihar Agencies' drug sent to Punjab for the twenty-year period was 1,207 maunds (99,318.8399 pounds). This is a two-decade annual average of only 60.35 maunds (4,965.941995 pounds).

Two other Royal Commission documents confirm the modest presence of the licit Bengal Excise drug in Punjab. Mr. J. F. Finlay (secretary to the Government of India, Department of Finance and Commerce) presents data from 1883/84 through 1892/93. The entries, all in seers, show no Bengal Excise imports for the period 1883/84 through 1885/86. The number of seers sent each year to Punjab from 1886/87 through 1892/93, like the Rivett-Carnac data mentioned above, was small (GBO [Finlay–Appendix IX] 1894a:II:350).

The second Royal Commission file concerning the status of Bengal Excise opium in Punjab has consumption (not quantity of imports) statistics from 1883/84 through 1892/93. The document indicates that no Bengal Excise opium was consumed legally in the province during 1883/84 through 1885/86. And only modest amounts were sold during each of the next seven years (1886/87–1892/93) (GBO [Walker] 1894:V:106).

The Finlay and Walker material reveals that only a modest amount of the legal Bengal commodity was circulating in Punjab. The quantity available for consumption was not in great demand.

14. The amount of Malwa opium consumed in Punjab province might be considerably more than an annual average of 60.35 maunds. Mr. H. Hastings, subdeputy opium agent for the Benares Agency, cites 572 chests of "Biscuit" opium exported to Punjab. This most likely occurred during 1894/95. He claims the figure represents an increase but provides no numbers for previous seasons. "Biscuit opium" is made from "inferior opium which is not good enough for China export, or from an admixture of Rubba and ordinary chik . . . " "Chik" is the common name in the region for crude opium. "Rubba," also called "dhoi" or "washings," is prepared by "soaking soiled opium bags in water and . . . inspissated either by boiling or by sun drying" (Hastings 1895:9).

15. The average annual production of opium in Punjab province from 1879/80 through 1889/90 was 1,460 maunds or 120,137.122 pounds. An 1892 Parliamentary Paper citing a total of 1,898 and 2,375 maunds for 1879/80 and 1880/81 respectively also notes these totals probably include "a large weight of poppy heads." The document's entry for 1886/87 specifies that 730 maunds were poppy heads (GBC [Consumption] 1892:62–63).

16. A contradiction might exist regarding Madras. In one document submitted to the Royal Commission on Opium, Mr. J. F. Finlay indicates that Madras produces none of its own opium. The opium agent at Indore city (located within the Central India Agency) fulfills the opium needs of Madras by supplying the Malwa product (GBO [Finlay–Appendix X] 1894b:II:357). Finlay might be referring to the Indore Opium Agent fulfilling the needs of the population of Madras city and its environs. A small amount of poppy cultivation yielding very meager quantities of the drug, however, was permitted within the larger Madras Presidency. All of it was consumed locally.

Statistics for native states throughout India from 1891/92 through 1898/99 are available. See IDRA 1898–1900. Volume II: Native States," 13th, 14th, and 15th editions. Also see GBO [Robertson–Appendix XI] 1894:IV:406–17 for cursory comments about production in the native states of Central India. Robertson tried to compile data from 1888. He admits that most states and entities within these states that cultivated poppy submitted no statistics. Furthermore, the material that was sent in had to be accepted with caution (GBO [Robertson–Appendix XI] 1894:IV:406].

17. For commentary submitted to the Royal Commission about illicit opium activity in Burma and adjoining regions of Northeast India, see GBO [Fryer] 1894:II:500–07.

18. The subdivisions comprising the Behar and Benares Opium Agencies are listed in GBO [Clarke] 1894:II:445–46. J. F. Richards (1981:69–82) provides a concise description of the relations of production in both Agencies. His article also chides academicians for ignoring the ideological significance of opium exports for the East India Company and the Government of India.

19. Each of these Bengal Excise chests contained one maund and twenty seers of the drug, a total of 123.4257 pounds (GBS [Godley] 1897:6; GBS [Watt] 1891:69). The standard equivalency was one maund weighing 82.2857 pounds and one seer equal to 2.057 pounds. The fractions above 140 pounds and 123 pounds are the weights of "leewa" used for packing opium cakes in "Provision" and Excise ("Abkari") chests. "Leewa" contained varying, but always small amounts of opium. Cake buyers often treated "Provision" chest "leewa" to maximize quantity of the smoking extract. Excise opium cake "leewa" also was frequently used because of the residual amount of opium it contained. The author's calculations include "leewa."

20. The Central India Agency consisted of the Indore Residency, the Gwalior Residency, and the Agencies of Bhopal, Bundelkhand (Bandelkhand), Bagelkhand (Baghelkand), Western Malwa, Bhopawar and Goona (Guna). A grand total of seventy-one opium-producing native states, or smaller administrative units within a native state, comprised the residencies and agencies of the larger Central India Agency. The Rajputana Agency consisted of Meywar (Mewar), the Western Rajputana States, Jeypore, Haroati & Tonk, and the Eastern States (GBO [Finlay–Appendix IX] 1894a:II:346–47; Watt [1908] 1966b:854).

Similar to Central India, each of these subdivisions consisted of opium-producing native states or smaller entities within a state. There were twenty-four native states, or subdivisions thereof, in the Rajputana Agency (GBO [Finlay–Appendix IX] 1894a:346–47). The "subdivisions" within a native state in Central India and Rajputana were land tenure systems known as "jagirdari" and "muafi." The terms designate tenure rights in land granted to citizens by the chief or ruling family of a native state. "Muafi" was any kind of land held revenue-free for either a fixed period or in perpetuity. In the British-controlled Ajmere (also spelled Ajmir or Ajmeer) district on the Malwa plateau, and in Gwalior (a large poppy-cultivating native state in Central India), a "jagir" or jagirdari was land granted either as a reward for military service or a charitable donation. Like "muafi" land, a recipient (jagirdar) ostensibly paid no taxes to the chief of the native state. See IDR 1904:18:xxviii, and H. H. Wilson [1855] 1968.

21. In 1895, H. Hastings says that a portion of what is called 'Malwa' does not originate "strictly in Malwa, [the location] being the country below the Vindhyans [hills] along both sides of the Nebadda [river]." Hastings provides no data for amounts produced other than observing that the drug, apparently from Nimar district, is of high quality due to less adulteration. 'Malwa opium' therefore included the product from the native states of the Central India and Rajputana Agencies, from Ajmere-Marwara, and latex from a small amount of poppy cultivated on land adjacent to the Malwa plateau.

22. The Government of India weighing station in Ajmir city shipped Malwa opium to Ghazipur in 1882/83 through 1888/89 and again in 1893/94 and 1894/95 (GBS [Godley] 1893:6; GBS [Godley] 1897:7).

23. The Ahmedabad station collected opium from Baroda State and Dungapore, a small native state in the Rajputana Agency. There were subsidiary scales in other locations. These places received small amounts of the Malwa drug. The Royal Commission on Opium document that mentions these subsidiary locations lumps their "pass-duty" statistics with data for Indore, Ajmir, and Ahmedabad (GBO [Finlay–Appendix IX] 1894a:II:347). The subsidiary stations were located in the cities of Rutlam (also appearing as Ratlam), Ujjain (sometimes cited as Ujain), Chitore, Dhar, Maundisaur (also cited as Maundsaur or Maundesur), Udaipur, and Jaora (GBO [Clarke] 1894:II:446; GBO [Griffin] 1894:I:105).

24. Malwa opium was also packed in half chests. Documents, however, cite amounts in chests, not half-chests (GBO [Clarke] 1894:II:446).

25. The reserve for both Bengal Excise and Malwa opium taxed at the weighing stations fluctuated from season to season depending upon quality of the season's poppy crop. Administrators of the Ghazipur and Patna opium factories held a modest number of Bengal Excise chests in reserve from 1884/85 through 1894/95. The average "[n]umber of chests remaining in store at close of [the] year" for the eleven-year period was 2,024. The highest season was 3,295 for 1885/86; the lowest was a mere 831 chests at the end of 1889/90 season. The number of chests held in "reserve" for the remaining years were 2,599 (1884/85), 2,715 (1886/87), 2,176 (1887/88), 1,370 (1888/89), 2,635 (1890/91), 1,515 (1891/92), 2,228 (1892/93), 1,665 (1893/94), and 1,816 (1894/95) (GBC [Statistical Abstract–No 43] 1896b:95).

The importance of revenue obtained from the exported drug required much more Provision opium to be held in "reserve." The average number of Bengal Provision (export) chests for the same period was 59,823. The greatest number was 92,455 chests at the end of the 1888/89 season; the lowest was 25,293 recorded for 1894/95 (GBC [Statistical Abstract–No 43] 1896b:95). There are, however, contradictory statistics regarding amounts of the Provision opium "reserve." Another document states that "the last 20 years...the reserve has once fallen to 24 chests, and has risen, in 1889, to 49,700 [and] [d]uring 1891–92 it was returned at 9,292 [chests]" (Great Britain. Parliament [East India] [Statement–Opium] 1891–92:245). Data for 1883/84 through 1892/93 also are provided in a table on page 346 of GBO [Finlay–Appendix IX] 1894a:II:344–54.

26. The Government of India's Department of Revenue and Agriculture [IDRA] compiled data for the native states as best it could. These appear in the series entitled *Agricultural Statistics*. The thirteenth edition, published in 1898, covered 1892/93 through 1896/97. This and later editions have separate volumes for British India and native states.

Gwalior is the only entry for the native states comprising Central India and Rajputana Agencies in the thirteenth edition, and disclaimers indicate British officials recognized the probable inaccuracy of this material. Earlier issues in the series have no data about native states. Statistics for 1892/93 through 1898/99 are found in IDRA 1898–1900. Volume II: Native States, 13th, 14th, and 15th editions.

27. The poppy-cultivating native states in India produced and exported opium before European arrival in the subcontinent. As dependence upon drug revenue from China and Southeast Asia increased, the East India Company attempted to regulate the manufacture and distribution of the native states' drug within the country and abroad (GBO [Clarke] 1894:II:446). Treaties negotiated between 1818 and 1828 were partially successful in minimizing competition. Malwa merchants responded by shipping as much drug as the market would bear from locations on the western coast over which the East India Company had no control. Merchants' ability to avoid entering British territory ended in 1843. An East India Company military force defeated soldiers loyal to the Maharajah of Sind. This event ended unrestricted access to the Portuguese ports of Daman and Diu, the major exporters of the Malwa drug before 1830. The conquest of Sind provided the East India Company with control of all routes from the interior of the country to Bombay and the western coast. The event enabled the Government of India to continue influencing the Malwa opium export trade well into the twentieth century. See Edward E. Thompson & G. T. Garratt ([1935] 1966), and Winther 1988:114–30.

The contents of treaties negotiated throughout India are in eight volumes compiled by Sir Charles Umpherston Aitchison ([1862–65, 1876] 1973). Treaties concerning the poppy-cultivating native states of Central India and Rajputana are discussed at length in the fourth, fifth, and sixth volumes.

Two sources in the Royal Commission on Opium volumes contain comments about regulations for these native states during the late nineteenth century. The first is an appendix, and two enclosures (appendices) within it. The source is GBO [Finlay–Appendix X] 1894b:II: 354–70. The material is "Text of Agreements Between the British Government and native states Under the Central India Agency" (Appendix B, page 359); [and] "Text of Agreements Between the British Government and native states Under the Rajputana Agency (Appendix B, p. 359). Both are in Appendix X "Arrangements with native states Regarding Opium."

The second source is GBO [Clarke] 1894:II:446. The item is "No. 1236–'93, dated the 4th December 1893. *From*: S. E. J. Clarke, Esq., Secretary, Bengal Chamber of Commerce. *To*: The Hon'ble H. J. S. Cotton, C.S.I., C.S., Chief Secretary to the Government of Bengal." Appendix XXVII.

28. The situation remained unchanged during the Royal Commission on Opium hearings. The significance of Watt's lament is that generalizations about acres of poppy cultivation and total amount of Malwa opium manufactured before the twentieth century are qualified. The same caution applies to per capita consumption of this drug in these native states, in the native states located on the Malwa plateau that did not produce opium, and for people anywhere in India. Henceforth, production and consumption figures for Malwa opium in the native states themselves are estimates based upon data available to the Government of India and its representatives during the 1890s. Calculations and estimates concerning per capita consumption of all licit and illicit opium in India introduced later in the chapter use this information. Data from documents published after the Royal Commission on Opium completed its work also is used.

29. One chest of Bengal Provision contained 140.143 pounds of opium. The corresponding amount for a chest of the Malwa drug was 140.25 pounds. For more details, see Tables III and IV in GBS [Godley] 1897:5–6. See GBO [Finlay–Appendix IX] 1894a:345 for additional confirmation and information regarding pounds of opium in one Provision chest.

30. Hastings' entries (1895:10) for each of these years are slightly higher than the Godley and Finlay listings. Hastings calculates totals from place of shipment within Malwa (from Indore, Maundsaur, and so forth) whereas Godley and Finlay cite the actual number of chests leaving Bombay harbor. The reason for the modest difference between the two sets of figures is that some of the Malwa drug each season was either stolen en route to Bombay or diverted for consumption within Bombay Presidency and Baroda State.

31. The average amount of Indian opium reaching foreign shores each year from 1885/86 through 1894/95 has to be calculated by combining pounds of Malwa and Bengal Provision. The slight difference in amounts of opium in one container of Malwa compared to one for Bengal Provision precludes using chests. The problem is which "chest" (Malwa or Bengal) to select in calculating quantity.

32. One Bengal Excise chest contained 123.4257 pounds of opium. Maunds are first converted to pounds and the amount divided by 123.4257. The result is the number of chests carried out several decimal points.

33. The two British India factories produced a twenty-year (1873/74–1892/93) grand total of 133,633 maunds. This figure represents almost 10,996,084.95 pounds of opium (the exact figure is 10,996,084.9481) for consumption within the country. The average yearly output was 6,681.65 maunds or slightly less than 549,804.25 pounds (the exact amount is 549,804.2474). The 549,804.25 pounds converts to a bit more than 4,454.5 Excise chests. The precise total is 4,454.5362. This is rounded off to the nearest tenth to simplify calculations presented at the end of the chapter.

The greatest amount of *Papaver somniferum Linn* manufactured in any one season for the twenty-year period was the 1890/91 tally of 10,335 maunds (approximately 850,422.75 pounds or 6,890.15 chests). This was exceptionally high. The season of lowest production was 1888/89: 4,372 maunds (a fraction more than 359,753 pounds or almost 2,914.75 chests).

The number of chests manufactured during this twenty-year period is calculated by converting maunds into pounds and then dividing the result by 123.4257 (the weight of opium in one Bengal Excise chest expressed in pounds). Column 3 ("Total [Maunds]") of table 7 indicates a two-decade grand total of 133,633 maunds. There are 82.2857 pounds in one maund, and these figures yield a total of 10,996,084.95 pounds (the exact quantity being 10,996,084.9481). This huge amount of opium is equivalent to the content of 89,090.7 chests (or 89,090.7238). These awkward calculations are unavoidable because British officials' used varying statistical formats. Some documents cite amounts in pounds, others in maunds or chests or both, and sometimes in seers.

34. The Government of India could not control the weather and officials had only embryonic awareness about the effects of most other environmental variables. The Benares and Bihar poppy crop might provide an adequate supply of the crude drug in one season. The next year might bring abundance or a shortfall. Periodically, the crop was a total failure in parts of each Agency. Starting in the 1870s, economic disruption created by these uncertainties prompted Benares and Bihar agency administrators to maintain a "reserve" for both Provision and Excise opium. The purpose of the program was to stabilize prices and guarantee availability of sufficient quantities of the drug to satisfy consumer demand at

home and abroad. Flexibility regarding the amount of opium to retain was essential for success. The Government of India had fixed the Provision reserve at a minimum of 30,000 chests. The actual amount fluctuated from year to year. Sometimes the variation was extreme. In 1890, for example, the number of chests was 49,705. By December 1893 the number had dropped to only 1,184 (GBO [Rivett-Carnac] 1894:II:321).

The reserve system also explains the discrepancy between amount of Excise opium manufactured by the Ghazipur and Patna factories and a higher figure supplied to Provincial governments during a single year. Including the domestic drug held over from a previous season or seasons satisfied demand in the provinces. One document indicates this occurred during nine of the twenty years from 1873/74 through 1892/93. The document also provides a useful discussion about the "reserve" system for "Provision" opium. See GBO [Rivett-Carnac] 1894:II:321–22. Data regarding the number of Bengal Excise chests held in reserve at the Ghazipur and Patna opium factories are in a preceding note. Also see J. F. Richards' comment about the creation of the reserve system in British India and some statistics (1981:68–69).

The provincial governments also established reserves to ensure availability of the Ghazipur and Patna excise drug distributed within their jurisdictions. A drastic, sustained increase in demand for either Bengal "Provision" or Excise opium made a commensurate raise in minimum reserves necessary. This provided insurance against disastrous crop failures.

One consequence of these arrangements is that figures for per capita consumption in a province or locale might appear to contradict the quantities cited for Ghazipur and Patna factory production of domestic opium. The figures also might contradict statistics concerning the actual distribution of the product to provinces, and the amount allotted to vendors from a provincial government for eventual sale among its citizens.

35. Exact provincial *distribution* numbers (for the twenty-year period) are as follows. The cumulative grand total is 10,377,749.055 pounds or 84,080.941453 chests. The annual average statistic is 6,305.925 maunds, or 518,887.45277 pounds, or 4,204.0470726 chests. The highest quantity distributed in any one year (the 1889/90 season) is 791,711.86255 pounds, or 6,414.4814455 chests. The smallest amount was in 1874/75; only 236,982.816 pounds, or 1,920.0443344 chests.

36. Godley's data for British India in 1881/82, 1886/87 and 1890/91 are higher than those cited by Rivett-Carnac. This remains true even after the amounts, which Godley specified for native states, are subtracted from "Total Quantity of Bengal Excise Opium Supplied to Provinces and native states." The smallest discrepancy between the Rivett-Carnac and Godley entries is 33.810691 chests (1890/91), the second is 58.3020545 (1886/87), and the biggest difference is 228.50283054 chests during 1881/82. The only explanation is that slightly different data were available to Godley and Rivett-Carnac.

37. The more precise figure supplied to British provinces from 1881/82 through 1890/91 was 4,204.047 chests or 518,887.4517 pounds. Godley uses seers (one seer is equivalent to 2.057 pounds) in his dispatch. Details for his entries expressed in seers with pound and chest equivalents are as follows. The grand total of Bengal Excise opium redistributed to native states in India from 1881/82 through 1890/91 was 53,720 seers (110,502.04 pounds or 895.29198538 chests). This is an annual average of 5,372 seers or 11,050.204 pounds or 89.5 chests per season (the exact figure is 89.529198538 chests).

38. Native states differed in how they reported acres of poppy cultivated and opium produced from landed estates within their jurisdiction. Gwalior is one example. A few jagirdars and other grantees of minor status might pay an annual or periodic collective

tax on all crops. Rare instances of forced payments were usually the result of infraction of law or etiquette. The severity of the transgression had not merited termination of landholding privileges. Nobody in the native states' administrative departments, however, was required to specify the percentage that opium contributed to the tribute. Hence, the British resident could never assume that data provided by the maharajah's officials were accurate. This is one reason for the discrepancy in the quantity and reliability of agricultural statistics available from British India and the native states before the late 1890s and the early twentieth century. Government publications for British territory have much information; the native state entries for crops and acreage are modest or nonexistent for the same years.

39. This grand total and average annual amounts are calculated using only figures in column 3 in table 6 for ten years (1883/84–1892/93), not twelve years. The reason is that Godley provides data for the last two years (1893/94 & 1894/95) (1897:1–7). He has no data about "Amount Diverted for Sale in British Territory and native states."

40. The greatest quantity of licit Malwa opium available for sale in any one season was 3,515.25 chests during 1891/92. The lowest amount was 2,856.75 chests in 1885/86 (GBO [Finlay–Appendix IX] 1894a:II:347).

41. The Ajmir weighing station periodically supplied the Ghazipur opium factory with a portion of the crude opium required for manufacturing Bengal Opium. This happened for twelve years during the period from 1881/82 through 1894/95. The drug from Ajmere district was shipped to Ghazipur in 1882/83 through 1888/89 and again in 1893/94 and 1894/95 (GBS [Godley] 1893:6; GBS [Godley] 1897:7).

42. George Watt has no table compiled by the Government of India that lists native states' yearly production of Malwa opium. His calculation is a generalization based upon two sources of information: British officials stationed in several native states and pass-duty transactions at the three weighing stations (GBS [Watt] 1891:38).

43. George Watt is unclear about the number of years involved although his phrase "it may be said" implies a long time or continually. The time is at least 1883/84 through 1890/91 and probably covers the entire thirty-year period (1860/61–1890/91). Three tables precede Watt's comments. The first one lists area under poppy cultivation in the Benares and Bihar Opium Agencies from 1860/61 through 1889/90. The other two tables, the "Extent of Cultivation and Total Produce in the Patna Agency," and "Extent of Cultivation and Total Produce in the Benares Agency," have data for only a seven-year period, from 1883/84 through 1889/90. His comments about average annual production in the native states of Central India and Rajputana, therefore, are appropriate for the entire thirty-year duration, or at least the seven-year period within it.

44. For comments about restrictions and other arrangements with the opium cultivating native states in the Central India and Rajputana Agencies, see GBO [Finlay–Appendix X] 1894b:354–56. Also consult IFCD [Meyer] 1900:2.

45. See GBS [Watt] 1891:37–8, GBO [Finlay–Appendix IX] 1894a:II:344, and GBS [Godley] 1897:30 for Benares and Bihar Agencies' poppy acreage for 1860/61 through 1894/95. Comments about the amount of crude opium that these agencies were capable of producing circa 1891 are found in GBO [Batten] 1894:I:133, and other locations in the Batten document.

46. H. Hastings (1895:10) illustrates the problem when declaring that "nothing seems known of the quantity of opium consumed locally." And he is silent about the amount available each year for clandestine shipment beyond the borders of the opium-producing native states. Hastings admitted the statistics for acreage under cultivation that these

poppy-growing entities submitted to the Government of India were the only data available and "not very reliable." His acreage figures are therefore low, as are the statistics for opium produced. British "pass duty" data for Malwa opium confirm the statement. The native states were shipping more opium overseas each year than the production figures that Hastings cites make possible for export. This underestimation also applies to consumption within the native states and for clandestine shipment to British India territories. The native states' compilation of pre-1894/95 statistics regarding poppy cultivation and opium manufacturing among their own people must be used with caution.

47. The exact amount is 548.57133333 chests of Malwa opium. One maund is 82.2857 pounds, and 935 maunds are equivalent to 76,937.1295 pounds. The last figure is the amount of opium in 548.57 chests of the Malwa product, with each chest containing 140.25 pounds of the drug.

48. See GBS [Godley] 1897:7 for amount of smuggled opium confiscated from 1885/86 through 1894/95.

49. The lack of accurate information about native states' opium activity was not a recent development. The 1831–32 Select Committee on the Affairs of the East India Company contains useful information about the problem of smuggling from Malwa. Three witnesses identify reasons for its post-1818 increase, including the ineffectiveness of treaties negotiated with native states. See GBR. Parliament [Stark] 1831–32:XI:9–23, GBR [Kennedy] 1831–32:XI:84–92, and GBR [Mills] 1831–32:XI:263–68. Amar Farooqui (1998) discusses Malwa smuggling from 1818 through 1831. Extensive use of archival data makes his effort the most complete discussion of the topic that is currently available for the period before 1832.

The 1871 Select Committee on East India Finance found that little had changed from the early 1830s. Smuggling remained a problem. And British observers now fully realized Malwa's potential for producing enormous amounts of opium over which they had little control. Sir Robert North Collie Hamilton, for example, was convinced that Malwa poppy cultivators could supply all opium exported from India if shipments of British Provision chests ceased (GBR. Parliament [Hamilton] 1871:(323):VIII:228. Reverend John Wilson told the Select Committee that the best fields in Malwa were used for poppy, and the "whole acreage in 1866–1867 . . . devoted to opium was 289,062 acres." The Reverend also read from a government document when commenting about Malwa's estimated production during 1866–1867 season. It was "estimated at 48,5000 chests of provision opium, and 3,523 chests of Abkari opium" (GBR. Parliament [Wilson] 1871:(323):VIII:343).

For readers unable to review the original Parliamentary papers, see IUP/PP (1977). Parts of the 1831–32 document (and the aforementioned witnesses) are in the IUP/PP. Volume 9: Colonies. East India. The 1871 Select Committee testimonies are found in IUP/PP. Volume 19: Colonies. East India.

50. The native state of Baroda near Bombay also had tracts of poppy on the Malwa plateau. The estimated production in 1891/92 was 1,367 maunds. Beginning in 1887, none of it had been sent overseas from Bombay. Baroda's residents consumed most of the yearly production. Some of it was occasionally sold to the Bombay provincial government. Baroda state imported 338 maunds of additional Malwa opium during 1891/92. The document does not specify if this shipment came from British India's Ajmir district or from a native state (GBO [Finlay–Appendix X] 1894b:355). Watt's discussion excludes statistics for Baroda's Malwa drug because the small annual amount is used locally.

51. Deepak Kumar says that six volumes in the series were available to the public from 1885 through 1893 (1995:250). Excerpts from George Watt's ten-volume series were

reprinted in an abridged single volume publication during 1908. The out-of-print 1908 edition was reprinted in 1966. The opium consumption data in the 1908 reprint is applicable to the period from 1860/61 through at least 1889/90, and perhaps for several additional seasons. In the early twentieth-century abridged edition, Watt does not indicate if material had been edited or updated to include statistics through 1907/08.

52. The exact number is 5.4242706872 grains of opium. It is small, and the amount of anarcotine is indeed very little.

53. The per capita consumption of opium for 265,473,431 people ingesting less than 2,500 maunds of opium (an amount smaller than 222,500 pounds) during 1890/91 cannot be calculated because Watt's "less than" is inexact. Assume this population did ingest 222,500 pounds, but also realize the resulting statistic for average per capita consumption is actually more modest. Population growth during each decade further complicates making a generalization. The British compiled no census for the *entire* country during the 1860s.

54. A typical opium eater, according to George Watt, consumed ten grains of opium per day whereas "20 grains would be a very full daily allowance" (1891:37–8). There are 7,000 grains (avoirdupois) in one pound. One ounce, therefore, is equivalent to 437.5 grains and one-tenth of an ounce is equal to 43.75 grains.

55. For a table citing average consumption in seers per 1,000 people during 1900/01, see "Appendix: General Statistics of Excise Opium Revenue" in IFCD [Meyer] 1902:28. The document cites average consumption per 1,000 population for twelve British territories. The latter are Assam (8.8), Bengal (1.2), United Provinces & Oudh (1.2), Punjab (2.6), Madras (.8), Bombay (2.5), Central Provinces (2.1), Burma (3.7), Coorg (.2), Hyderabad Assigned Districts (3.9), Ajmer[e]-Merwara (5.8) and Baluchistan (1.8). The number between parenthesis after each location is the average consumption in seers per 1,000 population. The figures most likely include Bengal Excise opium as well as the Malwa drug paying pass duty at the Malwa weighing stations. The data probably omit all smuggled opium from the native states comprising the Central India and Rajputana Agencies, from Nepal, and from other sources of the drug consumed in south Asia.

The entry for Punjab Province includes quantities for the Northwest Frontier Province. The Bombay Presidency entry has no data for native states located within its jurisdiction, and the statistics for Ajmer[e]-Merwara apply only to the municipal areas of the district(s). The table was prepared before the 1901 census data became available. The compiler, therefore, had to use figures obtained from the 1891 census. This suggests that natural population increase from 1891 through 1900/01 would have reduced several entries for the season of 1900/01 if statistics for the latter season had been available.

Several conclusions can be made about consumption of Excise opium in India during 1901/02. The people living in the twelve locations consumed a total of 34.2 seers (or 70.3494 pounds) of the drug during the season of 1900/01. This is an average of 2.8833 seers (or 5.9309481 pounds) per 1,000 population. The entry for Assam is much higher than any other province or location listed. Ajmer[e]-Merwara is much less but still considerably more than any other entry. In 1900/01, therefore, consumption of the drug was highly concentrated in widely separated parts of the country, these being the northeast and central-western part of India.

56. "Licit consumption" includes the Malwa product sent to Ajmir, Indore, and Ahmedabad because the drug eventually was consumed in South India and the Bombay Presidency. "Bengal Opium" (the Benares and Bihar drug) was shipped to locations in the northern part of the country. The table has entries for British territory throughout the subcontinent.

57. Watt obtained this information from an 1881 publication entitled *Papers Relating to Consumption of Opium in British Burma*. (Rangoon Press). He provides no additional bibliographic material for the document. See note *** under table 9: "Total Population Grouped by Provinces, with Average Yearly Consumption of Licit Opium Per Head" for statistics with Assam included and excluded from totals calculated for Bengal, Berar, Bombay, Sindh, Central Provinces, Madras, Punjab, and the Northwest Provinces and Oudh. Data for table 9 are taken from table I ("Tables Showing the Distribution by Districts, of the Opium Habit in British India") in GBO [Memorandum VIII] 1895:VI:178.

58. As mentioned in the preceding chapter, Sir William Roberts also said that 45 percent of Berar's annual mortality rate was the result of 'malarial fever.' The percentage for Madras Presidency was 38 percent (GBO [Roberts] 1895:109). Roberts does not cite specific numbers and Clarke excludes both locations from his calculations.

59. Statistics about identical topics found in Royal Commission on Opium documents or Parliamentary Papers occasionally differ. Table 9: "Total Population Grouped by Provinces, with Average Yearly Consumption of Licit Opium Per Head" and the Clarke document is an example. Clarke's total population for India is less than the tally given in table 9. The discrepancy is the consequence of different documents consulted in constructing tables. This illustrates that nineteenth-century Government of India demographic statistics must be used with caution. Differences do not invalidate generalizations, but it is important to emphasize that such statements are expression of trends, estimates, probabilities, and possibilities for this early era of census collection in South Asia.

Clarke's numbers (and Roberts' figures) warrant another precaution. The annual death rate statistics (at least for 1891/92) that Clarke cites in the column "Registered Mortality" is probably an underestimation. His number refers to *documented* fatalities. These are the deaths about which the Government of India was cognizant. Reports about people dying might have been commonplace in a highly populated area, or in a locale where British officials lived. Documentation was less common, and possibly of questionable reliability, when the presence of Government of India bureaucrats was minimal or nonexistent. An example of this might have been regions of rural Bengal. Therefore, Clarke's data for percentage of 'fever' deaths compared to total mortality also might be approximations, and an unavoidable understatement of reality in the subcontinent.

60. The correlation is valid only if accepting the Roberts and Clarke perspective about the nature of the disease and how to avoid dying from it.

61. The title of table III in Memorandum VIII is "Showing the Population under each Group of Average Consumption by Provinces, in relation to the Total Population of the Groups and the Provinces Respectively."

62. The title of Memorandum VIII is "Tables Showing the Distribution by Districts, of the Opium Habit in British India." Table III (page 184) in the memorandum is entitled "Showing the Population under each Group of Average Consumption by Provinces, in relation to the Total Population of the Groups and the Provinces Respectively." It has statistics for all ten British provinces. The table has separate entries for Assam, Bengal, Berar, Bombay, Sindh, Central Provinces, Madras, the Northwest Provinces, Oudh, and Punjab.

63. As discussed earlier, the Government of India's status quo was merely a reduction in the *rate* of growth in poppy cultivation. It did not entail, as the SSOT had assumed during the 10 April 1891 debate in Parliament, an actual *decrease* in acreage.

64. The annual average amounts of licit opium from Bengal, Malwa, Punjab, and the smuggled commodity from all sources, had kept mortality rates at the level stipulated by

Roberts and Clarke. Increasing the maximum and minimum number of chests manufactured, distributed, and consumed in future years for all kinds of opium would further reduce the number of deaths. For this to happen, more poppy plants had to be cultivated. This step would infuriate anti-opiumists despite Roberts' having provided an ostensible medical justification for doing so.

65. See Appendix D: "Anarcotine and Crude Opium Requirements (in pounds) using the three Alkaloid Extraction Ratios for More than One Million Sufferers." Appendix D gives amounts of opium needed for 1,500,000 to 4,000,000 victims stated in pounds rather than Bengal Excise chests (as in table 11). All fractions of Bengal Excise chests (each one containing 123.4257 pounds of opium) in table 11 are rounded off to the nearest hundredth.

66. The long title of table 10 is "Population and 'Fever' Mortality Statistics in Five British Provinces Compiled by Mr. S. E. J. Clarke, Secretary to the Bengal Chamber of Commerce, December 4, 1893 and Submitted to the Royal Commission on Opium."

67. The calculation is as follows: 3,050,000 people/x pounds = 3,000,000 people/16,842.21 pounds; 51,368,740,500.0 = 3,000,000/x; x = 51,368,740,500.0 divided by 16,842.21 pounds. x = 17,122.91 pounds. An alternative phrasing is if 3,000,000 victims need 16,842.21 pounds of anarcotine, then 3,050,000 victims require "x" (17,122.21) pounds.

68. The anarcotine requirement for 3,062,031 sufferers is calculated as follows. It is 16,842.21 pounds (for 3,000,000 people) plus whatever is needed for the remaining 62,031 individuals. The closest entry to the latter figure in column 2 of table 5 ("Estimate of Anarcotine and Crude Opium Requirements for Quotidian and Tertian Fever Patients Based upon Dr. A. Garden's 1859–1860 Ghazipur Experiment") is 68,400 "sufferers" needing 384 pounds of anarcotine (column 3) for a complete "cure" and "convalescence." Less alkaloid is required for 62,031 people. The difference between the 68,400 and 62,031 figures is 6,369. Calculating the anarcotine requirement for 6,369 people, and then subtracting this figure from the amount stipulated for 68,400 people, yields the quantity necessary for 62,031 people. There is no column 2 entry in table 5 for exactly 6,369; the nearest is 6,840 individuals who require 38.40 pounds of anarcotine (column 3) if they are morphia-intolerant. If 6,840 unfortunate souls need 38.40 pounds of the alkaloid, then 6,369 of them must obtain a total of 35.76 pounds.

These steps yield the 35.75 pounds of anarcotine required for the 6,369 patients is calculated as follows: 6,369 people/x pounds = 6,840 people/38.40 pounds; 244,569.60 = 6,840/x; x = 244,569.60 divided by 6,840 pounds and x = 35.76 pounds. An alternative phrasing is if 6,840 victims need 38.40 pounds of anarcotine, then 6,369 victims require "x" (35.76) pounds.

Deducting 35.76 from 384 comes to 348.24 pounds of the alkaloid for 62,031 victims. Adding this to the 16,842.21 pounds for 3,000,000 people and the amount of anarcotine which 3,062,031 morphia-intolerant 'malarial fever' victims require for a complete "cure" and "convalescence" increases to 17,190.45 pounds.

69. The exact amount of Bengal Abkari chests required for the extraction of sufficient anarcotine to treat 3,000,000 people is 15,951.74.

70. The 116.9:1 ratio calculation for Clarke's 3,062,031 documented victims is 3,062,031/x = 3,000,000/15,951.75; 48,844,753,004.2 = 3,000,000x; x = 16,281.58 Abkari chests (Table 12).

71. As previously cited in the chapter narrative, the greatest amount of Abkari opium produced in one season during the period from 1873/74–1892/93 was 6,890.15 chests in

1890/91. This was an exceptionally high number. The smallest production figure was less than 2,914 chests during the 1888/89 season. The administration could increase future annual Abkari production to a level matching the unusually high number during the 1890/91 season. But this would exacerbate the SSOT's displeasure regardless of the excuse. Changing production to the lowest figure (1888/89) decreases the amount of anarcotine available to prevent 'malarial fever' deaths. The least controversial, and most humane, alternative open to the Government of India was a production figure close to the twenty-year annual average of slightly more than 4,454.5 chests of the mother drug prepared for domestic consumption. The 116.9:1 ratio (table 12) results in 3,000,000 sufferers needing more than 358 percent of the average annual production figure for the period 1873/74–1892/93. The Clarke and Roberts' 3,062,031 statistic involves an increase of approximately 365.5 percent, the 3,500,000 number is about 418 percent, and for 4,000,000 people the amount is slightly less than 482 percent.

72. The 24:1 ratio calculation for Clarke's 3,062,031 documented victims is $3,062,031/x = 3,000,000/3,274.95$; $10,027,998,423.4 = 3,000,000x$; $x = 3,342.67$ Abkari chests (Table 13).

73. The Bengal Opium chest requirements for anarcotine extraction are compared to the twenty-year average annual production figure rather than the highest and lowest seasons during the period. The yearly average provides a more realistic assessment of amounts of the mother drug that had to be allocated for alkaloid extraction during each of the twenty seasons. The high and low figures are extremes. The rationale applies to the 116.9:1 and the 24:1 ratios. The 16:1 calculations found in Table 14 also are compared to the twenty-year average annual figure for the same reason.

74. Additional calculations expressed in pounds (not chests) are in Appendix D: "Anarcotine and Crude Opium Requirements (in pounds) Using the Three Alkaloid Extraction Ratios for More than One Million Sufferers."

75. The 16:1 opium/anarcotine ratio calculation for Clarke's 3,062,031 documented victims is $3,062,031/x = 3,000,000/2,813.20$; $6,685,332,282.30 = 3,000,000x$; $x = 2,228.44$ Abkari chests (table 14).

76. See Appendix E for an alternate format expressing the contents of tables 12, 13, and 14.

77. Roberts' proposal might be good news for British India's administration. But it was no help in China unless the alkaloid could be imported from India. The Chinese government had no extraction industry that could possibly meet the needs of its citizens who, like Indians, were susceptible to morphine toxicity. Dr. J. A. Otte describes the situation. He says that to

> be of value narcotine must be taken in doses of from two to five grains. This is about equal to from 40–200 grains of opium, as opium contains from one to ten percent. [sic] of narcotine. This is an amount never taken at one time, even by the pipe. Hence, we can safely conclude that opium is an antiperiodic of such feeble power that it may be excluded from the list. (1908:227)

Typical consumers in China endangered their lives if they relied upon smoking opium to obtain the dose(s) of narcotine that prevented them from the misery of Roberts' version of 'malaria.' That is a mild assessment of the consequences of his proposal. And, consuming 200 grains of the drug over a period of several days to obtain five grains of narcotine is a very precarious way to avoid death from an ethereal poison. The behavior would likely ensure the person's demise.

9
The Wider Context: Anglo-European Science and the Rhetoric of Empire

CONTRASTING EXPRESSIONS OF IMPERIALISM: ANTI-OPIUMISTS AND DEFENDERS OF THE TRADE

The events described in this book are not merely details of an arcane argument in the history of science during the nineteenth century. They reveal something more than the diagnostic and therapeutic sophistication of Anglo-European medicine. Many of the people mentioned in the chapters were motivated by a desire to dominate. Rhetoric aside, what they sought to control was not restricted to the natural environment or to "mother nature." And the quest was not just to conquer disease. These justifications sound noble, but they are self-serving. The passions, the accusations, and the exaggerations convey another message. These strong personalities wanted to dominate other people, and the populations to be ruled were not Anglo-European. They were Asian.

These antagonists, however, did not construe imperialism in the same way. And some of their ideas about the nature of proper conduct in a colonial milieu were incompatible. India is an example. At one level, the participants were arguing about the health of subjugated masses. At another, and more fundamental level, they were arguing about whose version of imperialism would prevail in the subcontinent.

There is another hint that these people were really arguing about ideology. It is the status of India's Ayurvedic and Tibb (sometimes spelled as Tibbi; also called Unani) medical beliefs in their arguments. It is reasonable to expect that the antagonists would select facts from these indigenous systems to enhance the credibility of what they were saying. And there were some facts that could have been cited.

The Government of India and its supporters claimed that opium was indispensable in the lives of the country's natives. It was consumed to prevent and to cure 'malaria.' The Ayurvedic tradition, however, does not support this contention. The drug was not prominent. It was occasionally prescribed for certain stages of diarrhea and dysentery, but little beyond that. In fact, "Hindu physicians never made much use of the sedative and pain-relieving properties of opium on the human organism" (Chopra 1928:401). And extensive references in the literature to the prophylactic and febrifugal capabilities of opium for either plasmodial malaria or the lumpers' 'malaria' are absent.

The anti-opiumists did not mention this contradiction prior to the Royal Commission hearings. Members of the SSOT and other people did not cite it when they testified, and it is virtually absent from SSOT post-Commission critiques. India had provided the anti-opiumists with a counterargument. They ignored it.

The pro-trade people were no different. They also made mistakes. Opium *was* prominent in Tibb medicine. This is not surprising. According to Bijan G. Banerjee and Ritula Jalota, this tradition was "built upon the ancient Greek medical concept of Hippocrates and Galen" (1988:25). They further identify the shared heritage. Greek medicine, they tell us

> was taken over [in India] during the early Islamic period . . . [and] [o]ver the decades and centuries, it has become almost indigenous. It is very much a variant of Galenic humoural doctrines. (Banerjee & Jalota 1988:25)

The intellectual compatibility of Tibb physicians and pro-traders extends beyond a debt to Galen. Practitioners of Tibb medicine believed that opium was "an antiperiodic and . . . recommended [it] especially in fevers of the intermittent type" (Chopra 1928:402). But here the concurrence ends, and the mistake begins.

The Tibb doctors dispensed opium to relieve pain that was associated with some kinds of paroxysms. This was the symptom management idea that the SSOT and its supporters frequently expressed during the Royal Commission hearings. Opium, they said, did not cure or prevent malaria; it alleviated discomfort. The drug was only an anodyne. Tibb physicians agreed. Nonetheless, some pro-traders construed relief from pain as freedom from disease. This sometimes prompted them to declare that native physicians supported their interpretation. They were wrong.

Other pro-trade advocates and Royal Commission witnesses occasionally mentioned the beliefs held by segments of India's native population. The instances are actually quite few. Chopra indicates who these witnesses were talking about, and why pro-traders also refrain from citing qualified Ayurvedic and Tibb physicians in defending the Government of India.

> [O]pium became very popular in India and rapidly fell into the hands of shopkeepers and itinerant quacks, who made use of it for all sorts of diseases and conditions, [but] its use in both the Ayurvedic and Tibbi systems was comparatively limited . . . [Furthermore] properly trained practitioners of the indigenous systems . . . do not give raw opium, but give it as a constituent of one of their preparations. (1928:402)

Relying upon quacks to support an agenda for noninterference in the opium commerce was not a strong argument. Furthermore, the Government of India was defending the custom of eating the drug by itself. The absence of this custom in the Ayurvedic and Tibb systems was no help. Furthermore, the modest stature of the drug in both traditions provided weak support for pro-opium advocacy.

So, pro-traders had little to gain from including the thoughts of India's people in the argument for opium eating in the country. The indigenous folk, in other words, were basically irrelevant.

The anti-opiumists were not so crass. Arrogance was tempered by ignorance. Their conviction about knowing the truth about opium precluded them from seeking support from the people of India. The truth that most of the anti-opiumists were concerned about was religious, not *Papaver somniferum Linn*. And they were not *seeking* support from India's natives; they wanted to *provide* it.

The Anti-Opiumists

Christian evangelists dominated the ranks of the SSOT and its antecedents. It was their mission to go forth and spread the word of God. They wanted to save souls. They sought to fill the spiritual vacuum in which 'natives' were immersed, and to which many of these people were oblivious. The heathens in Asia were doomed but did not know it, and it was the task of Christian missionaries to show them the path to salvation.

The evangelists did not condemn Great Britain's domination of India. And they did not reject the Anglo-European presence anywhere else in Asia. But, they were opposed to the harm being inflicted upon natives by the Government of India.

This "compassionate" imperialism, of domination in the guise of Christianity, would not bloom among people who would not, or could not, listen to truth. The evangelists knew that some Indian and Chinese natives were hostile to the message of Christ. Nothing would change their minds. They also believed that many other natives would listen yet could not. These people were sick; they were victims of unrestricted accessibility to a substance that polluted the soul, that destroyed the senses. The obstacle to salvation was the eating and smoking of opium. The missionaries blamed the drug, not their message's lack of appeal, for a failure to rescue many souls in Asia. Opium became a scapegoat. And so did the Government of India. The administration's domestic and export drug policy made consumption too convenient for too many people.

The antagonism of many of these anti-opiumists was not irrational. It was linked to their conception of human nature. People were weak. They were susceptible to sin. Strict guidance was needed to stay on the moral path, or to resume the trek to a proper life. Human existence was a never-ending battle, a constant struggle with temptation to stray from the straight road. And for some adamant anti-opiumists, the cultures of Asia were examples of moral corruption writ large. The duty of a good Christian was to protect these people from the eternal damnation they faced. And the missionaries considered themselves good people indeed.

Spiritual and Physical Suffering

The evangelists also knew that the people in Asia whom they were trying to convert suffered from disease. The SSOT and prior organizations were replete with people trained in Anglo-European medicine. The physicians wanted to alleviate discomfort and minimize mortality. For these dedicated laborers, a healthy native had possession of all of his or her physical and mental faculties. And people with these traits could, and would, appreciate the blessed logic of Christianity. So physical health went hand in hand with spiritual well-being. They complemented each other. An environment that had one but not the other was an impediment to saving souls.

Here is where the servants of God took issue with their antagonists as the decades of the nineteenth century unfolded. The SSOT's stance was unambiguous. Many medicines had a dual nature. Substances that protected and restored the physical and mental health of human beings could also harm them. Opium was a potent example. The drug preyed upon the inherent weakness of human beings, their predisposition to succumb to sin. It could be *safely* used *only* if availability was regulated. In the absence of such constraint, the virtues of opium became the vices of opium. And if the substance did not kill, it remained a poison to the human soul. The soul, that most precious entity, would remain forever beyond the capability of the Christian evangelist to salvage.

Morality as Science Versus Morality *and* Science

The SSOT argument was as much a blend of medical reality as it was a moral argument in the guise of science. At times the morality was hard to deny. The analogy between opium and alcohol is one example of the trait. At other times there was no masquerade, no deception, no pretense. The SSOT's warnings about opium consumption leading to moral degradation contained a truth that Anglo-European science was revealing to the public.

Morality as Science and the Opium/Alcohol Analogy

Obviously, both opium and alcohol did affect the psychology and physiology of a human being. This was not a new idea; it was conventional wisdom before the 1800s. And each substance *could* have deleterious consequences for any person if it was consumed in excess. But to say that consuming alcohol led to moral and physical decline was, at best, an exaggeration. And it was plainly false when anti-opiumists claimed this is what happened to a person who consumed opium. The substances were similar in some ways; they were not identical in all ways.

Although a few ardent evangelists continued to emphasize the alcohol/opium analogy, it was not a salient part of the SSOT critique. Other weapons were more potent. Part of the arsenal was the concept of addiction. Its acceptance among members of the medical community during the 1870s enhanced the credibility of some anti-opiumists' warnings. Anglo-Europeans' belated recognition that morphine and heroin were not benign substances also helped the cause. And an event that was just as significant had occurred decades earlier.

Morality and Science: The Underlying "Sameness" of Humankind

A major component of anti-opiumists' successful agitation in Great Britain was the momentous change in public perception about drug consumption. The reinterpretation began after 1830. The missionaries' dirge from Asia had been incessant; opium harmed natives physically and morally. It could even kill them. The problem now was not limited to the exotic "Oriental." This poison respected no national boundary. It was an equal-opportunity plague that was restricted to no particular race, religion, or location on earth. And it was harming English men, women, and children.

A person who declared that the consumption of opium does bad things to both Anglo-European and Asian populations was making a radical assertion. Proponents of the idea were, perhaps unknowingly, also suggesting that people in the West and the East were essentially the same. This notion contested the beliefs about people of certain religions, social classes, speaking certain languages, and so forth, as having an inherent attraction to the drug. These were the ideas that pro-trade activists used to defend the export and domestic policies of the East India Company and the Government of India. In other words, the Christian moralists did not accept the "racial" theory of drug use.

For many anti-opiumists, the color of a person's skin or hair, or other physical traits that people used to differentiate themselves from others, were irrelevant. Beneath these superficial differences there *really* is no difference. Each person is a bundle of potentials, expectations, and needs. And each individual has a soul that cries out for help. The use and abuse of opium in the East and West had revealed the fundamental sameness of everybody.

The Possibility of Asian People Becoming "Civilized"

If all human beings are "constructed" the same way, and if the Anglo-Europeans were "civilized," then Chinese and Indians could aspire to the same thing. But the transition required change, profound change. The accomplishments of Western people, especially in Great Britain, were not an accident. They did not just suddenly occur. They were the products of individuals who had embraced Christian beliefs, who behaved like Christians. The message to Asian people was unequivocal. They had to rid themselves of the spiritual constraints to which they were born. Christian morality and conduct, beliefs about the hereafter, and so forth, must replace the negativity of non-Christian beliefs. Nonoccidental traditions were shackles that Asian people had to cast off. Only then could they strive to a level of civilization that was comparable to Anglo-European societies.

And under no circumstance could the "unwashed" masses of Asia achieve anything if they were enslaved by passion, by sloth, by vice, by negligence, by a host of "bad" behaviors. This, unfortunately, was the plight of many people in China, India, and elsewhere in the East. The SSOT and its antecedents did not blame the victim; they blamed the entity and the agency responsible for the moral and physical misery. This was opium, the East India Company, and the Government of India.

Incompatible Missions?

The SSOT needed to create an environment in Asia that was inhabited by people who could think clearly. They had to be free from impediments that prevented them from accepting the truth that the Anglo-European evangelists were offering. One of the ways these moralists could fulfill their obligation to God was to prevent the Indian public from obtaining opium. This was extreme. It would deny help to needy people. The alternative was to strictly regulate accessibility. In the absence of such constraint, whatever medical benefit the substance offered would be lost. And any chance an Indian citizen had for becoming "civilized" was forfeited. "Civilization" required Christianity, and habituation to opium just might preclude the "acquisition" of both.

Saving souls was not the mission of British bureaucrats. Their duty was to protect, to augment the empire. The Government of India needed money and domestic political stability to achieve either goal. Defenders of the opium trade said that Indian people's accessibility to the drug was not a luxury; it was a necessity. Indulgence provided help for natives trying to cope with their miserable existence. Indulgence was natural because Indians *were* inherently different from more "civilized" people.

The SSOT disagreed. The most important help was Jesus, not the drug. The response of the British administration was the same as most people in India. It found the SSOT unappealing. The Government of India and its supporters used unconventional science, for lack of a better term, to get rid of the anti-opiumists. This is the paradox. The people who rejected the purported link between opium consumption and the prevention and cure of 'malaria' were splitters. Most of them were members of the SSOT. Other dissenters were not. But all of them were cognizant, in varying degrees, of current research in drug research and disease prevention. Their opponents were not. Nonetheless, the anti-opiumists lost the argument, and they lost the war. They were bearers of bad news. Sir William Roberts brought good tidings; he guaranteed positive things.

THE GOVERNMENT OF INDIA AND ITS DEFENDERS

The Political and Economic Benefits of Sir William Roberts' Proposals for the Provinces of British India

Provincial administrators had good reason to oppose the SSOT and its supporters. Curtailment of consumption guaranteed fewer sales, less cash in provincial treasuries, and diminished financial solvency. The amount of money lost posed a serious problem for a British Province having enclaves of high consumption, and for the native states within its jurisdiction, as well. In Punjab, for example, the added expense of preventing the inevitable increase in smuggling into the province and its native states promised to exacerbate financial difficulties already created by less revenue. The Government of India was obligated to address serious monetary shortfall in any of its provinces, and it was ultimately responsible for ameliorating citizen discontent. All of this meant that maintenance of the status quo regarding Excise opium was essential; any program leading to decreased use among the people of India had potentially precarious economic and political consequences.

Sir William Roberts' opium and anarcotine argument provided provincial administrators with a very attractive scenario. He offered them a medical justification for increasing, not just maintaining, current consumption of the mother drug and an opportunity to benefit from distribution of anarcotine among the citizenry. Many more people ingesting opium lessened the cost of treating sickness by rapidly restoring patients to health, and by preventing them from even becoming ill. Increased and unregulated sales of the drug to the public resulted in more money to further reduce expenses of health maintenance. A provincial treasury also kept the difference between the Ghazipur and Patna factories' selling price and what its citizens spent for the mother drug. And the availability of anarcotine, obtained at low cost through the Indian Medical Department or directly from the opium factory, increases the number of lives saved at minimal cost, especially if the 'efficient' 16:1 ratio governed the extraction process during the mid-1890s. Sir William Roberts' advocacy secured, and even enhanced, the financial well-being of each British province. It lessened the possibility of the central government having to assume the cost of administering these territories. This was not an insignificant benefit during the 1890s.[1]

The Political and Economic Benefits of Sir William Roberts' Proposals for the Government of India

Documents that indicate British India was exporting increasingly fewer Bengal opium chests after midcentury also identify the cause for the decline. It was the rise of indigenous poppy cultivation in China and competition from Turkish and Persian imports into that country. The Government of India met this challenge throughout the era by reducing manufacturing costs whenever possible. Another strategy was to periodically raise the price of each chest. This was feasible because the Chinese, especially inhabitants in the southern coastal cities, thought Bengal opium (prepared at the Patna factory) yielded the highest quality smoking extract. By the last decade of the century, a price increase to compensate for declining numbers of exported chests from Calcutta as well as Bombay was no longer feasible. Each increment made the less expensive and increasingly higher quality indigenous and non-Indian 'foreign' opium more attractive to Chinese consumers. The Government of India was in danger of pricing itself out of the market if it relied upon this tactic to compensate for the declining number of Provision chests leaving Bombay and Calcutta.

The Royal Commission on Opium volumes as well as books, articles, and documents published before its creation, are replete with dire warnings about the negative consequences of reducing or ending Indian opium exports. S. E. J. Clarke, for example, said India would suffer irreparable injuries, one of them being a revenue loss of £4,000,000 (GBO [Clarke] 1894:II:444). This guaranteed a budget deficit for British provinces and the central government in New Delhi. The revenue loss also ensured financial ruin for poppy cultivators and everybody else involved in opium commerce. Other problems ultimately attributed to the SSOT, and so often cited in the literature, include discontent, even rebellion, in all segments of the population. This population included the inhabitants and rulers of the quasi-independent native states. There also were warnings about increased smuggling throughout the country and from beyond its borders, and the strengthening of nationalists' calls for independence.

Equally sobering was the inevitable antagonism of people in Great Britain who would be forced to pay taxes to finance anti-opium activities. The hostility would be just as intense from that stratum of the Indian population ordered to help defray these costs.

Sir William Roberts' recommendations reduced the severity of these consequences by redirecting some of the opium that the Chinese no longer wanted. Each option implicit in his argument posited an alternate destination for cultivators' latex: a portion, possibly a very large portion, of their annual production was to be used for domestic consumption and anarcotine extraction. The Government of India now had morally correct and 'medically justified' programs that, if implemented, would minimize political and economic instability in the post-Royal Commission era. And most important, British India's administrators, not the SSOT, would decide how much *Papaver somniferum Linn* to redirect and the amount of poppy to cultivate. Both allotments, if any at all, would be determined by several factors. These were the numbers of 'malarial fever' victims in the country, the cost effectiveness of implementing relief programs, and the credibility accorded Sir William Roberts' argument by India's opium policy makers, members of Parliament, and influential commentators in various professions from around the world.

Late Nineteenth Century Western Medical Theory and Practice and Sir William Roberts' Portrayal of the Etiology, Clinical Course, and Therapeutic Treatment of "Malarial Fever"

The history of drugs, opium, disease, and malaria adumbrated throughout the book depicts a continuous struggle between competing interpretations. Old ideas, assumptions, and procedures grudgingly gave way to new thoughts, different presuppositions, and altered practices. It is understandable that anyone given the responsibility to resolve a mid-1890s controversy involving all interpretations might articulate a position combining provocative, new notions about one topic, and thoughts increasingly recognized in the western medical community as archaic about another. Sir William Roberts was such a person.

Roberts was not oblivious to seminal discoveries in Anglo-European research. He was cognizant of the specificity of drug action and that the individual components of a plant were the locus of physiological and psychological activity. He knew that *Papaver somniferum Linn* contained alkaloids and he appreciated the toxicity of morphine. This awareness also was expressed in his delineating the difference between the mother drug and anarcotine, a commonplace recognition very early in the 1800s. But his analysis evinced an ignorance of, or a reluctance to acknowledge, evidence accumulated during the nineteenth century and before the mid-1890s that had relegated the alkaloid to a position of secondary importance, if not insignificance, for disease therapy. The dearth of post-1850 documentation establishing the efficacy of anarcotine for 'malarial fever,' therefore, was no oversight by western researchers. It was indirect confirmation that allopathic medical practitioners and pharmacologists believed whatever utility the substance possessed did not include the prevention and cure of 'fever.'

Part of the reason explaining Roberts' enthusiasm for opium and anarcotine was the kind of evidence he heard and examined during his tenure on the Royal Commission. His evaluation was based almost exclusively upon the testimony of witnesses and documentation provided by the Government of India. Many witnesses were affiliated with officialdom in some capacity. They were reluctant to say anything that harmed British interests. However, a substantial number did do, as did individuals representing other occupations. They were articulating opinions about a scientific problem, and concerns about the political and economic ramifications of their utterances for India and Great Britain were not foremost in their minds. They were telling members of the Royal Commission what they either thought or knew to be true; not what they assumed the Government of India wanted them to say. Roberts acknowledged their reservations about capabilities of the drug and alkaloid, and he heard them expose contradictions in pro-opiumists' testimony. These revelations did not induce him to abandon a pre-Royal Commission conception of disease etiology, the clinical course of maladies, and therapeutic agents and procedures. And none of the verbal and written evidence dissuaded him from constructing an argument beneficial to the economic and political interests of the Government of India.

Roberts combined elements of miasmatic, environmental, and sanitation theory in elucidating the conditions conducive to human sickness. In India, proponents of sanitary theory emphasized filthy conditions created by human beings. In this case, it was Indian people. To these orientations Roberts added aspects of Hippocratic and Galenist notions of what specific individuals experienced when they succumbed to maladies. The historical literature presents these events as instances of excessive "heat," "humoral imbalance," and so forth. There was a proverbial grain of truth in each of these interpretations and a substantial dose of something other than accuracy as well. A nineteenth-century variant was Sir William Moore's nervous system disequilibrium. This Bombay physician's explanatory device was compatible with Sir William Roberts' pre-Royal Commission notions about factors that precipitated ill health.[2] For

Roberts and Moore, opium and anarcotine had the power to calm internal agitation and to prevent the condition from developing.[3] Add to this mixture Roberts' belief in the genetic, biological basis of societal "under-development" (or absence of "civilization,") and the inherent proclivity of a specific population (e.g., religion, caste) for, or avoidance of, particular "stimulants." Now include an abhorrence of vegetarianism. These, save for one more ingredient, were the wellspring of Sir William Roberts' 1895 analysis.

The last component in Roberts' evaluation was inconsistency in differentiating between a symptom of ill health and a malady responsible for the condition. Roberts occasionally expresses awareness of the distinction. He then ignores it by according credibility to oral and written evidence portraying elevated body temperature as a separate, distinct disease (a malady "unto itself"), rather than a manifestation of sickness traceable to diverse underlying causes. Roberts' entire opium and anarcotine argument is predicated upon this nosological confusion and vacillation. The man was not alone in mistaking symptom for disease; the linkage was prevalent in earlier times. It had, however, become less common among segments of western society as decades of the 1800s unfolded. And researchers' post-midcentury discoveries of discrete causes for various maladies that shared only overt manifestations had reduced this interpretation to almost anachronistic status among an increasing number of medical practitioners by the 1890s. Coupled with the gradual emergence of microbes such as plasmodia accepted as agents of infection, Roberts' proclivity to equate symptom management with disease cure is perplexing behavior for a person esteemed for careful research and astute statements predicated upon dispassionate analysis of facts.

Roberts' intellectual stance is difficult to defend considering what was known about disease symptom and causation during the 1890s. It is not when the Indian medical establishment's theoretical preferences and the political and economic imperatives of imperial rule are taken into account. Roberts' analysis, in short, did not challenge reigning orthodoxy about disease and how to prevent it. Contemporary commentators depict the collective mindset of high-ranking GOI public health and IMS officials as conservative and inimical to new ideas.

ROTTING VEGETATION, FILTHY HABITS, BUT NOT TINY BUGS

The principles and practices of nineteenth-century sanitary science, for example, continued to influence medical policy in India long after they had lost currency in Great Britain and continental Europe (Hume 1986:703–24; Kumar, A. 1998:36; Kumar, D. 1995:167; Worboys 1989:156). Furthermore, according to Anil Kumar, "formidable professional personalities in India during the nineteenth century" perceived vegetable decomposition to be the ultimate source of 'malaria' (1998:175). Other perspectives articulated from time to time were "subsoil theory, chill theory, drinking water theory and lunar theory" (Kumar, A. 1998:175). The least popular orientation among influential members of India's public health and medical bureaucracy was germ theory. This was peculiar: after Pasteur's discovery, people in the West accorded increasing credibility to the role of microbes in disease etiology whereas administrators in India consistently denigrated the idea. Mark Harrison (1994), Deepak Kumar (1995), Anil Kumar (1998), and Michael Worboys (1989) identify the factors responsible for an attitude described as ranging from indifference to hostility.

Legacy of the 1857 Uprising

One consequence of the 1857 Indian uprising against foreign occupation was increased British prejudice and contempt for indigenous ways of life (Harrison, M. 1994:49; Kumar, A. 1998:131). Feelings expressed earlier in the century about natives and climate being "fundamentally pathogenic" were exacerbated (Harrison, M. 1994:49).[4] The British administration reflected the attitudinal change. The pre-1857 reticence about Indian customs had been balanced by what Anil Kumar describes as "somewhat healthier westernizing utilitarian doctrines [shaping medical] policy in the 1830s" (1998:131). Negativity replaced optimism after the uprising. Disease causation, inextricably and ultimately linked to rotting vegetation, now had another component; it was the "filthy habits, and 'degenerate' life styles" of Indians themselves (Harrison, M. 1994:59). Sanitation, or lack of it, complemented putrefaction as modes of comprehending the etiology of misery in the subcontinent. The British confronted a monumental problem. The attempt to eliminate factors responsible for organic decay and miasma was easy compared to the difficult, probably impossible task, of changing the loathsome behavior of recalcitrant Indians. Something akin to institutional despair became part of the fabric of health policy in South Asia. Mark Harrison portrays the IMS approach to tropical disease in the post-1857 era as "stagnation" spawning "an attitude among medical officers in which innovation in theory and practice was distrusted and discouraged" (1994:49). His evaluation of the more inclusive IMS ideology and the behavior of its leaders is no less gloomy.

> The slowness of promotion with the IMS, the pervasive anti-intellectualism, and bitter internal conflicts, fostered a climate in which innovation in theory and practice was positively discouraged. Equally, the military orientation of the service and the narrow outlook of many of its officers encouraged fatalism and indifference to the plight of the Indian people." (Harrison, M. 1994:35)[5]

The IMS aversion to germ theory was, in part, a result of a change in attitude that occurred after the 1857 uprising. It involved policymakers and how they viewed India and its inhabitants. The British were xenophobic.[6] Microbes also represented a threat.

Status Integrity and the Subversive Significance of Germ Theory

The apathy and indifference pervading senior ranks of the IMS had profound consequences for health policy in the subcontinent. These officers, and other members of the Indian medical establishment, disparaged germ theory and bacteriology as irrelevant. They said the theory and the discipline revealed nothing about the origins of disease and nothing new about sanitation (Worboys, 1989:157; Kumar, A., 1998:176). The hostility of many of these people dates from the 1860s. It never abated.[7]

Another faction emerged in the early 1880s. This group, mostly clinicians and public health officials, initially doubted the existence of germs. As the decade passed and evidence supporting Laveran's objects accumulated, the group then insisted that a miniscule organism, if it did exist, still had no significance for comprehending the etiology of 'malaria.' Far more important work for solving the mystery had already been done and they were responsible for it. These skeptics thought they had "recast malaria in modern scientific and physiological terms as a paroxysmal fever, rescuing it from the vagaries of the sanitarians and miasmatists" (Kumar, A. 1998:184). The assumption was unwarranted. These people had taken a step toward a less amorphous classification of elevated temperatures and they were on the road to a more sophisticated nosology. But it was a small step and the trek was long. And as of 1893–1895, they still had far to go.

IMS and Government of India policy makers erred when they cited India's uniqueness to justify their partiality for putrefaction and sanitary science during the nineteenth century.[8] Something else was involved in their hostility to germ theory. Small bugs might endanger human life around the world, but in India these microbes also threatened the egos of people responsible for ameliorating misery. Alphonse Laveran's emphasis on a specific causal agent, according to Harrison, "was incompatible with the more holistic notions of disease causation associated with the 'natural historical' model, which continued to dominate medical thinking in India, long after it had become unpopular in Britain" (1994:57). Harrison's explanation for the contradiction merits full citation. 'Malaria,' he tells us

> had long been regarded [in India] as being at the 'noncontagious' end of the disease spectrum because of its apparent dependence on locality. Holistic concepts of disease causation were also difficult to dislodge because of their wider social and political significance. They underpinned traditional anti-malarial measures like the removal of vegetation from the immediate vicinity of European settlements. These measures probably did little to prevent disease, but at least served to comfort those who lived there—they were an art of the possible. Laveran's claim threatened to undermine the theoretical basis of existing preventive measures, and was also potentially damaging to medical men who had built their reputations as experts on malaria. (Harrison, M. 1994:57)

The presence of competing paradigms helps to explain how disease in India was defined during the nineteenth century. Contemporary scholars such as Harrison tell us that chauvinism and ego defense are just as important.

Sanitary Science and the Preservation of Health

The way to minimize the negative consequence of rotting vegetation was to avoid living in such locations. Separation and isolation became the mantra for

Europeans in India. Hill stations, cantonments, and civil stations were the result. The natives' filthy habits were to blame if occupants of these geographical enclaves still succumbed to 'malaria' or other diseases.[9] The British despaired about educating Indians to abandon entrenched behavior, and administrators were reluctant to impose nonindigenous practices upon a suspicious, if not hostile, populace (Kumar, A. 1998:161).[10]

It is therefore understandable that conservative personnel in the IMS and Government of India did not view Roberts' recommendation about opium eating with alarm. He proposed nothing new. He just wanted to increase the number of people who had a habit that purportedly dated from the distant past. Roberts' proposal was a low-cost, politically expedient alternative to far more expensive and potentially destabilizing programs to ameliorate misery in the subcontinent. Equally important, the assumptions about disease and therapy upon which his recommendations were based threatened the reputation of few people in power.

Sir William Roberts' acceptance of some witnesses' inclusive interpretation of 'malarial fever' permitted disparate maladies with similar overt manifestations such as pain or elevated body temperature, sometimes both, to be lumped into one category. This compartmentalization enabled these people to utter statements about curing diseases when they were actually referring to one phase of a specific malady. And Roberts was oblivious to research illuminating the diagnostic difficulties created by overt similarities among Kala-azar, enteric fever, and plasmodia-induced malaria.[11] The combination of alkaloids in Indian opium moderated the intensity or severity of the symptoms associated with the three afflictions, and so common in diverse other ailments. The mother drug then became an indispensable tool to alleviate suffering and preserve human life. The capability was especially important when the percentage of deaths in India attributed to 'malarial fever' was depressingly high. Roberts' medical evaluation ostensibly proved that continued ingestion of opium was one way to prevent deaths from increasing, and that more per capita and regional consumption might help to reduce the number of fatalities. His report also confirmed that anarcotine might resolve the problem of morphia toxicity for the far greater number of people who were unable to absorb enough of the mother drug to do any good.

Roberts' analysis was flawed. The assumptions that he made were moot. Many members of the western medical community did not accept them. He also seems to have been influenced by evidence that was biased. And the data that he used to write the evaluation supported his preconceived ideas about the cure and prevention of disease. With the exception of Henry Wilson, no member of the Royal Commission protested these limitations. The British administration simply ignored them.

The Government of India claimed that Roberts' report was an exhaustive study of the medical aspects of opium consumption in the country. The administration also said that his recommendations would play a major role in future drug policy. What occurred, or rather what did not happen, after 1895 belies both assertions.

Deception and SSOT Naiveté

Ant-opiumists made a serious mistake on 10 April 1891. They misconstrued what Sir James Fergusson told Parliament. Fergusson, the undersecretary for foreign affairs, claimed that the Government of India had always *wanted* to reduce its dependence upon the opium revenue. Furthermore, the administration had already taken steps "to reduce it, and they have diminished the area on which the poppy is grown" (Fergusson, quoted in Owen [1934] 1968:295).

The SSOT and its supporters were elated. They thought that the Government of India had finally acknowledged the righteousness of their cause. They also believed the administration's desire to decrease income from opium was a firm commitment to continue doing so in the future. They were wrong on both counts. Fergusson had misled them. He had not lied; he just had not told them the whole story. And the SSOT's naiveté, or stupidity, perhaps both, had precluded them from comprehending what the Government of India had actually done.

The Government of India's ostensible change of heart persuaded the SSOT to agree that the "deficiencies in the Indian budget might be made good by grants from the imperial treasury" (Owen [1934] 1968:295). From the perspective of the SSOT, inclusion of this provision in its 1891 resolution was innocuous. After all, Fergusson had confirmed the administration's future intentions. He also had identified steps already taken to honor the commitment. People would have to pay very little, perhaps nothing, because nonmedicinal opium as a source of income was becoming negligible. And it would soon be, the SSOT assumed, nonexistent.

Reality was far different. A series of poor seasons in the late 1880s had forced the Opium Department to increase poppy acreage. In 1891–1892 the Government of India halted the expansion, and announced "that henceforth the area under cultivation should not be increased by deliberate effort" (Owen [1934] 1968:295). The anti-opiumists concluded the administration was proclaiming a policy of "genuine reduction." They were wrong. The government's intervention "merely indicated that it was becoming sensitive to criticism and had determined, in the future, to give as little offense as possible" (Owen [1934] 1968:295).

The tactic succeeded. The key term was the phrase "not be increased by deliberate effort." It was a code word for stopping the "feverish expansion." A policy of "normal expansion" was now appropriate. The Bengal Opium Department was ordered to slow the rapid rate of increase in poppy cultivation. It did not, as anti-opiumists believed, halt it entirely. The administration's "definite policy of reduction" turned out to be a chimera. Beginning in 1891–1892, 100,000 more acres were added to the "area licensed for poppy cultivation" (Owen [1934] 1968:296; also see 313). Another commentator says that poppy acreage increased 50 percent between 1893 and 1900 (Brown, J. B. 1973:105).

In either case, Robert's program for *maintaining* 'malaria' mortality at current levels actually involved a formidable increase in drug production. This was the "do nothing policy." The amount of opium mandated by the options that might *reduce* the number of deaths also increased.

The Royal Commission on Opium generated much controversy when its recommendations were made public. Yet, no apologist used Roberts' proclamations about opium and 'malaria' to defend the administration's post-1895 drug policy. This suggests the Government of India did not believe *Papaver somniferum Linn* did what Roberts claimed it could do.

This is a bold statement, but other facts support it. Despite the 50 percent increase in poppy cultivation after 1895, no government document indicates that the reason for this expansion was to obtain the opium needed for the prevention and cure of 'malaria.' Roberts' recommendation is mentioned nowhere in the literature. His evaluation also had no effect upon drug commerce after 1895.

The drug's alleged prophylactic and febrifugal capability in India did not result in massive exports to millions of people in the world who undoubtedly suffered from the lumpers' version of the 'disease.' The China trade was waning and the Government of India needed money. The British administration had either made a mind-numbing mistake, or it knew that Roberts' opium and 'malaria' argument lacked credibility.

The Indian government's anarcotine policy after 1895 indicates the second interpretation is correct. Roberts' evaluation had provided the administration with an incentive to extract the alkaloid for India's many 'malaria' victims. It launched no such program. The man had also provided a justification to export anarcotine to people around the world who had the 'disease' but were susceptible to morphine toxicity. The profits for the Government of India were potentially huge. Decreased sales of the opium extract had created political and economic problems in India. Heeding Roberts' recommendation about anarcotine might have restored, even surpassed, the amount of revenue that had been lost. The Government of India disregarded the opportunity.

The Anglo-European research community virtually ignored Sir William Roberts' pronouncements about anarcotine. The definitive analysis of the alkaloid's effect upon 'malaria' was not undertaken until 1930. The investigators concluded that Roberts was wrong (Chopra, R. N. & R. Knowles 1930:5–13). Four years later, chemists concluded that the anarcotine available during most of the nineteenth century was indeed "impure" (Cooper & Hatcher 1934:419). The culprit, as discussed earlier, was incomplete extraction of other ingredients (active and inert) from the alkaloid. Roberts' enthusiasm about anarcotine, therefore, was unwarranted. Researchers had also established anarcotine's proper place in the western pantheon of useful substances (Chopra, Mukherjee, & Dikshit 1930:35–49). It was renamed noscapine.[12] The twentieth-century Anglo-European medical community classified it as a mild antitussive, a cough suppressant. The alkaloid that Sir William Roberts promoted as a preventive and cure of 'malaria' only reduces the severity of a nonspecific symptom. It relieves discomfort. Details about these topics, and related work, are found in appendix F: "Nineteenth- and Early Twentieth-Century Anarcotine/Narcotine Research and the Alkaloid's Irrelevance for 'Malaria' and 'Fever.'"

Thus far, the discussion has illuminated what Roberts' report *failed* to do. It *did not* prompt the Government of India to explore the potential of anarcotine for combating 'malarial fever.' It *did not* persuade administrators to resume anarcotine production for domestic use. And *no one* affiliated with the IMS or any other organization in the country argued for more per capita consumption of *Papaver somniferum Linn* in the post-Royal Commission era to prevent and cure 'disease.' Simply stated, the man's effort had little to do with science and a lot to do with the political economy of empire.

Roberts' *principal contribution* to the Government of India, and to British imperialism, was to *minimize* the SSOT as a factor in shaping domestic drug policy in South Asia after 1895. The anti-opiumists' insistence that consumption be restricted to legitimate (i.e., 'medical') use was turned against them. His evaluation portrayed all forms of ingestion, and quantities used for any purpose, as medicinal. Roberts had honored Sir Arthur Lyall's 1893 demand that the shrill, misguided moralists be silenced. They most certainly were. Martin Booth says the SSOT required "ten years to overcome the defeat" that had been inflicted by publication of the Royal Commission on Opium volumes and its recommendations to Parliament (1998:157). J. F. Richards agrees; the entire investigation "was so managed by the Government of India that the anti-opium groups were silenced for the next ten years" (1981:69). The SSOT continued to warn about drug consumption within South Asia. The concern went unheeded. The anti-opiumists withdrew to slowly resume agitation against the morality of India's continuing, albeit declining, drug trade with China.

In 1907 the Government of India signed an international agreement to end exports of opium to China by 1917. This was not an act of atonement. It did not signify that British administrators were admitting, albeit belatedly, the righteousness of the SSOT. The decision was pragmatic. India's rulers realized that Provision opium was destined to yield even less profit in the future (Reins 1991:114). Heightened competition from the less expensive Persian and Turkish drug available in the Empire made the decline inevitable. The ever-increasing amount of high-quality smoking extract opium manufactured by the Chinese themselves exacerbated the problem. Then there was increased awareness in the West, and in China, about the dangers of chronic dependence. Anglo-European science and the SSOT contributed to this public reeducation. The debilitating effects of opium indulgence had become a dominant theme in the rise of Chinese nationalism, and Great Britain was blamed for enslaving innocent Chinese citizens. This time the Protestant evangelists were not the only group protesting.

Members of Great Britain's Parliament did not seriously address the issue of opium consumption *within* India until the beginning of World War I. At this time the alliance with Germany ended Turkey's exports of high-morphine content opium to Great Britain, France, and other non-Axis powers involved in the conflict. There were discussions about possible curtailment of indigenous consumption. The Government of India took measures that bordered on desperation to increase the inherent morphine content of Indian opium to satisfy the needs of the military forces of Great Britain and its allies. This drama deserves a separate telling some other time.

RELIGION, SCIENCE, AND ANGLO-EUROPEAN IMPERIALISM

In 1990, John MacKenzie depicted imperialism as more than a set of political, economic, and military phenomena. He portrayed it as a "complex ideology" with "widespread cultural, intellectual, and technical expressions in the era of European world supremacy" (1990:viii). The Anglo-European encounter with disease in overseas colonies provides graphic illustrations of this ideological complex.

This study is one of an increasing number within a genre that explores the role of medical activity in extending British domination around the world. The book, however, differs from current literature. It is a response to MacKenzie's plea that more needs to be known about the "influence of scientific misconceptions on the practice of imperial rule" (1990:8). The misconception in this study consists of facts and fallacies about a drug, an alkaloid, and a disease. The antagonists introduced in these chapters describe human misery in India and how to alleviate it. They lament premature death in the subcontinent and gave instructions about how to prevent it. These people probably did believe they were arguing *only* about the welfare of India's people. But the passage of decades provides another interpretation of the volatile arguments that fill the book's pages.

The disagreement about the status of opium and anarcotine in preventing and curing 'malaria' was indeed an argument about Anglo-European medical science. But, what the participants said and how they said it also expressed the raison d'être of the British presence in south Asia, and whose interpretation of benevolent domination would determine the future of the Indian society. The anti-opiumists and Protestant evangelists lost the contest. The Government of India and its supporters won. The triumph was transient.

NOTES

1. Medicine became an issue in the rhetoric of empire at the end of the nineteenth century. The colonies of the imperial powers were in debt. The problem was exacerbated by the high cost of fighting diseases.

India was not exempt (Harrison, M. 1994:3). Michael Worboys claims that the cause of Great Britain's woes was the laissez-faire mentality that shaped pre-1895 colonial development. Administrators had incorrectly assumed that "market forces and individual initiative would . . . generate economic activity and development" (1990:166). By 1895, the inadequacy of the policy was obvious. Colonial companies were bankrupt and colonial governments were deeply in debt. Great Britain's response to the dismal situation demarcates the beginning of "constructive imperialism." This phase of British imperialism emphasized the creation of scientific institutions in its colonies and possessions. Their principal purpose was to preserve and to augment hegemony. Worboys says that the Imperial Institute of India was a classic example of the new policy (1990:166–67).

2. Mark Harrison (1994) offers a clue to the source of Sir William Moore's notion about nosology and predisposing factors for disease. One source might have been Edmund

Parkes. Parkes, who had spent several years in India, wrote a book about practical hygiene that "became the standard text for military medical men in Britain and the colonies in the 1860s, 70s, and 80s." Parkes claimed disease had two types of causes. The first group was attributes within the body ("predisposing"). The second category was external ("exciting"), and it consisted of "specific poisons created by "putrefying matter." Different poisons were responsible for different fevers: "material of vegetable origin" caused ague whereas "material of animal origin" was linked to enteric fever (Harrison, M. 1994:51–2).

The mode of 'fever' transmission varied. Enteric fever, for example, was "transmitted in the feces of a victim and contracted through ingestion of the infected matter [whereas] [c]holera was ascribed to the action of a 'specific agent,' transmitted in the stools of the victim, usually in contaminated water or food" (Harrison, M. 1994:52). As discussed in an earlier chapter, Sir William Moore believed that several factors contributed to the absence of health. These include poor diet, working in a damp and cold environment alternating with extreme heat, inadequate housing, and inappropriate clothing. The result was a person who, Moore hypothesized, was suffering from a type of ethereal imbalance, a form of internal disequilibrium. In Moore's version, a person with this constellation of attributes experienced a condition rendering the individual highly susceptible to one or more of the fevers that Parkes described.

3. Dane Kennedy's discussion of "tropical neurasthemia" and its "bewildering symptoms" helps to illuminate the thinking of Moore and Roberts. Kennedy is describing the characteristics that the two men portrayed as internal agitation and nervous system disequilibrium (1990:118–40).

4. See Deepak Kumar (1997:178) for helpful comments. British evaluations of Indian habits and medical practices were pejorative. Kumar discusses the status of bacteriology and epidemiology in their condemnations. The negative attitude explains why Royal Commission documents rarely mention the reasons why practitioners of indigenous medicine used, or did not use, opium. Pro-traders and SSOT activists might have found support for their respective opium and 'malaria' arguments if they had pursued the topic. They did not. Apparently, most participants in the Commission hearings viewed ideas about disease therapy that had non-Western roots as superstitious nonsense.

5. Anil Kumar and Mark Harrison address the topic. Harrison does it several times in his book. In the first chapter, he says that inertia and status anxiety pervaded the IMS, just as it did in other colonial services. Senior IMS officers discouraged innovation in theory and practice. The "military orientation of the IMS, and its lack of internal dynamism...[also] fostered fatalism about the plight of the Indian people" (Harrison, M. 1994:6). Harrison reiterates the theme in the second chapter. He claims that the "reluctance of most IMS officers to incorporate new scientific ideas [is] attributed to the internal problems of the service . . . and, in particular, its ethos of anti-intellectualism, its failure to reward or encourage innovation, and its increasing unpopularity with medical graduates in Britain" (1994:58).

Kumar (1998:131) illuminates the negative consequences of this mentality for Indians and Eurasians who aspired to enter British India's public health profession during the nineteenth century.

6. Xenophobia also was a factor explaining why the Government of India and the IMS were hostile to germ theory. In this case it was a reluctance to recognize that a foreigner had formulated a credible explanation of disease etiology. As late as 1894, British India's policy makers were especially loathe to give credit to French nationals such as Alphonse Laveran for his 1880 discovery of plasmodia. They also were reluctant to recognize Louis

Pasteur and his associates for their pioneering work during the 1860s (Harrison, M. 1994:57, 261 [footnotes 98, 99, 100]). Xenophobic inclinations might explain the British India administration's reaction to Robert Koch's confirmation of the cholera 'Comma' bacillus in Calcutta during 1883. This German researcher's discovery was a

> significant contribution to the germ theory of disease causation which had emerged in Western Europe in the 1860s; the studies like his and Pasteur helped to firmly establish the theory in the 1870s and 1880s. This modern scientific revolution in medicine challenged and ultimately triumphed over the earlier miasmatic theory. (Kumar, A. 1998:175)

Senior Government of India and IMS officials virtually ignored the discovery. Those who did react said that the event was irrelevant for understanding what caused disease and how to prevent it (Kumar, A. 1998:176; Kumar, D. 1995:167). A possible explanation is national chauvinism. The British in India simply did not like the idea of a foreigner making a seminal contribution to disease etiology on their own turf. The contention is speculative, albeit intriguing, and merits more study.

7. Harrison thinks the 1880 discovery of separate organisms "thought to cause enteric fever and malaria" initially "gave rise to more uncertainty in Indian medical circles" (1994:56). Most IMS officers, however, refused to accept any causal relation between the microbes and the diseases. Harrison says the skeptics included influential men in the Government of India hierarchy. He cites T. G. Hewlett, author of the *Report on Enteric Fever*, and Drs. T. R. Lewis and D. D. Cunningham. Lewis and Cunningham were "special scientific assistants to the Indian government" (Harrison, M. 1994:56). There is no mention of Hewlett, Lewis, or Cunningham changing their minds in the post-1880 era.

8. Mark Harrison (1994:36–47) describes eighteenth and early-nineteenth century European, especially English, beliefs. India is portrayed as being a unique repository of dangerous diseases and a fertile environment for the elaboration of racial theories of immunity.

9. Anil Kumar says the principles of sanitary science dictated the "physical placement of the European civil and military population in India." The British administration's use of the "criteria of soil, water, air and elevation . . . [to create] distinct areas of European residence like the 'cantonments,' civil station' and 'hill station.'" This led "to the development of a colonial mode of health and sanitation based upon the principle of social and physical segregation." One result of this mentality was that the "surroundings of the natives . . . remained the reservoirs of dirt, filth and disease" (1998:161).

10. The complaint continued into the twentieth century. Anil Kumar mentions a Sanitary Commissioner who "confirmed in 1921, [after] reviewing the period 1871–1921, that sanitary measures had hardly touched the population and that 'over fifty years of sanitary work in India' had produced complete failure" (1998:161). That kind of attitude prompted Ira Klein's 1973 contention about the IMS viewing "preventive medicine as 'a sham, a pretence'" (Klein, quoted in Kumar, A. 1998:161). And Michael Worboys says the cost of cholera vaccination was prohibitive. The procedure had to be limited to "troops, Europeans and Indian civil servants" (1989:157). The civilian Indian population received virtually nothing.

11. Malariologists in India were conscious of diagnostic problems during the 1890s and the twentieth century. But awareness did not prevent them from making mistakes. V. R. Muraleedharan describes the consternation of health officials when, in 1906, they discovered that Kala-azar was still being diagnosed as malaria in Madras (1991:109–10).

Mark Boyd (1949:1:3–25) provides an excellent review of medical treatises that failed to distinguish between fevers in general and the paroxysms later known to be exclusive to malaria.

Other efforts portray 'malaria' fevers as being different from ague. Nonetheless, commentators' ignorance about the role of plasmodia in the disease complicated categorization and treatment. Several scholars discuss the difficulties in separating the symptoms of malaria from nonmalaria afflictions during the period. For case studies that illustrate researchers' awareness of diagnostic difficulties during the 1890s, see deKorte (1900:178–81) and Plehn (1899:72–74, 121–123, 141–145). Hodgsen & Vardon (1926/7:779–84) describe the problem prior to the mid-1920s.

12. The word gnoscopine often is found in chemists' descriptions of narcotine/noscapine. Noscapine/narcotine signify the naturally occurring alkaloid. Gnoscopine is a "weakened" form; it has been processed to be fifty percent less "active" than narcotine/noscapine.

Appendix A
Opium Only Relieves Pain

Other witnesses mentioning opium and "malaria" are excluded from the chapter narrative. Several are cited only in endnotes. Their comments were either too brief or too general to determine if they were aware of the need to understand all factors accounting for the appearance, duration, and severity of the disease. All of them, however, rejected any contention that natives ingested opium for "malaria" regardless of how the term was defined. Some even rejected claims about the drug being consumed for any disease whatsoever in the locales for which they had expertise.

Reverend Cushing's negative attitude about opium was matched or exceeded by witnesses from East India, other regions in the country, and one person testifying about China. Cushing, cited in chapter 9 as having worked in Burma since 1867, had said some Rangoon and Shan State natives might view the drug as a pain reliever but nobody ever used it "directly" for "malaria" (GBOW [Cushing] 1894 II:196). Dr. William Gauld, a China veteran like Cushing, claimed the Chinese people he knew about never used opium as a preventive and only rarely construed it as a cure (GBOW [Gauld] 1894 I:60).

Fellow detractors were equally skeptical about Indian natives using the drug for any prophylactic or febrifuge purposes whatsoever. Reverend W. B. Phillips asserted that people in his part of Bengal never used it for either "fever" or "malarial fever" (GBOW [Phillips] 1894 II:40). Kali Sankur Sukul agreed, declaring that he had never even heard of patients in the "malarial tracts" of Bengal doing such a thing and he also had never met natives who had done so (GBOW [Sukul] 1894 II:269). And people in Calcutta city, according to Rai Lal Madhub Mookerjee Bahadur, a physician in private practice, rarely consumed opium as a prophylactic "against cold and malaria" (GBOW [Bahadur, R. L. M. M.] 1894 II:257).

Ram Dhurlabh Mazumdar from Assam said people in his locale never used the drug to prevent "malarious fevers" because physicians never prescribed it (GBOW [Mazumdar, R. D.] 1894 II:60). Doctors also never prescribed the substance as a "remedy for fever" in Gauhati, Assam, according to Satyanath Borah, a "pleader" in the region's legal profession. In fact, Borah had never even known any native consuming the substance to prevent sickness even when they had no access to physicians (GBOW [Borah] 1894 II:286). Lalit Mohun Lahiri, also associated with the Assamese legal profession, concurred. He had never heard of natives using or doctors prescribing the drug for "malarious fevers" (GBOW [Lahiri] 1894 II:289–90).

The American medical missionary Miss Carleton said that to the best of her knowledge, she had never met any person during her seven years in Umballa [Amballa], a city in the province of Punjab, who used the drug to prevent "fever" (GBOW [Carleton] 1894 III:169). Dr. Vishram Ramji Ghole, a private practitioner from Poona, a city southeast of Bombay, voiced a similar sentiment about residents in this urban area. In fact, Ghole declared, natives did not use the substance to prevent disease of any kind (GBOW [Ghole] 1894 IV:275). And in the native state of Dhrangadra in Kathiawar on the Western Coast, Darasha Hormaji Baria, listed as a "medical practitioner" for "Government or Native State," also said natives did not ingest opium as protection against "malaria" (GBOW [Baria] 1894 IV:141).

Another physician in private practice by the name of A. T. Bocarro told the Royal Commission that no evidence existed for natives taking the drug as a "malarial" prophylactic in Bombay itself and in adjacent locales. His colleague, Dr. Temulji Bhikaji Nariman, said there was minimal opium consumption in the city because there was not much "malaria" (GBOW [Bocarro] 1894 IV:270; GBOW [Nariman] 1894 IV:267–68). Nariman did not say enough to predict his attitude if the disease had been more prevalent in the city.

NOTE

See the Selected Bibliography for full citations concerning witnesses.

Appendix B

Opium Prevents and Cures Just About Everything, Including 'Malarial Fever,' 'Fevers,' and the Diverse Detrimental Consequences of 'Miasmatic Influences'

Twenty-seven more witnesses, in addition to those introduced in chapter 9, provided abbreviated comments about natives using opium to prevent or cure entries in the vague, inclusive category called "malarial disease," "miasmatic influences," "fever," and so forth. There was no concurrence among these witnesses about the actual diseases they were talking about, who engaged in the "opium habit" and the effects of consumption. Members of the Royal Commission also asked for no supplementary data or clarification from any of these people.

For many in this group, malaria was an amorphous entity, "invisible" to the eyes, ears, nose, and touch but devastatingly real in its effects upon the unfortunate. They construed opium as an all-purpose domestic remedy for ailments such as rheumatism, dysentery, chill, neuralgia, bronchitis, other ailments, and occasionally for all of them. Collectively, these individuals only demonstrated that people consumed the drug in various parts of the country for different ailments involving pain or elevated temperatures and sometimes for both.

Sir Joseph Fayrer and the Honorable A. S. Lethbridge did not identify what part of India they were referring to. Fayrer, a high-ranking official for the Government of India whose precise occupation when he testified is not specified in the Royal Commission volumes, and Lethbridge, the general-superintendent of the Thuggee and Dacoity Department as well as member of the Viceroy's Legislative Council, only mentioned that physicians and natives used the drug for "malarious diseases" (GBOW [Lethbridge] 1894:II:135; GBOW [Fayrer] 1894:I:110–11).

All other witnesses specified the locations prompting their comments. Sir Hugh Low cited Chinese miners, the poorest and most numerous category of laborers in the Malay States, using opium as "a prophylactic against miasma" (GBOW [Low] 1894:I:111). And Dr. George Dods, a physician at the British Naval Hospital in Canton for six years and then superintendent of the Hong

Kong jail for twelve years, said that Chinese natives occupying "marshy districts" told him they needed to smoke an extract of the drug in order to escape the always-present "fever" (GBOW [Dods] 1894:I:116).

Most of the remaining witnesses commented about areas in East India. See J. J. Driberg and Jaginnath Barooah for the status of opium among the natives of Assam (GBOW [Driberg] 1894:II:261–62; GBOW [Barooah] 1894:II:296). Mr. F. Bradley and D. M. Smeaton mentioned opium use among enclaves of people in Burma. Bradley, an apothecary and former civil surgeon in the Northern Shan States, had prescribed the drug with good results, whereas Sir James Lyall literally forced Smeaton to acknowledge something positive about the drug. The latter obliged and said that only forest workers in some districts ingested it to avoid "fever," a belief he thought was erroneous (GBOW [Bradley] 1894:II:194; GBOW [Smeaton] 1894:II:234). Nawab S. A. Hossein and Raja Peary Mohun Mookerjee said that Bengali natives took the drug for "medical purposes" (GBOW [Hossein] 1894:II:253; GBOW [Mookerjee] 1894:II:173). Surgeon-Captain W. E. H. Woodright also discussed Bengal. This medical officer for the 10th Bengal Lancers indicated that only some kinds of natives thought the drug was a prophylactic for "fever." They were the "Mahomedans and Dogra" soldiers in his regiment who also ingested the substance to alleviate dysentery, "bowel complaints generally," and lung complaints. Contact with these sepoys prompted Woodright to conclude that *Papaver somniferum Linn* was useful only in the "cold" stage of malaria, the shivering phase of a paroxysm (GBOW [Woodright] 1894:III:194).

Woodright is unusual in this category of witness because he seemed to be cognizant of the characteristic fever patterns associated with malaria's plasmodia, an observation not made by the Maharaja Durga Churn Law and T. N. Mukharji in their comments about opium use in the city of Calcutta. Law said that opium was "not used for purely pleasure or 'vicious' purposes because people view it as a remedy against what are called miasmatic influences" as well as "complaints arising from cold, bronchitis" and so forth (GBOW [Law] 1894:II:171). Mukharji chastised the anti-opiumists, especially missionaries, for having a "very unreasonable prejudice against opium." The substance, he declared, was a "poison" people needed to counteract something equally poisonous, this being "miasmatic effluvia" and "impure water" (GBOW [Mukharji] 1894:II:158).

Four witnesses mentioned the natives in Malwa and the Central Provinces, two locales within Middle India, who viewed opium as protection against "fever." Ram Krishna Mahipat talked about the situation in the native state of Dhar and Surgeon-Lieutenant Colonel R. Caldecott mentioned consumption among other Malwa inhabitants. Caldecott, in charge of the Political Agency of Western Malwa when he testified, said that Sikh soldiers in the Central India Horse used opium during his posting as commander of that military unit. He also had no doubt that Malwa natives looked upon the drug as an "alleviating remedy" and a "prophylactic" (GBOW [Caldecott] 1894 IV:94). Mahipat merely said the drug was "never productive of evil" and that the prohibition of opium consumption would result in much suffering for people with "malarial fever" (GBOW [Mahipat] 1894:IV:146).

The Central Provinces were represented by two witnesses: Brigade-Surgeon Lieutenant-Colonel J. B. Gaffney, civil surgeon for city of Jabbalpore and a former superintendent of jails for twenty-five years, and Kalidas Chaduri, a member of the legal profession whose title is "pleader." Gaffney only said that in the "Upper Godavery district, there was a prevalent belief that the use of opium was a protection against chills and malarial influences" whereas Chaduri had only heard about some people in "malarious localities" believing that opium was beneficial (GBOW [Gaffney] 1894:IV:339; GBOW [Chaduri] 1894:IV:344).

Dr. R. N. Khory commented about Muslim residents of Bombay and J. P. Marzban mentioned natives in Kathiawar. The third witness commenting about the status of opium for Western Coast locations was Khan Bahadur Dossabhai Pestonji, who described himself as "an honorary assistant surgeon to His Excellency the Viceroy." This assistant surgeon from Surat, a city halfway between Kathiawar and Bombay, talked about the indigenous inhabitants of this urban area. Khory said the drug was used to prevent the appearance as well as the recurrence of "fever." It also warded off other afflictions. Pestonji only said that the drug was "used as a prophylactic in malarial districts against fevers, chills and rheumatism" (GBOW [Khory] 1894:IV:259; GBOW [Pestonji] 1894:IV:272–73). Marzban, editor and publisher of native newspapers, declared that "men of influence and position, as a rule, take opium" but there was a "prevalent belief that the use of the drug is a sure preventive of malarious fevers and other diseases" (GBOW [Marzban] 1894:IV:348). And G. B. Prabhakar, a resident of Bombay with experience in Kathiawar, believed that opium was a preventive yielding "considerable beneficial results" for "dyspepsia, diarrhoea, dysentery, malarial fever, cold, rheumatism, neuralgia, and diabetes" (GBOW [Prabhakar] 1894:IV:272).

North India and South India were each represented by one person, whereas three witnesses provided comments based upon their experiences in two or more regions of the country. F. B. Mulock, deputy commissioner of the city of Lucknow in the United Provinces of North India as well as a "district officer," had noticed that "the vast majority of consumers" ingesting opium "in small doses" seemed to "work all the better, and are reported to enjoy a marked immunity from malarial fever and bowel complaints, such as dysentery" (GBOW [Mulock] 1894:III:97). Reverend H. F. Laflamme, a Canadian Baptist missionary laboring in Ganjam district of the Telegu-speaking part of South India, did not agree. He admitted that opium seemed to do some good in "malarious districts" but natives in his locale still had mixed opinions about the drug. Many thought it was "good for a fever with chill" and opium addicts swore it was a "protective against fever," a position nonaddicts ridiculed as a weak excuse for continued use (GBOW [Laflamme] 1894:IV:355–56).

Thirty-four years of experience in Bihar (North India) and Calcutta (East India) as planter, officer, and various other occupations prompted T. M. Gibbon to say that natives he had known did believe "opium is a preventive against chills and malarial influences" (GBOW [Gibbon] 1894 II:151). Surgeon-Major C. Henderson was slightly more informative and definitely more enthusiastic. In India since 1880, he had been stationed in such places as Madras (South India), the Central Provinces (Middle India), Burma, and Point Blair on the remote Andaman Islands (both East India). These assignments had "quite convinced" Henderson that opium was "an inestimable boon, having no appreciable effect other than beneficial" for people ingesting moderate amounts of the drug (from '5 to 30 grains per day') because it alleviated and prevented many "chronic afflictions." Henderson also asserted it was "undisputed, and in my opinion there is a strong probability of its possessing the property commonly attributed to it, viz., of acting as a prophylactic in certain diseases such as malaria" (GBOW [Henderson] 1894:IV:368). Compared to Henderson, the enthusiasm of Brigade-Surgeon Lieutenant-Colonel Purves was modest. Purves had been in India for only two years. His first posting, in the NWP, was followed by stints in Assam and Bengal. Assamese natives first told him about the drug being a "prophylactic against disease" but he had rejected the idea. He later changed his mind, becoming convinced that it relieved "fever and the complications from malaria" such as dysentery and rheumatism (GBOW [Purves] 1894:II:83).

NOTE

See the Selected Bibliography for full citations concerning witnesses.

Appendix C

Cinchona Cultivation and Quinine Production in South Asia During the Nineteenth Century

The British rulers of India in the 1800s knew the value of quinine. They also wanted to manufacture it. Impatience, incompetence, and nature prevented them from doing it. This changed early in the next century.

The bark that had been introduced to Anglo-European society in 1620 came from Peru, Bolivia, Ecuador, and Columbia. It was stripped (often clandestinely) from several species of the tree and shipped back home. The bark was then pulverized and dispensed as a powder or infusion. (Grier 1937:94; Howard, Bernard 1931:7).

The native people of these regions did not take kindly to their bark being exported. Supplies, therefore, were unstable. This became a crucial issue after 1820. The isolation of quinine was followed by Anglo-Europeans' increased demand for the alkaloid. They needed the bark; the problem was how to ensure that it would be there.

The French, English, and Dutch responded to the challenge. So did the Belgians and Americans. Commencing in the early 1860s, botanical expeditions from these countries smuggled cinchona seeds and small plants out of South America. The material was replanted in regions that were assumed to have compatible climates and other environmental characteristics. The assumptions were incorrect. The Belgians failed in the Congo, the Americans were unsuccessful in California, and the French made a futile attempt in Indochina and in Algeria. The English planted seeds in Jamaica to no avail (Fitzgerald 1968:802; Shaw 1935:4).

These efforts failed, in part, because of ignorance. By 1895, botanists had identified sixty-five species of cinchona trees. They also knew that only a few species had sufficient inherent quinine to make cultivation worthwhile. Furthermore, these species had different environmental requirements for successful growth and maturity (Holmes 1930:832). The Europeans, Americans, and planters in Jamaica did not know that cultivating cinchona was a science.

The British rulers of India had more success. The government opened its first plantation in the Nilgiri Hills during 1861. Private owners in the region and in the Palnai Hills of Travancore, did the same thing. And in 1865, plantations were established at Hakgala (Ceylon), in Coorg, and then at Wainad (Mysore), Darjeeling (Sikkim), and the Karen Hills of Burma (Howard, Bernard 1931:11–12; Shaw 1935:4). Except for Darjeeling and Sikkim, all plantations at this time were in South India.

DUTCH AND ENGLISH CINCHONA POLICY: A STUDY IN CONTRASTS

In the early 1860s, the Dutch began investing much time and money on cinchona research. They were determined to identify the species that were amenable to hybridization. Their goal was to create a tree that was capable of yielding substantial amounts of quinine under conditions unique to their plantations in Java. Dutch patience was rewarded; by 1879 the substance obtained from the bark of their Cinchona Calisaya, variety Ledgeriana, dominated the international quinine market (Gramiccia 1988:154–57, 161; Howard, Bernard 1931:13).

The Government of India had achieved nothing similar. Few species of the tree could tolerate the climate. Most trees were from the species called Succiruba and Officinalis. Both of them were quinine-deficient.

Mismanagement compounded the problem. One British expert writing in 1879 identified administrative ineptitude as the principal reason for failed attempts to raise the average quinine content of indigenous cinchona bark (Gramiccia 1988:154, 159, 175). In Java, he observed, the Dutch were

> wisely thinning out the inferior trees and allowing the best to develop themselves. In British India, on the contrary, they are acting in a way that is as consistent with common sense to believe that by fusing together a half-crown and a penny, one could produce a sovereign, as to believe that by blending inferior qualities one could induce the C. Ledgeriana, the best by far, of all. (John Eliot Howard, quoted in Gramiccia 1988:160)

The miscalculation that John Eliot Howard complained about began in the early 1860s. Managers of Government of India plantations, as well as those operated by private entrepreneurs, had been destroying the large amount of alkaloids that remained in bark after the extraction of quinine. There was no demand for these residual components within the country and elsewhere (Gramiccia 1988:160).

The administration's indifference to cinchona's other alkaloids changed after 1865. A commission was established to evaluate the results of a crude experiment. The test indicated that the bark material routinely discarded after quinine's removal was equally effective in combating fever. This bark material contained cinchonidine, cinchonine, and quinidine. It was then distributed to medical personnel in the Calcutta, Bombay, and Madras Presidencies. They were told to test the efficacy of each alkaloid. The contingent from Madras reported the three hitherto undervalued substances were scarcely, if at all, inferior to quinine as therapeutic agents (Gramiccia 1988:160). The Calcutta and Bombay personnel said essentially the same thing.

This convinced the Government of India that quinine was not indispensable to eliminate malaria in the subcontinent and anywhere else in the world. The quinine-deficient trees in South Asia had some value after all. The British administration proceeded to manufacture large quantities of a purportedly effective febrifuge. It was a mixture of the bark's abundant three alkaloids and its meager amount of quinine (Gramiccia 1988:161). Production continued during the latter part of the 1860s, through the 1870s, and the first part of the next decade. The product was cheap and widely available. The cost per dose came to "about one-sixth of that of quinine sulphate on the market [and] was sold at each post office throughout India at the price of about a halfpenny" (Gramiccia 1988:161).

Anyone in India who still wanted quinine had to look elsewhere. Most of what they obtained was produced in England from imported Javanese bark (Gramiccia 1988:162; Grier 1937:103). They were wise to do so. Physicians in India would eventually conclude that the admixture of cinchona alkaloids was not very effective in preventing or curing malaria victims. Giving only one of them to a patient was a different story.

Government of India policy makers had been partially correct; cinchonidine, cinchonine, and quinidine did have "similar specific febrifugal effect" (Gramiccia 1988:159). The problem was that the cost of extracting the alkaloids separately in a form that was appropriate for therapeutic use was high. It added greatly to their price when the proven merit of quinine was considered (Gramiccia 1988:159; Shaw 1935:6–7).

It was the Government of India's reluctance to pay for proper extraction procedures that had prompted John Eliot Howard's criticism in 1879. And for the remainder of the nineteenth century, cost effectiveness precluded attempts to retrieve whatever inherent quinine its trees possessed. Tests conducted in Java revealed the problem that had confronted British authorities. The bark from Succiruba, the dominant species in the Indian subcontinent, had about 8 percent alkaloids. Half of it was cinchonidine. Quinine content was 1.5 percent. And that was the good news. All types of cinchona that grew in India produced bark that contained a mere 0.5–2.0 percent of quinine. The other alkaloids amounted to only 3–4 percent (See Shaw 1935:6 for tests conducted in 1905).

The lesson learned too late was that the Government of India circa the 1860s had invested money and hope in a project with little chance of success. The species of cinchona that were able to survive in South Asia were inherently low in quinine. These trees also yielded only modest amounts of other alkaloidal substances that had medicinal value. Nevertheless, the problem was not insurmountable if the welfare of Indian citizens was the principal interest of British authorities. It was not.

Opium was the reason why the Government of India refused to bear the cost of producing sufficient quinine for its suffering population. It viewed the manufacture of cinchona febrifuge as protection from the potential volatility of the India-China opium trade. Sir Clements Markham, the man responsible for introducing cinchona cultivation to South Asia in 1859, included a footnote that conveyed the official attitude. The comment appears in his 1880 volume.

> It has been suggested by a writer in the *Pall Mall Gazette* of September 18, 1880, that China will hereafter be among the largest and most constant customers for cheap febrifuge alkaloids from British India. From the vast tracts of country in China where rice is cultivated, fever is never absent. Opium is now employed as the medicine easiest to be had and the cheapest. If chinchona [sic] alkaloids would come into competition with opium, and obtain the preference by their lower price, the immense superiority of chinchona [sic] over opium as a febrifuge would produce a revolution in the Chinese consumption of the two drugs. By this process a solution would be found for the dangers and uncertainties of the large opium revenue of India, and for the perplexing moral questions connected with it (Markham 1880:440 [footnote]).* *[* The original spelling of cinchona was "chinchona." The first "h" was unintentionally dropped when the substance first appeared in Europe. "Cinchona" is the version most often found in contemporary popular and scientific literature.]*

There were, therefore, several reasons for the British to continue production of the cinchona admixture. They believed that their product, despite manufacturing difficulties and its inherent quinine deficiency, did do something to prevent and cure a devastating disease. Its effect might be modest, but it was better than nothing. They also realized, as early as the 1860s, that the export of prodigious amounts of Indian opium might end. Indigenous poppy cultivation in China was increasing, and the Turkish and Persian drug, were potential threats to profits. Since malaria also plagued the Chinese, this population's reliance upon the Indian cinchona febrifuge guaranteed restoration of at least some of the British revenue lost from the controversial overseas sales of opium.

What appeared to be beneficial for sufferers around the world then evolved into a disaster for victims of malaria in South Asia. According to Grier, the

> rivalry between India and Java from about 1885 resulted in enormous overproduction [of bark] and a tremendous fall in price, causing disaster to scores of Indian planters, and the uprooting and destruction of most of the Indian plantations soon after 1890 in favour of more profitable crops. On the other hand, the scientific cultivation by Dutch growers, supported by the Dutch government, enabled them to continue cultivation of the tree . . . and to hold on during a period of twenty years of bitter competition and low prices. (Grier 1937:102; see also Howard, Bernard 1931:15–16; and IMG 1918:265)

Grier is essentially correct. The abundance of Dutch Ledgeriana quinine during the late 1870s did intensify competition between the two producers. The cost of quinine declined drastically in 1880. It was inexpensive until the beginning of World War I (Gramiccia 1988:164 [figure 17], 165; also see APA 1892:40:742 for fluctuations from 1823 through 1891).

The Government of India began to manufacture quinine for domestic use in 1890. The amount produced each year was modest. This continued for almost a decade and a half. Research that was designed to lower the cost of procuring quinine from Indian bark, as well to increase the inherent amount of all cinchona alkaloids in each tree, was underway by 1905 (Shaw 1935:8–16). And in 1929, according to Bernard Howard, the cinchona plantations and alkaloid manufacturing industry in India could easily supply the world's consumption of quinine. The amount was 600 hundred tons per annum (Howard, Bernard 1931:19).

Howard was too optimistic. Less than a decade later, James Grier reported that India manufactured only thirty percent of "its own requirements, while only 10 percent of the total quantity consumed in the British Empire is produced in British territory" (1937:103).

This brief review of cinchona cultivation and quinine production in nineteenth-century India reveals the Government of India was aware of the splitters' definition of malaria. Furthermore, it had identified quinine as an effective preventive and cure for the malady. It also was unable to extract sufficient quinine from the tree that grew in South Asia. Yet, it was increasing amounts of inexpensive Dutch quinine from Java that terminated its attempts to produce a cinchona febrifuge. The Government of India, however, did not resume narcotine extraction to compete with the Dutch product. And the most likely reason why it refrained from doing so was because informed people in the administration knew that the opium alkaloid did not do the thing that opium's defenders claimed that it did during the Royal Commission hearings.

INFORMATION ABOUT CINCHONA CULTIVATION AND QUININE PRODUCTION IN INDIA AVAILABLE TO THE PUBLIC DURING THE NINETEENTH AND EARLY TWENTIETH CENTURIES

There was abundant information available to the reading public circa the 1890s and early twentieth century concerning quinine and other cinchona alkaloids. There also were extensive commentaries about their efficacy for malaria. See the excellent nontechnical discussions in the *EB* [1893] 1894 "Quinine" 20:184–86, and *EB* 1911 "Malaria" 17:461–65. The 1911 article contains the opinions of Ronald Ross and Patrick Manson. They discuss the effective dosage levels of quinine as a malaria prophylactic and febrifuge. Frederick A. Flückiger's 1884 *The Cinchona Barks* is another example of his meticulous scholarship. The trait characterizes his 1879 book about *Papaver somniferum Linn* as well as articles he published before and after 1884. John Eliot Howard's 1869–1876 *The Quinology of the East India Plantations* is pioneering. It is the first detailed identification of the numerous species of cinchona to be published in the western world. Howard includes the types of cinchona that were introduced to India during the period. Colored plates of the different species make Howard's volume unique.

Two publications by Sir George King were also available to the reading public after 1870. The first item is the 1876 *A Manual of Cinchona Cultivation in India*. See C. H. Wood's description of the process that was followed for manufacturing cinchona febrifuge at the Sikkim plantations, and King's two annual reports (1875–1876) about cinchona cultivation in India.

The second King item is the 1880 *A Manual of Cinchona Cultivation in India*, second edition. It is a technical presentation of numerous facets of the country's struggling cinchona industry.

A contrast to King's 1880 effort is Sir Clements Robert Markham's 1862 *Travels in Peru and India: While Superintending the Collection of Chinchona* [sic] *Plants and Seeds in South America, and their Introduction into India*. Although biased, this very readable book illuminates the difficulties that plagued the preliminary stage of introducing cinchona cultivation to South Asia. This volume supplements his 1880 volume cited above.

THE FUTURE OF CINCHONA CULTIVATION AND QUININE PRODUCTION IN SOUTH ASIA AFTER 1895

Several sources discuss the prospects of quinine production and cinchona cultivation in India and South Asia in the post-1895 era. They also provide statistics. See Andrew Thomas Gage's 1918 *Report on the Extension of Cinchona Cultivation in India*. Equally informative is Sir George Watt's article entitled "Cinchona." It is found in his *The Commercial Products of India. Being an Abridgement of "The Dictionary of Economic Products of India"* ([1908] 1966:302–10). There is also the A. Wilson (T. J. Mirchandani [joint author]) 1940 publication. It is their *Report on the Prospects of Cinchona Cultivation in India*. Imperial Council of Agricultural Research. Miscellaneous Bulletin No. 29 (second edition). The authors describe the future of cinchona cultivation in India just before the beginning of World War II, and consequences of the possible cessation of quinine shipments from the Dutch East Indies and Java.

CINCHONA ACREAGE IN INDIA 1894/95–1908/09

Statistics for cinchona acreage from 1894/95 through 1898/99 in Bengal, Madras, Coorg, and Mysore (the provinces of British India where trees were planted), are found in IDR 1900 "No. 3–Area (in acres) under Crop, and Specification of Crops, in each Province in British India and in Mysore." *Agricultural Statistics of India for the Years 1894–95 to 1898–99*. 15th Issue. Part I. British India. 102–04. Subsequent issues of these reports contain amounts for later periods. The twenty-fifth issue, for example, has data for 1904/05 to 1908/09. See IDR 1910 "No. 3. Area (in acres) under Crops, and Specification of Crops, in each province in British India." *Agricultural Statistics of India for the Years 1904/05–1908/9 to 1898–99*. 25th Issue. Part I. British India. 114–15, 120, 122.

OTHER TWENTIETH-CENTURY CINCHONA PUBLICATIONS

The material published during the twentieth century is voluminous. Some of it was reviewed for this Appendix. A fraction of the material has been cited. See Gabriele Gramiccia 1987 "Notes on the Early History of Cinchona Plantations." *Acta Leidensia*. 55:5–13 for useful historical material. The data supplements her 1988 publication ("Notes on the Early History of Cinchona Plantations." *Acta Leidensia*. 55:5–13).

Five essays that review the history of cinchona in the East Indies are in the 1945 *Science and Scientists in the Netherlands Indies* (edited by Peter Honig and Frans Verdoran). The essays address the formidable physical and financial difficulties that confronted the Dutch. The authors provide many details about the challenge in growing trees in Java that contained sufficient quinine to realize a profit after deducting expenses and other factors. Some of this material is germane to the British experience in India during the 1860s and 1870s, as are Parliament's session [GBS] and command papers [GBC] that appeared periodically during the second half of the nineteenth and early twentieth centuries.

NOTE

See the Selected Bibliography for full citations about witnesses who discussed cinchona and quinine during the Royal Commission on Opium hearings.

Appendix D

Anarcotine and Crude Opium Requirements (in Pounds) Using the Three Alkaloid Extraction Ratios for More than One Million Sufferers

Appendix D provides pound equivalents for the opium chest requirements found in table 11.
Column 2: Pounds of Anarcotine Needed for 1,500,000 to 4,000,000 people.
Columns 3–5: Crude Opium Requirements (in Pounds) Using the Three Ratios.

1	2	3	4	5
Number of Sufferers	Their Anarcotine Needs (lbs.)	Garden's 116.9:1 Ratio (lbs.)	Garden's 24:1 Ratio (lbs.)	Roberts' 16:1 Ratio (lbs.)
1,500,000	8,421.10**	984,427.17	202,106.52	134,737.68
2,000,000	11,228.14	1,312,569.57	269,475.36	179,650.24
2,500,000	14,035.17**	1,640,711.96	336,844.20	224,562.80
3,000,000	16,842.21	1,968,854.35	404,213.04	269,475.36
3,500,000	19,649.24**	2,296,996.74	471,581.88	314,387.92
4,000,000	22,456.28	2,625,139.13	538,950.72	359,300.48

***Note:* The anarcotine requirement for the three numerical categories of sufferers is rounded off to the nearest hundredth. The original totals (8421.105 for 1.5 million people, 14,035.175 for 2.5 million, and 19,649.245 for 3.5 million) are used to calculate the crude opium requirement in each of the three ratio columns.

Space limitations require rounding off all crude opium requirements under the 116.9 ratio column to the nearest hundredth. Original numbers carried out an additional one or two decimal places are: 984,427.1745 pounds (1.5 million people); 1,312,569.566 pounds (2 million people); 1,640,711.9575 (2.5 million people); 1,968,854.349 (3 million people); 2,296,996.7405 (3.5 million people); and 2,625,139.132 (4 million people).

Appendix E

Alternative Format for Contents of Tables 12, 13, and 14

TITLE OF TABLES 12, 13, AND 14

"Quantity of Bengal Abkari (Excise) Opium Chests Required to Extract Sufficient Anarcotine for 'Cure' and 'Convalescence' of Four Groups of 'Malarial Fever' Sufferers. Entries Are Expressed as Percentage of Bengal Chests Prepared for Domestic Consumption During the 20-Year Period from 1873/74 to 1892/93"

ORIGINAL DATA

Bengal Abkari Production Figures for 20-Year Period (1873/74–1892/93)
Average Annual Production = 4,454 chests (fraction more than)
Highest Single Season = 6,890.15 chests (1890/91)
Lowest Single Season = 2,914 chests (fraction less than) (1888/89)

116.9:1 Ratio

3 million = 15,951.74 Bengal Abkari chests
[Approximately 350 percent greater than the Average Annual Abkari Production, from 1873/74 through 1892/93 for the 116.9:1 ratio and 3 million victims]

3,062,031 = 16,281.58 Bengal Abkari chests (Clarke & Roberts' victims)
[Approximately 366 percent greater than the Average Annual Abkari Production, from 1873/74 through 1892/93 for the 116.9:1 ratio and Clarke's 3,062,031 victims]

3.5 million = 18,610.36 Bengal Abkari chests.
[Approximately 418 percent greater than the Average Annual Abkari Production, from 1873/74 through 1892/93 for the 116.9:1 ratio and 3.5 million victims]

4 million = 21,456.28 Bengal Abkari chests
[Approximately 482 percent greater than the Average Annual Abkari Production, from 1873/74 through 1892/93 for the 116.9:1 ratio and 4 million victims]

24:1 Ratio

3 million = 3,274.95 Bengal Abkari chests
[Almost 74 percent (exactly .73528289178) of the Average Annual Abkari Production, from 1873/74 through 1892/93 for the 24:1 ratio and 3 million victims.]

3,062,031 = 3,342.67 Bengal Abkari chests (Clarke & Roberts' victims)
[Slightly more than 75 percent of the Average Annual Abkari Production, from 1873/74 through 1892/93. The exact calculation is .75048720251 or a fraction more than 75 percent for the 24:1 ratio and Clarke's 3,062,031 million victims.]

3.5 million = 3,820.77 Bengal Abkari chests
[Almost 86 percent of the Average Annual Abkari Production, from 1873/74 through 1892/93; the exact calculation is .85782891783 percent for the 24:1 ratio and 3.5 million victims]

4 million = 4,366.60 Bengal Abkari chests
[A fraction more than 98 percent of the Average Annual Abkari Production, from 1873/74 through 1892/93; the exact calculation is .98037718904 percent for the 24:1 ratio and 4 million victims]

16:1 Ratio

3 million = 2,183.30 Bengal Abkari chests
[Almost 50 percent (exactly .49018859452) of the Average Annual Abkari Production, from 1873/74 through 1892/93 for the 16:1 ratio and 3 million victims]

3,062,031 = 2,228.44 Bengal Abkari chests (Clarke & Roberts' victims)
[Slightly more than 50 percent (exactly .50032330489) of the Average Annual Abkari Production, from 1873/74 through 1892/93 for the 16:1 ratio and Clarke's 3,062,031 million victims]

3.5 million = 2,547.18 Bengal Abkari chests
[A fraction more than 57 percent (exactly .57188594522) of the Average Annual Abkari Production, from 1873/74 through 1892/93 for the 16:1 ratio and 3.5 million victims]

4 million = 2,911.07 Bengal Abkari chests
[The figure represents more than 65 percent (exactly .65358554109) of the Average Annual Abkari Production, from 1873/74 through 1892/93 for the 16:1 ratio and 4 million victims]

Appendix F

Nineteenth- and Early Twentieth-Century Anarcotine/Narcotine Research and the Alkaloid's Irrelevance for 'Malaria' and Fever, and Subsequent Research

Morphine, codeine, and narceine were the opium alkaloids most in demand in the western market at the end of the 1800s. This continued during the early years of the twentieth century. Other than the references cited in the first chapter, researchers paid little attention to the physiological and psychological effects of anarcotine/narcotine in human beings. And what these people concluded was that the substance was of minor therapeutic significance. Improvements in extraction technology during the twentieth century, combined with more discoveries about the mother drug's ingredients, eventually altered the alkaloid's status. Anarcotine/narcotine was renamed noscapine (gnoscopine) (Sim 1965:59). Its principal use is described below.

The "career" of this opium alkaloid raises a question. Sir William Roberts cites India data from 1838–39, and 1859–60 (O'Shaughnessy, Palmer, and Garden). But was there anything else about the alkaloid that might have explained his enthusiasm? Was there any pre-1895 research that contradicted declarations about the alkaloid's lack of narcotic or "therapeutic" capability?

THE SURGEON-GENERAL'S *INDEX-CATALOGUE*

A bibliographic serial published by the office of the United States Surgeon-General (SG) provides a partial answer. This author examined all articles that are cited in the following paragraphs. The Surgeon General's multivolume *Index-Catalogue* cites very few publications from the early nineteenth century to the 1893 creation of the Royal Commission on Opium. Narcotine is mentioned in only four issues through 1906. The 1896 publication repeats the entries found in the 1880 publication.

The 1880 issue of the *Index-Catalogue* has only two entries under narcotine. The first is Dr. Garden's 1860 experiment in India. Palmer's work during 1859 is unmentioned. The second entry is E. H. Janes 1862:149. He mentions the anarcotine/'malaria' work in south Asia.

The 1888 edition of the serial cites eight articles. Five are English language publications, and two are French. One is German. Only one of the English language publications discusses the effects of narcotine on the human "constitution." This is W. Tully's description of the appropriate techniques for documenting the effects of the alkaloid (1833:37, 56). The three-page German article by J. F. H. Albers (1862:144–146) is a brief discussion of dispensing narcotine for sickness in general. All other publications describe the chemical composition of the alkaloid, not its effects upon the physiology and psychology of human beings.

The surgeon-general publications cite nothing else for anarcotine/narcotine until 1906. This volume has four listings. One of them is Sir William Roberts' 1895 medical report to the Royal Commission on Opium. Two citations are German articles. Both were published in 1903. The first work analyzes the derivatives from narcotine. The second work examines how high temperature affects the alkaloid's composition.

The last article cited is A. C. Crawford and A. R. L. Dohme (1902:472–78). It is a review of anarcotine/narcotine research from the early 1800s to 1902. The authors say that most experimenters tested the alkaloid using nonhuman animals (dogs, cats, roosters, pigeons, rabbits, frogs, and guinea pigs). Considering the time span involved, research involving human subjects is negligible. Crawford and Dohme mention Palmer's recognition about the alkaloid lacking narcotic properties. They also credit him for renaming it anarcotine (1902:472). The authors say nothing about Palmers' 1860 narcotine/malaria experiment in India, and they do not mention Dr. Garden's continuation of the research.

Crawford and Dohme cite the conclusions of Magendie and other early nineteenth-century investigators. For example, an 1825 article by Bailly indicates that "small doses . . . are inactive in man, while large ones, 3–3.5 Gm. induce merely headache and slight nausea; after a dose of 7 Gm. one of his cases merely experienced slight giddiness" (Crawford & Dohme 1902:472).

All articles after 1825 indicate the same thing: the alkaloid has mild effects when administered in small to moderate amounts. Larger doses produce only transitory, harmless, and relatively inconsequential effects. The Crawford and Dohme generalization is based upon their examination of documents from 1827, 1856, 1875, 1896, and several sources with no publication date cited. Their comments also suggest that anarcotine/narcotine's effects upon human physiology and psychology was a remarkably minor topic of interest as the 1800s unfolded. According to Crawford and Dohme, there are no citations (except the 1896 document) that investigate the alkaloid's effects upon human circulation, respiration, alimentary canal, urinary organs, and elimination (1902:474–78).

The Crawford and Dohme discussion about the use of anarcotine/narcotine for the splitters' idea of 'malaria,' as well as the lumpers' version of the plasmodia-linked malady, is brief and revealing. The alkaloid was not used extensively as a preventive or cure for one of the world's worst diseases (no matter how it was defined.) The authors conclude that the "general action" of "pure narcotine" for any disease is modest. It only ameliorates symptoms.

> Daily doses of from 0.12 Gm. have been used for migraine associated with malaria, and the only untoward symptom has been some weakening of the pulse (Semaine med. 1896, No. 14, quoted by Kunkel Handb. d. Toxikol. v.2, p.820). The usual dose for intermittent fever cases is given as from 1.5 grains. (Crawford and Dohme 1902:473)

Sir William Roberts' is the only source that Crawford and Dohme cite for the intermittent fever dose. They conclude the review by declaring that there are

> no reasons to believe that small doses of narcotine are injurious. Any unpleasant action the undenarcotized tincture of opium may have is probably due to other so-called odorous principles, and it does not reenforce the action of morphine. We have found no practice of the toxic effect claimed for narcotine by Ebert in his paper published this month. (Crawford and Dohme 1902:478)

The Crawford and Dohme review leaves no doubt: anarcotine/narcotine is only useful for temporary relief from a severe headache. Furthermore, the only citation ostensibly "proving" that it prevents and cures 'malaria' is Roberts' own 1895 report. Empirical evidence that supports the man's evaluation is virtually nonexistent. Roberts was enthusiastic about a substance that actually had inconsequential physiological and psychological consequences for human beings. The most positive thing that could be said about the substance was that it was not harmful if used in moderation.

THE 1899 CRITIQUE OF ANDREW DUNCAN

The *Index-Catalogue* missed one important nineteenth-century publication. The article further justifies why the Anglo-European response to Sir William Roberts' assessment of anarcotine in the prevention and cure of 'malaria' was, at best, indifference.

A reevaluation of the alkaloid's purported febrifugal (curative) and prophylactic (preventive) capabilities appeared in 1899. Andrew Duncan, a physician, published the results of a study conducted in India during the three years before his departure from the country. Duncan examined fifteen "remedies" used to cure or prevent 'malaria'/malaria. He concluded that quinine was, by far, the best of the fifteen febrifuges. Duncan mentions Sir William Roberts' enthusiasm about narcotine/anarcotine. But Duncan was unimpressed by what he actually observed. The alkaloid only ranked fourth. His comments suggest that anarcotine/narcotine occupied this status because its continued administration to sufferers repressed their symptoms over the course of treatment. Quinine, however, effected a "complete cure faster," although the symptoms of some people clearly were different from the individuals who were given anarcotine/narcotine. Having established the alkaloid's power to *cure*, Duncan proceeds to examine its ability to *prevent* the disease.

Duncan says that 'preventive' experiments were performed in India during 1886, 1887, 1889, 1896, and 1897, but he gives no bibliographic detail. The researchers had tested fewer substances. He compares the remedies common to all investigators, including his 1899 effort. They were "quinine, quinetan, cinchona febrifuge, cinchonidine, arsenic, 'atees,' and narcotine" (1899:66).

The five experiments, and Duncan's 1899 observations, portray anarcotine/narcotine as slightly more effective than ingesting nothing at all. In other words, the alkaloid seems to provide psychological relief; potential victims *think* they are avoiding sickness. The physiological benefits are virtually nonexistent. Sir William Roberts did not mention the 1886, 1887, and 1889 critiques in his 1895 medical report for the Royal Commission.

Duncan ends the article with a solid endorsement of the best-known cinchona alkaloid.

> In the curative treatment of malarial fever no drug has yet been found to supersede quinine. It is especially valuable in severe cases when administered by enema. In the preventive treatment, as far as India is concerned, quinine again holds the field. (1899:67)

A word of caution applies to Duncan's analysis. He provides few details about patients' symptoms. This suggests that some of his test subjects might have had the disease associated with plasmodia. Other people might have been victims of the lumpers' version of 'malaria'. In either case, anarcotine/narcotine was an unimpressive febrifuge and prophylactic.

One more nineteenth-century article should to be mentioned. Nusserwanji Surveyor (1896:839) describes his anarcotine experiment using dogs and mice. He began his research in India immediately after publication of the Royal Commission on Opium volumes. His conclusions do not confirm Roberts' assessment, and what he found applies to nonhuman subjects.

ANGLO-EUROPEAN ANARCOTINE/NARCOTINE RESEARCH DURING THE TWENTIETH CENTURY (POST-1902)

The definitive examination of Roberts' drug, alkaloid, and disease scenario was published slightly more than three decades after Duncan's critique. Ram Nath Chopra and R. Knowles (1930:5–13) concluded that (1) opium and anarcotine/narcotine did not prevent or cure plasmodial malaria (falciparum, vivax, ovale, and malariae); and (2) the role of the mother drug and the alkaloid in other afflictions called 'malaria' was fever suppression and symptom management. And in 1989, Winther demonstrated how Roberts was able to conclude that the mother drug and its alkaloid prevented and cured either version of the disease. The alkaloid's peculiar effects on the sick person's consciousness of "illness" are isolated and described in this preliminary analysis.

Twentieth-century research has produced an enormous literature about opium and its components (Krueger et al. 1943). Alkaloid extraction technology was perfected. For most of the twentieth century, noscapine (anarcotine/narcotine) has been classified as a mild antitussive (Bickerman 1962:353–68; Chopra, Lieut. Col. R. N., et al. 1930:35–49; Cooper & Hatcher 1934:411–20; Idänpään–Heikkilä 1968:201–16; Karlsson, et al. 1990:275–79; Kasé 1968:363–419; Mourey, et al. 1992:619–26; Nayak, et al. 1965:191–94; Tsunoda & Yoshimura 1979:181–82; Vedsö 1961b:119–28; Wade 1977:1249–50; Winter 1954:99–108). The antitussive status is now debated (Empey, et al. 1979:393–97; Pawetczyk, et al. 1976:69–76). Recent experiments also indicate that this cough suppressant might have another capability. It reduces the size of cancer tumors in laboratory animals. There is a possibility that it might do the same thing in human beings (Gatehouse, et. al. 1991:279–83; *Science News* 1998:168; Ye, et al. 1998:1601–06). And some works also temper earlier pronouncements about the alkaloid's benign nature (Karlsson, et al. 1988:195–203; Lasagna, et al. 1961:33–4; Mitchell, I. et al. 1991:479–86; Vedsö 1961a:154–64). This work suggests that Roberts' recommendations, if they had been heeded in 1895, would have been unexpectedly harmful to the victims of 'malaria' who required prolonged, repeated exposure to the alkaloid.

NOTE

See the Selected Bibliography for full citations.

Tables

Table 1. Occupational Category of Witnesses with Opium and Malaria Testimony

Occupational Category	Witnesses with Opium & Malaria Testimony	Total in Category
Medical Practitioners Employed by Government or Native States	49	81
Medical Practitioners (Private)	31	65
Medical Missionaries	9	15
Christian Missionaries & Catechists	9	47
Officials, Divisional & District	9	51
Representatives of Associations	8	52
Landowners & Tenants	6	88
Opium & Excise Officials	6	14
Chiefs & Officials of Native States	5	87
Merchants, Bankers, Mill Owners & Shopkeepers	4	83
Lawyers & Pleaders	2	27
Officials Attached to Government	4	14
Planters	3	27
Pensioned Officials	1	12
Journalists	1	8
TOTAL	149 *	671 **

* Witnesses from six occupational categories provided no information germane to opium and 'malaria.' The categories were "Political Officers," "Military Officers," "Military Pensioners," "School Masters, Professors, and Teachers," "Religious Teachers (non-Christian)," "Miscellaneous," a group consisting of "Civil Engineer, Labour Contractor, Municipal Commissioners, Actuary, Writer, College Students [and] Without Occupation." ([GBO] Great Britain. Royal Commission on Opium. ["Index to Witnesses Examined by the Commission"] 1895:VII:223–29).

** This is the total number of people in all categories from which opium and 'malaria' witnesses were selected according to pages 223–29 of the "Index to Witnesses Examined by the Commission."

Table 2. Patients Receiving Anarcotine During the Two Periods of Dr. Garden's Nine-Month Study

Category of Patient	"Virulent" Fever Period [10 Oct.–Dec. 1859 through January 1860]	"Non-Virulent" Period [Feb. to 10 June 1860]	Total(s)
Jail Hospital	173	65	238 (Jail)
Police Hospital	352	94	446 (Police)
Total(s)	525	159	684 (Both)

Table 3. Condensation of Statistics in Dr. Garden's Table 4: "Shewing [sic] the Number of Paroxysms After the First Administration of Anarcotine with Percentage"

Number/ Fevers	Quotidian (150)		Tertian (37)		Totals (187)	
	Number/ Patients	% of 150 Patients	Number/ Patients	% of 37 Patients	Number/ Patients	% of 187 Patients
0	39	26.00%	3	8.10%	42	22.46%
1 to 3	72	48.00%	26	70.26%	98	52.40%
4 to 6	25	16.66%	5	13.50%	30	16.04%
7 to 9	9	5.99%	2	5.41%	11	5.87%
10 to 12	5	3.22%	1	2.70%	6	3.20%
Totals	150	99.87%*	37	99.97%*	187	99.97%*

* *Source:* Percentages for the three categories are not rounded off to 100%. See page 405 of Dr. A. Garden 1860 "Report on Anarcotine." *Indian Annals of Medical Science.* 7:400–18.

Table 4. Statistics in Dr. Garden's Table 5: "Shewing [sic] Average Amount of Anarcotine Taken Before and After Cessation of Fever According to the Numbers of Paroxysms"

Fevers After Initial Dose	Quotidian (150)		Tertian (37)		Totals (187)	
	Before Cure (grains)	Before Conval.* (grains)	Before Cure (grains)	During Conval.* (grains)	Before Cure (grains)	During Conval.* (grains)
0	6.19	15.20	5.00	14.16	6.15	16.40
1	10.17	12.18	17.54	19.37	12.13	14.10
2	15.70	16.69	26.40	10.45	18.80	14.80
3	19.26	12.83	32.37	5.75	22.02	11.30
4	33.20	17.50	41.30	13.30	35.25	14.30
5	33.60	24.45	151.00	39.00	44.45	25.70
6	43.60	18.90	150.00	150.00	58.80	37.70
7	60.00	27.30	0.00	0.00	60.00	27.30
8	49.60	13.30	93.00	19.50	60.80	17.07
9	50.00	14.00	0.00	0.00	50.00	14.00
10	37.00	40.00	0.00	0.00	57.00	40.00
11	64.00	23.00	82.00	27.00	68.50	24.00
12	72.00	18.00	0.00	0.00	72.00	18.00
Avg. Total	19.37 grains	15.8 grains	39.5 grains	18.3 grains	22.7 grains	16.3 grains

Source: Adapted from Dr. A. Garden. 1860 "Report on Anarcotine." *Indian Annals of Medical Science.* 7:407 [Table 5].

* "Convalescence is abbreviated to "Conval." Garden uses the heading "Before Convalesence" for Quotidian data and "During Convalescence" for the Tertian and "Totals" columns. He gives no explanation for the change.

Table 5. Estimate of Anarcotine and Opium Requirements for Quotidian and Tertian Fever Patients Based upon Dr. A. Garden's 1859–1860 Ghazipur Experiment*

*Columns 4–6: Opium Requirements Using the Three Ratios.

1 684 People Multiplied by	2 Number of Sufferers	3 Their Anarcotine Needs (lbs.)	4 Garden's 116.9:1 Ratio (lbs.)	5 Garden's 24:1 Ratio (lbs.)	6 Robert's 16:1 Ratio (lbs.)
0	684	3.84	448.34	92.16	61.44
2	1,368	7.68	897.79	184.32	122.88
3	2,052	11.52	1,346.69	276.48	184.32
5	3,420	19.20	2,244.48	460.80	307.20
10	6,840	38.40	4,488.96	921.60	614.40
20	13,680	76.80	8,977.92	1,843.20	1,228.80
30	20,520	115.20	13,466.88	2,764.80	1,843.20
40	27,360	153.60	17,955.84	3,686.40	2,457.60
50	34,200	192.00	22,444.80	4,608.00	3,072.00
100	68,400	384.00	44,889.60	9,216.00	6,144.00
200	136,800	768.00	89,779.20	18,432.00	12,288.00
300	205,200	1,152.00	134,668.80	27,648.00	18,432.00
350	239,400	1,344.00	157,113.60	32,256.00	21,504.00
400	273,600	1,536.00	179,588.40	36,864.00	24,576.00
450	307,800	1,728.00	202,003.20	41,472.00	27,648.00
500	342,000	1,920.00	224,448.00	46,080.00	30,720.00
600	410,400	2,304.00	269,337.60	55,296.00	36,864.00
700	478,800	2,688.00	314,227.20	64,512,00	43,008.00
800	547,200	3,072.00	359,116.80	73,728.00	49,152.00
900	615,600	3,456.00	404,006.40	82,944.00	55,296.00
1,000	684,000	3,840.00	448,896.00	92,160.00	61,440.00
1,250	855,000	4,800,00	561,120.00	115,200.00	76,800.00
1,461.998*	1,000,000*	5,614.07*	656,285.18	134,737.76	89,825.17

* *Note:* 1,461.9983 multiplied by 3.84 lbs. = 999,999.99 people. This is rounded off to 1,000,000 "fever" sufferers. Multiply 1,461.9983 by 3.84 to calculate the probable anarcotine consumption of 1 million people. This is 5,614.0734 lbs. The opium requirements of 1 million individuals using Garden's 116.9:1 ratio is 656,285.18 lbs and the needed amount using the 24:1 ratio is 134,737.76 lbs. Sir William Roberts' 16:1 ratio produces a figure of 89,825.174 lbs, or 89,825.17 lbs. All opium requirements for the group of 1,000,000 people in the table are to the nearest hundredth.

Table 6. Bengal and Malwa Opium Exports*

Year	Exports from Calcutta [Bengal Provision] (chests)	Exports from Bombay [Malwa] (chests)	Total (chests)
1883/84	—	38,245.5	—
1884/85	—	38,686	—
1885/86	51,054	36,901.5**	87,955.5**
1886/87	54,616	41,222.5**	95,838.5**
1887/88	56,385	33,711	90,096
1888/89	57,358	30,431	87,789
1889/90	55,985	29,181	85,166
1890/91	55,597	28,156	85,753
1891/92	56,773	30,786 **	87,559 **
1892/93	48,149	27,268.5**	75,417.5**
1893/94	43,593	27,246	70,839
1894/95	39,778	29,056	68,834
Total	519,288	390,891	835,214
Average Annual Export	51,928.8 (10 years)	32,574.25 (12 years)	83,521.4 (10 years)

* The source for table 6 is page 6 of [GBS] Great Britain. [East India] [Godley] 1897. "Table IV. "Quantities of Opium Exported from India to China and other Countries during the Ten Years 1885–86 to 1894–95" in: "Return Showing for the Last Ten Years the Acreage under Poppy in India; the Amount of Advances to the Cultivators for Crude Opium; and the Quantity of Opium Produced in the Factories, Distinguishing between the Behar and Benares Agencies" [and] "Also the Quantity Exported to China and other Countries; the Quantity of Malwa and other Opium purchased by the Indian Government; and the Quantity which in any other way came under the Cognizance of the Indian Government" (66). LXIII. 1–7.
Column 3 entries are also found on page 347 of [GBO] Great Britain. Royal Commission on Opium [Finlay]. 1894a. "Opium Produced or Consumed in India." [Presented by Mr. Finlay to the Government of India, Department of Finance and Commerce]. Appendix IX. *In Minutes of Evidence Taken Before the Royal Commission on Opium between 18 November and 29 December 1893; with Appendices.* Volume II. Part 2. [C–7397] 344–54.
** The 1894a Finlay document does not round off fractions of a chest to the nearest highest figure for any year. Bombay/Malwa entries for several years, therefore, differ slightly from the 1897 document. The 1897 Godley source entries for 1885/86 and 1886/87 are 36,902 and 41,223 respectively. Finlay's calculations for these years are used in this table. There are two other discrepancies. The first is a difference of 1 chest for the 1891/92 entries. The 1897 document cites 30,785 chests whereas the 1894a Finlay material indicates 30,786. The second pertains to 1892/93. Finlay lists a total of 27,268.5 chests but the 1897 Godley source indicates only 27,235. The compilers provide no explanation for the difference. Finlay's data is preferred in both cases because the document is used extensively in the following discussion about the production, distribution, and consumption of Malwa opium in India and exports from the region. Column 4 entries for 1885/86, 1886/87, 1891/92, and 1892/93 also reflect this preference. Godley's 1897 numbers are 87,956; 95,839; 87,558 and 75,384 chests respectively. The amounts cited for these years in column 4 been adjusted to reflect the inclusion of Finlay's data in column 3.

Table 7. Statement Showing Quantities of Excise Opium Manufactured at the Bihar and Benares Agencies and the Quantities Supplied to the Several Local Governments during the Last 20 Years. *, **

Year	Quantity of Bengal Excise Opium Manufactured at Each Agency (maunds)		Total (maunds)	Qty. of Bengal Excise Opium Supplied to Brisith India (maunds)
	Bihar	Benares		
1873/74	5,011	768	5,779	4,775.5
1874/75	4,016	1,812	5,828	2,880
1875/76	5,453	1,108	6,561	5,240.5
1876/77	4,298	1,523	5,821	5,221
1877/78	3,795	1,083	4,878	5,603
1878/79	3,876	2,185	6,061	6,095
1879/80	4,020	2,997	7,017	6,426.5
1880/81	5,284	719	6,003	5,981
1881/82	3,956	2,055	6,011	6,206
1882/83	3,240	2,632	5,872	6,864.5
1883/84	1,837	5,356	7,193	6,600
1884/85	3,991	5,856	9,847	7,221
1885/86	2,653	4,102	6,755	6,188.5
1886/87	931	5,143	6,074	6,393
1887/88	3,289	2,876	6,165	6,795.5
1888/89	1,698	2,674	4,372	5,478.5
1889/90	1,913	5,920	7,833	9,621.5
1890/91	5,030	5,305	10,335	7,674
1891/92	5,097	2,637	7,734	6,619
1892/93	2,996	4,498	7,494	8,234.5
Total Maunds for 20-Year Period	72,384 (maunds)	61,249 (maunds)	133,633 (maunds)	126,118.5 (maunds)
Avg. Maunds/Yr. (maunds)	3,619.2 (maunds)	3,062.45 (maunds)	6,681.65 (maunds)	6,305.925 (maunds)

* Statistics (in maunds) and title of table are taken from J. H. Rivett-Carnac. "Statement F–Table I," page 327. Conversions cited below are calculated using 1 maund = 82.2857 lbs. and 1 Bengal Excise = 123.4257 lbs. Rivett-Carnac does not provide figures for "Total Maunds for 20-year Period" and "Average Maunds Per Year." The numbers are the author's calculations.

** *Source:* [GBO] Great Britain. Royal Commission on Opium [Rivett-Carnac]. 1894. "Statement F–Table I." In "Note on the Supply of Opium" [Presented by Mr. J. H. Rivett-Carnac, C.I.E.] Appendix V. In *Minutes of Evidence taken before the Royal Commission on Opium between 18 November and 29 December 1893; with Appendices.* Volume II. [C–7397]. 319–30. The listed destinations are Bengal, NWP and Oudh, Central Provinces, Assam, Burma, and Punjab.

Table 8. Chests of Malwa Opium Weighed/Taxed at All Stations and Number of Chests Manufactured for Sale in British Territory and Native States *, **

Year	Total Malwa Opium at Indore (Central India Agency)— Chests	Total Malwa Opium at Ajmir (Rajputana Agency)— Chests	Total Malwa Opium at Ahmedabad (Bombay)— Chests	Total Malwa Opium at All Stations Per Season— Chests	Diverted or Weighed for Sale in British Territory & Native States—Chests
1883/84	40,275.00	186.250	882.5	41,343.75	2,865.75
1884/85	40.688.50	146.200	350.5	41,165.20	2,875.70
1885/86	40,516.50	.600	—	40,517.06	2,856.75
1886/87	42,299.00	—	209.5	42,508.50	2,837.00
1887/88	38,416.50	—	482.0	38,943.50	2,969.50
1888/89	31,936.25	14.000	281.5	32,231.75	3,077.25
1889/90	32,079.00	187.333	68.5	32,335.00	3,293.00
1890/91	31,617.00	387.500	115.5	32,120.00	3,291.50
1891/92	34,269.75	392.000	89.5	34,751.25	3,515.25
1892/93	30,152.00	430.000	79.0	30,661.00	3,348.00
Total Chests for Ten Years	321,602.19	1,743.883	2,558.5	366,577.01	30,929.70
Avg. Chests per Season	32,160.219	174.3883	255.85	36,657.701	3,092.97

* *Note:* Table 8 expresses all fractions of chests in the original document as decimal points. The original document has no rows entitled "Total Chests for 10 Years" and "Average per Season." The author calculated these entries.

** *Source:* These are data is found on page 347 of [GBO] Great Britain. Royal Commission on Opium [Finlay] 1894a. "Opium Produced or Consumed in India." [Presented by Mr. Finlay to the Government of India, Department of Finance and Commerce]. Appendix IX. In *Minutes of Evidence Taken Before the Royal Commission on Opium between 18 November and 29 December 1893; with Appendices.* Volume II. [C–7397]. 344–54. The Indore weighing station distributed Malwa opium to the Madras Presidency, Hyderabad Assigned Districts, and Mysore. Ahmedabad supplied Bombay and the Ajmir station sent some Malwa opium to Punjab province and periodically forwarded chests to the Ghazipur factory ([GBO] Great Britain. Royal Commission on Opium [Batten] 1894:I:Appendix I:135–36).

Table 9. Total Population Grouped by Provinces, with Average Yearly Consumption of Licit Opium Per Head*

Province	Population (1891)	Average Yearly Consumption of Licit Opium per Head, 1892/93 (grains)
Assam	5,433,199	141.4
Bengal	71,069,643**	15.0
Berar	2,897,491	91.0
Bombay	15,985,270	47.0
Sindh	2,871,774	44.0
Central Provinces	10,046,546	34.0
Madras	35,630,440	14.0
Northwest Provinces and Oudh	46,905,085	18.0
Punjab	20,860,913	42.0
Total Population of British India (1891)	211,700,361	***

* Adapted from Table I, page 178 of [GBO] Great Britain. Royal Commission on Opium. [Memorandum VIII]. 1895. "Tables Showing the Distribution by Districts, of the Opium Habit in British India." Memorandum VIII. In *Final Report of the Royal Commission on Opium. Part I.* The Report with Annexures. Volume VI. [C-7723]. 178–84.

** The entry for Bengal Province excludes people inhabiting the "hill tracts in North Lushai, Chittagong, and Angul" ([GBO] Great Britain. Royal Commission on Opium. [Memorandum VIII]. 1895:VI:178).

*** The total number of grains for the nine British Provinces is 446.4. The average consumption per Province (not per capita) is slightly more than 49.65 grains per year (the exact number is 49.655555556 grains). Excluding Assam statistic reduces the grand total 305 grains, an average of almost 33.9 grains per province (the exact figure is 33.888888889).

Table 10. Population and 'Fever' Mortality Statistics in Five British Provinces Compiled by Mr. S.E.J. Clarke, Secretary to the Bengal Chamber of Commerce, 4 December 1893 and Submitted to the Royal Commission on Opium

Province	1891 Population Appendix XXVII (p. 445)	Registered Mortality # of Deaths in Province	Registered Mortality % of Province Population	Mortality from "Fever" # of Deaths in Province	Mortality from "Fever" % of Total Register Mortality
Assam	5,634,258	150,156	2.66%	75,965	50.59%
Bengal	70,368,267	1,896,261	2.69%	1,333,395	70.31%
Central Provinces	9,516,146	287,395	3.02%	177,358	61.71%
Northwest Provinces/Oudh	43,722,745	1,460,732	3.34%	1,033,059	70.72%
Punjab	20,553,982	598,789	2.91%	442,254	73.85%
TOTAL:	149,795,398 [a]	4,393,333	2.93%	3,062,031	69.69%

Note: [a] The figure of 149,795,398 out of 287,223,431 total population in 1891 is based on Clarke's numbers for "British Territory" (221,172,952 people) and "Native Territory" (66,050,479 people). ([GBO] Great Britain. Royal Commission on Opium [Clarke] 1894:II:Appendix XXVII:447).

Table 11. Anarcotine and Bengal Excise Opium Requirements Using the Three Ratios for More than One Million Sufferers*

Column 2: Pounds of anarcotine needed for 1.5–4 million people.
Columns 3–5**: Crude opium requirements using the three ratios with each Bengal Excise (Abkari) chest containing 123.4257 lbs. of opium.

1 Number of "Malarial Fever" Sufferers in Five British Provinces	2 Their Anarcotine Requirement (pounds)	3 Garden's 116.9:1 Ratio (# of Bengal Excise chests req.)	4 Garden's 24:1 Ratio (# of Bengal Excise chests req.)	5 Robert's 16:1 Ratio (# of Bengal Excise chests req.)
1,500,000	8,421.10*	7,975.87	1,637.47	1,091.65
2,000,000	11,228.14	10,634.49	2,183.30	1,455.53
2,500,000	14,035.17*	13,293.11	2,729.12	1,819.42
3,000,000	16,842.21	15,951.74	3,274.95	2,183.30
3,500,000	19,649.24*	18,610.36	3,820.77	2,547.18
4,000,000	22,456.28	21,268.98	4,366.60	2,911.07

* *Note:* Each entry in column 2 is the amount of anarcotine required for the complete "cure" and "convalescence" of the number of victims listed in column 1. The anarcotine requirement for three numerical categories of sufferers has been rounded off to the nearest hundredth. The original totals (8421.105 for 1.5 million people; 14,035.175 for 2.5 million; and 19,649.245 for 3.5 million) were used to calculate the crude opium requirement in each of the three ratio columns.
** For data in columns 3–5 (Table 11) converted to pounds, see Appendix D: Anarcotine and Crude Opium Requirements (in pounds) using the Three Alkaloid Extraction Ratios for More than One Million Sufferers.

Table 12 [116.9:1 Ratio]: Quantity of Bengal Abkari (Excise) Opium Chests Required to Extract Sufficient Anarcotine for 'Cure' and 'Convalescence' of Four Groups of 'Malarial Fever' Sufferers. Entries Are Expressed as Percentage of Bengal Chests Prepared for Domestic Consumption During the Twenty-Year Period from 1873/74 to 1892/93.*

Opium to Anarcotine Extraction Ratio	Number of "Malarial Fever" Sufferers	# of Bengal Abkari Opium chests REQUIRED to Extract Sufficient Anarcotine for the Complete "Cure" and "Convalescence" of Patients Entered in Column 2 Using Extraction Ratio Cited in Column 1 (116.9:1)	Column 3 Entries Expessed as % of Avg. Annual Production of Bengal Abkari Chests (approx. 4,454.5 chests) Prepared for Domestic Consumption From 1873/74 Through 1892/93 and Comments
116.9:1	3,000,000	15,951.74	More than 358% greater than the Average Annual Abkari Production, from 1873/74 through 1892/93 for the 116.9:1 ratio and 3 million victims.
116.9:1	3,062,031 [Clarke & Roberts]	16,281.58	Approximately 365.5% greater than the Average Annual Abkari Production, from 1873/74 through 1892/93 for the 116.9:1 ratio and Clarke's 3,062,031 victims.
116.9:1	3,500,000	18,610.36	Approximately 418% greater than the Average Annual Abkari Production, from 1873/74 through 1892/93 for the 116.9:1 ratio and 3.5 million victims.
116.9:1	4,000,000	21,456.28	Approximately 482% greater than the Average Annual Abkari Production, from 1873/74 through 1892/93 for the 116.9:1 ratio and 4 million victims.

* *Data: Bengal Abkari Production Figures for Twenty-year Period (1873/74–1892/93):*
Average Annual Production = 4,454.5 chests (fraction more than)
Highest Single Season = 6,890.15 chests (1890/91)
Lowest Single Season = 2,914 chests (fraction less than) (1888/89)

Table 13 [24:1 Ratio]: Quantity of Bengal Abkari (Excise) Opium Chests Required to Extract Sufficient Anarcotine for 'Cure' and 'Convalescence' of Four Groups of 'Malarial Fever' Sufferers. Entries Are Expressed as Percentage of Bengal Chests Prepared for Domestic Consumption During the Twenty-Year Period from 1873/74 to 1892/93. *

Opium to Anarcotine Extraction Ratio	Number of "Malarial Fever" Sufferers	# of Bengal Abkari Opium chests REQUIRED to Extract Sufficient Anarcotine for the Complete "Cure" and "Convalescence" of Patients Entered in Column 2 Using Extraction Ratio Cited in Column 1 (24:1)	Column 3 Entries Expressed as % of Avg. Annual Production of Bengal Abkari Chests (approx. 4,454.5 chests) Prepared for Domestic Consumption From 1873/74 Through 1892/93 and Comments
24:1	3,000,000	3,274.95	Figure represents more than 73.5% (.7352) of the Average Annual Abkari Production, from 1873/74 through 1892/93 for the 24:1 ratio & 3 million victims
24:1	3,062,031 [Clarke & Roberts	3,342.67	Figure represents slightly more then 3/4 of the Average Annual Abkari Production, from 1873/74 through 1892/93. Calculation is .7504, a fraction more than 75% for the 24:1 ratio and 3.5 million victims.
24:1	3,500,000	3,820.77	Figure represents almost 86% of the Average Annual Abkari Production, from 1873/74 through 1892/92. Calculation is close to .8577 for the 24:1 ratio and 3.5 million victims.
24:1	4,000,000	4,366.60	Figure represents a fraction more than 98% of the Average Annual Abkari Production, from 1873/74 through 1892/93. Calculation is .9803 for the 24:1 ratio and 4 million victims.

* *Data: Bengal Abkari Production Figures for Twenty-year Period (1873/74–1892/93):*
Average Annual Production = 4,454.5 chests (fraction more than)
Highest Single Season = 6,890.15 chests (1890/91)
Lowest Single Season = 2,914 chests (fraction less than) (1888/89)

Table 14 [16:1 Ratio]: Quantity of Bengal Abkari (Excise) Opium Chests Required to Extract Sufficient Anarcotine for 'Cure' and 'Convalescence' of Four Groups of 'Malarial Fever' Sufferers. Entries Are Expressed as Percentage of Bengal Chests Prepared for Domestic Consumption During the Twenty-Year Period from 1873/74 to 1892/93. *

Opium to Anarcotine Extraction Ratio	Number of "Malarial Fever" Sufferers	# of Bengal Abkari Opium chests REQUIRED to Extract Sufficient Anarcotine for the Complete "Cure" and "Convalescence" of Patients Entered in Column 2 Using Extraction Ratio Cited in Column 1 (16:1)	Column 3 Entries Expressed as % of Avg. Annual Production of Bengal Abkari Chests (approx. 4,454.5 chests) Prepared for Domestic Consumption from 1873/74 through 1892/93 and Comments
16:1	3,000,000	2,183.30	Figure represents more than 49% (.4901) of the Average Annual Abkari Production, from 1873/74 through 1892/93 for the 16:1 ratio and 3 million victims.
16:1	3,062,031 [Clarke & Roberts	2,228.44	Figure represents slightly more than 50% (.5003) of the Average Annual Abkari Production, from 1873/74 through 1892/93 for the 16:1 ratio and Clarke's 3,062,031 victims.
16:1	3,500,000	2,547.18	The figure represents a fraction more than 57% (.5718) of the Average Annual Abkari Production, from 1873/74 through 1892/93 for the 16:1 ratio and 3.5 million victims.
16:1	4,000,000	2,911.07	The figure represents more than 65% (.6535) of the Average Annual Abkari Production, from 1873/74 through 1892/93 for the 16:1 ratio and 4 million victims.

* Data: Bengal Abkari Production Figures for Twenty-year Period (1873/74–1892/93):
  Average Annual Production = 4,454.5 chests (fraction more than)
  Highest Single Season = 6,890.15 chests (1890/91)
  Lowest Single Season = 2,914 chests (fraction less than) (1888/89)

Selected Bibliography

BOOKS/ARTICLES

Aitchison, Sir Charles Umpherston, compiler. [1862–1865] 1876, 1973. *A Collection of Treaties, Engagements, and Sunnuds, Relating to India and Neighbouring Countries.* n.p.: Savielle and Cranenburgh, Bengal Printing Co., Ltd. Reprint (1876). Foreign Office Press. Reprint (1973) Kraus Reprints of Nendeln, Lichenstein.

Albers, J. F. H. 1862. "Veber Narcotin und Aesculin und Ihre Anwendung in Krankenheit." *Deutsche Klinik (Berlin)*. 14:144–56.

Alcock, Sir Rutherford. 1881. "Opium and Common Sense." *Nineteenth-Century* 10: July–December: 854–68.

American Journal of Medical Science. 1839. "Preparation of Pure Narcotine." 25:248–49.

American Pharmaceutical Association. Proceedings of the American Pharmaceutical Association. 1892. "Quinine–Fluctuation of Price, 1823 Through 1891." 40:742.

———. 1896. "Papaveraceae." Proceedings of the American Pharmaceutical Association. 44:609–13.

Anglo-Oriental Society for the Suppression of the Opium Trade. 1875–76. *The Friend of China; the Organ of the Anglo-Oriental Society for the Suppression of the Opium Trade.*

Austin, Gregory A. 1978. *Perspectives on the History of Psychoactive Substance.* Rockville, Md.: National Institute on Drug Abuse.

Banerjee, Bijan G., and Ritula Jalota. 1988. *Folk Illness and Ethnomedicine.* New Delhi: Northern Book Centre.

Barbier, M. André. 1947. "L'extraction des opiacés: Vingt-cinq ans de pratique industrielle dans le traitement de l'opium." *Annales Pharmaceutiques Francaises.* 5:2:121–40.

Bass, C. C. 1915. "The Present Status of the Prevention of Malaria." *American Journal of Tropical Disease and Preventive Medicine.* 2:12:735–37.

———. 1915–1916. "A Method of Concentrating Malaria Plasmodia for Diagnostic and Other Purposes." *American Journal of Tropical Disease and Preventive Medicine* 15: July–June:298–303.

———. 1926. "The Influence of Malaria on the Progress of Civilization." *Southern Medical Journal* 19:12 (December):851–56.
Battley, Richard. 1823/24a. "On the Constituent Parts of Opium." *Lancet* 2:277–91.
———. 1823/24b. "Mr. Battley's Second Letter on the Components of Opium." *Lancet* 2:631–33.
Beattie, Hilary J. 1969. "Protestant Missions and Opium in China, 1858–1895." East Asian Research Center. *Harvard University Papers on China*. 22A (May):104–33.
Beckett, G. H., and C. R. Wright. 1875. "On Narcotine, Cotarnine, and Hydrocartonine." *Journal of the Chemical Society of London*. New Series. xiii:537–85.
Berridge, Virgina. 1977a. "Fenland Opium Eating in the Ninteenth Century." *British Journal of Addiction*. 275–84.
———. 1977b. "Our Own Opium: Cultivation of the Opium Poppy in Great Britain, 1740–1823." *British Journal of Addiction*. 90–4.
———. 1978. "Victorian Opium Eating: Responses to Opiate Use in Nineteenth Century England." *Victorian Studies* 21:437–61.
Berridge, Virginia, and Griffith Edwards. 1981. *Opium and the People; Opiate Use in Nineteenth-Century England*. New York & London: St. Martins Press.
Bhattacharya, Sabyasachi. 1971. *Financial Foundations of the British Raj. Men and Ideas in the Post-Mutiny Period of Reconstruction of Indian Public Finance, 1858–1872*. Simla: Indian Institute of Advanced Study.
Bickerman, Hylan A. 1962. "Clinical Pharmacology of Antitussive Agents." *Clinical Pharmacology and Therapeutics* 3:353–68.
Birdwood, Sir George. 1865. *Catalogue of the Vegetable Products of the Presidency of Bombay; including a List of the Drugs Sold in the Bazaars[sic] of Western India*. 2nd ed. Bombay: Education Society's Press.
———. 1881. "Letter to the Editor" *The Times* (London). December 26:1.
———. 1882a. "The Opium Question." *The Times* (London). Friday, January 20:3.
———. 1882b. "Two Letters Addressed to the Editor of the 'Times,' December 26, 1881, and January 20, 1882, Respectively, by Sir George Birdwood, C. S. I., M.D." Appendix 3. In *Truth About Opium, being a Refutation of the Fallacies of the Anti-opium Society and a Defence of the Indo-China Opium Trade*. Ed. William H. Brereton. 230–43. London: W. H. Allen.
Blyth, J. 1843–45. "On the Composition of Narcotine, and Action of Some of Its Products of Decomposition by the Action of Bichloride of Platinum." *Memoirs of the Chemical Society of London*. 2:33–39.
Booth, Martin. 1998. *Opium. A History*. New York: St. Martin's Press.
Boyd, Mark F. 1949. "Historical Review." In *Malariology*. Ed. Mark F. Boyd. 1:3–25. Philadelphia and London: W. B. Saunders.
Brecher, Edward. 1972. "Effects of Opium, Morphine, and Heroin on Addicts." In *Licit and Illicit Drugs*. Edited by E. M. Brecher. 21–32. Boston: Little, Brown & Co.
Brereton, William H., ed. 1882. *Truth about Opium; Being a Refutation of the Fallacies of the Anti-Opium Society and a Defence of the Indo-China Opium Trade*. 2nd ed. London: W. H. Allen.
Bridgeman, Elijah Coleman, and S. Wells Williams. [1831/32–51] 1968. *The Chinese Repository*. 20 Vols. Canton. Reprint. Klaus Reprints.
Brill, Henry. 1969. "Recurrent Patterns in the History of Drug Dependence." In *Drugs and Youth: Proceedings of the Rutgers Symposium on Drug Abuse*. (1st, 1968). Eds. J. R. Wittenborn, Henry Brill, and Jean Paul Smith. 8–25. Springfield, Ill.: Charles E. Thomas.

British and Foreign Medical Review. 1839. "Abstract." 8:263:839.* [*Abstract of 1838 article entitled: 'Quotidian of Nine Months' Duration Cured by Narcotine.' *Indian Journal of Medical and Physical Science*.]

British Medical Journal. 1899. "Obituary: Sir William Roberts." 1:August 29:1063–66.

Brough, J. C. 1868–69. "Note on Narcotine and Products of Its Decomposition." *The Pharmaceutical Journal and Transactions* 10:4:211–14.

Brown, G. H., comp. 1955. "Roberts, Sir William." In *Munk's Roll; Lives of the Fellows of the Royal College of Physicians of London, 1826–1925*. 14:146–47. London: The College.

Brown, J. B. 1973. "Politics of the Poppy: The Society for the Suppression of the Opium Trade, 1874–1916." *Journal of Contemporary History* 8:3 (July): 97–111.

Bryant, Robert J. 1988. "The Manufacture of Medicinal Alkaloids from the Opium Poppy—A Review of a Traditional Biotechnology." Paper presented at a Meeting of the Fine Chemicals Group of the SCI, held in Birmingham on 11 November 1987. *Fifth Society of Chemical Industry Process Development Symposium. Chemistry No. 5*, 7 March 1988. 146–53.

Buckland, Charles Edward (ed.) [1906] 1969a. "Sir George Birdwood." *Dictionary of Indian Biography*. 43. Reprint. New York: Greenwood Press.

———. [1906] 1969b. "Fanshawe, Sir Authur Upton." *Dictionary of Indian Biography*. 143. Reprint. New York: Greenwood Press.

———. [1906] 1969c. "Lyall, Sir James Broadwood." *Dictionary of National Biography*. 257. Reprint. New York: Greenwood Press.

———. [1906] 1969d. "Sir William James Moore." *Dictionary of Indian Biography*. 298. Reprint. New York: Greenwood Press.

Burnes, James. 1839. *A Narrative of a Visit to the Court of Sinde; a Sketch of the History of Cutch, from its first connexion [sic] with the British Government in India till the conclusion of the treaty of 1819; and some remarks on the medical topography of Bhooj*. Edinburgh: R. Cadell.

Burton, Antoinette. 1994. Burdens of History. *British Feminists, Indian Women, and Imperial Culture, 1865–1915*. Chapel Hill, N.C.: University of North Carolina Press.

Carlson, Eric T., and Meribeth M. Simpson. 1963. "Opium as a Tranquilizer." *American Journal of Psychiatry* 120: July–June: 112–17.

Chadhuri, Binod Bhushan. 1970. "Growth of Commercial Agriculture." Part II. *Indian Economic and Social History Review* 7:2 (June):211–51.

Chaudhuri, R. N. 1954. "Tropical Medicine—Past and Present." *British Medical Journal* 2: 423–29.

———. (ed.) 1971. *The Economic Development of India: Under the East India Company 1814–1858*. Cambridge: Cambridge University Press.

Chopra, Lieut.-Col. R. N. 1928. "The Present Position of the Opium Habit in India." *Indian Journal of Medical Research* 16:2 (October):389–440.

Chopra, Lieut.-Col. R. N., B. Mukherjee, and B. B. Dikshit. 1930. "Narcotine: Its Pharmacological Action and Therapeutic Uses." *Indian Journal of Medical Research* 18:1 (July):35–49.

Chopra, Ram Nath, and R. Knowles. 1930. "The Action of Opium and Narcotine in Malaria." *Indian Journal of Medical Research* 18:1 (July):5–13.

Clausen, John A. 1968. "Drug Addiction: Social Aspects." In *International Encyclopedia of the Social Sciences*. Ed. David L. Sills. 4:298–304. New York: Macmillan.

Collis, Maurice. 1947. *Foreign Mud: Being an Account of the Opium Imbroglio at Canton in the 1830's and the Anglo-Chinese War that Followed*. New York: Knopf, London: Faber & Faber.

Cooper, Nathaniel and Robert Hatcher. 1934. "A Contribution to the Pharmacology of Narcotine." *The Journal of Pharmacology & Experimental Therapeutics* 51:411–20.

Cousland, P. B. 1896. "Some Observations on the Opium Habit." *China Medical [Missionary] Journal* 10:1:19–23.

Crafts, Dr. and Mrs. Wilbur Fisk, and Mary and Margaret Leitch. 1911. *Intoxicating Drinks & Drugs in All Lands and Times, a Twentieth Century Survey of Temperance, Based on a Symposium of Testimony from 100 Missionaries and Travelers*. 11th rev. ed. Washington, D.C.: International Reform Bureau.

Crawford, A. C., and A. R. L. Dohme. 1902. "Contributions to the Pharmacology of Narcotine." *Proceedings of the American Pharmaceutical Association*. Baltimore, Maryland. 1:472–78.

Crawfurd, John. 1856. *A Descriptive Dictionary of the Indian Islands & Adjacent Countries*. London: Bradbury & Evans.

Crellin, J. K. 1968. "The Dawn of the Germ Theory: Particles, Infection, and Biology." In *Medicine and Science in the 1860s*. Ed. F. L. N. Poynter. 57–76. London: Wellcome Institute of the History of Medicine.

Day, Horace B. 1868. *The Opium Habit; with Suggestions as to the Remedy*. New York: Harper & Row.

deKorte, W. E. 1900. "Typhoid or Malarial Fever." *The Journal of Tropical Medicine* February:178–81.

DeQuincey, Thomas. 1822. *Confessions of an English Opium Eater*. London: Taylor & Hessey.

Dickens, Charles. 1870. *The Mystery of Edwin Drood*. London: Chapman & Hall.

Dictionary of National Biography: The Twentieth Century. With Index. 1927. "Brassey, Thomas." 62–3. London: Oxford University Press, & Humphrey Milford.

———. *Dictionary of National Biography. Twentieth Century 1912–1921*. 1938. "Birdwood, Sir George Christopher Molesworth." 46–7. London: Oxford & London.

Dott, D. B. 1876. "The Variation in Strength of the Opium Preparations." *The Pharmaceutical Journal and Transactions*. 3rd Series. 8: September 16:239–40.

Doyle, Arthur Conan. 1892. "The Man With the Twisted Lip." In *Adventures of Sherlock Holmes*. Story 6:126–52. New York: Harper Brothers.

Draper, Henry Napier. 1885. "The Opium and Morphine Dose of the Pharmacopoeia." *The Pharmaceutical Journal and Transactions* December 26:546–47.

Duncan, Andrew. 1899. "The Comparative Value of Certain Drugs in the Treatment of Malaria Fever." *The Journal of Tropical Medicine* October. 65–7.

Eatwell, W. C. B. 1851–52. "Selections from the Records of the Bengal Government on the System of Cultivating the Poppy and of Preparing Opium in the Benares Opium Agency; With a Brief Sketch of the Constitution of the Department." *The Pharmaceutical Journal and Transactions* 11:269–71, 306–11, 359–64.

———. 1852. "Observations on the Cultivation of the Poppy and the Manufacture of Opium in British India, More Especially of Benares, Taken Chiefly from a Report to the Bengal Government." *American Journal of Pharmacy* 24:118–33.

Edmonds, F. H. 1900. "Malaria and Pregnancy." *The Journal of Tropical Medicine* May: 259–60.

Eisenlohr, L. E. S. 1934. *International Narcotics Control*. London: George Allen & Unwin.

Empey, D. W.; L. A. Laitinen; G. A. Young, C. E. Bye, & D. T. D. Hughes. 1979. "Comparison of the Antitussive Effects of Codeine Phosphate 20 mg, Dextomethorpen 30 mg and Noscapine 30 mg using Citric Acid-Induced Cough in Normal Subjects." *European Journal of Clinical Pharmacology* 16:393–97.

Encyclopaedia Britannica. [1893] 1894. "Quinine." 20:184–86. Chicago: The Werner Company. Reprint. R. S. Pearce.

———. 1911. "Malaria." 11th ed. 17:461–65. Cambridge: Cambridge University Press.

———. 1911 "Opium." 11th ed. 20:130–37. Cambridge: Cambridge University Press.

Etkin, Nina L. 1979. "Indigenous Medicine Among the Hausa of Northern Nigeria: Laboratory Evaluation for Potential Therapeutic Efficacy of Antimalarial Plant Medicinals." *Medical Anthropology* 3:4:401–29.

Etkin, Nina L., and Paul J. Ross. 1983. "Malaria, Medicine, and Masks: Plant Use Among the Hausa and Its Impact on Disease." In *The Anthropology of Medicine: From Culture to Method.* Ed. Lola Romanucci-Ross, et al. 231–59. South Hadley, Mass.: Bergin & Garvey.

Fay, Peter Ward. 1976. *The Opium War, 1840–1842.* New York: W. W. Norton.

Farooqui, Amar. 1998. *Smuggling as Subversion: Colonialism, Indian Merchants and the Politics of Opium.* New Delhi: New Age International.

Fitzgerald, William J. 1968. "Evolution of Use of Quinine in Treatment of Malaria." *New York State Journal of Medicine* 68:6 (March 15):800–02.

Flückiger, Frederick A. 1875. "Examination of Some Specimens of Opium." *The Pharmaceutical Journal and Transactions* 5:April:845.

———. 1879. "Note on the Estimation of Morphine in Turkey Opium." *The Pharmaceutical Journal & Transactions* 10:254–55

———. 1884. *The Cinchona Barks.* London: Churchill.

Flückiger, Friedrich A., and Daniel Hanbury. 1879. *Pharmacographia. A History of the Principal Drugs of Vegetable Origin, Met with in Great Britain and British India.* 2nd ed. London: MacMillan & Co.

Foster, Arnold. 1896. "The Report of the Opium Commission." *China Medical [Missionary] Journal* 10:1:1–16.

Gage, Andrew Thomas. 1918. *Report on the Extension of Cinchona Cultivation in India.* Calcutta: Government Printing Office.

Garden, Dr. A. 1860. "Report on Anarcotine." *Indian Annals of Medical Science.* 7:400–18.

Gatehouse, D. G., G. Stemp, S. Pascoe, P. Wilcox, J. Hawker, & D. J. Tweats. 1991. "Investigations into the Induction of Aneuploidy and Polyploidy in Mammalian Cells by the Anti-Tussive Agent Noscapine Hydrochloride." *Mutagenesis* 6:4:279–83.

Giles, J. M. 1899. "A Description of the Culididæ Employed by Major R. Ross, I. M. S., in His Investigations on Malaria." *The Journal of Tropical Medicine* October: 62–5.

Gramiccia, Gabriele. 1988. *The Life of Charles Ledger (1818–1905). Alpacas and Quinine.* Hampshire & London: Macmillan Press.

———. 1987 "Notes on the Early History of Cinchona Plantations." *Acta Leidensia* 55:5–13.

Grant, Kevin. 2001. "Christian Critics of Empire: Missionaries, Lantern Lectures, and the Congo Reform Campaign in Britain." *The Journal of Imperialism and Commonwealth History* 29:2 (May):27–58.

Great Britain. Parliament [East India] [Statement–Opium]. 1891–92. "Opium." In *Statement Exhibiting the Moral and Material Progress and Condition of India and the Nine Preceding Years.* London: H. M. Stationery Office. 244–49.

Grier, J. 1937. *A History of Pharmacy.* London: Pharmaceutical Press.

Guiart, J. 1900. "The Recent Discoveries of Paludism." *The Journal of Tropical Medicine* July: 300–05.

Harrison, Gordon A. 1978. *Mosquitoes, Malaria & Man. A History of the Hostilities Since 1880.* New York: Dutton.

Harrison, Mark. 1994. *Public Health in India. Anglo-Indian Preventive Medicine. 1859–1914*. Cambridge & New York: Cambridge University Press.

Hastings, H. 1895. *Opium in Malwa*. Calcutta: Bengal Secretariat Press.

Haynes, Douglas. 2001. *Imperial Medicine. Patrick Manson and the Conquest of Tropical Disease*. Philadelphia: University of Pennsylvania.

Hayter, Aletha. 1968. *Opium and the Romantic Imagination*. Berkeley: University of California.

Hehir, Lieut.-Col. Patrick. 1913. *Hygiene and Disease in India, a Popular Handbook*. 3rd ed. Madras: Higginbothams.

———. Major-General Patrick. 1927. *Malaria in India*. London: Humphrey Milford and Oxford University.

Henry, T. A. 1929. "The Vegetable Alkaloids: Introduction." in *Allen's Commercial Organic Analysis*. 5th ed. Ed. C. Ainsworth Mitchell. 1–47. Philadelphia: P. Blakiston's & Co.

Hess, Albert G. 1965. *Chasing the Dragon. A Report on Drug Addiction in Hong Kong*. Amsterdam: North Holland.

Hodgson, Lieutenant-Colonel E. C., and A. C. Vardon. 1926–27. "A Preliminary Note on a Quick and Simple Test for the Differentiation of Malaria from Kala-Azar, Enteric and Other Fevers." *Indian Journal of Medical Research* 14:779–84.

Holmes, E. M. 1891. "The Opium Used in Medicine." *The Pharmaceutical Journal and Transactions* September 26:352–53.

Holmes, E. M. 1894. "Opium." *Encyclopaedia Britannica*. 9th ed. 17:787–95. New York: Henry G. Allen.

———. 1930. "Three Hundred Years of Cinchona. A Short Account of the Discovery and Application of Peruvian Bark Since its First European Use in 1630." *The Chemist and Druggist*. June 28:827–32.

Honig, Peter, and Frans Verdoran, eds. 1945. *Science and Scientists in the Netherlands Indies*. New York: Board for the Netherlands, Indies, Surinam, and Curaçao.

Howard, Bernard. 1931. *Some Notes on the Cinchona Industry*. London: Institute of Chemistry of Great Britain and Ireland.

Howard, John Eliot. 1869–76. *The Quinology of the East India Plantations*. London: L. Reeve & Co.

Hume, Jack. 1986. "Colonialism and Sanitary Medicine: The Development of Preventive Health Policy in the Punjab, 1860–1900." *Modern Asian Studies* 20: 703–24.

Idänpään-Heikkilä, J. E. 1968. "Studies on the Fate of 3H-Noscapine in Mice and Rats." *Annales Medicinae Experimentals et Biologiae Fenniae*. 46:201–16.

Impey, Dr. Elijah. 1848. *A Report on the Cultivation, Preparation and Adulteration of Malwa Opium. And Appendix*. Bombay Opium Department. Bombay: The Times Press.

India, Department of Finance and Commerce. 1891. "No. 14A.–Account of Opium Revenue, for the Year ended 31st March 1890." *Revenue Accounts of the Government of India for the Years 1889–90*. Calcutta: Government Printing Office. 30–31, 35.

India, Department of Revenue. 1900. "No. 3–Area (in acres) under Crop, and Specification of Crops, in each Province in British India and in Mysore." *Agricultural Statistics of India for the Years 1894–95 to 1898–99*. 15th Issue. Part I. British India. 102–04. Calcutta: Government Printing Office.

———. 1904. *Agricultural Statistics of India for the Years 1897–98 to 1901–02*. 18:xxviii. Calcutta: Government Printing Office.

———. 1910 "No. 3. Area (in acres) under Crops, and Specification of Crops, in each province in British India." *Agricultural Statistics of India for the Years 1904/5–1908/9*

to *1898–99*. 25th Issue. Part I. British India. 114–15, 120, 122. Calcutta: Government Printing Office.
India, Department of Revenue and Agriculture. 1898–1900. *Agricultural Statistics for the Years [1892/93 through 1898/99]*. Volume II: Native States. 13th, 14th, and 15th editions. Calcutta: Government Printing Office.
India, Finance and Commerce Department [Meyer]. 1900. *Memorandum on Excise Administration in India So Far as It Is Concerned with Opium*. Compiled by W. S. Meyer, Indian Civil Service. Simla: Government Central Printing Office.
———. [Meyer]. 1902. "Appendix: General Statistics of Excise Opium Revenue." *Memorandum on Excise Administration So Far as It Is Concerned With Opium*. Compiled by W. S. Meyer. Simla: Government Central Printing Office.
Indian Journal of Medical and Physical Science. 1838. "Quotidian of Nine Months' Duration Cured by Narcotine." Volume 3. New Series. 710–11.
Indian Medical Gazette. 1908. "Malaria and Empire Decay." 43:January:21–6.
Indian Medical Gazette. 1918. "The Quest for Quinine." 13:July:261–66.
Indian Medical Record. 1895. "The Consumption of Opium in India. A Critique of the Memorandum Presented by Sir William Roberts, M.D., F. R. S. as Medical Member of the Late Royal Commission on Opium, 1893–94." *Henry Morse Stephens Collection Pamphlets on India*. 3:1–51.
Inglis, Brian. 1975. *The Forbidden Game: A Social History of Drugs*. New York: Charles Scribner's Sons.
Jaffe, Jerome H., and William R. Martin. 1985. "Opioid Analgesics and Antagonists." In *The Pharmacological Basis of Therapeutics*. 7th ed. Ed. Alfred Goodman Gilman, Louis S. Goodman, Theodore W. Rall, and Ferid Murad. 491–531. New York: Collier.
Janes, E. H. 1862. "Anarcotine as an Antiperiodic." *American Medical Times, New York* 4: 149.
Jarcho, Saul. 1970. "A Cartographic and Literary History of the Word Malaria." *Journal of the History of Medicine* 25: 31–39.
———. 1980. "Discussion: Some Ancient and Medieval Statements about Fever [and] Evolution of the Concept of Certain Individual Fevers." In *Times, Places and Persons; Aspects of the History of Epidemiology*. Ed. Abraham M. Lilienfeld. 132–38. Baltimore: Johns Hopkins University Press.
Jetson, T. W. 1832/33. "Employment of Narcotine in Ague." *Lancet* (London) 1: 41.
Johnson, Bruce. 1975. "Righteousness Before Revenue: The Forgotten Moral Crusade Against the Indo-Chinese Opium Trade." *Journal of Drug Issues* 5:4 (Fall):304–26.
Johnston, James. 1854. *The Chemistry of Common Life*. New York: D. Appleton & Co.
Jones, William Henry S. 1909. *Malaria and Greek History*. Manchester: The University Press.
Journal of the American Medical Association. 1887. "Opium in Fevers." 8: March 5:265–66.
Journal of the Indian Medical Association. 1980. "Hundred Years of Malarial Research." 74:8 (April):156–57.
Karlsson, Mats O., Bengt Dahlström, & Anders Neil. 1988. "Characterization of High-Affinity Binding Sites for the Antitussive [3H] Noscapine in Guinea Pig Brain Tissue." *European Journal of Pharmacology* 145: 195–203.
Karlsson, M. O., B. Dahlström, S.-A. Ecknäa, & A. Tufvesson Alm. 1990. "Pharmacokinetics of Oral Noscapine." *European Journal of Clinical Pharmacology* 39:275–79.
Kasé, Y. 1968. "Evaluation of Antitussive Agents." In *Selected Pharmacological Testing Methods*. Volume 3. Ed. Alfred Burger. 363–419. New York: Marcel Dekkers.

Kennedy, Dane. 1990. "The Perils of the Midday Sun: Climatic Anxieties in the Colonial Tropics." In *Imperialism and the Modern World*. Ed. John M. MacKenzie. 118–40. Manchester and New York: Manchester University Press.

King, Sir George. 1876. *A Manual of Cinchona Cultivation in India*. Calcutta: Government Printing Office.

———. 1880. *A Manual of Cinchona Cultivation in India*. 2nd ed. Calcutta: Government Printing Office.

Kitchen, S. F. 1949. "Falciparum Malaria." In *Malariology*. Ed. Mark F. Boyd. 2:995–1016. Philadelphia and London: W. B. Saunders.

———. 1949. "Vivax Malaria." In *Malariology*. Ed. Mark F. Boyd. 2:1027–45. Philadelphia and London: W. B. Saunders.

Knab, Frederick. 1913. "The Species of Anopheles That Transmit Human Malaria." *American Journal of Tropical Disease and Preventive Medicine* 1:1(July):33–43.

Kramer, John C. 1977. "Heroin in the Treatment of Morphine Addiction." *Journal of Psychedelic Drugs* 9: 3:193–98.

Krueger, Hugo, Nathan B. Eddy, and Margaret Sumwalt. 1943. "Morphine." Part I, and "Other Alkaloids." Part II. In *The Pharmacology of the Opium Alkaloids*. Supplement no. 165. Public Health Reports. Washington, D.C.: U.S. Government Printing Office.

Kumar, Anil. 1998. *Medicine and the Raj. British Medical Policy in India 1835–1911*. Walnut Creek, Calif.: AltaMira Press.

———. 1995. *Science and the Raj. 1857–1905*. Delhi: Oxford University Press.

———. 1997. "Unequal Contenders, Uneven Ground: Medical Encounters in British India, 1820–1920." In *Western Medicine as Contested Knowledge*. Ed. Andrew Cunningham and Bridie Andrews. 172–90. Manchester: Manchester University Press.

Kuo, Pin-chia. 1935. *A Critical Study of the First Anglo-Chinese War, with Documents*. Shanghai: The Commercial Press, Ltd.

Kurland, Alfred A. 1978. *Psychiatric Aspects of Opiate Dependence*. West Palm Beach, Fla: CRC Press.

Lancet. 1839. "Abstract" 2:606* [*Of 1838 article entitled: 'Quotidian of Nine Months' Duration Cured by Narcotine.' *Indian Journal of Medical and Physical Science*.]

———. 1882. "The Opening of Parliament: The Opium Question." February 11:233–34.

Lancisi, Giovanni Maria. 1717. *De Noxiis Paludum Effluvis Eorumque Remedis (Noxious Emanations of Swamps and Their Cures.)* Libri duo. Auctore Jo: Maria Lancisio, Roma, Jo Mariae Salvioni.

Lasgna, Louis, Albert H. Owens, Jr., Bruce I. Shnider, & G. Lennard Gold. 1961. "Toxicity After Large Doses of Noscapine." *Cancer Chemotherapy Reports*. No. 15, December. 33–4.

LaWall, Charles H. 1927. *The Curious Lore of Drugs and Medicines. (Four Thousand Years of Pharmacy.)* Garden City, N.Y.: Garden City Publishing Company.

Leach, D. J. 1899. "The Life and Work of Sir William Roberts." *The Medical Chronicle*. 11:157–88.

Leake, Chauncey D. 1975. *An Historical Account of Pharmacology to the Twentieth Century*. Springfield, Ill.: Charles E. Thomas.

Lockhart, William. 1861. *The Medical Missionary in China. A Narrative of Twenty Years Experience*. 2nd ed. London: Hurst & Blackett.

Lodwick, Kathleen Lorraine. 1976. *Chinese, Missionary, and International Efforts to End the Use of Opium in China, 1840–1916*. Ph.D. Dissertation. Department of History, University of Arizona.

Lomax, Elizabeth. 1973. "The Uses and Abuses of Opiates in Nineteenth-Century England." *Bulletin of the History of Medicine* 47: 167–76.
Lowes, Peter D. 1966. *The Genesis of International Narcotics Control.* New York: Arno Press; Geneva: Droz.
Lyons, Albert S., and R. Joseph Petrucelli. 1978. *Medicine. An Illustrated History.* New York: Harry N. Abrams.
Macht, David I. 1915a. "Action of the Opium Alkaloids, Individually and in Combination with each Other, on the Respiration." *Journal of Pharmacological & Experimental Therapeutics* 7: 339–73.
———. 1915b. "The History of Opium and Some of Its Preparations and Alkaloids." *The Journal of the American Medical Association* 64:6 (February 6):477–81.
———. 1917a. "The Action of Opium and Some of Its Alkaloids on the Digestive Tract." *American Journal of Medical Science* 154: 874–83.
———. 1917b. "On the Comparative Effects of the Opium Alkaloids Individually and in Combination with Each Other on the Gall Bladder." *Journal of Pharmacological and Experimental Therapeutics* 9: 472–81.
Macht, David, and S. Issacs. 1917. "The Effect of Morphine and Opium on Psychological Reaction Time." *Journal of Pharmacological & Experimental Therapeutics* 9: 351–52.
Malcolm, Sir John. 1823. *India. A Memoir of Central India. Including Malwa and Adjoining Provinces With the History and Copious Illustrations of the Past and Present Condition of That Country.* Volume 1. London: Kingsbury, Parbury & Allen.
Marcovich, Anne. 1988. "French Colonial Medicine and Colonial Rule: Algeria and Indochina." In *Disease, Medicine and Empire: Perspectives on Western Medicine and the Experience of European Expansion.* Eds. Roy MacLeod and Milton Lewis. 103–08. New York and London: Routledge.
Markham, Sir Clements Robert. 1862. *Travels in Peru and India: While Superintending the Collection of Chinchona Plants and Seeds in South America, and their Introduction into India.* London: J. Murray.
———. 1880. *Peruvian Bark. A Popular Account of the Introduction of Ch[sic]inchona Cultivation Into British India[;] 1860–1880.* London: John Murray, Albermarle Street.
Martin, Robert Montgomery. 1847. *China; Political, Commercial, and Social; in an Official Report to Her Majesty's Government.* Volumes 1 & 2. London: Madden; [Volume 2: James Madden].
Matheson, Donald. 1856. *What Is the Opium Trade?* (bound with Robert Alexander, *The Rise and Progress of British Opium Smuggling*). Edinburgh: T. Constable.
Matthews, Leslie G. 1962. *History of Pharmacy in Britain.* Edinburgh and London: E. & S. Livingstone.
Matthiessen, A., and G. C. Foster. 1863/4, 1867, 1868, 1869, 1870. "Researches into the Chemical Constitution of Narcotine, and of Its Products of Decomposition." *Philosophical Transactions of the Royal Society of London.* 1863/64 (cliii:345); 1867; 1868 (clvii:687); 1869, 1870 (clix:66).
Maxwell, J. Preston. 1899. "Phagocytosis in Malarial Fever (Quartan)." *The Journal of Tropical Medicine* November: 90–91.
Miskel, James F. 1973. "Religion and Medicine: The Chinese Opium Problem." *Journal of the History of Medicine and Allied Sciences* 27: 3–14.
Mitchell, I. DeG. Mitchell, J. B. Carlton, M. Y. W. Chan, A. Robinson, & J. Sunderland. 1991. "Noscapine-Induced Polyploidy in Vitro." *Mutagenesis* 6: 6:479–86.

Mitchell, Sally, ed. 1988. "Opium." In *Victorian Britain. An Encyclopedia.* 559–60. New York & London: Garland.

Moore, Sir William James. 1870. "Famine and Fever in Rajputana." *Indian Medical Gazette.* n.p.

———. 1870. "On the Value of Quinine." *Indian Medical Gazette.* n.p.

———. 1874. "Diagnosis of Indian Fevers." *The Indian Annals of Medical Science.* n.p.

———. 1875. Annual Report. Superintendent-General of Dispensaries and Vaccination in Rajpootana. *Selection from the Records of the Government of India, Foreign Department No. 108, of 1875.* n. l.

———. 1876. "Malaria versus Recognisable Causes of Disease." *Indian Medical Gazette.* n.p.

———. 1878a. "Marwar—The Land of Death." *The Indian Annals of Medical Science* 20: 497–530.

———. 1878b. "Remarks on Remittent and Intermittent Fevers, and Their Complications." *The Indian Annals of Medical Science* 20: 1–95.

———. 1880. "The Opium Question." *Indian Medical Gazette* September 1: 225–30; October 1:257–64.

———. 1882a. "Is the Habitual Use of Opium in Moderation Injurious?" *Transactions of the Bombay Medical Society.* Bombay: Bombay Medical Society. n.p.

———. 1882b. *The Other Side of the Opium Question. Article 1.* London: J. A. Churchill.

———. 1886a. "A Letter to the Editor of the Times of India, Being a Reply to a Critique on 'The Other Side of the Opium Question'." *The Times of India.* (Bombay).

———. 1886b. *A Manual of the Disease of India; with a Compendium of Disease Generally.* 2nd ed. London: J. & A. Churchill.

———. 1892a. "The Errors of Anti-Opiumists." *The Provincial Medical Journal* (Leicester) 11: February:58–63.

———. 1892b. "Malaria and Its Remedies." *The Provincial Medical Journal* (Leicester) 11: 638–40.

———. 1892c. "Opium: Its Use and Abuse." *Medical Reporter* 1 (December 1): 224–29.

———. 1893. "Opium as a Preventive of Ague." *British Medical Journal* 2 (December 2): 1196.

———. 1894a. "Opium." *Medical Reporter* 3: 89–95.

———. 1894b. "Opium." *The Provincial Medical Journal* (Leicester) 13: 15–21.

———. 1895. "The Adulteration of Opium." *The Provincial Medical Journal* (Leicester) 14:9.

———. 18?. "Masked Malarial Fever." *The Indian Annals of Medical Science.* n.p.

———. 18?. "On Fever." *The Indian Annals of Medical Science.* 21:n.p.

Moorhead, Helen Howell, and Harold Tobin. 1933. "Opium Problem." In *Encyclopaedia of the Social Sciences.* Ed. Edwin R. A. Seligman. 11:471–76. New York: MacMillan.

Mouat, Dr. F. J. 1892. "The Ethics of Opium and Alcohol." *Lancet* April 30: 959–61.

Mourey, Robert J., Ted M. Dawson, Roxanne K. Barrow, Anne E. Enna, & Solomoon H. Snyder. 1992. "[3H] Noscapine Binding Sites in Brain: Relationship to Indoleamines and the Phosphoinositide and Adenylyl Cyclase Messenger Systems." *Molecular Pharmacology* 42: 619–26.

Muirhead, William. 1870. *China and the Gospel.* London: J. Nisbet.

Muraleedharan, V. R. 1991. "Malady in Madras: The Colonial Government's Response to Malaria in the Early Twentieth Century." In *Science and Empire. Essays in the Indian Context (1700–1947).* Ed. Deepak Kumar. 101–112. Delhi: Anamika Prakashan.

Musto, David F. 1973. *The American Disease. Origins of Narcotic Control.* New Haven & London: Yale University Press.

MacCulloch, John. 1830. *An Essay on the Remittent and Intemittent Diseases, Including Generically, Marsh Fever and Neuralgia. Comprising Under the Former, Various Anomolies, Obscurities, and Consequences, and Under a New Systematic View of the Later, Treating of Tic Douloureux, Sciatica, Headach[e], Ophthalmia, Toothach[e] Palsy, and Many Other Modes and Consequences of This Generic Disease.* Philadelphia: Carey & Lea.

MacGowan, D. J. 1859. "Note on Chinese Opium." *Transactions of the China Branch of the Royal Asiatic Society.* 6:41–7.

MacGregor, Sir William. 1900. "An Address on Some Problems of Tropical Medicine." *Journal of Tropical Medicine* October: 63–71.

MacKenzie, John M. 1990. "Introduction." In *Imperialism and the Natural World.* Ed. John M. MacKenzie. 1–14. Manchester: Manchester University Press.

Nayak, K. P., E. Broachmann-Hanssen, & E. Leongway. 1965. "Biological Disposition of Noscapine. 1. Kinetics of Metabolism, Urinary Excretikon, and Organ Distribution." *Journal of Pharmaceutical Science* 54: 191–94.

Newman, R. K. 1989. "India & the Anglo-Chinese Opium Agreements, 1907–14." *Modern Asian Studies* 23:3 (July): 525–60.

Nuttall, George. 1900. "Upon the Part Played by Mosquitoes in the Propagation of Historical and Critical Study." *The Journal of Tropical Medicine* 2:March: 198–200; 2:April: 231–33; 2:May: 245–47; 2:June: 275–77; 2:July: 302–07; 3:August: 11–13.

O'Brien, Robert, and Sidney Cohen. 1984. *The Encyclopedia of Drug Abuse.* New York: Facts on File.

O'Shaughnessy, W. B. 1838. "On Narcotine as a Substitute for Quinine in Intermittent Fevers." *American Journal of Medical Science* 25:194–95.

Otte, J. A. 1896. "The Influence of the Opium Habit on Malarial Infection." *China Medical [Missionary] Journal* 22:4 (July):225–29.

Owen, David Edward. [1934] 1968. *British Opium Policy in China and India.* New Haven, Conn.: Yale University Press. Reprint. Archon Books.

Parssinen, Terry M. 1983. *Secret Passions, Secret Remedies. Narcotic Drugs in British Society 1820–1930.* Philadelphia: Institute for the Study of Human Issues.

Paton, William. 1924. *Opium in India.* Calcutta: National Christian Council of India, Burma, and Ceylon.

Pawetczyk, Ewaryst, Mario Zajac, & Barbara Matlak. 1976. "Kinetics of Autoxidation of Narcotine in Aqueous Solutions." *Polish Journal of Pharmacology and Pharmacy* 28: 69–76.

Peters, Dolores. 1981. "The British Medical Response to Opiate Addiction in the Nineteenth Century." *The Journal of the History of Medicine and Allied Sciences* 36: 455–88.

Plehn, Albert. 1899. "On Tropical Anæmia, and Its Relations to the Latent and to the Manifest Forms of Malarial Infection." *The Journal of Tropical Medicine* October: 72–4; December: 121–23; January: 141–45.

Publications and Information Directorate. 1966. *"Papaver Linn." The Wealth of India. A Dictionary of Indian Raw Materials and Industrial Products.* VII:N–Pe:231–48. New Delhi: Publications and Information Directorate.

Puri, I. M. 1949. "Anophelines of the Oriental Region." In *Malariology.* Ed. Mark F. Boyd. 483–505. Philadelphia and London: W. B. Saunders.

Reins, Thomas D. 1991. "Reform, Nationalism and Internationalism: The Opium Suppression Movement in China and the Anglo-American Influence, 1900–1908." *Modern Asian Studies* 25:1: 101–42.

Richards, J. F. 1981. "The Indian Empire and Peasant Production of Opium in the Nineteenth Century." *Modern Asian Studies* 15:1: 59–82.

Richmond, Phyllis A. 1980. "The Germ Theory of Disease." In *Times, Places, and Persons; Aspects of the History of Epidemiology*. Ed. Abraham M. Lilienfeld. 84–93. Baltimore: The Johns Hopkins University Press.

Roberts, Sir William. 1865. *A Practical Treatise on Urinary and Renal Disease, including Urinary Deposits*. London: Walton & Maberly.

———. 1877. "The Doctrine of Contagium Vivum and Its Appplication to Medicine." *British Medical Journal* 77 (August 11):168–73.

———. 1885a. "On Feeding the Sick." Address in Therapeutics Delivered Before the British Medical Association at Cardiff, 1885. *British Medical Journal* 2: 188–92.

———. 1885b. *Lectures on Dietetics and Dyspepsia, delivered at the Owens College School of Medicine in February and March, 1885*. London: Smith, Elder. [1886. 2nd ed. London: Smith, Elder.]

———. 1890. "On Some Points in Dietetics." Address Delivered at the Opening of the Current Session of the Manchester Medical Society, Manchester, England. *British Medical Journal* 2: 883–85.

———. 1891. *Collected Contributions on Digestion and Diet*. London: Smith, Elder. [1897. 2nd ed.]

———. 1895. "On Anarcotine, a Neglected Alkaloid of Opium." Address Delivered at the Opening of the Section of Pharmacology and Therapeutics at the Annual Meeting of the British Medical Association at London, 1895. *British Medical Journal* 2: 405–06.

Rowntree, Joshua. 1895. *The Opium Habit in the East: A Study of the Evidence Given to the Royal Commission on Opium*. Westminster: P. S. King & Son; Scarborough: E. T. W. Dennis, The Westboro Press; London: Society for the Suppression of the Opium Trade.

Russell, Paul Farr. 1943. "Malaria and Its Influence on World Health." *Bulletin of the New York Academy of Medicine* 19:9 (September): 599–630.

Schlittler, Emil, 1950. "Isoquinoline Alkaloids." In *Thorpe's Dictionary of Applied Chemistry*. 4th ed. Ed. Jocelyn Field Thorpe. 4:359–66. London: Longmans, Green & Co., Ltd.

Science News. 1998. "Stopping Coughs . . . and Cancer?" March 14:168.

Scott, Henry Harold. 1939. *A History of Tropical Medicine: Based on the Fitzpatrick Lectures Delivered Before the Royal College of Physicians of London, 1937–38*. Baltimore: Williams and Wilkins.

Scott, James Maurice. 1969. *The White Poppy: A History of Opium*. London: Heineman.

Scott, John. 1877. *Manual of Opium Husbandry, for the Use of Officers in the Government Agencies of Behar and Benares*. Calcutta: Bengal Secretaries Press.

Sewall, J. G. 1870. "Opium Eating and Hypodermic Injection." *The Medical Record* 4:May: 137.

Shaw, George Elliott. 1935. *Quinine Manufacture in India*. Seventeenth Streatfield Memorial Lecture, 1934. n.p. The Institute of Chemistry of Great Britain and Ireland.

Sim, Stephen. 1965. "Alkaloids of the Isoquinoline Group." *Medicinal Plant Alkaloids. An Introduction for Pharmacy Students*. 2nd ed. Toronto: University of Toronto Press. 54–65.

Sonnedecker, Glenn. 1963. *Emergence of the Concept of Opiate Addiction*. Madison, Wis.: American Institute of the History of Pharmacy.
Spangenberg, Bradford. 1976. *British Bureaucracy in India*. Columbia, Mo.: South Asia Books.
Squibb, Edward R. 1860. "Opium as a Therapeutic Agent." *American Journal of Pharmacy* 32: 115–20.
Stelle, Charles Clarkson. 1981. *Americans and the China Opium Trade in the Nineteenth Century*. New York: Arno Press.
Stenton, M., and S. Lees, eds. 1978a. "Mowbray, Sir Robert Gray Cornish." *Who's Who of British Members of Parliament* 2 (1886–1918): 260. Sussex, England: Harvester Press.
———. 1978b. "Wilson, Henry Joseph." *Who's Who of British Members of Parliament* 2 (1886–1918): 377. Sussex, England: Harvester Press.
Stephen, Sir Leslie, and Sir Sidney Lee, eds. 1921–22. "Roberts, Sir William." *Dictionary of National Biography* 22–Supplement: 1171–72. London: Oxford University Press; London: Humphrey Milford.
Sternberg, George Miller. 1884. *Malaria and Malarial Diseases*. New York: Wood.
SG. Surgeon-General (U.S.) 1880. "Narcotine." In *The Index-Catalogue of the Library of the Surg'n-General's[Sic] Office U.S. Army*. Volume I. "A-Berlinsky". 1st Series. 297.
———. 1888. "Narcotine." In *The Index-Catalogue of the Library of the Surg'n-General's [Sic] Office U.S. Army*. Volume IX. "Medicine (Popular)–NY Welt." 1st Series. 631.
———. 1896. "Narcotine." In *The Index-Catalogue of the Library of the Surg'n-General's [Sic] Office U.S. Army*. Volume I. 365.
———. 1907. "Narcotine." In *The Index-Catalogue of the Library of the Surg'n-General's [Sic] Office U.S. Army*. Volume XI "Mo-Nyström." 2nd Series. 327.
Surveyor, Nusserwanji. 1896. "Report on Anarcotine." *British Medical Journal* 2:September 26: 839.
Talbott, John H. 1970. *A Biographical History of Medicine. Excerpts and Essays on the Men and Their Work*. New York and London: Grune and Stratton.
Taylor, Frank O. 1929. "Opium Alkaloids." In *Allen's Commercial Organic Analysis*. 5th ed. Edited by C. Ainsworth Mitchell. 7:655–758. Philadelphia: P. Blakiston's & Co.
Terry, Charles E. 1931. "Drug Addiction." In *Encyclopaedia of the Social Sciences*. Edited by Erwin R. A. Seligman. 5:242–52. New York: Macmillan.
Terry, Charles E., and Mildred Pillens. 1928. *The Opium Problem*. New York: Committee on Drug Addictions [and] Bureau of Social Hygiene.
Thayer, William Sydney. 1897. *Lecture on the Malarial Fevers*. New York: Appleton & Co.
Thin, George. 1899. "The Etiology of Malarial Fever." *The Journal of Tropical Health* August: 1–6.
Thompson, Edward E., and G. T. Garratt. [1935] 1966. *Rise and Fulfillment of British Rule in India*. London: Macmillan. Reprint. Allahabad: Central Book Depot.
Thorne, Susan. 1999. *Congregational Missions and the Making of an Imperial Culture in Nineteenth-Century England*. Stanford: Stanford University Press.
Thorpe, Jocelyn Fried. 1950. "Quinoline." and "Isoquinoline Alkaloids." In *Thorpe's Dictionary of Applied Chemistry*. 4th ed. Ed. Jocelyn Field Thorpe. 10: Plagioclase–Sodium: 347–66. London: Longmans, Green & Co., Ltd.
Tinling, J. F. B. 1870. *The Poppy Plague and England's Crime*. London: Elliot Stock.
Tod, Lieutenant-Colonel James. [1829, 1832, 1914] 1971. *Annals and Antiquities of Rajast'han or the Central and Western Rajpoot States of India*. 2 vols. London: Kegan & Paul. Reprint. Delhi: K. M. N. Publishers.

Tsunoda, N, & H. Yoshimura. 1979. "Metabolic Fate of Noscapine. II. Isolation and Identification of Novel Metabolites Produced by C-C Bond (Leverage)." *Xenobiotica* 9:3:181–82.

Tully, William. 1832. "Results of Experiments and Observations on Narcotine." *Boston Medical and Surgical Journal* 7: No. 1 (Wednesday, August 15):1–12, No. 3, (Wednesday, August 29): 37–44, No. 4 (Wednesday, September 6):56–63.

———. 1833. "Experiments for the Purpose of Determining the Operation of Narcotine Upon the Human System, in a State of Health." *Boston Medical & Scientific Journal* VII: 37, 56.

Turner, F. Storrs. 1876. *British Opium Policy and its Results to India and China*. London: Simpson Low, Marston, Searle & Rivington.

University of Chicago Press. 1982. *The Chicago Manual of Style. Thirteen Edition, Revised and Expanded. For Authors, Editors, and Copywriters*. Chicago and London: The University of Chicago Press.

V. W. B. 1927. "Brassey, Thomas." In *The Dictionary of National Biography: The Twentieth Century. With Index*. Ed. Sir Leslie Stephen, and Sir Sidney Lee. 62–3. Oxford University Press/London: Humphrey Milford.

Vedsö, Sven. 1961a. "Absorption and Excretion of Noscapine." *Acta Pharmacologica et Toxicologica* 18: 157–64.

———. 1961b. "The Determination of Noscapine (Narcotine) in Plasma and Urine." *Acta Pharmacologica et Toxicologica* 18: 119–28.

Wade, Ainley (editor). 1977. "Noscapine." In *Martindale. The Extra Pharmacopoeia*. Incorporating Squire's Companion. 27th ed. London: The Pharmacological Press. 1249–50.

Warshaw, Leon. 1947. *Malaria, the Biography of a Killer*. New York: Rinehart.

Watt, Sir George. [1908] 1966. *The Commercial Products of India. Being an Abridgement of 'The Dictionary of the Economic Products of India.'* London: J. Murray. Reprint. New Delhi: Today & Tomorrow Printers.

Watt, Sir George. [1908] 1966a. "Cinchona." In *The Commercial Products of India. Being an Abridgement of 'The Dictionary of Economic Products of India.'* 302–10. London: J. Murray. Reprint. Delhi: Today & Tomorrow Printers.

———. [1908] 1966b. "Papaver and Opium." In *The Commercial Products of India. Being an Abridgement of 'The Dictionary of Economic Products of India.'* 845–61. London: J. Murray. Reprint. New Delhi: Today & Tomorrow Printers.

Watt, Henry E., and R. G. Johnson. 1949. "Opium." In *Thorpe's Dictionary of Applied Chemistry*. 4th ed. Ed. Jocelyn Field Thorpe. 9 (Oils, fatty-Pi.):98–116. London: Longmans, Green, and Company, Ltd.

Webster's New Intercollegiate Dictionary. 1975. Springfield, MA.: G. & C. Merriam Company.

Weil, Andrew, and Winifred Rosen. 1983. "Narcotics." In *Chocolate to Morphine. Understanding Mind-Active Drugs*. Boston: Houghton Mifflin. 80–92.

Wilde, Oscar. 1890. *The Picture of Dorian Gray*. New York: J. H. Sears.

Willoughby, Westel W. 1925. *Opium as an International Problem; the Geneva Conferences*. Baltimore: Johns Hopkins University Press.

Wilson, A. (T. J. Mirchandani [joint author]). 1940. *Report on the Prospects of Cinchona Cultivation in India*. Imperial Council of Agricultural Research. Miscellaneous Bulletin No. 29. 2nd ed. Delhi: Manager of Publications.

Wilson, H. H. [1855] 1968. *A Glossary of Judicial and Revenue Terms, and of Useful Words Occurring in Official Documents Relating to the Administration of the Government of India.* W. H. Allen: London. Reprint. 2nd ed. Delhi: Munshilal Manoharlal.

Winchester, A. M., and Thomas R. Mertens. 1983 *Human Genetics.* 4th ed. Columbus, Ohio: Charles E. Merrill.

Winter, Charles A. & Lars Flataker. 1954. "Antitussive Compounds: Testing Method and Results." *The Journal of Pharmacology and Experimental Therapeutics* 112: 99–108.

Winther, Paul C. 1988. "British Policy in the Period of Incomplete Monopoly: The Pre-1848 India-China Opium Trade." *Annals of the 27th Annual Meeting of the Southeast Conference, Association for Asian Studies.* 114–30. 14–16 January. Charlotte, N.C.: University of North Carolina, Charlotte.

———. 1989. "Physiology, Alkaloids and the Indian Empire: British Conceptualization of Opium Eating and Malaria Eradication from 1776 to 1907." Paper presented to the panel *Misery in Service to the Empire: British Response to Disease in Colonial India and Malaya.* 41st Annual Meeting of the Association for Asian Studies, March 1989. Washington, D.C.

———. 1990. "To Adulterate or Not to Adulterate. That is the Question: Models of the Mysterious Powers of Opium and the China-India Drug Trade, 1750–1910." Paper presented at the *Third International Congress on Traditional Asian Medicine,* 4–7 January, Bombay, India.

Woodland, John. 1882–23. "Report on the Strength of Commercial Samples of Tincture and Liquid Extract of Opium." *The Pharmaceutical Journal and Transactions* September 30: 275–76.

Wootton, A. C. [1910] 1972. *Chronicles of Pharmacy.* 2 vols. London: MacMillan. Reprint. Tuckahoe, N.Y.: U.S. Pharmaceutical Corporation.

Worboys, Michael. 1989. "British Colonial Medicine and Tropical Imperialism: A Comparative Perspective." In *Dutch Medicine in the Malay Archipelago 1816–1942.* Articles Presented as a Symposium Held in Honour of Prof. D. de Moulin. 30 September 1989. Eds. G. M. van Heteren, A. de Knecht-van Ekelen, and M. J. D. Poulissen, 153–67. Amsterdam and Atlanta: Rodopi.

———. 1990. "The Imperial Institute: The State and the Development of the Natural Resources of the Colonial Empire, 1887–1923." In *Imperialism and the Natural World.* Eds. John M. MacKenzie. 164–86. Manchester: Manchester University Press.

Wormley, T. G. 1859–60, 1860. "Notes on Some of the Chemical Reactions of Narcotine and Meconic Acid." *Ohio Medical & Surgical Journal.* 1859/60:xii:277–85. Also in *Chemical News* (London). 1860:ii:158, 170.

Wright, C. R. Alder. 1876. "New Derivatives from the Opium Alkaloids." *The Pharmaceutical Journal and Transactions* 7:245–46.

Who Was Who, 1897–1915. 1935. "Wilson, Henry Joseph (M.P.)." 1:771. London: Adam & Charles Black.

Who Was Who, 1916–1928. 1929a. "Brassey, Sir Thomas Allnutt." 2:120–21. London: Adam & Charles Black.

———. 1929b. "Lyall, Sir James Broadwood." 2:63. London: Adams & Charles Black.

Ye, Keqiang, Yong Ke, Nagalaksmi Keshava, John Shanks, Judith A. Knapp, Rajeswar R. Tekmal, John Petros, & Harish C. Joshi. 1998. "Opium Alkaloid Noscapine Is an Antitumor Agent That Arrests Metaphase and Induces Apoptosis in Dividing Cells." *Proceedings of the National Academy of Science [Cell Biology]* 95: 1601–06.

Parliamentary Papers

Items from the *Royal Commission on Opium* [GBO] are entered according to volume. Entries within one volume are listed alphabetically by the bracketed name (or title of document). For example, in Volume I, [Batten] is cited before [Griffin] although [Griffin] is located earlier in the volume. Other sections in the Select Bibliography for Parliamentary Papers use the same format. The sections are *Reports of Standing and Select Committees* [GBR], and the *Irish University Press Series of British Parliamentary Papers* [IUP/PP].

Material from the British Parliament's *Command Papers* [GBC], and its "ordinary" *Session Papers* [GBS] is entered by year, and alphabetically (name or document title between brackets) within one year.

Some sources in the *Royal Commission on Opium* [GBO] volumes are difficult to find. The following citation style helps to locate them in the voluminous literature.

Material that G. M. Gregory sent to the Royal Commission describes the experience of W. J. Palmer, and associates such as T. W. Sheppard, with alkaloid extraction problems and manufacturing at Ghazipur during 1858–1860 and subsequent years. The Palmer and Sheppard documents (including one table compiled by Gregory) are in [GBO] Great Britain. Royal Commission on Opium. 1894. "Correspondence No. 291C–787, Regarding the use of Narcotine as a Febrifuge." Appendix III. Proceedings. In *Appendices Together with Correspondence on the Subject of Opium with the Straits Settlements and China, etc*. Volume V. [C-7473]. 76-83. A Palmer, Sheppard, etc. document *within* Appendix III of Volume V is identified by the name Gregory followed by an enclosure number, both within brackets. The enclosure number is the specific Palmer, Sheppard, etc. document.

Documents in the Gregory material (Appendix III) are listed in the [GBO] Select Bibliography according to their actual location in volume V. This means that enclosure 169 appears before enclosure 2.

And an example of the format in all chapters for citing a document submitted by Gregory (Appendix III) is: (GBO [Gregory–Enclosure 169] 1894:V:68).

GREAT BRITAIN. ROYAL COMMISSION ON OPIUM

GBO. Great Britain. Royal Commission on Opium. 1894. *First Report of the Royal Commission on Opium; with Minutes of Evidence and Appendices*. Volume I. [C-7313]. London: Printed for Her Majesty's Stationery Office. By Eyre and Spottiswoode.

Volume I

———. Royal Commission on Opium [Anti-Opium Society]. 1894. "Memorial presented by the Anti-Opium Society in November 1892." Appendix III. 162–65.

———. Royal Commission on Opium [Batten]. 1894. "The Opium Question. Paper read by Mr. G. M. H. Batten before 'The Society of Arts,' on the 24th March 1891." Appendix I. 133–46.
———. Royal Commission on Opium [Court of St. James/Lord Kimberley]. 1894. "Royal Commission on Opium. Court of Saint James, September 2, 1893." v(a3)–vi.
———. Royal Commission on Opium [Edkins]. 1894. "Historical Notes on Opium and the Poppy in China." [by Dr. Edkins]. Appendix II. 146–61.
———. Royal Commission on Opium [Griffin]. 1894. "Testimony of Sir Lepel Griffin, 15 September 1893." 105–09.
GBO. Great Britain. Royal Commission on Opium. 1894. *Minutes of Evidence taken before the Royal Commission on Opium between 18 November and 29 December 1893; with Appendices*. Volume II, Parts 1 & 2. [C–7397]. London: Printed for Her Majesty's Stationery Office. By Eyre and Spottiswoode.

Volume II

GBO. ———. Royal Commission on Opium [Appendices I–L]. 1894. "Appendices I–L." iv (Names of appendices that appear in II:Part 2:313–664).
———. Royal Commission on Opium [British Indian Association]. 1894. "The Humble Memorial of the British Indian Association; Dated 23rd August 1893; submitted by Narendra Krishna and Raj Kumar Sarvahikaril." Appendix I. Part 1. 313.
———. Royal Commission on Opium [Brown]. 1894. "Memorandum by the Chairman of the Calcutta Missionary Conference on Mr. Lyall's Note on the Memorial of the Calcutta Missionary Conference." Appendix IV. Part 1. 318–19.
———. Royal Commission on Opium [Calcutta Medical Society]. 1894. "The Effects of the Habitual Use of Opium on the Human Constitution. Supplement to the 'Medical Gazette' for August 1892." Submitted by the Calcutta Medical Society. Appendix XXI. Part 2. 407–25.
———. Royal Commission on Opium [Calcutta Missionary Association]. 1894. "The Memorial of the Calcutta Missionary Conference; Dated 21st September 1893." Appendix II. Part 1. 314–15.
———. Royal Commission on Opium [Clarke]. 1894. "No. 1236–'93, dated the 4th December 1893. *From*:: S. E. J. Clarke, Esq., Secretary, Bengal Chamber of Commerce. *To*: The Hon'ble H. J. S. Cotton, C.S.I., C.S., Chief Secretary to the Government of Bengal." Appendix XXVII. [received from the Secretary to the Government of Bengal]. Part 2. 439–52.
———. Royal Commission on Opium [Cobb]. 1894. "Testimony of Surgeon-Major D. Cobb." Part 1. 84–85.
———. Royal Commission on Opium [Edwards]. 1894. "'Opium Eating,' by the late Dr. Vincent Edwards [Extracted from the Indian Medical Gazette of 1 August 1877]." Appendix XXIV. Part 2. 436–37.
———. Royal Commission on Opium [Finlay]. 1894a. "Opium Produced or Consumed in India." [Presented by Mr. Finlay to the Government of India, Department of Finance and Commerce]. Appendix IX. Part 2. 344–54.
———. Royal Commission on Opium [Finlay]. 1894b. "Text of Agreements Between the British Government and Native States Under the Central India Agency." [Appendix B.] 359. [AND] "Text of Agreements Between the British Government and Native States Under the Rajputana Agency." [Appendix C.] 359. In Arrangements with Native States Regarding Opium. Appendix X. Part 2. 354–70.

———. Royal Commission of Opium [Fryer]. 1894. "Memorandum on the Smuggling of Opium into Burma. [Handed in by Mr. Fryer, Chief Commissioner of Burma, at Rangoon]." Appendix XLI. Part 2. 500–07.

———. Royal Commission on Opium [Lyall]. 1894. "Note on the Memorial Submitted by the Missionary Conference to His Excellency the Viceroy in Council regarding Opium, dated 21st September." Appendix III. Part 1. 315–18.

———. Royal Commission on Opium [Phillips]. 1894. "W. D. Phillips; Before the Royal Commision on Opium. Thursday, November 30th, 1893." Part 1. 319.

———. Royal Commission on Opium [Rice]. 1894. "Testimony of Surgeon Major-General Rice." Part 1. 11–15.

———. Royal Commission on Opium [Rivett-Carnac]. 1894. "Note on the Supply of Opium" [Presented by Mr. J. H. Rivett-Carnac, C.I.E.]. Appendix V. Part 1. 319–335.

———. Royal Commission on Opium [Spence]. 1894. "No. 13 (Confidential), dated 11th April 1882. *From*: W.D. Spence, Esq., Her Britannic Majesty's Acting Consul, Ichang, *To*: The Assistant Secretary to the Government of India, Finance and Commerce Department." Appendix XII. Part 2. 383–88.

GBO. Great Britain. Royal Commission on Opium. 1894. *Minutes of Evidence Taken Before the Royal Commission on Opium from 3rd to 27th January 1894*. Volume III. [C–7419]. London: Printed for Her Majesty's Stationery Office. By Eyre and Spottiswoode.

Volume III

No citations. Volume III contains only witness testimony. *See* Royal Commission on Opium: Witnesses.

GBO. Great Britain. Royal Commission on Opium. 1894. *Minutes of Evidence Taken Before the Royal Commission on Opium from 29th January to 22nd February 1894*, with Appendices. Volume IV. [C–7471]. London: Printed for Her Majesty's Stationery Office. By Eyre and Spottiswoode.

Volume IV

GBO. Royal Commission on Opium [Government of Madras–Appendix XIX]. 1894. "Abstracts of Evidence of Witnesses Who Were Tendered for Examination by the Government of Madras, But Not Examined by the Royal Commission." Appendix XIX. 448–54.

———. Royal Commission on Opium [Hendley–Appendix I]. 1894. "'Summary of Operations on Opium' by Surgeon Lieutenant-Colonel Hendley, C.I.E." Appendix I. 376–81.

———. Royal Commission on Opium [Hendley–Appendix II]. 1894. "Analysis (handed in by Surgeon Lieutenant-Colonel Hendley, C.I.E.) of the Cases of 4,409 opium eaters in Jeypore, showing the causes which led to their use of the drug in 1893." Appendix II. 381–82.

———. Royal Commission on Opium [Huntly–Appendix IX]. 1894. "'Data of a Hundred Cases of Opium Eating Recorded by Dr. Huntly [handed in by Dr. Huntly. See A. 21, 298.]" Appendix IX. 404.

———. Royal Commission on Opium [Jehangir–Appendix XXII]. 1894. "Extract from 'Lives of Bombay Opium Smokers,' by Mr. Rustomji Jehangir." Appendix XXII. 485–95.

———. Royal Commission on Opium [Robertson]. 1894. "Testimony of Lieutenant-Colonel D. Robertson, 6 Feburary 1894." 87–90.

Selected Bibliography

———. Royal Commission on Opium [Robertson–Appendix X]. 1894. "Questions Regarding Opium Issued by Lieut.-Colonel D. Robertson to the Durbars of the Native States in Central India." Appendix X. 405–06.

———. Royal Commission on Opium [Robertson–Appendix XI]. 1894. "Statistics regarding Opium in the Native States in Central India with Prefatory Note by Lieutenant-Colonel D. Robertson." Appendix X. 406–17.

———. Royal Commission on Opium [Robertson–Appendix XIII]. 1894. "Abstracts of Evidence of Witnesses tendered for Examination from the Native States in Central India but not examined by the Royal Commission." Appendix XIII. 417–24.

GBO. Great Britain. Royal Commission on Opium. 1894. *Appendices; together with Correspondence on the Subject of Opium with the Straits Settlements and China, etc.* Volume V. [C–7473]. London: Printed for Her Majesty's Stationery Office. By Eyre and Spottiswoode.

Volume V

GBO. Royal Commission on Opium [Gregory]. 1894. "Correspondence No. 291C–787, Regarding the Use of Narcotine as a Febrifuge." From G. M. Gregory, Esq., Sub-Deputy Opium Agent, Ghazipur, to J. P. Hewlett, Esq., C.I.E., Secretary Royal Opium Commission. Appendix III. 76–83.*

[* Enclosures listed according to order of appearance (page number) in Appendix III of Volume V.]

Enclosure 79: Letter dated 16 December 1858 from W. J. Palmer to H. C. Hamilton, Benares Opium Agent, Ghazipur. 77.

Enclosure 103: Letter dated 13 April 1859 from W. J. Palmer to G. Osborne, Sub-Deputy Opium Agent, Gorakhpur. 77.

Enclosure 169: Letter dated 15 November 1859 from W. J. Palmer to H. C. Hamilton, Benares Opium Agent, Ghazipur. 77–78.

Enclosure 192: Letter with Appendix dated 14 February 1860 from W. J. Palmer to J. Forsyth, Director-General Medical Department, Calcutta. 78–81.

Enclosure 2: "On the Preparation of Narcotine and Morphia" undated document by T. W. Sheppard, Principal Assistant, Benares Opium Agency. 81.

Enclosure 74: Letter dated 7 October 1875 from T. W. Sheppard, Principal Assistant, Benares Opium Agency, to the Benares Opium Agent. 81–2.

Enclosure 175: Letter dated 27 March 1877 from T. W. Sheppard, Principal Assistant, Benares Opium Agency, to the Benares Opium Agent. 82.

[Statement] "Statement showing the Quantity of Narcotine issued to the Medical Department before 1878," and "Statement of Narcotine supplied from 1876 to January 1894." Tables submitted by G. M. Gregory, Sub-Deputy Opium Agent of the Benares Opium Agency, Ghazipur to the Royal Commission on Opium, February 14, 1894. 82.

———. Royal Commission on Opium [Her Majesty's Minister in China]. 1894. "Questions regarding Opium Consumption and Opium Revenue in China, issued by the Royal Commission on Opium, through Her Majesty's Minister in China" Appendix XXVI. 212–343.

———. Royal Commission on Opium [Singapore, Penang, and Hong Kong]. 1894. "Questions Issued by the Royal Commission on Opium regarding Opium Consumption and Opium Revenues in the Colonies and Dependencies of Singapore, Penang, and Hong Kong." Appendix XXV. 145–212.

———. Royal Commission on Opium [Walker]. 1894. "Memorandum on the System of Excise on Opium in the Punjab, with Details of Consumption, etc." [Handed in by Mr. T. Gordon Walker, Commissioner of Excise in the Punjab]. Appendix IX. 101–06.

GBO. Great Britain. Royal Commission on Opium. 1895. Part I. The Report, with Annexures. In *Final Report of the Royal Commission on Opium*. Volume VI. [C–7723]. London: Printed for Her Majesty's Stationery Office. By Eyre and Spottiswoode.

Volume VI

GBO. ———. Royal Commission on Opium [Baines]. 1895a. "On the Course of the Movement in England against the Opium Trade, with especial reference to the Action taken in connexion with it in Parliament." Memorandum VI. By the Secretary (J. A. Baines). Part I. The Report, with Annexures. 163–71.

———. Royal Commission on Opium [Baines]. 1895b. "The Government Policy in Regard to the Supply of Bengal Opium." Memorandum VI. By the Secretary (J. A. Baines). Part I. The Report, with Annexures. 172–77.

———. Royal Commission on Opium. [Final Report]. 1895. "The Report, with Annexures." Part I. 1–97.

———. Royal Commission on Opium [Memorandum VIII]. 1895. "Tables Showing the Distribution by Districts, of the Opium Habit in British India." Memorandum VIII. The Report with Annexures. Part I. 178–84. Table I: "Average Yearly Consumption of Licit Opium Per Head, 1892–93." 178–80. Table II: "Showing the Districts of British Provinces arranged according to their Average Annual Consumption of Licit Opium per Head." 181–83. Table III: "Showing the Population under each Group of Average Consumption by Provinces, in relation to the Total Population of the Groups and the Provinces Respectively." 184.

———. Royal Commission on Opium [Roberts]. 1895. "On the General Features and the Medical Aspects of the Opium Habit in India; by Sir William Roberts, M.D., F.R.S." Memorandum I. Part 1. The Report, with Annexures. 99–119.

———. Royal Commission Opium [Wilson–Minute of Dissent]. 1895. "Minute of Dissent, by Mr. Henry J. Wilson, M. P. with Notes and Appendix" Annexure IV. Part I. The Report, with Annexures. 137–52.

———. Royal Commission Opium [Wilson–Note A. to par. 2]. 1895. "Note A. to par. 2.–Resolution of the House of Commons (30 June 1893) Which Led to the Appointment of the Commission." B.–Notes to Mr. Wilson's Dissent. Annexure IV. Part I. The Report, with Annexures. 152–60.

———. Royal Commission Opium [Wilson–Appendix C]. 1895. "Memorandum on the Attitude of the Authorities in India." Note C.–Appendix to Mr. Wilson's Dissent in Annexure IV. Part I. The Report, with Annexures. 161–62.

GBO. Great Britain. Royal Commission on Opium. 1895. Part II. Historical Appendices; together with an Index of Witnesses and Subjects, and a Glossary of Indian terms Used in the Evidence and Appendices. *Final Report of the Royal Commission on Opium*. Volume VII. [C–7723–1]. London: Printed for Her Majesty's Stationery Office. By Eyre and Spottiswoode.

Volume VII

GBO. Royal Commission on Opium [Glossary]. 1895. "Glossary of Indian Terms Used in the Evidence and Appendices." Appendix G. Part 2. Historical Appendices Together With an Index of Witnesses, and a Glossary of Indian Terms Used in the Evidence and Appendices. 314–20.

———. Royal Commission on Opium [Occupation]. 1895. "Index to Witnesses Examined by the Commission: Part II–Race and Occupation. In Appendix E: Index of Witnesses Examined. Part II. Historical Appendices Together With an Index of Witnesses, and a Glossary of Indian Terms Used in the Evidence and Appendices. 223–29.

Great Britain. Parliament. Command Papers

GBC. Parliament [Consumption]. 1892. *Consumption of Opium in India*. [C.–6562]. LVIII. 1–109.

———. Parliament [Statistical Abstract–No. 42]. 1896a. "No. 42–Amount of Opium Revenue and Charges; in Tens of Rupees." *Statistical Abstract Relating to British India from 1885–86 to 1894–95*. 30th Number. [CD–828]. 95. London: Eyre and Spottiswoode.

———. Parliament. [Statistical Abstract–No. 43]. 1896b. "No. 43–Number of Chests of Bengal Opium Sold for Export and Issued to Excise and Medical Departments, and Number of Chests Paying Duty in Bombay." *Statistical Abstract Relating to British India for the Year 1885–86 to 1894–95*. 30th number. [CD–828]. 95. London: Eyre and Spottiswoode.

———. Parliament [Statistical Abstract–Population]. 1904. "Population of British Territory, Gross Revenue and Expenditure, Surplus or Deficit and Debt for 25 Years." Appendix A. *Statistical Abstract Relating to British India from 1893–94 to 1902–03*. 38th Number. [CD–2299]. 58. London: Eyre and Spottiswoode.

Great Britain. Parliament. Reports of Standing and Select Committees

GBR. Great Britain. Parliament. 1831–32. *Minutes of Evidence Taken Before the Select Committee on the Affairs of the East India Company; and Also an Appendix and Index*. Volume XI. Session 1831–32. No. 735–III. Revenue. Ordered, by the House of Commons, to be Printed 16 August 1832.
[Kennedy]. "Testimony of Langford Kennedy." 8 February 1832. 55–61, 84–92. *See also* IUP/PP.
[Mill]. "Testimony of James Mill." 28 June 1832. 263–67. *See also* IUP/PP.
[Stark]. "Testimony of Mr. Hugh Stark." 14 & 16 February 1832. 9–35. *See also* IUP/PP.
———. Parliament. [Report]. 1871. *Report from the Select Committee on East India Finance; with the Proceedings of the Committee, Minutes of Evidence, Appendix and Index*. (363). Volume II. Ordered, by the House of Commons, to be printed 18 July 1871.
[Hamilton]. "Testimony of Sir Robert North Collie Hamilton." 16 May 1871. 226–31. *See also* IUP/PP.
[Wilson]. "Testimony of Reverend John Wilson." 16 June 1871. 339–47. *See also* IUP/PP.

Great Britain. Parliament. Session Papers

GBS. Great Britain. East India (Opium) [Watt]. 1891. "RETURN of an Article on Opium by Dr. Watt, Reporter on Economic Products with the Government of India, recently written by him, and intended to be published in the Sixth Volume of the Dictionary of Economic Products of India" (Submitted by A. Godley, Under Secretary of State, India Office, July 30, 1891). (384). LIX. 3–79.

———. East India (Opium) [Godley]. 1893. Showing the Quantity (in seers) of Bengal Excise Opium Manufactured at the Patna and Ghazipur Factories, the Quantity Supplied to Local Governments and Administrations, including the Native States under their Political Control, and the Balance remaining in Stock in the several Provinces for each of the Ten Years from 1881–82 to 1890–91," in "The Quantity of Bengal and Malwa Opium Disposed in Each such Year (1) to each of the Provincial Excise Administrations, and (2) to the Native States which are Supplied with Opium by the Indian Government"; "And, the Quantity of Bengal and Malwa Opium in Stock at the close of each such Year for Consumption in India." Despatch No. 207 of 1892. 46:1–7, and "Returns Showing the Quantity (1) of Behar and Benares OPIUM manufactured, and (2) of Malwa OPIUM purchased, for Sale in India during each of the past Ten Years." Enclosure in Despatch No. 207 of 1892. (39). 46:7.

———. East India [Godley]. 1897. "Table III. QUANTITY of Opium Manufactured in the Government Factories in the Years 1885-86 to 1894–95." *and* "Table IV. QUANTITIES of Opium Exported from India to China and other Countries during the Ten Years 1885–86 to 1894–95."

Table III and Table IV are in "Return showing for the Last Ten Years the Acreage under Poppy in India; the Amount of Advances to the Cultivators for Crude Opium; and the Quantity of Opium Produced in the Factories, distinguishing between the Behar and Benares Agencies," and "Also the Quantity Exported to China and other Countries; the Quantity of Malwa and other Opium purchased by the Indian government; and the Quantity which in any other way came under the Cognizance of the Indian Government." LXIII. (66). 1–7.

Irish University Press. British Parliamentary Papers

IUP/PP. Irish University Press Series of British Parliamentary Papers. Shannon: Irish University Press. Colonies. East India. Volumes 1–4, 7, 9, 11, 19.

IUP/PP. [1831–32] 1971. *Minutes of Evidence Taken Before the Select Committee on the Affairs of the East India Company with Appendix and Index [III Revenue]. 1831–32.* Volume 9.

[Kennedy]. "Testimony of Mr. Langford Kennedy." 25 February 1832; 8 March 1832. 55–61, 84–92. *See also* GBR.

[Mill]. "Testimony of Mr. James Mill." 28 June 1832. 263–67. *See also* GBR.

[Stark]. "Testimony of Mr. Hugh Stark." 14 February 1832:9–23; 16 February 1832:24–35. 9–35. *See also* GBR.

———. [1871] 1971. *Report from the Select Committee on East India Finance With Proceedings[,] Minutes of Evidence[,] Appendix[,] and Index[.] 1871.* Volume 19.

[Hamilton]. "Testimony of Sir Robert North Collie Hamilton." 16 May 1871. In *Volume II* (363). 226–31. *See also* GBR.

[Wilson]. 1871. "Testimony of Reverend John Wilson." 16 June 1871. In *Volume II* (363). 339–47. See also GBR.

Royal Commission on Opium Witnesses

GBOW. ROYAL COMMISSION ON OPIUM. WITNESSES (VOLUMES I–IV)

The people listed below testified before the Royal Commission on Opium in England and India. They either volunteered information or were asked about the relationship between opium eating and the prevention or cure of 'malaria.' Their responses are the content of Chapter 9: "Witnesses' Perspectives About Why People in India Eat Opium," Chapter 10: "Witnesses' Observations About Who Eats Opium in India," and Appendices A and B. Three witnesses cited in the book provided information about the drug or the disease, but not about the relationship between the two. They are Sir Lepel Griffin (Volume I: 105–09); Surgeon-Major Cobb (Volume II, Part 1: 84–85); and Lieutenant-Colonel D. Robertson (Volume IV: 87–90). Bibliographic information for the three is cited in the [GBO] Royal Commission on Opium section of the selected bibliography. The chapter entitled "Sir William Roberts' Evaluation of the Opium and 'Malaria' Evidence" contains Cobb's material. The Griffin and Robertson comments are introduced in the "The Anti-Opiumists' Nightmare" chapter. Volumes V–VII contain no witnesses providing information about the opium and 'malaria' connection.

VOLUME I

GBOW. Great Britain. Royal Commission on Opium. 1894. *First Report of the Royal Commission on Opium; with Minutes of Evidence and Appendices.* Volume I. [C–7317].
Adams, Reverend Joseph Samuel, 23–9
Birdwood, Sir George, 77–80
Dods, Dr. George, 116–17
Fayrer, Sir Joseph, 110–11
Gauld, Dr. William, 59–61
Lay, H. N., 81–6
Low, Sir Hugh, 111
Maxwell, Dr., 17–23
Moore, Surgeon-General Sir William J., 71–4
Mouat, Dr. F. J., 75–7
Partridge, Deputy Surgeon-General W. F., 124–28
Pringle, Brigade-Surgeon R., 52–56

VOLUME II

GBOW. Great Britain. Royal Commission on Opium. 1894. *Minutes of Evidence taken before the Royal Commission on Opium between 18th November and 29th December 1893; with Appendices.* Volume II. Parts 1 & 2. [C–7397].
Ali, Munshi Rahmat, 301–02
Bahadur, Prince Wala Kadar Syed Husain Ali Mirja, 247
Bahadur, Rai Lal Madhub Mookerjee, 255–58
Bardalai, Babu Madhav Chandra, 302–05
Barooah, Jaginnath, 296–99
Borah, Satyanath, 286–88
Bose, Dr. Juggo Bundo, 90–2
Bose, Dr. Kailas Chunder, 87–90
Bose, Khurgeshur, 99–100
Bradley, F., 193–94
Crombie, Surgeon-Lieutenant-Colonel A., 75–81
Cushing, Reverend Dr., 195–98
Dantra, Surgeon-Major, 209–12
Datta, Atool K., 311–12
Dobson, Surgeon-Major Edwin F. H., 282–85
Driberg, J. J., 261–62
Evans, Reverend T., 46–51
Ferris, Dr. G. R., 105–08
Gibbon, T. M., 150–52
Haviland, R. C., 291–93
Hmyin, Maung Hpo, 204–06
Hossein, Nawab S. A., 253–54
Johnstone, Surgeon-Lieutenant-Colonel Hugh, 207–08
Krishna, Maharajah Bahadur Sir Narendra, 169–70
Kirkpatrick, Reverend M. B., 217–21
Lahiri, Lalit Mohun, 288–91
Law, Maharaja Durga Churn, 171–72
Lethbridge, Honorable A. S., 135–38
Lyall, The Honorable D. R., 63–7
Maynard, Dr. Surgeon-Captain Frederic Pinsent, 69–70
Mazumdar, Ram Dhurlabh, 60–3
Mookerjee, Raja Peary Mohun, 172–74
Morison, Dr. Donald, 100–05
Mukharji, T. N., 158–59
Naik, Sudan Chunder, 110–12
Peal, S. E., 153–55
Phillips, Reverend W. B., 38–43
Purves, Brigade-Surgeon Lieutenant-Colonel, 83–4
Rice, Surgeon Major-General, 11–15
Roy, Dr. Ram Moy, 114–17

Roy, Sita Nath, 43–6
Russell, Surgeon-Lieutenant-Colonel E. G., 84
Ryland, W. H., 156–58
Sircar, Nil Ratan, 162–65
Smeaton, D. M., 225–40
Sukul, Kali Sankur, 269–71
Surbadhicari, Dr. Surji Coomar, 92–93
Tull Walsh, Surgeon Captain J. H., 85–6
Wallace, Dr. James Robert, 117–21
Westmacott, E. V., 127–31

VOLUME III

GBOW. Great Britain. Royal Commission on Opium. 1894. *Minutes of Evidence taken before the Royal Commission on Opium from 3rd to 27th January 1894.* Volume III. [C–7419].
Anderson, Surgeon-Major J., 113–15
Barry, Surgeon-Major D. F., 115–17
Bielby, Dr. Elizabeth, 215–17
Browne, Surgeon-Major S. H., 237–38
Brownrigg, F. W., 117–20
Carleton, Miss, 169
Chatterjee, Pares Nath, 37–9
Clark, Dr. H. Martyn, 191–93
Condon, Brigade Surgeon J. H., 180–84
Gregory, G. M., 88–95
Griffiths, Dr. R. Glyn, 274–75
Hooper, Brigade Surgeon-Lieutenant Colonel W. R., 102–04.
Jennings, Surgeon Captain S.E., 158–60
Khan, Raja Muhammad Salamat, 72
Little, Surgeon-Major S., 160–62
Mazumdar, Dinnonath, 32–4
Mulock, F. B., 96–101
Mulroney, Surgeon-Major T. R., 162–64
Newton, Reverend F. J., 199–201
Scott, Reverend T. J., 106–08
Singh, Raja Udai Pratap, 101–02
Singh, Assistant-Surgeon Soorjee Narain, 39–41
Stoker, T., 275–81
Tyler, Sir John, 109–10.
Valentine, Reverend Colin S., 292–97
Wace, A. A., 5–10
Walker, T. Gordon, 235–37
Woodright, Surgeon Captain W. E. H., 194

VOLUME IV

GBOW. Great Britain. Royal Commission on Opium. 1894. *Minutes of Evidence taken before the Royal Commission on Opium from 29th January to 22nd February 1894, with Appendices*. Volume IV. [C–7471].
Adams, Surgeon-Major A., 38–40
Arnot, Brigade-Surgeon Lieutenant-Colonel James, 211–12
Bahadur, Assistant Surgeon Mohammed Osman Sahib, 244–46
Baria, Darasha Hormaji, 141
Bartholomeusz, Surgeon Lieutenant-Colonel M. L., 306–07
Benjamin, Joseph, 172–74
Bhikaji, Dr. Hari, 187–88
Blaney, Dr. Thomas, 291–92
Bocarro, A. T., 270–71
Caldecott, Surgeon-Lieutenant Colonel R., 94
Cama, Manekji D., 268–70
Chaduri, Kalidas, 344–45
Chitnavis, The Honorable Gangadhar Rao, 367
Cook, Surgeon Colonel H., 214–15
da Cunha, Dr. J. Gerson, 261–63
da Gama, Dr. J. A., 266–67
Freeman Underwood, Dr. M. C., 328–30
French-Mullen, Surgeon-Major D., 47–48
French Mullen, Brigade Surgeon Lieutenant-Colonel T., 65–66
Gaffney, Brigade-Surgeon Lieutenant-Colonel J. B., 338–39
Ghole, Vishram Ramji, 274–75
Gimlette, Surgeon-Major, 95–97
Girdharlal, Rao Bahadur Dulerai, 199–200
Gubbay, E. S., 232–33
Henderson, Surgeon-Major C., 368–69
Hendley, Surgeon Lieutenant-Colonel T. H., 8–13
Huntley, Dr. William, 58–64
Kale, Appaji Govindrao, 192–93
Khan, Mirza Husain, 238
Khory, Dr. R. N., 259–61
Khote, Anant Gangadhar, 115–21
King, Surgeon Major W. G., 242–43
Kirtikar, Surgeon-Major K. R., 304–06
Laflamme, Reverend H. F., 353–57
Lal, Mansukh, 300–03
Lisboa, Dr. J. C., 263–64
MacKenzie, The Honorable T. D., 279–287
Maconochie, A. F., 130–33
Mahipat, Ram Krishna, 146
Marzban, J. P., 348–49
Mayne, Surgeon-Lieutenant Colonel, 239–42
Nanavati, B. H., 273–74
Nariman, Dr. Temulji Bhikaji, 267–68

Nassarvanji, Dr. Edalji, 264–65
Parakh, Surgeon Major D. N., 215–17
Pestonji, Khan Bahadur Dossabhai, 272–73
Porteus, Colonel A. W., 255–56
Prabhakar, G. B., 271–72
Prautch, Reverend A. W., 294–98 *
Quayle, Surgeon-Major D. A., 340
Shah, Assistant Surgeon Tribhovandas Motichand, 188–92
Singh, Kunwar Jaswant, 156–57
Sturmer, Surgeon-Major A. J., 243–44
Vaidya, Chintamanrao Vinayak, 110–11
Vurgese, G. T., 253–55
Weir, Surgeon-Lieutenant Colonel T. S., 222–24
Wilkie, Reverend J., 164–65
Yajnik, The Honorable Javerilal Umiashankar, 225–28
*See Prautch in "Errata." Volume VII. Part II. [C–7723], 324.

Index

Abkari opium. *See* Excise opium
abstinence, 50, 63, 66, 77, 87, 198–99n2, 299–302
Adams, A., 178–79
Adams, Joseph Samuel, 164, 196–97
addiction to morphine, 64–68, 74nn28–31, 77
addiction to opium, 7–8;
    alcoholism vs., 47–48, 54, 63, 73n20, 77, 112n2 (*see also* alcohol-opium analogy);
    British awareness of, 68–69;
    British indifference to, 38–39, 52, 70–71n4;
    in China:
        anti-opiumists on, 37, 49–50, 60–61;
        Chinese on, 13, 34;
        pro-trade activists on, 51, 89–95, 112n3, 131;
    cures for, 50–51, 54, 67, 74n27, 74n32;
    disease model of (*see* disease model of addiction);
    in India, 89, 232;
    inheritance of acquired characteristics and, 54
addiction therapists, 68, 85
Addison, Joseph, 103
adulteration of opium, 19, 24, 32n28, 34, 72n14

Agra Medical Missionary Training Institute, 186, 189
Agricultural Statistics, 313–14n26
ague, 29n15, 124, 154n10, 243–44, 341–42n11
Aitchison, Sir Charles Umpherston, 87, 314n27
Ajmere-Merwara opium, 284, 285
Albemarle, Lord, 56
Albers, J. F. H., 364
Albright, Arthur, 75
Alcock, Sir Rutherford, 60–61, 80
alcoholism, 47–48, 54, 63, 73n20, 77, 109, 112n2
alcohol-opium analogy:
    anti-opiumists on, 61;
    British officials on, 52, 88, 89, 91–92, 97–98;
    in Great Britain, 44;
    Indian officials on, 106;
    members of Parliament on, 101;
    missionaries on, 108, 326–27;
    physicians on, 47–48, 51, 79, 103–4;
    William Roberts on, 143–45
Alexander, Joseph Grundy, 82, 150, 220
Ali, Munshi Rahmat, 206
alkaloids of opium, 19–26, 30–32nn18–26. *See also* anarcotine; laudanum; morphine; narcotine

Allbutt, Thomas Clifford, 65, 77
Allen, Nathan, 49
allopathic medicine, 138–39, 161, 218–20, 221, 265
American Baptist Missionary Union, 60, 164
American Journal of Medical Science, 244
American Methodist Episcopal Church, 221
American Philosophical Society, 63
amul-pani, 311n12
anarcotine:
  extraction ratios for, 274–77, 306–8, 309–10nn1–8, 321–22nn65–76, 357, 359–61, *377–80*;
  Ghazipur experiments and, 245–64, 270–71nn14–24, *370–72*;
  Government of India and, 277–80;
  research on, 363–67. See also narcotine
Anderson, J., 182, 183, 191, 194
Anglican Anti-Opium Committee, 84
Anglo-European, 26n2
Anglo-Oriental Society for the Suppression of the Opium Trade. *See* SSOT
Annals and Antiquities of Rajast'han (Tod), 129
anodyne, opium as, 161–74, 199–200nn7–13, 324, 343–44;
  in East India, 164–65, 170–72;
  in Middle India, 162–64, 169;
  in South India, 168, 174;
  on Western Coast, 167–68, 172–74;
  in West India, 165–67, 169–70
Anstie, Francis, 112n2
anthrax, 139
anti-opiumist, 70n1
anti-opiumist organizations, 7, 55, 83. *See also* SSOT
anti-opiumists:
  aftermath of First Opium War and, 45, 51, 54, 73n20;
  aftermath of Second Opium War and, 67–70, 74n33;
  Chinese as, 7, 13, 36;
  influence in British Parliament, 6–7, 33, 82–83;
  medical defense of opium and, 4–5, 26, 40;
  as members of British Parliament, 7, 46–47, 55–56, 59, 75, 98;
  missionaries as, 35–38, 48–51, 58–59, 70nn1–2, 73n16, 73n24;
  rhetoric of, 323–39;
  Sir Rutherford Alcock and, 60–61, 80;
  vision of imperialism, 2–3, 5;
  William James Moore on, 125–26, 128
Anti-Opium Urgency Committee, 84
antisocial behavior:
  alcohol consumption and, 48, 61, 97;
  anti-opiumist arguments about, 7, 54, 64, 68;
  pro-trade arguments about, 93;
  xenophobia about, 69
aphrodisiac, 79–80, 112n3, 233
apologists for opium trade, 6, 7, 36, 52
Arnot, James, 219
arsenic, 34, 183, 186, 242, 244, 270n11
Atterbury, B. C., 268n2
Ayurvedic medicine, 217, 323–25

Baber, Colborne, 81, 86
Baer, A., 229n3
Bahadur, Mohammed Osman Sahib, 174
Bahadur, Rai Lal Madhub Mookerjee, 343
Bahadur, Wala Kadar Syed Husain Ali Mirja, 199n3
Balaram, Ebrahim, 236
Banerjee, Bijan G., 324
Banner of Asia, 185
Baptist Missionary Society, 46
Bardalai, Babu Madhav Chandra, 218
Bareilly Theological Seminary, 221
Baria, Darasha Hormaji, 344
Barogir, Kisimgu, 236
Barooah, Jaginnath, 346
Barry, D. F., 179, 182, 216
Bartholomeusz, M. L., 167–68
Basham, Dr., 48
Batten, G. M.:
  on opium consumption, 294, 295;
  pro-trade arguments of, 84–95, 113nn5–10;
  on smuggling, 292–93;
  Society of the Arts and, 126, 128, 292;
  on William James Moore, 152–53n3

Battley, Richard, 23, 24, 31–32n26
Beattie, Hilary, 2
Beauperthy, Louis, 29n14
Bellews, Dr., 154n12
Benares Opium Agency, 248, 270n13, 281–84, 287, 289, 312n18, 317n43, 317n45
Bengal opium. *See* Provision opium
Benjamin, Joseph, 195
Bennett, Risdon, 76
Benzylisoquinoline group, 20
bhang, 157, 198n1
Bhikaji, Hari, 216
Bielby, Elizabeth, 188–89, 232
Bihar Opium Agency, 248, 281–84, 287, 289, 312n18, 317n42, 317n44
Binz, Karl, 28n12
Birdwood, Sir George:
  as defender of opium trade, 76, 79–80, 102, 112n1, 115–16, 128–33, 135, 152–53nn2–3;
  at Grant Medical College, 116, 169;
  Lancet critique of, 133–34;
  on opium as food, 129, 132–33, 174–75, 177, 180;
  William James Moore on, 126
"Biscuit" opium, 311n14
black markets, 58
Blaney, T., 188
bleeding, 41
blistering, 41
Blyth, 21
Bocarro, A. T., 344
Bombay College of Medicine, 195
Bombay Medical Services, 219
Booth, Martin, 27n7
Borah, Satyanath, 229n5, 344
Bose, Juggo Bundo, 170–71, 188, 214–15
Bose, Kailas Chunder, 176, 217–18, 229–30n9
Bose, Khurgeshur, 209–10, 214
Bowring, John, 55
Boyd, Mark, 15, 341–42n11
Boyle, William, 23
Bradley, F., 346
Brahmo Samaj New Dispensation Church, 217
Braithwaite, Rachel, 83

Brassey, Sir Thomas Allnut, 135–38, 149–50, 155n20, 237, 245;
  Final Report and, 265;
  interrogation by, 160:
    on consumption of opium, 205;
    on narcotine, 191, 193–94;
    on opium as anodyne, 165, 167;
    on opium as food, 175–76, 177;
    on opium/'malaria' correlation, 211–13, 224, 226–27;
    on quinine, 183, 185, 186–87
Brassey's Naval Annual, 137
Brereton, William H., 80, 86
Bridgeman, E. C., 36
Bright, Mr., 55
Bright (colleague of John Crawford), 29n14
Britain's Opium Harvest (Braithwaite), 83
British Empire, 3
British hegemony, 4, 26n2
British Indian Association, 106–7, 110
British Medical Association, 69, 141, 201n14
British Medical Journal, 79, 141, 266
British officials:
  as anti-opiumists, 49, 60–61, 73n17;
  in China, 89–91;
  in India, 51, 79, 87–89, 113n7;
  as pro-trade activists, 36–37, 52–53, 80;
  Royal Commission and (*see* Royal Commission on Opium)
Brodie, Sir Benjamin, 46, 56, 107, 109
Broomhall, Benjamin, 83, 112–13n4
Brough, J. C., 21
Brown, H. J., 268n2
Brown, J. B., 2–3, 27n7, 107–10
Browne, S. H., 192, 194, 201n16
Brownrigg, F. W., 205, 214
Bruce, C. A., 61
Brunton, Dr., 107, 109
Burma, 61, 79, 83, 87, 97, 99, 101–2, 164
Burnes, James, 130
Byramji Medical School, 172

Caine, W. P., 136
"cake opium," 280–81, 286, 310n9, 312n19
Calcutta Medical College, 192, 201n16

Calcutta Medical Society, 102–4, 113–14n12, 176, 217, 224, 242–43, 270n10
Calcutta Missionary Conference, 107–8, 109–10
Caldecott, R., 229n4, 346
calomel, 40–41
Cama, Manekji D., 176
Cameron Prize, 140
Campbell, Sir George, 80
Campbell, Mr., 89
canal irrigation, 204–5, 208
Canterbury, Archbishop of, 78
Carleton, Miss, 200n8, 229n8, 344
Catalogue of the Vegetable Products of the Presidency of Bombay (Birdwood), 129
Caventou, 25–26
Celli, Angelo, 15
Central India Agency, 284–85, 287, 289–93, 312–13n20, 313–14n26, 314n27, 317nn43–44
Chaduri, Kalidas, 347
chandoo shops, 126
chandul, 126
Chapman, J., 243, 245
Chatterjee, Pares N., 192, 194
Chaudhuri, R. N., 17, 29–30n16, 309n3
Chefoo convention, 78, 81, 97, 112–13n4
The Chemistry of Common Life (Johnston), 53
chemists, 41, 57–58, 63, 72n10, n11, n139
Chevers, Norman, 165
chìk, 311n14
"chill" theory, 116–24, 127–28, 154n12, 179, 182, 183, 227
China Inland Mission, 83, 112–13n4
China Medical [Missionary] Journal, 271n26
Chinese officials:
as anti-opiumists, 49, 50, 61, 73n17;
opposition to drug trade, 34, 48;
pro-trade arguments about, 81
Chinese Recorder, 3
The Chinese Repository (Bridgeman and Williams), 36
Chitnavis, Gangadhar Rao, 206
cholera, 17, 40, 71n7, 139, 340–41n6, 341n10

Chopra, Ram Nath, 366
chorodynomania, 77
Christianity:
as cure for addiction, 50–51, 74n27;
opium associated with, 3, 48, 53, 60, 73n16, 88
Christian Union for the Severance of the Connection of the British Empire with the Opium Traffic, 83, 112–13n4
Christison, Sir Robert, 42, 50, 54, 103, 130
Chuckravarti, D., 104
Church of England, 75
cinchona, 25–26, 30–31n22, 154–55n15, 193, 270n15, 310n6, 310n8, 349–55;
Royal Commission testimony on, 158, 184, 209
The Cinchona Barks (Flückiger), 353
cinchonidine, 25
cinchonine, 25
Civil War (U.S.), 65
Clark, H. Martyn, 165, 210
Clarke, S. E. J., 27–28n8, 299–308, 320–22nn59–72, 330, *377*
class affiliation with opium, 74n31;
in China, 50, 59;
in Great Britain, 42, 54, 71n5
coarnine, 31n25
Cobb, R., 232, 268n1
codamine, 30n18
codeine, 20, 22, 30n18
Coleridge, Samuel Taylor, 38, 70–71n4
Collected Contributions on Digestion and Diet (Roberts), 146
colonies. *See* periphery, colonial
commerce. *See* India-China opium trade
The Commercial Products of India (Watt), 354
Condon, J. H., 184, 191, 194, 210
Confessions of an English Opium-Eater (DeQuincey), 38
Conservative Party, British, 59, 83
consumption (disease), 71n7
consumption of opium:
in China, 5, 34, 37, 39, 49, 51, 53, 322n76;
in Great Britain, 6, 39–44, 47–48, 62, 68–69, 72nn12–14;
in India:
anti-opiumists on, 61, 73n23;

British attitudes toward, 6, 7, 35;
  pro-trade activists on, 87–88,
    281–308, 311nn12–14,
    317–20nn42–57;
  Royal Commission testimony on,
    203–28, 228–30nn1–9, 376;
  in Java, 34;
  in United States, 64–65, 71n5, 73n25,
    74n27. See also ingestion of opium;
    opium eating
contagion theories, 116, 118
Cook, H., 178
Cooper, Thomville T., 59–60
Copleston, Mr., 87
cotarnine, 21, 30–31n22
Cousland, P. B., 271n26
Crafts, Wilbur F., 1–2, 73n24
Crawford, A. C., 364–65
Crawford, John, 29n14
Crawfurd, John, 52, 86, 130
Crombie, A., 102–4, 186–87, 219,
  229–30n9, 235
Cross, Viscount, 83, 84, 87, 95
Crudeli, 117
Crumpe, Samuel, 38–39
crytopine, 30n18
Cuboni, 117
Cushing, Reverend, 164, 343

dacoity, 61, 73n22
da Cunha, J. Gerson, 188, 218
da Gama, J. A., 188
Dane, R. M., 88
Dantra, Surgeon-Major, 188
Datta, Atool K., 223–24, 229n7
Day, Horace, 74n27
death rates. See mortality rates
defenders of trade. See pro-trade activists
Delafield, 28n12
delirium tremens, 71n7
delivery modes, 24–25, 70–71n4
de Mas, Sinibaldo, 52–53, 86
*De Noxiis Paludum Effluviss Eorumque
  Remediis* (Lancisi), 28–29n12
DeQuincey, Thomas, 38, 69, 70–71n4, 92,
  103
Derby, Lord, 55
Derosnè, Charles Louis, 21, 245
Desai, Haridas Viharidas, 172, 176

dhoi, 311n14
diabetes, 71n7, 201n17
"Diagnosis of Indian Fevers" (Moore),
  153n4
diarrhea, 34, 41, 201n17, 232, 324
Dickens, Charles, 69
*The Dictionary of the Economic Products
  of India* (Watt), 294
Dictionary of the Malay Archipelago
  (Crawfurd), 130
dietary supplement, opium as. See food,
  opium as
Dietetics and Dyspepsia (Roberts), 212
diphtheria, 139
"Discussion on the Effects of the Habitual
  Use of Opium on the Human
  Constitution," 229–30n9
disease/drug correlation. See
  drug/disease correlation
disease model of addiction, 66, 67, 76,
  112n2, 119–20
Dobbs, William, 43
Dobson, Edwin F. H., 178, 189–90
Dods, George, 345
Dohme, A. R. L., 364–65
dosage:
  of anarcotine, 250–52, 260–62,
    271nn22–23, 274–75;
  delivery modes and, 64;
  opium abuse and, 42, 43
Dott, D. B., 22
Dover's Powder, 23, 50
Downing, Charles Toogood, 47–48
Doyle, Arthur Conan, 69
Driberg, J. J., 346
dropsy, 71n7
drug/disease correlation, 4–5, 12, 22,
  28n11, 69, 345–48;
  in Royal Commission testimony:
    contrived theory of, 220–28,
      229–30nn6–9;
    ingestion of opium and, 157–58,
      198–99nn2–3;
    'malarious regions' and, 203–20,
      228–30nn1–5;
    William Roberts on, 231–42, 269nn3–6,
      299–308, 320–21nn58–64, 322n76
druggists. See pharmacists
drug ingestion. See ingestion of opium

drug trade. *See* India-China opium trade
Duff, Thomas W., 268n2
Duncan, Andrew, 365–66
Durham, Bishop of, 75
Dutch cinchona policy, 350–53
dysentery, 34, 71n7, 163, 180, 201n17, 232, 324
dyspepsia, 201n17

East India Company:
 drug policy of, 2, 5–6, 34, 37, 55, 314n27;
 in early decades of India-China opium trade, 35–36;
 employees of, 130;
 opium exports as revenue source for, 8–9, 27nn6–7, 312n18
eating opium. *See* opium eating
Eatwell, W. C. B., 52, 86, 109, 130
Edinburgh Committee for the Suppression of the Indo-Chinese Opium Traffic, 55, 84
Edkins, Dr., 90, 113n9
Edmonds, F. H., 229n3
Edwards, Vincent, 93, 126, 235
Egyptian physicians, 16
elephantiasis research, 117
Elgin, Lord, 58
Elliot, Dr., 79
Elliott, Sir Charles, 87
encephalitis, 29–30n16
English Methodist Free Church, 90
environmental variables of disease, 14–16, 28n11, 29n15, 121–24, 125
Erlenmeyer, Albrecht, 66
"The Errors of the Anti-Opiumists" (Moore), 128, 154–55n15
ethnicity affiliation with opium, 69, 74n31
Etkin, Nina L., 229n3
Eucomen, 77–78
euthanasia, 43
Evans, Mr., 243
Evans, T., 226–27
Evershed, Arthur, 64
Excise opium, 8, 28n9, 284, 311n13, 312n19, 313n25;
 anarcotine and, 306–8, 321–22nn66–77, 359–61, *377–80*;
 native consumption of, 286–88, 315–17nn33–38, *374*;
 revenues from, 10–11, 27–28nn8–9
exploitation, 3, 36

Facts and Evidence Relating to the Opium Trade with China (Fry), 48
fallacies, 14–26
"Famine and Fever in Rajputana" (Moore), 153n4
Fanshawe, Arthur Upton, 136, 178, 212–13, 222
Fayrer, Sir Joseph, 345
febrifuge:
 for 'malaria,' 18;
 narcotine as, 190, 193, 194, 277, 280;
 opium as, 160, 162;
  anti-opiumist arguments about, 177–78, 211, 266;
  Ayurvedic medicine and, 324;
  native physicians on, 216, 222;
  pro-trade arguments about, 227;
  in South India, 168, 174;
  in West India, 165–66, 169;
  William Roberts on, 237;
 quinine as, 182, 310n6;
febrile diseases, 119–20
feminists, middle-class British, 26n3
The Fens (England), 43, 57, 68–69, 72n13, 73n26, 137, 155n16, 234
Fergusson, Sir James, 96, 336
Ferris, G. R., 176, 189
'fever.' *See* 'malarial fevers'
fevers, 15–18, 25, 29–30nn15–16, 32n31, 41, 71n7, 88;
 William James Moore on, 117–24, 153n4, 153–54nn9–14;
 William Roberts on, 139–40
Ffrench-Mullen, D., 183,
Ffrench-Mullen, T., 189
Finlay, J. F., 286, 311n13, 315n30
First Opium War. *See* Opium War, First
Fitzpatrick, Sir Dennis, 108
Flückiger, Frederick, 22, 31n23, 353
folk beliefs, 115, 222, 323, 340n4
food, opium as:
 George Birdwood on, 129, 132–33;
 Royal Commission testimony on, 158, 174–80, 220–21, 227;

William James Moore on, 124, 127;
    William Roberts on, 232
food preferences, 140–48
Forsyth, J., 247–48, 249
Foster, Arnold, 271n26
Foster, Mr., 126
Fowler, Sir Robert, 96
Francis, Mr., 278, 310n7
Franco-Prussian War, 74n29
Freeman Underwood, M. C., 169
Frerichs, T., 28n12
Friend of China, 75, 76
Friends' Anti-Opium Committee for
    Suffering, 83–84
Fry, William S., 46, 48

Gaffney, J. B., 347
Gage, Andrew Thomas, 354
Galen, 14
galenicals, 23, 24, 40
Galpin, F., 90
Gamgee, Arthur, 76
ganja, 97, 104, 113n11
Garden, A., 245–46, 252–64,
    270–71nn17–24, 274–78,
    309nn3–5, 310n7, 364,
    370–72
Garrod, Dr., 107, 109
Gauld, William, 185, 196–97, 343
gender affiliation with opium, 71n5, 215,
    229nn3–4
genetic heritage, 90–91, 229n4
genetic structure, 24
German researchers, 65, 77
germ theory of disease, 15–18, 28–29n12,
    29–30n16, 116–17, 139, 332–38,
    340–41nn5–8
Ghazipur experiments, 245–64,
    270–71nn14–24, 274–78, 309nn3–5,
    370–72
Ghole, Vishram Ramji, 344
Ghosh, Jaganath, 104
Gibbon, Dr., 247
Gibbon, T. M., 347
Gimlette, Surgeon-Major, 177
Girdharlal, R. B. D., 172
Gladstone, 45, 79, 96, 98, 105, 110–11,
    114n13
gnoscopine, 22, 30n18, 342n12

Godley, Arthur, 97, 286, 287, 315n30,
    316nn36–37
Golgi, Camillo, 15
Gooeve, Mr., 243–45
Gordon, Dr., 154n12
gout, 71n7
Government of India, 108–10;
    drug policy of, 4–5, 70n2, 214, 220,
        229n6, 329–30, 336–38;
    opium exports as revenue source for,
        8–11, 27–28nn7–8, 312n18, 313n25;
    production of anarcotine and, 277–80,
        310nn7–8;
    production of opium and (*see* poppy
        cultivation);
    questionnaires on opium use, 86–87,
        89, 113n6;
    quinine production and, 350–53;
    Royal Commission and, 11, 13, 86,
        110–11, 137, 138, 144, 210;
    witnesses and, 149–52, 159–60, 212
        (*see also* Indian Medical Service
        personnel);
    SSOT and, 76, 79, 81, 82, 96–97,
        99–100, 101, 105–6
Graham, Sir James, 45
Gramiccia, Gabriele, 355
Grant, Dr., 248
Grant Medical College, 116, 169, 176, 195,
    196
Great Britain. Board of Trade, 46
Great Britain. Parliament, 265;
    anti-opiumist influence on, 4, 7–8, 33,
        70n1 (*see also* SSOT);
    debates:
        1830–1833, 36–38;
        1843, 46–47;
        1857–1860, 55–59;
        from 1875 to early 1880s, 78–79;
        1889 (May), 82–83;
        1892 (August), 98–101;
        1893 (30 June), 104–6
    First Opium War and aftermath, 44–47,
        52, 55;
    Second Opium War and aftermath,
        55–64;
    Select Committee (1830–1833), 35,
        36–38, 70n2;
    Select Committee (1857), 55;

416   *Index*

Select Committee (1871), 60–62, 80.
    See also Royal Commission on
    Opium
Great Britain. Parliament. House of Lords,
    45, 56, 78
Greek disease therapy, 14, 16, 17, 29n13
Green, Mr., 244–45
Gregory, D. M., 192–93, 194, 245, 274
Gregory, G. M., 277, 310nn6–7
Gregory–Robertson system, 30–31n22,
    274, 309n2
Grier, James, 352–53
Griffiths, R. Glyn, 186
grocers, 41, 69, 71n8, 72n11
Gubbay, E. S., 207–8
Gupta, Pundit Modoosoodona, 243
Gurney, Samuel, 46

Halford, Sir Henry, 46
Hamilton, H. C., 247–48
Hamilton, R. N. C., 60
Handy, Hast, 39
Hansard, 78
Hansbury, Thomas, 75
Hare, Mr., 268n2
Harrison, Mark, 333–34, 339–40n2,
    340–41nn5–8
Hart, Sir Robert, 90
Harvey, Charles, 23
Hastings, H., 311n14, 313n21, 315n30
Hastings, Warren, 35
Haviland, C., 199–200n7
Haynes, Douglas, 29n15
hemp, 91, 113n11, 198n1
Henderson, C., 347–48
Hendley, T. H., 169–70, 235–36
herbal medicines, 34, 38, 41
"heroic treatments," 40–41
heroin, 74n32
"hill tracts," 297
Hind, Mr., 61
Hmyin, Maung Hpo, 211
Hobson, Dr., 55
Homeopathic Medical Society
    (Philadelphia, Pa.), 224
homeopathy, 40–41, 138–39, 146–47, 218
home remedies, 38, 41, 42, 50
Honig, Peter, 355
Hooper, W. R., 207, 208

Hossein, Nawab S. A., 346
House of Commons. *See* Great Britain,
    Parliament
Howard, Bernard, 353
Howard, John Eliot, 350–51, 353
humoral theory of disease, 14–15, 17–18
Huntly, William, 167, 181–82, 190–91,
    194, 200n9, 210, 227
Hurst, R. W., 268n2
hydrocartinine, 30n18
hydropaths, 40–41
hypodermic injections. *See* subcutaneous
    hypodermic injections

illegal opium trade, 34, 35, 36, 315n30.
    See also smuggling
immorality of drug trade, 6, 12, 13, 44,
    70n1, 79
Imperial government of China, 7, 34
imperialism, 2–3, 5, 8–11, 13,
    26–28nn2–9, 323–39, 339n1
Impey, Elijah, 32n28, 51, 130, 309n1
imports of opium:
    into China (*see* India-China opium
        trade);
    into Great Britain, 40, 41, 42, 62,
        72n12, 73n15, 73n25;
    into United States, 73n25
Index-Catalogue, 363–65
India, Government of. *See* Government of
    India
India-China opium trade, 1–3, 5–8,
    322n77;
    aftermath of First Opium War and, 46,
        73n15;
    aftermath of Second Opium War and,
        67–70;
    anti-opiumist arguments about, 34,
        48–49, 53–54 (*see also* SSOT);
    British Parliament debates on (*see*
        Great Britain. Parliament);
    early decades of, 35–36, 90, 113n9;
    end of, 13, 338;
    India's dependence upon, 10, 35, 36,
        314n27;
    morphine-deficient opium and, 22,
        31n24;
    pro-trade defense of, 51–54, 92;
    Second Opium War and, 58

The Indian Annals, 153n4
Indian Medical Gazette, 153n4, 201n14, 226
Indian Medical Record, 226, 234–35, 266
Indian Medical Service personnel;
  inertia of, 333–34, 340–41nn5–7;
  "medical opium" and, 280–81;
  Royal Commission testimony of, 159, 160, 163, 164, 176, 183, 188, 191, 221;
  William Roberts on, 242, 264. *See also* names of individual witnesses
"Indian Mutiny" (1857–58), 191, 201n15
Indian Register and Directory, 225
indifference to opium addiction, 38–39, 52, 70–71n4
infant mortality rates, 43, 63, 72nn13–14
ingestion of opium;
  alcohol consumption vs. (*see* alcohol-opium analogy);
  contradictory accounts about, 52–54, 56, 73n18;
  by literary celebrities, 38, 69, 70–71nn3–4;
  problem with, 23–25, 31–32nn26–30;
  research on, 19–20, 21;
  Royal Commission on, 11–12, 18–19, 197. *See also* opium eating; opium smoking
inheritance of acquired characteristics, 54
injections. *See* subcutaneous hypodermic injections
insanity, 104, 233
insect vectors, 16, 29nn13–14
insurance, life, 41–42
Irish Home Rule, 105
irrigation canals, 204–5, 208
isoquinoline family, 20, 30n19, 31n23

"jagirdari," 312–13n20
Jalota, Ritula, 324
Janes, E. H., 364
Jardine & Matheson Co., Ltd., 44
Jeffreys, Julius, 50
Jehangir, Rustomji, 236
Jennings, S. E., 221–22
John, Griffith, 100
Johnston, James, 53, 58–59
Johnstone, Hugh, 171–72, 187–88

Journal of Medical Science, 50
Journal of the Society of Arts, 80

kala-azar, 199–200n7, 335, 341–42n11
Kale, Appaji Govindrao, 218–19
Kelsch, Achille, 28n12
Kennedy, Dane, 340n3
Kerr, Norman, 76, 77, 102, 112n2
Khan, Mirza Husain, 208
Khan, Raja Muhammed Salamat, 199n3
Khory, R. N., 347
Khote, Anant Gangadhar, 185, 209, 216, 217
Kimberley, Lord, 81, 98, 100–101, 105
King, Albert Freeman Africanus, 29n14
King, Charles W., 34
King, Sir George, 354
King, W. G., 168
Kirkpatrick, M. B., 164, 221
Kirtikar, K. R., 173
Klebs, 117
Knowles, R., 366
Koch, Robert, 15, 116, 340–41n6
Krishna, Narendra, 106, 206
Kubla Khan (Coleridge), 38
Kumar, Anil, 340n5, 341nn9–10
Kumar, Deepak, 318–19n51, 340n4
Kung, Prince, 60–61

laboring classes. *See* working class
Lady Aitchison's Hospital (Lahore, West India), 188–89
Laehr, S., 66
Laflamme, H. F., 347
Lahiri, Lalit Mohun, 196–97, 229n5, 344
Laing, Samuel, 91
Lal, Amrita, 104
Lal, Mansukh, 185, 210
Lancet, 133–34
Lancisi, Giovanni Maria, 16, 28–29n12, 29n14, 117
lanthopine, 30n18
latex, 19, 24, 27–28n8, 32n28, 49, 70–71n4, 310n10
laudanidine, 30n18
laudanine, 30n18
laudanum:
  cause of death and, 41, 43, 56, 63;
  criminal offenses and, 53;

labeling of, 57;
    opium eating and, 23, 70–71n4;
    William Roberts on, 234
laudonosine, 30n18
Laveran, Alphonse, 15, 17, 18, 28–29n12, 334, 340–41n6
Law, Durga Churn, 346
Lawall, Charles, 22
Lay, H. N., 177
Lectures on Dietetics and Dyspepsia (Roberts), 140
"leewa," 312n19
Leitch, Margaret, 1–2, 73n24
Leitch, Mary, 1–2, 73n24
Lethbridge, A. S., 199n3, 345
Levinstein, Edward, 66–67, 112n2
Lewis, Malcolm, 53
Liberal Party, British, 75, 83, 96, 98
licenses for poppy cultivation, 82, 83, 88, 89, 95, 99–100, 104
licorice, 50
Lin, Commissioner, 44–45
Lisboa, J. C., 195, 196
Lister, Joseph, 139, 147
literary celebrities, 38, 69, 70–71nn3–4
Little, S., 50, 166–67
lobbying, 8, 58, 81
Lodwick, Kathleen, 3, 112n3
London Missionary Society, 46, 100
longevity argument, 42, 50, 51, 93, 130
Lord Mayor of London, 78
Low, Sir Hugh, 345
Lowry, J. H., 268n2
lumpers, 159, 161, 162, 174, 200n11, 209, 215, 219, 229–30n9, 235, 324
"lunatic asylums," 168, 182, 207, 237
Lyall, D. R., 108–11
Lyall, Sir James Broadwood, 135–38;
    interrogation by, 160, 346;
    on opium as anodyne, 164;
    on opium as food, 176, 177;
    on opium/'malaria' correlation, 205, 208–9, 211, 216, 218
Lyons, Dr., 154n12

MacDonnell, Sir Anthony Patrick, 106
MacFarland Company (Edinburgh, Scotland), 30–31n22
MacGowan, D. J., 50–51

Macht, David, 31–32n26
MacKenzie, Alexander, 99, 101–2
MacKenzie, John, 339
MacKenzie, T. D., 176, 208–9
MacNamara, Dr., 154n12
Maconochie, A. F., 175
MacPherson, Dr., 51
Madras Medical College, 174
Magendie, Francois, 21, 22, 40, 364
Maharajah of Sind, 27n6, 313–14n27
Mahipat, Ram Krishna, 346
malaria:
    causes of, 14–17, 28–30nn11–16;
    cures for, 12, 13, 17–18, 25–26;
    in periphery, 26n2;
    pro-trade arguments about, 4. *See also* 'malarial fevers'
"Malaria and Its Remedies" (Moore), 154–55n15
'malarial fevers,' 17–18, 345–48;
    anarcotine/narcotine research and, 363–67;
    anarcotine production and, 277–80, 306–8, 310n6, 321–22nn68–77;
    Ghazipur experiments and, 246–64, 274–78;
    Royal Commission testimony on, 159–61;
    consumption of opium and, 194–97, 201n17, 203–28, 228–30nn1–9;
    narcotine and, 190–94;
    opium as anodyne for, 162–74, 200–201n13;
    quinine and, 181–90;
    W. B. O'Shaughnessy on, 242–45, 270n11;
    William James Moore on, 120–29;
    William Roberts on, 234–40, 269n6, 320n58, 330–32
"malarial poison" hypothesis, 117–28, 153–54nn6–13
malaria/opium correlation. *See* drug/disease correlation
"Malaria versus Recognisable Causes of Disease" (Moore), 153n4
'malarious regions,' 159, 160, 189, 203–28, 234–40. *See also* environmental variables of disease

Malcolm, Sir John, 130
Malwa opium, 284–85, 313–15nn22–29;
　consumption of, 282, 288–97, 311n14, 317nn42–51;
　export of, 27–28n8, 31n24, 70n2, 83, 94–95, 285–86, 289–91, 315nn30–31, 317nn40–41, *373, 375*;
　Royal Commission testimony on, 208;
　smuggling of, 288, 292–93, 317nn48–49;
　William Roberts on, 241, 269n7
Manning, Cardinal, 78
Mansfield, R. W., 268n2
Manson, Patrick, 29n14, 117, 353
A Manual of Cinchona Cultivation in India (King), 354
A Manual of Diseases in India (Moore), 116, 124, 126, 127, 153nn4–5
"The Man with the Twisted Lip" (Doyle), 69
Mar, Earl of, 41, 43, 50
Marchiafava, Ettore, 15, 117
Margary, Consul, 132
Markham, Sir Clements, 352, 354
Marshall, Captain, 243, 245
Martin, R. M., 73n17
"Marwar—The Land of Death" (Moore), 153n6
Marzban, J. P., 347
"Masked Malarial Fever" (Moore), 153n4, 154n10
Materia Medica, 24
Matheson, Donald, 53
Maxwell, Dr., 184–85, 210
Maynard, Frederic Pinsent, 188, 191, 194
Mayne, Surgeon Lieutenant-Colonel, 191, 194, 201n14
Mayo, Lord, 62
Mazumdar, Dinnonath, 163, 217
Mazumdar, Ram Dhurlabh, 184, 344
McKibbin, W. K., 60
Meadows, Thomas Taylor, 73n17
Meckel, Heinrich, 28n12
meconidine, 30n18
meconin, 31n25
Medhurst, W. H., 37, 55

medical defense of opium:
　in British Parliament, 56;
　in opposition to SSOT, 79, 86, 93, 102–4, 113n10;
　Royal Commission and, 4–5, 12. *See also* drug/disease correlation
medical evidence against opium, 59, 68, 74n33;
　in British Parliament, 46–47, 56;
　Calcutta Missionary Conference and, 107;
　SSOT and, 76, 85
Medical Missionary Association, 184, 210
"medical opium":
　production of, 280–83, 310–11nn11–15;
　pro-trade rebuttal of, 94–95, 98, 135;
　SSOT and, 83
medical profession, Anglo-European:
　Calcutta Medical Society and, 102–4;
　during early decades of India-China Opium Trade, 38–44, 71nn6–7, 72n13;
　after First Opium War, 46, 47–48, 52–54, 56;
　in *Lancet* critique of pro-trade activists, 133–34;
　Royal Commission and, 221 (*see also names of witnesses*);
　after Second Opium War, 58;
　SSOT and (*see* SSOT). *See also* science, Anglo-European
Medical Times and Gazette, 77
Melbourne, Lord, 45
Memoir of Central India (Malcolm), 130
memorialists. *See* anti-opiumists
memorials:
　of British Indian Association, 106, 110;
　of Calcutta Medical Society, 102, 113–14n12;
　of Calcutta Missionary Conference, 108–10;
　of SSOT, 79, 83–84, 87, 97, 98–102, 104, 228–29n2
meningitis, 29–30n16
merchants:
　American, 34;
　British, 44, 59, 62, 75, 78;
　Chinese, 78;

Dutch, 34;
Indian, 32n28
Merck process, 245
"metropolis," 26n2
metropolitan science, 28n11, 30n21
Meyer, W. S., 10–11
miasmatic causation, 14–17, 29n15, 160, 345–48;
  Royal Commission testimony on, 208–9, 229n4;
  William James Moore on, 116, 118, 119
microbes, malarial, 14–15, 28–29n12
microbial theory, 117
misconceptions, medical, 4, 13, 339;
  about heroin, 74n32;
  about ingestion of opium, 23–24, 32n30;
  about narcotine, 21
missionaries, 1–3, 6, 26n1, 73n24;
  in early decades of India-China opium trade, 35–39, 70n1;
  after First Opium War, 46, 48–51, 55, 73n16;
  hypocrisy and, 3, 48, 53, 60, 73n16, 88;
  Royal Commission and, 150–51;
  after Second Opium War, 58–59, 60–61; *See also* anti-opiumists; SSOT
Mitchell, James K., 29n14
Mohr process. *See* Thiboumery and Mohr process
Moir, D. M., 104
Montgomery, Robert, 49
Mookerjee, Raja Peary Mohun, 346
Moore, Sir William James:
  as defender of opium trade, 102, 113n10, 115–29, 135, 152n1, 152–55nn3–18;
  George Birdwood on, 130, 131, 132;
  Lancet critique of, 133–34;
  on opium as food, 124, 127, 174–75, 177, 180;
  Vincent Edwards on, 235
Moore, Sir William, 331–32, 339–40nn2–3
moral and physical degeneration;
  in China, 37–38, 50, 90–91;
  in India, 8
moral deficiency, 39, 47, 54, 64–67, 74n31

moral opposition to opium;
  during early decades of India-China Opium Trade, 5, 6;
  after First Opium War, 48–51, 73nn15–16;
  Royal Commission and, 2–3, 11–12;
  SSOT and, 326–27
Morison, Donald, 211–13, 219, 221
morphia/morphine, 20, 21–24, 30n18, 30–31nn22–23, 31n26;
  export to western markets and, 241, 280, 310n10;
  extraction of, 274–75, 277, 309n2, 310n6;
  infant mortality rates and, 43;
  injections of, 64–67, 74nn28–32;
  in patent medicines, 78;
  reexportation of, 73n25
"morphine eater," 70–71n4
morphine epidemic, 67
Morphine Group, 20
morphinomania, 77
mortality rates, 72nn13–14;
  in Great Britain, 43, 63, 67, 73–74n26;
  in India, 205, 239, 249–50, 254–55, 269n5, 302–5, 377;
Morton, Thomas, 25
mosquitoes, 28–29n12
mother drug;
  addiction to (*see* addiction to opium);
  alkaloids in, 20, 102, 127–28, 247, 274–75, 309nn1–2, 310n6 (*see also* Ghazipur experiments);
  death by, 64;
  eating of, 21, 23, 24, 31–32n26;
  Indian domestic sales of, 10;
  as stimulant, 40;
  William Roberts on, 273
Mouat, F. J., 97–98, 157, 201n16
Mowbray, Robert Gray Cornish, 135–36, 175, 226
Muirhead, William, 60
Mukharji, T. N., 346
Mulock, F. B., 198–99n2, 347
Mulroney, T. R., 179, 222–23
Muraleedharan, V. R., 341n11
murder, 60, 61, 73–74n26
The Mystery of Edwin Drood (Dickens), 69

Naik, Sudan Chunder, 206, 217
Nanavati, B. H., 172–73, 191, 193–94
Napier, Lord, 37
narceine, 22, 30n18, 30–31n22
narcotic addiction, 77
narcotine, 4, 20, 21–22, 23, 25, 30n18, n21, 30–31n22, 31n23, n25, 342n12, 363–67;
  Royal Commission testimony on, 158, 190–94, 201n16, 227;
  W. B. O'Shaughnessy on, 242–45, 270nn10–13;
  William James Moore on, 123, 127, 154–55n15, 155n18;
  William Roberts on, 241–42, 269nn8–9. See also anarcotine
Nariman, Temulji Bhikaji, 195, 344
Narrative of a Visit to the Court of Sinde (Burnes), 130
Nassarvanji, Edalji, 196–97, 198n2
National Christian Anti-Opium Convention, 84
National Righteousness, 83, 106
National Righteousness, 112n4
"Native Christians," 200–201n13
native physicians, 217–19, 222, 224–26, 229n5, 229–30n9, 323–25, 340n4. *See also names of individual physicians*
native states of India:
  consumption of opium in, 286–97, 315–18nn32–47;
  economies of, 28n9;
  poppy cultivation in, 5–6, 27n6, 35, 83, 282–85, 312n16, 312–13nn20–21, 313–14n25, n27–28
neuralgia, 64, 201n17
Newton, F. J., 182–83, 186
Nineteenth Century, 80
nonalkaloids, 19
nonconformists, 75
"nonmedical use" classification of opium, 76, 82, 281
noscapine, 22, 342n12, 367
nosology, 16, 17, 227
Nott, Josiah Clarke, 29n14

O'Brien, Mr., 243
occupational categories of witnesses, 159, 199n4

O'Connell, Dr., 154n12
"Offences Against the Person Act," 53
officinal capitals, 23, 24
Oldham, Dr., 154n12
"On Fever" (Moore), 153n4
"On Narcotine as a Substitute for Quinine in Intermittent Fevers" (O'Shaughnessy), 270n10
"On the Value of Quinine" (Moore), 153n4
opianic acid, 21, 30–31n22
opianine, 30n18
opiomania, 77
opium. *See* mother drug
opium abuse:
  in China, 50, 92–93;
  in Great Britain, 7, 11, 40, 42, 69, 72n13. *See also* addiction to opium
"Opium and Common Sense" (Alcock), 80
opium consumption. *See* consumption of opium
opium dens, 69, 83, 88, 89, 92
"opium eater," 70–71n4
opium eating:
  in China, 60, 73n18;
  pro-trade arguments about, 80, 130, 132–33;
  research on, 19–20, 23, 24, 31–32n26, 50;
  Royal Commission testimony on, 11–12, 18–19, 32n30, 175;
  Select Committee on, 60. *See also* ingestion of opium
"opium habit," 297–99, 303–4
The Opium Habit; with Suggestions as to the Remedy (Day), 74n27
opium/malaria correlation. *See* drug/disease correlation
opium production. *See* poppy cultivation
"The Opium Question" (Batten), 84, 113n5
"The Opium Question" (Birdwood), 128
opium smoking:
  anti-opiumist arguments about, 37, 49–51, 55, 59;
  in China, 5, 22, 34, 37, 48, 58–59, 81;
  in India, 83, 88, 89, 236;

pro-trade arguments about, 80–81, 86, 109, 112n3;
  by George Birdwood, 130–32, 175;
  by William James Moore, 126, 131;
  Royal Commission testimony on, 164, 175. *See also* ingestion of opium
opium trade. *See* India-China opium trade
Opium War, First, 27n6, 44–46;
  aftermath of, 46–47, 73n15
Opium War, Second, 55–59, 62
oral ingestion. *See* ingestion of opium
Orphine, 77–78
Osborne, G., 250
O'Shaughnessy, R., 243–44, 245, 270n12
O'Shaughnessy, W. B.:
  legacy of, 242–45, 246–47, 248, 270nn10–12, 270n15, 310n10;
  longevity argument of, 51, 93;
  Royal Commission testimony about, 192, 201n16, 211;
  William James Moore on, 127
Osler, William, 15
The Other Side of the Opium Question (Moore), 134
Otte, J. A., 271n26, 322n76
overindulgence. *See* opium abuse
oxynarcotine, 22, 30–31n22

pain relief, 41, 158, 161–74, 326
Palmer, W. J., 245–52, 269n8, 270nn14–19, 271n22, 274–78, 364
Palmerston, Lord, 37, 46, 59
papaveramine, 30n18
papaverine, 20, 30n18
Papaverine Group, 20
Papaver somniferum Linn. See mother drug
Papers Relating to Consumption of Opium in British Burma, 320n57
Paracelsian essences, 23, 24
paradigms, fading, 14–26, 26n2
Parakh, D. N., 173
parasites, 15
Parkes, Edmund, 339–40n2
Parkinson's disease, 29–30n16
Partridge, W. P., 213
pass-duty transactions, 285, 289
Pasteur, Louis, 15, 17, 116, 139, 147
patent medicines, 41, 63, 71–72nn8–11, 77

Patna Medical School, 206
Peal, S., 218
Pease, Sir Arthur, 75, 136;
  interrogation by, 172, 175, 176, 185, 189, 209
Pease, Edward, 75
Pease, Sir Joseph, 75, 78, 81, 82, 95–97, 98, 104–5
Peel, Sir Robert, 45, 47
Pegg, James, 49
Pelletier, 25–26
Pereira, Dr., 54, 56, 107, 109, 110, 130
periphery, colonial, 26n2, 28n11, 29n15, 30n21
Persian opium, 9, 13
Pestonji, Khan Bahadur Dossabhai, 347
Pestonji Jehangir, Rustomji, 228–29n2
petitions, anti-opium, 84, 90, 95–96, 99
pharmaceutical industry, 22, 31n24, 71n8
Pharmaceutical Journal, 57, 86
Pharmaceutical Society, 57–58
pharmacists, 41, 57–58, 62, 63, 72n11, n14, 139
pharmacologists, 85
Pharmacy Act, 56–58, 63, 69, 74n29, 82, 83, 94, 99
phenethrane family, 20, 30n19
Phillips, W. B., 110, 343
physicians. *See* medical profession, Anglo-European; native physicians
Piaget, Sir James, 153n7
The Picture of Dorian Gray (Wilde), 69
Planck, Dr., 154n12
plasmodia, 15, 17, 18;
  malarial, 25, 29–30nn15–16, 341–42n11;
  Ayurvedic medicine and, 324;
  in Royal Commission testimony, 158, 164, 167, 183, 201n17, 214, 219, 229n4;
  William James Moore on, 120, 124
Pliny, 132
poison, opium labeled as, 56–57, 59, 63, 107, 109
poisoning, opium, 53, 58, 63, 73–74n26, 109;
  of children, 43, 63, 72n14, 232;
  by injection, 65
Poisons (Christison), 130
poppies, syrup of, 57, 63

poppy cultivation, 3, 7–8, 26n2;
  adulteration techniques during, 19, 24, 32n28;
  in China, 9, 13, 78, 81, 92;
  in Great Britain, 38, 71n7;
  in India, 5–6, 13, 35, 68, 78, 281–308, 310–22nn10–77;
  termination or restriction of:
    anti-opiumists on, 46, 49, 68, 78–79, 82–83, 88, 97, 99–100, 104;
    pro-trade activists on, 94–95, 101–2
poppy heads, 311n12, 311n15
poppyhead tea, 42
Porteus, C. A., 208
Pottinger, Sir Henry, 36–37, 47, 86
Prabhakar, G. B., 201n17
A Practical Treatise on Urinary and Renal Disease (Roberts), 139
Prautch, A. W., 213–14, 228–29n2
prescriptions for opium:
  in Great Britain, 71n7;
  in India, 176, 215–20, 229n5
Pringle, Robert, 76–77, 166–67, 177–78, 182, 185
privatization, 82
Problems of Empire; the Case for Devolution (Brassey), 137
prohibition of liquor. *See* Temperance Movement
prophylactic:
  for cholera, 236;
  cinchona as, 25;
  for 'malaria,' 17–18;
  narcotine as, 190–94, 280;
  opium as, 160, 162, 175;
    A. A. Wace on, 205;
    Ayurvedic medicine and, 324;
    contrived theory of, 220–28;
    D. M. Smeaton on, 199n6;
    Donald Morison on, 211–12;
    in East India, 164, 171, 200n8;
    Henry Wilson on, 265–66;
    native physicians on, 217–19;
    Robert Pringle on, 178;
    on Western Coast, 172–73;
    in West India, 165–66, 169;
    William James Moore on, 153–54n9;
    William Roberts on, 237;
  quinine as, 180–90, 310n6;

proprietary medicines, 41, 71–72nn8–11
prostitutes, 53
Protestant missionaries. *See* missionaries
protopine, 30n18
pro-trade activists:
  aftermath of Second Opium War and, 68, 74n33;
  in British Parliament, 62;
  in defense of opium, 51–54, 135;
  rebuttal of SSOT arguments, 79–81, 84–95, 102–4, 113nn7–9;
  rhetoric of, 323–39;
  Royal Commission and, 4, 26, 32n30, 138, 144, 227;
  sexual appetite argument of, 79–80, 112n3;
  views on imperialism, 2
Provision opium, 8, 284, 312n19;
  adulteration of, 24, 32n28;
  export of, 9, 10–11, 285–86, 313n25, 315nn29–31, *373*;
  termination of sale of, 100
pseudomorphine, 30n18
psychiatry, 71n6
Purves, Brigade-Surgeon, 348
pyrexia, 16, 121, 154n11
Pyridinphenethrane family, 20

quack medicine, 217
Quaker reformers, 6, 7, 55, 75, 82. *See also* SSOT
quality control technology, 19
Quayle, W. A., 163–64
Questionnaires:
  Government of India, 86–87, 89, 113n6;
  on opium/'malaria' correlation, 232, 235–39, 268n2, 269n4
quinidine, 25
quinine, 25–26, 30–31n22;
  Andrew Duncan on, 365–66;
  in Ghazipur experiments, 247, 270n15;
  Government of India and, 310n6, 310n8;
  production of, 349–55;
  Royal Commission testimony on, 158, 163, 180–90, 209, 218, 227;
    in East India, 184–85;
    in North India, 182–83, 185–86;

in South India, 183–84;
on Western Coast, 185;
in West India, 183, 185–86;
W. B. O'Shaughnessy on, 243–45;
William James Moore on, 123, 153–54n9, 154–55nn14–15
The Quinology of the East India Plantations (Howard), 353

racial theory, 39, 48, 90–91, 207, 327–28, 340n8
Raffle, Sir Stamford, 129
Rajputana Agency, 284–85, 287, 289–93, 312–13nn20–21, 313n23, 313–14nn26–27, 317nn43–44
Rana of Udaipur, 35
red poppies, syrup of, 57
reexportation, 62, 72n12, 73n25
Reins, Thomas D., 28n10
religious affiliation with opium, 74n31, 204–5
"Remarks on Remittent and Intermittent Fevers" (Moore), 153–54n9
Renaissance disease therapy, 14, 16, 23
Report on the Cultivation, Preparation, and Adulteration of Malwa Opium (Impey), 130
Report on the Extension of Cinchona Cultivation in India (Gage), 354
Report on the Prospects of Cinchona Cultivation in India (Wilson), 354
resolution (SSOT), 45, 83–84, 95–97, 99–100, 111
rheumatism, 71n7, 163, 201n17
rhoeadine, 30n18
Rice, Surgeon-General, 127, 155n17, 163, 189–90
Richards, J. F., 312n18
Richards, Vincent, 93
Richardson, Benjamin Ward, 76–77, 266
Richthofen, Baron, 81, 86
Ringer, Dr., 107, 109
Rivett-Carnac, J. H., 282, 287, 310–11n11, 311n13
robbery. *See* theft
Roberts, Sir William, 135–48, 155nn21–22, 212;
Final Report of:
on anarcotine, 193, 260–68, 270n10, 270n13, 270n15, 273–80, 310n6, 364–66;
on opium consumption, 158, 214, 296, 299–302, 329–30;
on opium/'malaria' correlation, 231–42, 269nn3–6, 299–308, 320–21nn58–64, 322n76, 336–38;
interrogation by, 160;
on narcotine, 191, 192;
on opium as anodyne, 166, 168, 169, 170;
on opium as food, 175–78;
on opium/'malaria' correlation, 194, 195, 217, 219, 222, 224–26;
on quinine, 186, 188–89
Robertson, D., 236–37, 312n16
Robertson-Gregory system, 30–31n22, 274
Roman physicians, 14, 16, 29n13
Ross, Ronald, 29n14, 353
Rowntree, Joshua, 70n2, 271n26
Rowntree, William, 60
Roy, Debendra Nath, 104
Roy, Ram Moy, 104, 175, 220
Roy, Sita Nath, 206
Royal College of Physicians, 76, 140
Royal Commission on Alcohol, 54
Royal Commission on Opium, 11–14;
British Indian Association and, 106–7;
composition of, 135–48;
creation of, 4, 98, 105–6, 111–12;
Final Report of, 1, 2, 5, 21, 231–68, 270–71nn10–26, 273, 314n28;
itinerary in India, 149–52;
opium revenues during, 8, 9, 10, 286, 315n31;
pro-trade arguments about, 32n30;
pro-trade arguments and, 18–19, 85–86;
witnesses, 77, 128–29, 149–52, 157–61, 198–99nn1–6, *369 (see also names of individual witnesses)*;
on narcotine, 30n21, 190–94, 201nn14–16;
on opium as anodyne, 161–74, 199–201nn7–13;
on opium as food, 158, 174–80, 220–21, 227;

on opium/'malaria' correlation, 194–98, 203–28, 228–30nn1–9;
on quinine, 180–90
Royal Society of Arts. *See* Society of the Arts
Rubba, 311n14
Ruffles, Stamford, 34
rural-urban connection, 214–15, 298–99
Russell, E. G., 176–77
Russell, George, 98
Ryland, W. H., 206

Sanitary Commissioner's Report (1892), 205
sanitation theory, 14, 28n11, 334–35, 341n9–11
Sarvadhikari, Rajkumar, 106
scarlet fever, 139
science, Anglo-European, 3–4;
ingestion of opium and, 23–25, 31–32nn26–30;
malaria and, 14–18, 28–30nn11–16;
narcotine and, 21–22, 30n21, 30–31n22;
opium and, 18–20, 30–31nn18–25;
quinine and, 25–26;
rhetoric of empire and, 323–39, 339n1
Science and Scientists in the Netherlands Indies (Honig and Verdoran), 355
Scott, T. J., 221
Seaman, Valentine, 39
Second Opium War. *See* Opium War, Second
sedation, 21, 22, 39–40, 43, 44, 71n7, 72n14
Select Committee on East India Finance, 60–62, 80
Select Committees. *See* Great Britain, Parliament
self-medication:
in Great Britain, 38, 41, 58;
in India, 216
Sen, Boyle Chunder, 104
Sen, Koylash Chunder, 104
Sewall, J. G., 65–66
sexual appetite argument, 79–80, 112n3, 233
Shaftesbury, Lord, 46–47, 55–56, 59, 75, 79

Shah, Tribhovandas Motichand, 179–80
Sheppard, T. W., 270n13, 277, 310n6
Singh, Kunwar Jaswant, 216
Singh, Sir Laksmiswar, 135–36
Singh, Soorjee Narain, 206, 210, 214
Singh, Raja Udai Pratap, 214
Sircar, Nil Ratan, 210–11
slave trade, 55
smallpox, 71n7, 120
Smeaton, D. M., 199n6, 346
Smith, Dr., 243
Smith, George, 48–49, 61
Smith, Samuel, 82
Smith, W. G., 71n5
Smith, W. H., 96
smoking. *See* opium smoking; tobacco smoking
smuggling, 47, 282–83, 288, 292–93, 302–3, 312n17, 317nn48–49, 320–21n65
Smyrna opium, 241
Society for the Study and Cure of Inebriety, 77, 102, 112n2
Society for the Suppression of the Opium Trade. *See* SSOT
Society of Friends, 55
Society of the Arts, 80, 84, 94–95, 126, 129, 292
Spence, W. Donald, 80–81, 85, 86
spleens, enlarged, 165, 212, 217, 242–43, 245
splitters, 161, 162, 174, 215, 219, 235, 310n6
spontaneous generation debate, 139, 147
SSOT (Society for the Suppression of the Opium Trade), 7–8, 27n7, 45–46, 75–78;
British Indian Association and, 106–7;
British Parliament and, 78–79;
India as target for activism, 82, 112–13n4;
"medical use" argument of, 83, 135;
pro-trade rebuttal of, 79–81, 84–95, 102–4, 109, 113nn7–10;
resolution and memorials of, 79, 83–84, 87, 95–102, 104, 111, 228–29n2;
response to pro-trade argument, 81, 95–98, 299;

rhetoric of, 325–26, 336–38;
  Royal Commission and, 12, 13, 19, 138, 144, 146, 220, 221, 222;
  witnesses for, 149–51, 166;
  William James Moore on, 154–55n15;
  William Roberts on, 232–34
Stafford, Augustus, 56
Stanhope, Lord, 45
Stanton, Lord, 45
Stark, Hugh, 37, 70n2
Statistical Abstracts, 9, 27–28n8
Staunton, Sir George, 45, 47
Stewart, Sir Mark, 78
Stiles, Thomas, 137
stimulant/sedative argument, 21, 31–32n26, 39–40, 43–44, 71n5
Stoker, T., 183, 207
Strachey, Sir John, 27n7
strychnine, 153–54n9
Sturmer, A. J., 183–84, 222
subcutaneous hypodermic injections, 24–25;
  of morphine, 64–67, 74nn28–30;
  of quinine, 153–54n9
suicide, 56, 73–74n26, 233
Sukul, Kali Sankur, 184, 229nn5–6, 343
Surbadhicari, Surji Coomar, 191, 194, 204–5, 206, 214
Surveyor, Nusserwanji, 366
Sydenham, Thomas, 25
Sym, Mr., 61
symptoms, 16, 18, 29–30n16
syphilis, 71n7

tariffs, 47, 81
taxation:
  in Great Britain, 63, 96, 100, 101, 105, 150;
  in India, 6, 27n6, 82, 90, 150, 284–85, 313n25
Taylor, A. S., 58
Taylor, Frank O., 22, 31n25
tellurian causation, 14–15, 17–18, 208–9
Temperance Movement, 42, 43–44, 77, 143–45
thebaine, 20, 30n18, 43
theft, 53, 60, 61, 73n22
thermometers, 140
Thiboumery and Mohr process, 245

Thin, Dr., 183–84
Tibb medicine, 323–25
The Times (London), 57, 76, 79, 128, 180
Tinling, J. F. B., 61, 70n2, 73n17
Tipper, Henry, 53
tobacco smoking, 34, 79, 109, 130
Tod, James, 35, 129
Torti, Francisco, 25
toxicity, 65, 74n28, 109, 250, 279
Travels in Peru and India (Markham), 354
treaties, 285, 314nn27–28
Treaty of Nanking (1842), 46
Treaty of Tientsin (1860), 58, 59, 78
Trevor, A. C., 89
tritopine, 30n18
"tropical neurasthenia," 340n3
Truth about Opium (Brereton), 80, 86
Tull Walsh, J. H., 164–65
Tully, W., 364
Turkish opium, 9, 13, 22, 40, 70n2
Turner, F. Storrs, 75
Tyler, Sir John, 170, 186, 200n12
typhoid fever, 17, 120, 139, 154n10

Unani medicine, 217
United States. Civil War, 65
urban-rural connection, 214–15, 298–99

vaids, 216, 217
Vaidya, Chintamanrao Vinayak, 176
Valentine, Colin S., 186, 189
Valentine, Dr., 108
vector theory, 16, 29nn13–14, 183
Verdoran, Frans, 355
Victoria, Queen, 135, 141, 148
Viharidas, Haridas, 135–36, 218
Vurgese, G. T., 200–201n13

Wace, A. A., 205–6, 220, 228n1, 234, 269n3
Wade, Sir Thomas, 108
Walker, T. Gordon, 176, 204–5, 206, 208, 214, 311n13
Wallace, James Robert, 165, 200n8, 224–26, 229n8

Watt, George:
  on cinchona, 354;
  on opium consumption, 294–96, 298, 311n12, 318–19n51, 320n57;
  on opium production, 281, 285–86, 291–92, 314n28, 317nn42–43;
  pro-trade arguments of, 97;
  on revenues from opium exports, 28n9
Webb, Alfred, 95–96, 105
weights and measurements, 275–76, 309nn3–4
Weir, T. S., 167
Wesleyan Missionary Society, 46
"western," 26n2
Westmacott, E. V., 209, 210
Westminster Medical Society symposium, 47–48
What Is the Opium Trade? (Matheson), 53, 73n19
Whigs, 45
White, Anthony, 46
whooping cough, 71n7
Wilde, Oscar, 69
Wilkie, J., 162, 182, 185
Williams, S. Wells, 36
Wilson, A., 354
Wilson, Dr., 61, 73n23
Wilson, Edward, 64
Wilson, Henry Joseph, 135–38, 149, 150;
  Final Report and, 265–66, 271n25;
  interrogation by:
    on opium as food, 175, 176, 178;
    on opium/'malaria' correlation, 205–6, 209–10, 211, 213, 214, 217, 218, 221, 224–26, 229–30n9;
    on quinine, 185, 188, 189
Wilson, H. H., 198n1
Wilson, John, 53, 317n49
Winchester, Dr., 60, 126
Winther, Paul, 366
Woman's Anti–Opium Urgency Committee, 83
Women's Medical College (Philadelphia, Pa.), 200n8
Wood, C. H., 354
Wood, George Bacon, 63–64, 65
Woodright, W. E. H., 194–95, 346
Worboys, Michael, 339n1, 341n10
working class, 42–43, 44, 47–48, 63, 73n15
Wright, C. R. Alder, 22, 30–31n22
Wunderlich, 140

xantholine, 30n18
xenophobia, 69, 333, 340–41n6

Yajnik, Javerilal Umiashankar, 201n13
yellow fever, 17
Yung Cheng, Emperor of China, 34

About the Author

Paul C. Winther holds a doctorate from Cornell University. He teaches anthropology at Eastern Kentucky University in Richmond, Kentucky.

He has published several articles and presentations discussing the chemistry of opium and its alkaloids. He is at work on a second and third book. The second manuscript is entitled *Clay Pots and Asian History: Opium Adulteration and British Domination of the Nineteenth-Century Asian Drug Trade*. The third manuscript is *Drinking "History": The Intriguing Evolution of the Gin and Tonic*.

The author's other research interest stems from his experience in the erstwhile Gwalior State, now a part of Madhya Pradesh, India. The topic is dacoity (banditry) in the region known as the Chambal River Valley. He has published articles about the structure of dacoity, the logic of kidnapping, and folk perceptions of killing and "personhood."

His nonacademic interests are many. He is a board member and treasurer of Appalachia—Science in the Public Interest (ASPI). This organization encourages the adoption of "appropriate technology" in rural Appalachia. Appropriate technology involves the use of nonfossil fuels as energy sources. He is also a community activist, especially about the issue of homelessness and the daunting problems confronting the working poor of the region, the state, and the country. The author and his wife, Monique, an attorney, live in Lexington, Kentucky.